The Diagnosis and Treatment of Alcoholism

The Diagnosis and Treatment of Alcoholism

Second Edition

Edited by:

Jack H. Mendelson, M.D.
and
Nancy K. Mello, Ph.D.

McGraw-Hill Book Company

*New York   St. Louis   San Francisco   Auckland
Bogotá   Hamburg   Johannesburg   London   Madrid
Mexico   Montreal   New Delhi   Panama   Paris
São Paulo   Singapore   Sydney   Tokyo   Toronto*

Library of Congress Cataloging in Publication Data
Main entry under title:

The Diagnosis and treatment of alcoholism.
  Includes bibliographies and index.
  1. Alcoholism. 2. Alcoholism—Treatment.
I. Mendelson, Jack H. (Jack Harold), 1929–
II. Mello, Nancy K. [DNLM: 1. Alcoholism—diagnosis.
2. Alcoholism—therapy. 3. Social Environment.
WM 274 D536]
RC565.D46 1985   616.86′1   84-19358
ISBN 0-07-041477-7

ISBN 0-07-041477-7

The editors for this book were Thomas H. Quinn and Stephan O.
Parnes, the designer was Christine Aulicino, and the production
supervisor was Teresa F. Leaden. It was set in Times Roman by
Achorn Graphics.

Printed and bound by R. R. Donnelley & Sons Company.

*Preparation of this text
was made possible by a grant
from the
Distilled Spirits Council
of the United States, Inc.,
Washington, D.C.*

Contents

The Diagnosis and Treatment of Alcoholism

CHAPTER 1

Diagnostic Criteria for Alcoholism and Alcohol Abuse

Jack H. Mendelson, M.D.
Professor of Psychiatry, Harvard Medical School
Codirector, Alcohol and Drug Abuse Research Center
McLean Hospital
Belmont, Massachusetts

Nancy K. Mello, Ph.D.
Professor of Psychology in the Department of Psychiatry,
Harvard Medical School
Codirector, Alcohol and Drug Abuse Research Center
McLean Hospital
Belmont, Massachusetts

I. INTRODUCTION

Alcohol abuse and alcoholism are major public-health problems in the United States and virtually all other industrial nations. There is also evidence that alcohol-related problems are increasing in many Third World nations and societies where alcohol abuse has been relatively uncommon until recent times. Although exact data for the incidence and prevalence of alcoholism in the United States remains unknown (case findings and survey information have limited accuracy, due, in part, to continued stigmatization of persons with alcohol-related problems), it is estimated that over 10 million American adults have major alcohol-related disorders which directly impact upon another 5 to 10 million people.

The perception of alcohol abuse and alcohol dependence as disease entities has been a relatively recent occurrence in American medicine.

Traditionally, alcoholism has been viewed as a legal and moral transgression, and physicians often were unwilling to treat patients with alcohol problems. Once it was determined that alcohol abuse can result in addiction, i.e., physical dependence upon and tolerance for alcohol's effects, it was possible to regard alcoholism as a medical problem. Although it has long been known that chronic alcohol abuse may result in adverse medical consequences (cf. Seixas, Williams, and Eggleston, 1975), treatment often did not include attention to the underlying drinking problem.

Most disease processes result from an interaction between the host, the environment, and the agent, rather than from one specific factor (Mendelson, 1975). It is useful to think of alcoholism within the framework of this medical model because factors which are specific only to alcohol, to the individual, or to the environment cannot adequately account for the initiation or the perpetuation of alcohol abuse problems. Rather, a series of complex interactions between these factors appears to determine the expression of the resulting behavior disorder (Mello and Mendelson, 1978).

The diagnosis of alcoholism has always been complicated by inconsistent attitudes and imprecise standards for what constitutes a drinking problem. The stigma usually associated with alcoholism has led to denial by the patient, the family, and the physician alike. It would be misleading to suggest that these issues have been resolved and that the criteria for differential diagnosis to be described are universally accepted. However, as more objective information concerning alcohol problems accumulates, the discord diminishes. Gradually, the bastions of once unchallenged beliefs are crumbling in the face of an unrelenting assault of empirical data.

This chapter relies upon some commonly accepted standard sources for the diagnosis of alcohol problems. Specific aspects of this material are discussed in the context of recent clinical research findings wherever possible. For the convenience of the reader, terms used in this chapter are based upon categories taken from the *Diagnostic and Statistical Manual* of the American Psychiatric Association. The terminology derived from this source is also related to nosology and criteria developed by the World Health Organization expert groups as described in the *Manual on Drug Dependence* edited by Kramer and Cameron (1975) for the World Health Organization.

The term "alcoholism" serves as a convenient shorthand for describing a series of complex behavior disorders which emerge as a concomitant of excessive or inappropriate use of alcohol by individuals with varying risk susceptibilities in heterogeneous environmental situations. The nosological designation of "alcoholism" is no more or less precise than specification of disorders such as arthritis, angina, or anemia. Alcoholism, like these disorders, consists of a congery of pathophysiological and behavioral antecedents, concomitants, and consequences. There are both "hard" and "soft" signs and symptoms associated with alcoholism as there are with virtually all other biomedical and biobehavioral derangements. Moreover, alcoholism, a chronic disease, is rarely a stable phenomenon, and transitional patterns which indicate proximity either to remission or to recrudescence are common and often unpredictable. Diagnostic precision is often compromised, not only by evanescent changes within the inflicted individual and/or the environmental context in which their problem is manifest, but also by the demands of contemporary science which simultaneously strives both for reductionism and for elaboration of the nomenclature of disease.

Inadequate definitions of alcoholism have often been cited as the primary reason for lack of success in developing adequate epidemiological, diagnostic, prognostic, and even prevention endeavors. But it could be argued that the corollary is true. More information is needed about the epidemiological and natural history of alcohol-related disorders in order to formulate more adequate definitions of classes and subclasses of disease, a process analogous to the success achieved in the diagnostic nosology of formerly generic entities such as diabetes.

II. DEFINITIONS AND DIAGNOSTIC CRITERIA

A. WHO Diagnostic Criteria

The World Health Organization (WHO) Expert Committee has recommended that the term "alcoholism" be abandoned and replaced by the phrase "alcohol-type drug dependence." The WHO definition of this disorder is as follows:

> Drug dependence of the alcohol type may be said to exist when the consumption of alcohol by an individual exceeds the limits that are accepted by his culture, if he consumes alcohol at times that are deemed inappropriate within that culture, or his intake of alcohol becomes so great as to injure his health or impair his social relationships.

Comparison of the WHO and the APA definition (which follows) illustrates an important difference in emphasis. The World Health Organization relies primarily on cultural criteria to define alcoholism, whereas the American Psychiatric Association stresses damage to personal health and impairment of social and occupational function.

In justification of its approach, the World Health Organization comments:

Since the use of alcoholic beverages is a normal or almost normal part of the cultures of many countries, dependence on alcohol is usually apparent as an exaggeration of culturally accepted drinking patterns and the manifestations of dependence vary accordingly in a characteristic fashion with the cultural mode of alcohol use. For example, in North America and countries in Northern Europe, alcohol is frequently taken in concentrated forms as an aid to social intercourse so that dependence on alcohol in these countries is usually characterized by heavy consumption of strong spirits during short periods of the day, by a tendency to periodic drinking, and by overt drunkenness. In some countries, on the other hand, alcohol is customarily consumed as wine, usually with meals. In these countries dependence on alcohol is characterized by the drinking of wine throughout the day and by a relatively continuous intake of alcohol in this manner and by relatively little overt drunkenness.

These comments illustrate one of the major problems with definitions of alcoholism which involve primarily cultural criteria. There is an enormous variation in acceptable drinking practices both within and between countries. This problem can be resolved, in part by defining alcoholism in terms of objective pharmacological criteria of addiction, tolerance, and physical dependence, rather than in terms of its social consequences. However, the criterion of physical dependence is necessarily restricted to a late stage in the disease process of alcoholism.

B. Diagnostic Criteria of the American Psychiatric Association, DSM-III

1. Essential Features

Alcohol abuse is a pattern of pathological use for at least a month that causes impairment in social or occupational functioning.

Alcohol dependence is a pattern of pathological alcohol use or impairment in social or occupational functioning due to alcohol, and either tolerance or withdrawal. Alcohol dependence has also been called alcoholism.

2. Diagnostic Criteria for Alcohol Abuse

Pattern of pathological alcohol use: need for daily use of alcohol for adequate functioning; inability to cut down or stop drinking; repeated efforts to control or reduce excess drinking by "going on the wagon" (periods of temporary abstinence) or restricting drinking to certain times of the day; binges (remaining intoxicated throughout the day for at least two days); occasional consumption of a fifth of spirits (or its equivalent in beer or wine); amnesic periods for events occurring while intoxicated (blackouts); continuation of drinking despite a serious physical disorder that the individual knows is exacerbated by alcohol use; drinking of nonbeverage alcohol.

Impairment in social or occupational functioning due to alcohol use; e.g., violence while intoxicated, absence from work, loss of job, legal difficulties (e.g., arrest for intoxicated behavior, traffic accidents while intoxicated), arguments or difficulties with family or friends because of excessive alcohol use.

Duration of disturbance of at least one month.

3. *Diagnostic Criteria for Alcohol Dependence*

Either a pattern of pathological alcohol use or impairment in social or occupational functioning due to alcohol use.

Pattern of pathologic alcohol use: need for daily use of alcohol for adequate functioning; inability to cut down or stop drinking; repeated efforts to control or reduce excess drinking by "going on the wagon" (periods of temporary abstinence) or restricting drinking to certain times of the day; binges (remaining intoxicated throughout the day for at least two days); occasional consumption of a fifth of spirits (or its equivalent in wine or beer); amnesic periods for events occurring while intoxicated (blackouts); continuation of drinking despite a serious physical disorder that the individual knows is exacerbated by alcohol use; drinking of nonbeverage alcohol.

Impairment in social or occupational functioning due to alcohol use: e.g., violence while intoxicated, absence from work, loss of job, legal difficulties (e.g., arrest for intoxicated behavior, traffic accidents while intoxicated), arguments or difficulties with family or friends because of excessive alcohol use.

Either tolerance or withdrawal:

Tolerance: need for markedly increased amounts of alcohol to achieve the desired effect, or markedly diminished effect with regular use of the same amount.

Withdrawal: development of alcohol withdrawal (e.g., morning "shakes" and malaise relieved by drinking) after cessation of or reduction in drinking.

The diagnostic criteria for *alcohol dependence,* or *alcoholism,* in DSM-III are relatively specific because pharmacological criteria of tolerance and physical dependence (withdrawal) are clearly defined and unambiguous. Diagnostic criteria for *alcohol abuse* are less specific and less well defined. Although the frequency-of-intoxication criterion used in DSM-II has been abandoned, it has been replaced by a duration-of-drinking criterion in DSM-III. Selection of an arbitrary period of continuous or episodic use of alcohol for "at least one month" was probably achieved by committee consensus. However, it is obvious that episodic drinking for one month has no intrinsic advantage over episodic drinking once each month in establishing an unequivocal diagnosis of alcoholism. The criteria specified for social complications of alcohol use, psychological dependence, and pathological patterns of use described in DSM-III present similar problems. For some, these criteria may appear exceedingly stringent; for others, the same criteria may be too diffuse.

C. National Council on Alcoholism: Diagnostic Criteria

Whereas the American Psychiatric Association has provided criteria for the identification of advanced drinking problems, the National Council on Alcoholism (NCA) has attempted to identify signs and symptoms which are more likely to occur early and late in the illness (NCA, 1972). One advantage of these criteria is that they guide the physician in the differential diagnosis of alcohol problems on the basis of reasonably objective signs and symptoms which have been shown to be clinically valid. A simplified summary of the NCA criteria appears in Table 1. These criteria attempt to distinguish among three kinds of data: physiological; clinical; and behavioral, psychological, and attitudinal. Certain signs and symptoms, designated as 1 under Diagnostic Level in Table 1, are classic signs of alcoholism. Other signs and symptoms, designated as 3 in Table 1, are common in alcoholic individuals but are insufficient to define the condition as unique.

D. Summary

Criteria for the diagnosis of alcohol abuse are imprecise and ambiguous, and it is often difficult to diagnose this disorder with certainty in its early stages. Advanced alcoholism is associated with several specific signs and symptoms including tolerance for and physical dependence upon alcohol. Since these criteria are common to many forms of drug addiction, the American Psychiatric Association has now included alcoholism and alcohol abuse among the substance use disorders.

A number of factors contribute to the ambiguities and problems involved in the differential diagnosis of alcoholism. In addition to inconsistent social criteria for defining a drinking problem, alcohol abusers may have no overt symptoms of any psychological or physiological disorder other than excessive alcohol intake. Since alcoholics tend to regard their disorder as associated with some form of social stigma, they often tend to deny or minimize symptoms of alcohol dependence. Frequently an alcohol-related problem is detected within the context of evaluation of a medical disorder. Illnesses which are frequently associated with alcohol-related problems include alcoholic hepatitis and cirrhosis, acute gastritis, acute pancreatitis, and chronic disorders of the peripheral nervous system. Chronic nutritional disorders may also be associated with alcohol abuse and include poor dietary intake and malabsorption syndromes induced by the effects of ethanol on the gastrointestinal tract (Mendelson, 1975). The combination of excessive drinking and poor diet may culminate in the genesis of disorders of the central and peripheral nervous system (Victor, 1975; Dreyfus, 1974).

III. TEMPORAL DEVELOPMENT OF ALCOHOL PROBLEMS

The onset of problem drinking is insidious, and the progression to alcohol addiction usually requires several years. Variability in patterns of drinking and types of alcoholic beverage consumed further complicate the diagnosis of alcohol problems. For example, some people may begin drinking beer during early adolescence and progress to consumption of large quantities of distilled spirits. Detection of an alcohol-related problem may not occur until late in the third or fourth decade of life. However, other people may begin drinking large quantities of alcohol, and the first evidence of withdrawal signs and symptoms may appear within two to three years (Mello and Mendelson, 1976). Still others may never drink beer or distilled spirits but drink large quantities of wine daily. This pattern of wine drinking is quite common in European countries, such as France and Italy, and is becoming more common in the United States.

Sufficient consumption of alcohol in any beverage form may result in physical dependence on alcohol (Mello and Mendelson, 1977). Alcohol intake may be steady and uninterrupted, as often occurs in abuse of wine, or it may be intermittent and aperiodic, as occurs in binge or weekend drinking by those who abuse distilled spirits. Episodic drinking sprees may be interspersed with intervals of relative sobriety or abstinence. There is no convincing evidence that beer or wine protect the excessive drinker against alcoholism because of the relatively low alcohol content. Moreover, equivalent amounts of beer, wine, and distilled spirits (1.3 g/kg/alcohol) have been shown to produce equivalent impairment on sensory, motor, and physiological measures (Kalant et al., 1975).

The prognosis for problem drinkers is far more encouraging than was once believed. Rapid spontaneous remission or gradual disappearance of

Table 1
NCA Criteria for the Diagnosis of Alcoholism

PHYSIOLOGICAL CRITERIA		CLINICAL CRITERIA	
Criterion	Diagnostic Level*	Criterion	Diagnostic Level*
A. *Physiological Dependency*		B. *Clinical: Major Alcohol-Associated Illnesses*	
1. Physiological dependence as manifested by evidence of a *withdrawal syndrome* when the intake of alcohol is interrupted or decreased without substitution of other sedation. It must be remembered that overuse of other sedative drugs can produce a similar withdrawal state, which should be differentiated from withdrawal from alcohol.		Alcoholism can be assumed to exist if major alcohol-associated illnesses develop in a person who drinks regularly. In such individuals, evidence of physiological and psychological dependence should be searched for.	
		Fatty degeneration in absence of other known cause	2
(a) Gross tremor (differentiated from other causes of tremor)	1	Alcoholic hepatitis	1
(b) Hallucinosis (differentiated from schizophrenic hallucinations or other psychoses)	1	Laennec's cirrhosis	2
		Pancreatitis in the absence of cholelithiasis	2
		Chronic gastritis	3
(c) Withdrawal seizures (differentiated from epilepsy and other seizure disorders)	1	Hematological disorders:	
		Anemia: hypochromic, normocytic, macrocytic, hemolytic with stomatocytosis, low folic acid	3
(d) Delirium tremens. Usually starts between the first and third day after withdrawal and minimally includes tremors, disorientation, and hallucinations.	1	Clotting disorders: prothrombin elevation, thrombocytopenia	3
		Wernicke-Korsakoff syndrome	3
		Alcoholic cerebellar degeneration	2
2. Evidence of *tolerance* to the effects of alcohol. (There may be a decrease in previously high levels of tolerance late in the course.) Although the degree of tolerance to alcohol in no way matches the degree of tolerance to other drugs, the behavioral effects of a given amount of alcohol vary greatly		Cerebral degeneration in absence of Alzheimer's disease or arteriosclerosis	1
		Central pontine myelinolysis } diagnosis only	2
		Marchiafava-Bignami's disease } possible postmortem	2
		Peripheral neuropathy (see also beriberi)	2

Criterion	Diagnostic Level*
between alcoholic and nonalcoholic subjects.	
(a) A blood alcohol level of more than 150 mg without gross evidence of intoxication.	1
(b) The consumption of one-fifth of a gallon of whiskey or an equivalent amount of wine or beer daily for more than one day, by a 180-lb individual.	1
3. Alcoholic "blackout" periods. (Differential diagnosis from purely psychological fugue states and psychomotor seizures.)	2
Toxic amblyopia	3
Alcohol myopathy	2
Alcoholic cardiomyopathy	2
Beriberi	3
Pellagra	3

BEHAVIORAL, PSYCHOLOGICAL, AND ATTITUDINAL CRITERIA

Criterion	Diagnostic Level*
All chronic conditions of psychological dependence occur in dynamic equilibrium with intrapsychic and interpersonal consequences. In alcoholism, similarly, there are varied effects on character and family. Like other chronic relapsing diseases, alcoholism produces vocational, social, and physical impairments. Therefore, the implications of these disruptions must be evaluated and related to the individual and his pattern of alcoholism. The following behavior patterns show psychological dependence on alcohol in alcoholism:	
1. Drinking despite strong medical contraindication known to patient	1
2. Drinking despite strong, identified, social contraindication (job loss for intoxication, marriage disruption because of drinking, arrest for intoxication, driving while intoxicated)	1
3. Patient's subjective complaint of loss of control of alcohol consumption	2

*Diagnostic Level 1. Classical, definite obligatory. A person who fits this criterion must be diagnosed as being alcoholic. Diagnostic Level 2. Probable, frequent, indicative. A person who satisfies this criterion is under strong suspicion of alcoholism although other corroborative evidence should be obtained.
Diagnostic Level 3. Potential, possible, incidental: These manifestations are common in people with alcoholism, but do not by themselves give a strong indication of its existence. They may arouse suspicion, but significant other evidence is needed before the diagnosis is made.

alcohol-related problems may occur in a significant number of individuals. Surveys of American drinking practices and problems have revealed that approximately 20% of all those who report alcohol-related problems which affect their social function, or health, or both, state that these problems are no longer present three years following their initial report (Cahalan, 1970). Thus, there seems to be a large turnover rate in individuals with alcohol-related problems, and it is not correct to assume that an inevitable downward course will occur. The notion that alcoholism is a condition that cannot be "cured" has led some physicians to adopt a nihilistic attitude toward treatment. Reluctance to treat alcoholics is often balanced by an unqualified enthusiasm for a particular treatment modality. However, the therapeutic zealot should recognize that the efficacy of any form of psychiatric intervention must be evaluated against expected rates of spontaneous remission. Some alcoholics are able to return to social drinking. The time-honored notion that abstinence is the only possible therapeutic goal for the alcoholic patient must be evaluated on an individual basis (cf. Mello, 1975; Vaillant, 1983).

In summary, alcoholism should be considered as a chronic disorder with aperiodic remissions and relapses which cannot be explained by existing biomedical data. Alcoholism is similar to other chronic medical disorders in that it may improve, remain stable, or become worse. As is also the case with most behavioral disorders, the patient's economic, intellectual, and personal resources are often a major determinant of outcome with or without therapeutic intervention.

IV. CLINICAL CHARACTERISTICS OF ALCOHOL ABUSERS

There is no "typical" alcoholic, and problem drinkers are as heterogeneous as any other group with a complex behavior disorder. No specific personality type, family history, social-economic situation, or stressful experience has been found to predict uniquely the development of alcohol problems (cf. Mello and Mendelson, 1978; Mello, 1983). There is recent evidence that genetic factors may increase the risk for the development of alcohol problems (Goodwin, 1976). Children of an alcoholic parent were found to be more likely to develop alcohol problems than controls. Moreover, some biological factors seemed to predispose to alcoholism more strongly than exposure to an alcoholic parent figure during childhood (cf. Goodwin, 1976, for review).

There are no unique or specific mental-status findings for patients with alcohol abuse or alcohol addiction problems examined during sobriety. Most patients with alcohol-related problems do not present evidence of disturbances in appearance, ideation, cognitive processes, memory function, judgment, and insight when they are not drinking. However, a history of alcohol abuse may often be associated with a variety of organic brain syndromes which have been described in greater detail in the medical literature (Dreyfus, 1974; Victor, 1975). Severe derangements in mental status, particularly cognitive processes and memory function, may be observed in individuals who have a history of alcohol abuse in association with evidence of Wernicke-Korsakoff disorders.

A. Alcohol Intoxication

Grossly intoxicated individuals usually have evidence of facial flushing, nystagmus, dysarthria (thickening and slurring of speech), and ataxia. In addition, many intoxicated individuals tend to become more boisterous, belligerent, and dysphoric; and impairment of psychomotor skills, attention, and memory also occurs. Although most states have established blood alcohol values which define legal limits for alcohol intoxication (usually between 80 and 100 mg/100 ml of blood), these values do not always correlate well with actual behavior. This is particularly true for heavy drinkers who have developed a high degree of tolerance for alcohol. Most social drinkers will show significant signs of intoxication at blood levels between 100 and 150 mg/100 ml and will be grossly intoxicated at levels above 200 mg/100 ml. Stupor and coma may occur at levels above 300 mg/100 ml. Alcohol addicts who have adequate liver function and who have developed a high degree of tolerance will not show such impairments. For example, alcohol addicts with blood ethanol levels between 200 and 300 mg/100 ml can perform quite accurately in tasks requiring psychomotor skills and good cognitive and memory function (Mello and Mendelson, 1978). Therefore, it is important for the physician to remember that signs of obvious alcohol intoxication commonly observed in social drinkers with minimal alcohol tolerance may not occur in alcohol abusers who have developed considerable tolerance for alcohol.

Diagnostic criteria specified in DMS-III for alcohol intoxication are:

A. Recent ingestion of alcohol (with no evidence suggesting that the amount was insufficient to cause intoxication in most people).

B. Maladaptive behavioral effects, e.g., fighting, impaired judgment, interference with social or occupational functioning.

C. At least one of the following physiological signs:
1. slurred speech
2. incoordination
3. unsteady gait

      4. nystagmus
      5. flushed face
   D. At least one of the following psychological signs:
      1. mood change
      2. irritability
      3. loquacity
      4. impaired attention
   E. Not due to any other physical or mental disorder.

DSM-III also lists a disorder described as Alcohol Idiosyncratic Intoxication. Diagnostic criteria for this disorder is specified as:

   A. Marked behavioral change, e.g., aggressive or assaultive behavior that is due to the recent ingestion of an amount of alcohol insufficient to induce intoxication in most people.
   B. The behavior is atypical of the person when not drinking.
   C. Not due to any other physical or mental disorder.

B. Alcohol Withdrawal

Alcohol withdrawal signs and symptoms can exist in isolation or occur in combination. Clinical signs and symptoms of the alcohol withdrawal syndromes are listed in Table 2. The most common withdrawal syndrome includes tremulousness which is usually associated with the subjective feeling state of apprehension and anxiety. The onset of tremulousness usually begins 6 to 24 hours following cessation of drinking and most frequently involves the tongue and distal portions of the upper extremities. Tremor is coarse in character and is often accentuated when the patient attempts to maintain extension of the fingers or protrude the tongue. Tremulousness may persist up to 72 hours and is usually accompanied by mild tachycardia and hypertension, hyperreflexia, sweating, insomnia, and anorexia. The tremulous state is most frequently a self-limited condition and spontaneous recovery usually occurs without any specific medication or treatment (Victor and Adams, 1953; Mello and Mendelson, 1977).

Although the common abstinence syndrome usually occurs after cessation of drinking, it is important to remember that the alcohol withdrawal states can also occur when blood ethanol levels are still relatively high. There is evidence that some withdrawal symptoms occur when blood alcohol levels begin to fall from a high sustained level (Victor and Adams, 1953; Mello and Mendelson, 1970, 1972). For example, a fall from a blood alcohol level of 200 to 100 mg/100 ml may be accompanied by mild tremor and anxiety. Hence, some patients are able to control severity of alcohol withdrawal states by reinstitution of drinking.

Alcohol-related *seizure disorders* usually begin 12 to 48 hours following cessation of drinking. Seizures may occur in persons with otherwise normal clinical EEGs and appear to be unrelated to epilepsy (Victor, 1968). Seizures are of the grand mal type without a preceding aura. A postictal confusion state of short duration is not uncommon. Seizure disorders are usually preceded by the onset of tremulousness. Seizures may recur during a period of 24 to 96 hours following cessation of drinking, but such seizures are usually isolated and rarely proceed to *status epilepticus.*

Hallucinations may be associated with the common abstinence syndrome and are usually present in the most severe abstinence syndrome, delirium tremens. Hallucinations may be either visual, auditory, or both in combination. The hallucinatory experiences may be disturbing and frightening to the patient, but pleasant or amusing hallucinations may also occur. However, it now appears that hallucinations are not uniquely associated with alcohol withdrawal. Recent studies have shown that alcohol addicts may also experience transient visual and auditory hallucinatory experiences during intoxication when there is no evidence of other alcohol withdrawal signs or a past history of psychotic illness (Wolin and Mello, 1973). Hallucinatory phenomena during both acute intoxication and alcohol withdrawal usually remit spontaneously.

Delirium tremens, a term often erroneously applied to all alcohol withdrawal states, is a rare but potentially lethal condition (Victor and Adams, 1953; Mello and Mendelson, 1977). Delirium tremens usually occurs abruptly, 73 to 96 hours following cessation of drinking, and is usually preceded by the more benign withdrawal states described above. Delirium tremens is characterized by disorientation and confusion, vivid hallucinations, severe tremor and agitation, fever and sweating, tachycardia, increased blood pressure and respiratory rate, insomnia, anorexia, and other signs and symptoms of a serious debilitating illness. The hallmark of this syndrome is confusion and disorientation in association with severe tremulous states. Severity of disorientation is such that patients cannot accurately report time or place. Confusion is characterized by memory disorders which involve both recent and remote events. Patients with delirium tremens are seriously ill and require immediate hospitalization and medical treatment.

C. Alcohol-related Amnestic Disorders and Dementia

The *Diagnostic and Statistical Manual*-III of the American Psychiatric Association specifies the following diagnostic criteria for the *amnestic syndrome.*

A. Both short-term impairment (inability to learn new information) and long-term memory impairment (inability to remember information that was known in the past) are the predominant clinical features.

Table 2
Clinical signs and symptoms of the alcohol withdrawal syndrome[a]

	Early or Partial Withdrawal	Common Abstinence Syndrome	Alcoholic Epilepsy or "Rum Fits"	Delirium Tremens
Time course Onset (after last drink)	8–16 h[d]	6–8 h	12–48 h (only after several weeks continuous drinking)	(abrupt) 73–96 h
Peak Usual duration Symptom progression	Until next drink if abstinent	24 h 48–72 h 5% develop delirium tremens	36 h 30% develop delirium tremens	24–72 h 1% mortality[f]
Blood alcohol levels Defining signs and symptoms which differentiate the 4 syndromes	0–100 mg/100 ml[b,d] Mild tremulousness Nausea	to Zero Tremor[g] Sweating Nervous and startle-prone Flushed face Conjunctival injection Mild tachycardia[g]	Zero Grand mal seizures (in bursts of 2–6)	Zero Confusion and disorientation Delusions Vivid hallucination Tremor Agitation Insomnia Autonomic hyperactivity Fever Sweating Tachycardia Mydriasis

Additional common signs and symptoms	Early morning drink
	"Anxiety"[d]
	Agitation[d]
	Tachycardia[d]
		Nausea[g]
		Vomiting[g]
		Anorexia[g]
		Nystagmus[c]
		Hyperreflexia[c]
		Mild disorientation[g]
		Nightmares[g]
		Illusions[g] 25%
		Hallucinations[g]
		  visual (83.4%)
		  auditory
		  mixed 16.6%
		Insomnia[g]
		Sleep fragmentation[e,g]
			Distractible
			Suggestible

Estimated incidence in alcoholics		80%	5%

[a] All data from Victor and Adams, 1953, and Victor, 1966, unless otherwise indicated.
[b] Reported by Isbell et al., 1955.
[c] Reported by Mendelson, 1964.
[d] Reported by Mello and Mendelson, 1970c, 1972.
[e] Reported by Mello and Mendelson, 1970b.
[f] Reported by Tavel et al., 1961.
[g] Also observed during intoxication by the authors.
Reprinted with permission of the publisher.

    B. No clouding of consciousness as in delirium, intoxication or general loss of intellectual abilities as in dementia.

    C. Evidence from the history, physical examination or laboratory tests of a specific organic factor that is judged to be etiologically related to the disturbance.

The alcohol-related amnestic syndrome associated with Wernicke's encephalopathy has been well described in the clinical literature. This disorder is characterized by derangement of memory function, confusion, ophthalmoplegia, nystagmus, and ataxia. The major cause of Wernicke's encephalopathy is thiamine deficiency associated with poor dietary intake plus maldigestion and malabsorption during protracted consumption of large amounts of alcohol. A more chronic form of memory disorder associated with antecedent alcohol use is Korsakoff's disease, but it is important to note that this disorder may occur in the absence of any history of alcohol abuse or alcoholism. It is often impossible to predict the duration of persistence of alcohol amnestic disorder or degree of severity of derangement of memory function following cessation of alcohol use and resumption of normal dietary intake. In some instances rapid remission of the amnestic disorder occurs, while in other cases severe impairment of memory function may persist throughout life.

The diagnostic criteria for *dementia* in DSM-III is as follows:

    A. Loss of intellectual abilities of sufficient severity to interfere with social and occupational functioning.

    B. Memory impairment.

    C. At least one of the following:

    1. Impairment of abstract thinking as manifested by concrete interpretation of proverbs, inability to find similarities and differences between related words, difficulty in defining words or concepts, and other similar tasks.

    2. Impaired judgment.

    3. Other disturbances of higher cortical function such as aphasia (disorder of language due to brain dysfunction), apraxia (inability to carry out motor activities despite intact comprehension and motor function), agnosia (failure to recognize or identify objects despite intact sensory function), "constructional difficulty" (e.g., inability to copy three-dimensional figures, assemble blocks, or arrange sticks in specific designs).

    4. Personality change, i.e., alteration or accentuation of pre-morbid traits.

    D. State of consciousness not clouded (i.e., does not meet the criteria for delirium or intoxication although these may be superimposed).

    E. Either (1) or (2):

    1. Evidence from the history, physical examination, or laboratory tests of a specific organic factor that is judged to be etiologically related to the disturbance.

2. In the absence of such evidence an organic factor necessary for the development of this syndrome can be presumed if conditions other than organic mental disorders have been reasonably excluded and if the behavioral change represents cognitive impairment in a variety of areas.

In dementia associated with alcoholism there is usually a history of prolonged, heavy intake of alcohol prior to the onset of dementia, and symptoms usually persist many weeks or months following cessation of alcohol intake. Although the course and severity of alcohol-related dementia may show wide variation, the appearance of moderate to severe dementia following prolonged episodes of drinking has ominous significance. Most individuals afflicted with severe dementia associated with alcohol abuse or alcoholism often require prolonged periods of custodial care, and remissions are frequently transient and unpredictable.

There remains considerable controversy about the exact causation of alcohol-related dementia. Undoubtedly poor nutritional intake and intercurrent illness associated with problem drinking have a role in causation. It is also possible that large amounts of ethanol ingested over long periods of time may cause direct damage to the central nervous system. However, evidence for this phenomena has not been unequivocally demonstrated in either experimental animal studies or clinical investigation with humans.

V. CONCLUSIONS

Diagnostic criteria for alcoholism and alcohol abuse are in a continuing state of evolution. This process reflects a transition in emphasis from moral and legal to biomedical and public health concerns. Yet within this transition process, a number of traditional concerns have been incorporated into more enlightened conceptualizations. Most diagnostic conceptualizations have abandoned circular definitions of alcoholism and alcohol abuse (e.g., craving and loss of control). On the other hand, a number of shibboleths persist: for example, "pathological intoxication" (described as Alcohol Idiosyncratic Intoxication in DSM-III), a phenomenon which has never been clearly documented under experimental conditions. Yet "pathological intoxication" is commonly used as a legal defense to explain various "pathological" behaviors.

Most diagnostic criteria still try to define alcohol abuse quantitatively, i.e., how much alcohol was consumed for how long. Given the considerable variability in drinking patterns, the value of this quasi-quantitative approach is open to question. Since the term "abuse" denotes some aspect of deviant behavior, and since social norms influence the quality of deviance, societal issues will continue to have a strong impact upon the construction of diagnostic criteria for alcohol abuse.

At a more basic level, lack of consensus regarding diagnostic criteria for alcoholism and alcohol abuse is in part due to lack of adequate information about biological and behavioral aspects of alcohol-related disorders. For example, it is not uncommon for alcohol-induced aggression and sexual behavior to be attributed to a phenomenon of "disinhibition." This notion appears to assume that humans are basically aggressive, belligerent, and continually sexually aroused. The disinhibition hypothesis asserts that alcohol releases basic drives or interferes with judgment about controlling these drives. Yet there is no experimental evidence to suggest that "disinhibition" is a basic underlying mechanism, and the hypothesis is not strongly supported in clinical or experimental animal studies with alcohol or other central nervous system depressants.

Finally, although alcoholism and drug abuse have traditionally been regarded as distinct and separate disorders, it now appears that there may be many commonalities in the expression and maintenance of drug-related problems which transcend the pharmacological differences between the abused drugs. Moreover, it can no longer be assumed that alcoholics abuse alcohol to the exclusion of all other agents (Freed, 1973). Alcoholism is not necessarily different from or unrelated to other forms of drug abuse. Polydrug use and abuse is an increasingly common occurrence which greatly complicates the diagnosis and treatment of drug-related problems (Bourne, 1975; Benvenuto et al., 1975). The identification of common processes in the addictive disorders and the development of maximally effective forms of treatment are among the challenges of the next decades.

In summary, professionals who have to make decisions about the presence or absence of alcohol abuse for their patient or client must make a series of complex judgments. These judgments involve behavioral and medical as well as social factors. Indeed, an adequate disease conceptualization of alcoholism and alcohol abuse emphasizes the interaction between the individual who uses alcohol, the pharmacological properties of alcohol, and the social or environmental context in which alcohol is used. Rigid diagnostic criteria for alcohol abuse are not possible or potentially beneficial for patients. An appreciation that alcohol abuse exists when alcohol use is associated with impairment of health and social functioning is a useful general thesis. Critical clinical assessment of pharmacological factors, tolerance, and physical dependence remain the clearest criteria for establishing an unequivocal diagnosis of alcoholism or alcohol dependence.

REFERENCES

American Psychiatric Association, 1980, *Diagnostic and Statistical Manual of Mental Disorders,* Third Edition, Task Force on Nomenclature and Statistics of the American Psychiatric Association, Washington, D.C.

Benvenuto, J. A., Lau, J., and Cohen, R., 1975, Patterns of nonpiate/polydrug abuse: Findings of a national collaborative research project, in *Problems of Drug Dependence,* Proceedings of the 37th Annual Scientific Meeting, Committee on Problems of Drug Dependence, National Academy of Sciences–National Research Council, Washington, D.C., pp. 234–254.

Bourne, P. G., 1975, Polydrug abuse—Status report on the federal effort, in *Developments in the Field of Drug Abuse,* National Drug Abuse Conference, Cambridge, Mass. (E. Senay, V. Shorty, and H. Alksen, eds.), pp. 197–207; Schenkman Publishing Co., Cambridge, Mass.

Cahalan, D., 1970, *Problem Drinkers,* p. 202, Jossey-Bass, Inc., San Francisco.

Cahalan, D., Cisin, I. H., and Crossley, H. M., 1969, *American Drinking Practices: A National Study of Drinking Behavior and Attitudes,* Monograph No. 6, Rutgers Center of Alcohol Studies, New Brunswick, N.J.

Dreyfus, P. M., 1974, Diseases of the nervous system in chronic alcoholics, in *The Biology of Alcoholism,* vol. 3, *Clinical Pathology* (B. Kissin and H. Begleiter, eds.), pp. 265–290, Plenum Press, New York.

Freed, E. X., 1973, Drug abuse by alcoholics: A review, *Int. J. Addict.,* 2:451–473.

Goodwin, D., 1976, *Is Alcoholism Hereditary?,* p. 171, Oxford University Press, New York.

Isbell, H., 1955, Craving for alcohol, *Quart. J. Stud. Alc.,* 16:38–42.

Kalant, H., LeBlanc, A. E., Wilson, A., and Homatidis, S., 1975, Sensorimotor and physiological effects of various alcoholic beverages, *Canad. Med. Ass. J.,* 112:953–958.

Knupfer, G., 1966, Some methodological problems in the epidemiology of alcoholic beverage usage: Definition of amount of intake, *Amer. J. Public Health,* 2:237–242

Kramer, J. F., and Cameron, D. C. (eds.), 1975, A manual on drug dependence, p. 107, World Health Organization, Geneva.

Mello, N. K., 1975, A semantic aspect of alcoholism, in *Biological and Behavioral Approaches to Drug Dependence* (H. D. Cappell and A. E. Leblanc, eds.), pp. 73–85, Addiction Research Foundation of Ontario, Ontario, Canada.

Mello, N. K., 1983, Etiological theories of alcoholism, in *Advances in Substance Abuse, Behavioral and Biological Research,* vol. 3 (N. K. Mello, ed.), pp. 271–312, JAI Press, Greenwich, Conn.

Mello, N. K., and Mendelson, J. H., 1970. Experimentally induced intoxication in alcoholics: A comparison between programmed and spontaneous drinking, *J. Pharmacol. Exp. Ther.,* 173:101–116.

———, 1972, Drinking patterns during work contingent and non-contingent alcohol acquisition, *Psychosom. Med.,* 34(2):139–164.

———, 1976, The development of alcohol dependence: A clinical study, *McLean Hosp. Jrnl.,* 1(2):64–88.

———, 1977, Clinical aspects of alcohol dependence, in *Drug Addiction I, Hand-*

book of Experimental Pharmacology (W. R. Martin, ed.), pp. 613–666, Springer-Verlag, Berlin.

————, 1978, Alcohol and human behavior, in Handbook of Psychopharmacology, volume XII, section III, Chemistry, Pharmacology and Human Use (L. L. Iversen, S. D. Iversen, and S. H. Snyder, eds.), pp. 235–317, Plenum Publishing Corporation, New York.

Mendelson, J. H. (ed.), 1964, Experimentally induced chronic intoxication and withdrawal in alcoholics, Quart. J. Stud. Alc., Suppl. 2.

Mendelson, J. H., 1975, Alcohol abuse and alcohol-related illness, in The Cecil-Loeb Textbook of Medicine (P. B. Beeson and W. McDermott, eds.), pp. 597–602, W. B. Saunders Company, Philadelphia.

National Council on Alcoholism, 1972, Criteria for the Diagnosis of Alcoholism, Amer. J. Psychiat., 129(2):127–135.

Seixas, F. A., Williams, K., and Eggleston, S. (eds.), 1975, Medical Consequences of Alcoholism, Ann. N. Y. Acad. Sci., 252:399.

Tavel, M. E., Davidson, W., and Batterton, T. D., 1961. A critical analysis of mortality associated with delirium tremens: Review of 39 fatalities in a 9 year-period, Amer. J. Mod. Sci., 242:18–29.

Vaillant, G. E., 1983, The Natural History of Alcoholism. Causes, Patterns, and Paths to Recovery, Harvard University Press, Cambridge, Mass.

Victor, M., 1966, Treatment of alcoholic intoxication and the withdrawal syndrome: A critical analysis of the use of drugs and other forms of therapy, Psychosom. Med., 28:636–650.

————, 1968, The use of drugs in the treatment of the alcohol withdrawal syndrome, in Psychopharmacology. A Review of Progress 1957–67 (D. H. Efron, ed.), PHS Publ. No. 1836, pp. 829–833, U.S. Government Printing Office, Washington, D.C.

————, 1975, Nutrition and diseases of the nervous system (including psychiatric disorders, Progress in Food and Nutrition Science, 1(3):145–172.

Victor, M., and Adams, R. D., 1953, The effect of alcohol on the nervous system, Res. Publ. Ass. Nerv. Ment. Dis., 32:526–573.

Wolin, S. J., and Mello, N. K., 1973, The effects of alcohol on dreams and hallucinations in Alcoholism and the Central Nervous System (F. A. Seixas and S. Eggleston, eds.), Ann. N.Y. Acad. Sci., 215:266–302.

CHAPTER 2

Medical Complications of Alcoholism

Mark A. Korsten, M.D.
Assistant Professor of Medicine, Mt. Sinai School of Medicine (CUNY)
Staff Physician at the Veterans Administration Medical Center
Bronx, New York

Charles S. Lieber, M.D.
Professor of Medicine and Pathology, Mt. Sinai School of Medicine (CUNY)
Director, Alcoholism Research and Treatment Center,
Veterans Administration Medical Center
Bronx, New York

Medical complications of alcoholism constitute an on-going challenge to health professionals in many diverse fields. A vast and growing literature has been generated by these illnesses, and an exhaustive review of this subject would require far more space than available in this volume.

Instead, we offer here a somewhat abbreviated review of the pathogenesis and clinical relevance of these conditions. Where possible, we delineate the relative pathogenetic roles of alcohol and malnutrition in these disorders. In addition, we specify those diseases which are not caused directly by alcohol but instead are linked secondarily to alcohol-induced damage in other systems. Alcoholic liver injury plays a major role in this respect. For example, altered hepatic metabolism has been implicated in hematologic dysfunction (macrocytic and sideroblastic anemias), plays a key role in a variety of endocrinologic imbalances (glucose homeostasis and gonadal function), and may adversely affect nutritional status by altering the activation or degradation of essential nutrients. Since many of the metabolic complications of alcoholism can be traced to the hepatic breakdown of ethanol, we begin by summarizing the pathways by which alcohol is metabolized and the imbalances that may result from its oxidative disposal.

I. ETHANOL OXIDATION: PATHWAYS AND REGULATION

A. Pathways

A major pathway for hepatic disposition of ethanol is alcohol dehydrogenase (ADH). This enzyme is found in the cell sap (cytosol) and catalyzes the conversion of alcohol to acetaldehyde. In this reaction, cofactor nicotinamide adenine dinucleotide (NAD) is also converted to its reduced form (NADH) (Figure 1A). In the absence of exogenous alcohol, substrates for this enzyme system include certain steroids (Okuda and Takigawa, 1970) and fatty acids (Bjorkhem, 1972). Multiple forms of ADH exist which are determined by three structural gene loci ADH, ADH_2 and ADH_3 (Smith et al., 1973). The various ADH types differ in terms of pH optima, activity, and population frequency (vonWartburg et al., 1965; Stamatoyannopoulos et al., 1975).

The net result of ADH-mediated ethanol oxidation is the generation of reducing equivalents in the cytosol (NADH) and acetaldehyde. The production of NADH shifts the redox potential of the cytosol and is responsible for a variety of metabolic abnormalities (Figure 2). Enhanced production of lactic acid and hyperlactacidemia is a reflection of the in-

A. $CH_3CH_2OH + NAD^+ \xrightarrow[\text{ADH}]{} CH_3CHO + NADH + H^+$

B. $CH_3CH_2OH + NADPH + H^+ + O_2 \xrightarrow[\text{MEOS}]{} CH_3CHO + NADP^+ + 2H_2O$

C. $NADPH + H^+ + O_2 \xrightarrow[\substack{\text{NADPH} \\ \text{Oxidase}}]{} NADP^+ + H_2O_2$

   $H_2O_2 + CH_3CH_2OH \xrightarrow[\text{Catalase}]{} 2H_2O + CH_3CHO$

Figure 1
Pathways of ethanol oxidation: (A) Alcohol dehydrogenase (ADH). (B) The microsomal ethanol oxidizing system (MEOS). (C) The combination of NADPH oxidase and catalase.

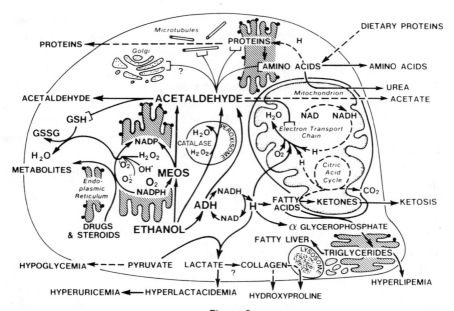

Figure 2
Metabolism of ethanol in the hepatocyte and schematic representation of its link to fatty liver, hyperlipemia, hyperuricemia, hyperlactacidemia, and ketosis. (From Lieber, 1982.)

creased NADH/NAD ratio and has been implicated in the pathogenesis of gouty attacks (vide infra). The increased NADH/NAD ratio also impairs gluconeogenesis and favors triglyceride accumulating in the liver. Both these effects are described in greater detail elsewhere in this review.

Non-ADH systems are involved in ethanol breakdown. The importance of non-ADH pathways in ethanol oxidation is suggested by the following observations: (1) Substantial ethanol metabolism persists despite inhibition of ADH activity (by pyrazole) both in vivo (Lieber and DeCarli, 1972) and in vitro (Papenberg et al., 1970; Lieber and DeCarli, 1970; Grunnet et al., 1973; Matsuzaki and Lieber, 1975); (2) the persistence of significant ethanol oxidation in a strain of deermice that lacks ADH activity (Burnett and Felder, 1980; Shigeta et al., 1982); and (3) the increased rate of the blood ethanol elimination in rats and baboons (Feinman et al., 1978; Salaspuro and Lieber, 1977; Pikkarainen and Lieber, 1980) at high blood levels of ethanol. A constant elimination rate would be expected once ADH activity was saturated provided atypical (high-Km) ADH is not present (it is known to be absent in the rat and baboon).

The microsomal fraction of the hepatocyte is capable of ethanol oxidation when supplied with NADPH and O_2 (Figure 1B); this microsomal ethanol oxidizing system, or MEOS, constitutes an important non-ADH pathway for ethanol disposal. Several lines of evidence support its in vivo role in ethanol metabolism: (1) Ethanol feeding results in a proliferation of the smooth endoplasmic reticulum (the in vivo counterpart of the microsomal fraction) in both rats (Iseri et al., 1966) and man (Lane and Lieber, 1966). This observation suggested that, in addition to its oxidation by ADH in the cytosol, ethanol was metabolized by microsomal constituents. (2) The in vitro Km for MEOS (8–10mM) is much higher than that of ADH (0.26–2.0mM) and agrees well with the corresponding value of the pyrazole-insensitive pathway in vivo (Lieber and DeCarli, 1972). Therefore, although ADH remains the main pathway for ethanol metabolism at low blood levels, as much as 80% of ethanol metabolism could proceed via a non-ADH pathway at high ethanol concentrations (Thieden, 1971).

Other possible pathways of ethanol oxidation are indicated in Figure 1. Catalase is capable of oxidizing ethanol in vitro in the presence of an H_2O_2-generating system, but its activity in this respect is limited by the rate of H_2O_2 generated rather than the amount of catalase per se. Since H_2O_2 production by the liver is only 2% of the rate of ethanol oxidation (3–3.6 μmol/hr/g liver vs. 180 μmol/hr/g), and since catalase inhibition (using aminotriazole) does not significantly depress ethanol oxidation, it appears unlikely that this pathway plays a major role in vivo or constitutes an important non-ADH pathway (Feytmans and Leighton, 1973; Lieber and DeCarli, 1972; Roach et al., 1972).

B. Regulation and Induction of Ethanol Metabolism

The major rate-limiting factor in ADH-mediated ethanol metabolism does not appear to be the level of ADH activity per se. Instead, elimination velocity depends on the availability of the cofactor NAD and the cell's capacity to dissociate the ADH-NADH complex and reoxidize NADH (Theorell and Chance, 1951). In part, the ability of the cell to reoxidize NADH depends on the transfer of NADH into the mitochondria where reoxidation takes place. The entry of NADH into the mitochondrial matrix requires a number of "shuttle" systems (the mitochondrial membrane is impermeable to NADH), and this step, at least during fasting, may ultimately determine the rate of which ethanol is eliminated (Cederbaum et al., 1977). In the fed state, the concentrations of shuttle substrates are higher; this permits increased NADH reoxidation and a higher rate of ethanol oxidation.

Chronic consumption of alcohol results in an increased rate of ethanol metabolism (Kater et al., 1969; Lieber and DeCarli, 1970; Ugarte et al., 1972), but the reason for this augmentation remains controversial.

Chronic intake of ethanol does not increase ADH activity but may actually decrease it (Ugarte et al., 1967; Salaspuro et al., 1981). Moreover, the activity of mitochondrial shuttles is not found to be increased by chronic intake of ethanol (Cederbaum et al., 1973). Another proposed mechanism that might spur ADH dependent ethanol oxidation involves enhanced ATPase activity and the development of a hypermetabolic state (Israel et al., 1973, 1975). Increased hepatic oxygen consumption is predicted by this hypothesis; it has been found by some (Israel et al., 1973; Thurman et al., 1976) but not all (Cederbaum et al., 1977; Gordon, 1977; Shaw et al., 1977) investigators.

The fact that pyrazole does not fully reverse the enhanced ethanol metabolism that follows chronic ethanol consumption is strong evidence for the involvement of non-ADH pathways (Lieber and DeCarli, 1970; Salaspuro et al., 1975). In this respect, MEOS activity in alcoholics is significantly increased by chronic ethanol consumption (Mezey and Tobon, 1971; Kostelnik and Iber, 1973) and, at least in animals, chronic ethanol consumption results in the appearance of a form of P-450 (a key constituent of MEOS) with unique spectral and catalytic properties (Joly et al., 1977; Ohnishi and Lieber, 1977; Koop et al., 1982).

II. HEPATIC COMPLICATIONS OF ALCOHOLISM

These are probably the most common and potentially most serious of the medical complications associated with alcoholism. The magnitude of the problem is revealed in a single vital statistic from the City of New York: cirrhosis of the liver is now the third cause of all deaths in the age groups 25 to 65.

A. Alcoholic Steatosis

1. Clinical Features of Alcoholic Fatty Liver

Fatty liver (steatosis) in the alcoholic is a silent and reversible condition. On physician examination, the liver is enlarged, smooth, and nontender. Liver enzymes such as the AST and ALT correlate poorly with the degree of steatosis or may even fall in the normal ranges (Devenyi et al., 1970). By light microscopy, fat is found within intracytoplasmic vacuoles with displacement of the nucleus. Ultrastructurally, there is dilatation of the endoplasmic reticulum and distortion of mitochondrial architecture. Histologic features at this early stage of alcoholic liver injury may have predictive value. In particular, it has been proposed that perivenular fibrosis in patients with steatosis is a precirrhotic lesion (Van-

Waes and Lieber, 1977a). This concept evolved from studies in the alcohol-fed baboon; pericentral fibrosis occurred at the fatty liver stage in those animals progressing to cirrhosis but was not detected in baboons that remained purely steatotic. These observations in the baboon were recently confirmed in a prospective human study (Nakano et al., 1982). With continued drinking, steatotic patients with perivenular fibrosis were far more likely to show progression of fibrosis than patients without this lesion. This transition took place in the absence of documentation of classic alcoholic hepatitis, suggesting that alcoholic hepatitis is not an absolute requirement for such progression. Perisinusoidal fibrosis is commonly associated with perivenular fibrosis (Van Waes and Lieber, 1977a, Nakano and Lieber, 1982) and has also been promoted as an early indication of poor prognosis (Nasrallah et al., 1980).

2. Pathogenesis of Alcoholic Fatty Liver

Early human and animal studies suggested that malnutrition was the key factor in the production of alcoholic fatty liver. The steatosis occurring in Kwashiorkor supported the impression that the injurious effects of alcohol were indirect and due to supplantation of dietary nutrients.

This concept of alcoholic fatty liver has not withstood critical experimental evaluation. Despite adequate nutrition, alcohol was found to induce the accumulation of intracytoplasmic lipid in alcoholic (Lieber et al., 1963; Lieber et al., 1965) and nonalcoholic volunteers (Rubin and Lieber, 1968). These alterations were not prevented by dietary supplementation of protein and choline. The mechanisms responsible for fat accumulation during chronic consumption of alcohol have been studied in rats where dietary factors can be closely controlled. It is now well established as a result of such animal experiments that the steatogenicity of ethanol is mediated by the increased NADH/NAD ratio that occurs during ethanol oxidation (vide supra, Fig. 2). In essence, reducing equivalents derived from ethanol oxidation are utilized for oxidative phosphorylation. This decreases citric cycle requirements for 2-carbon fragments and secondarily suppresses fatty acid oxidation (the major source of such 2-carbon fragments, viz. acetate). Finally, the increased NADH/NAD ratio also raises the concentration of α-glycerophosphate, an action that favors hepatic triglyceride accumulation by trapping fatty acids (Johnson, 1974). Lowering O_2 tension to the level prevailing in the perivenular zone exacerbates the ethanol-induced redox change (Jauhonen et al., 1982). By contrast, after prolonged exposure to alcohol, the redox change produced by an acute dose of ethanol is attenuated (Domschke et al., 1974; Salaspuro et al., 1981); such attenuation may explain why fat accumulation does not increase indefinitely despite continued alcohol abuse.

3. Treatment

As in all medical sequelae of alcoholism, abstinence and improved nutrition are the most urgent therapeutic goals. Dietary restriction of fat may be helpful (but has not been carefully studied), as may the administration of anabolic steroids. Long-term use of anabolic steroids has not been universally beneficial (Fenster, 1966) and is potentially harmful, given their androgenic and cholestatic potential. Fat mobilization may be delayed if steatosis is extreme or is complicated by obesity.

B. Alcoholic Hepatitis

1. Clinical Features

Defined clinically, alcoholic hepatitis is an illness that presents with jaundice, fever, anorexia, and right upper quadrant pain. Defined pathologically, alcoholic hepatitis is characterized by parenchymal and portal infiltration with polymorphonuclear leukocytes, steatosis, cholestasis, and sometimes intracytoplasmic clumping of hyaline-like material (Mallory bodies). A dissociation between the clinical and pathological pictures is not unusual. Indeed the pathological picture of alcoholic hepatitis is often found in relatively asymptomatic patients (Galambos, 1972). The mortality rate in alcoholic hepatitis is between 1.5% and 8% in individuals ill enough to require hospitalization but well enough to permit liver biopsy (Harinasuta and Zimmerman, 1971). Poor prognostic signs include a prolonged prothrombin time and ascites.

In patients with more severe illness, alcoholic hepatitis may occasionally mimic the findings in extrahepatic biliary obstruction (Mikkelsen et al., 1968). A variety of diagnostic modalities (CAT scan, ultrasonography, endoscopic retrograde cholangiography, percutaneous transhepatic cholangiography) now permit accurate differentiation between intra- and extrahepatic cholestasis in such patients.

The serum levels of ALT and AST correlate poorly with clinical or histologic evidence of disease severity. However, the serum level of glutamate dehydrogenase (GDH) may be more useful as an index of necrosis and inflammation (VanWaes and Lieber, 1977b) as may the AST/ALT ratio (DeRitis et al., 1972; Cohen and Kaplan, 1979). The AST/ALT ratio is greater than 1 in 55% of patients with alcoholic hepatitis and apparently reflects the levels of these enzymes in the liver parenchyma (Matloff et al., 1980).

2. Pathogenesis

The pathogenesis of alcoholic fatty liver is discussed above and includes the respective roles of malnutrition and metabolic effects of ethanol. Similar controversy has surrounded the progression of liver disease beyond the fatty stage. In the baboon, however, dietary deficiency is not a prerequisite for the development of inflammation and necrosis (Lieber et al., 1975). The role played by immunologic factors in the development and progression of alcoholic hepatitis has been investigated. Loss of delayed hypersensitivity, inhibition of PHA-stimulated lymphocyte transformation, and depletion of peripheral blood T lymphocytes have been detected in patients with alcoholic hepatitis. Finally, lymphocytes from baboons and patients with alcoholic liver injury have been shown to be cytotoxic against rabbit hepatocytes (Lue et al., 1979). The latter was also observed in patients with alcoholic hepatitis (Cochrane et al., 1977; Facchini et al., 1978). Of course, it remains to be shown that these immunologic factors are primary events rather than changes secondary to liver injury.

3. Treatment

Alteration in drinking habits is the cornerstone of therapy. Long-term (seven-year) survival increases from 50% to 80% when intake of alcohol is eliminated or moderated (Galambos, 1974). The role of corticosteroid therapy is still unresolved; steroids may be effective therapy in a subgroup of patients with hepatic encephalopathy, but this has not been a universal finding (Depew et al., 1980). Similar uncertainty pertains to use of propylthiouracil (PTU). The rationale for the use of PTU is based on the hypermetabolic hypothesis of Israel and co-workers (see above). However, the beneficial effects reported by Orrego et al. (1979) were not confirmed by Halli et al. (1982), and the use of PTU requires further evaluation.

C. Alcoholic Cirrhosis

1. Clinical Features

Cirrhosis becomes symptomatic at an average age of 50, usually after prolonged and heavy drinking. It is estimated that a 70-kg man who drinks approximately 210 g/day of alcohol for 20 years has a 50% risk of developing cirrhosis (Lelbach, 1975), and neither the type of beverage nor dietary factors seem to alter this probability. The most common signs of uncomplicated cirrhosis are weight loss, weakness, and anorexia (Ratnoff and Patek, 1942). Primary physical findings in cirrhosis include jaundice and hepatomegaly. Signs that may be present as secondary or tertiary manifestations of cirrhosis include splenomegaly, ascites, asterixis, testicular atrophy, gastrointestinal hemorrhage, edema, spontaneous peritonitis, gynecomastia, spider angiomata, palmar erythema, and Dupuytren's contracture. These and other complications of cirrhosis are covered more fully in subsequent sections of this review.

Apart from hypoalbuminemia and hyperglobulinemia, liver-function tests may be only minimally abnormal in cirrhosis. Serum electrophoresis often reveals a broad elevation of the beta and gamma globulins (so-called β-γ bridging) and there may be depression or even absence of alpha and prebeta lipoprotein bands (Sabesin et al., 1977; Borowsky et al., 1978).

The pathological picture depends on the duration of the cirrhosis. Fine, uniform nodularity of the liver is found early, but the liver may assume an irregular appearance (resembling postnecrotic cirrhosis) as the duration of the cirrhosis lengthens. Microscopically, degrees of steatosis, inflammation, cholestasis, and siderosis (iron deposition) may coexist with fibrous tissue. Scar tissue distorts the hepatic architecture by forming bands of connective tissue joining portal and central zones. Hemodynamically, cirrhosis results in a decrease in both total and effective hepatic blood flow. Total blood flow is reduced by extrahepatic portosystemic shunts, and effective circulation is limited by neovascularization of connective tissue septae and collagenization of the subsinusoidal space (Disse's space). As a result of these changes in hepatic vasculature, the blood supply to the hepatic parenchyma becomes tenuous and minor decrements in cardiac output or blood volume may result in pronounced deterioration of hepatic function.

2. Pathogenesis

Once again, the major issue in the pathogenesis of alcoholic cirrhosis has been the relative roles played by alcohol and malnutrition. As noted before, early studies suggested the primacy of malnutrition in the production of alcoholic liver injury. However, at least in the baboon, it is now clear that prolonged administration of ethanol may result in cirrhosis despite adequate nutrient intake (Lieber and DeCarli, 1974). In these studies liquid diets were employed, and the intake of alcohol reached 50% of total calories; nonalcohol calories of the diet were provided by protein (36% of total nonalcohol derived energy), fat (42%), carbohydrate (22%), and the diet was supplemented with minerals and vitamins (choline, in particular was given at twice the level recommended for the baboon). More recently, similar studies have been reported in the monkey (French et al., 1983; Mezey et al., 1983). The monkey diet differed from the baboon diet only in terms of the choline and folic acid content. The choline content of the monkey diet was four times that in the baboon diet, while the folic acid content was about one-half. Under these conditions, monkeys develop nonprogressive alterations in mitochondria ("megamitochondria") and fatty liver after 48 months of alcohol. However, none of the animals demonstrated necrosis, inflammation, or fibrosis. The importance of choline in the diet is still unsettled since monkeys fed ethanol and a low choline (100 mg) diet also failed to develop cirrhosis (Rogers et al., 1981). Moreover, a fivefold increase in dietary choline failed to prevent alcohol-induced fibrosis in the baboon (Lieber et al., 1984). Clearly, species may differ in their susceptibility to ethanol toxicity and their propensity to drink alcohol.

Alcoholic hepatitis has been considered to be the sole initiating factor in the progression to cirrhosis, but this view may require revision. In European and Japanese alcoholics and in baboons chronically fed alcohol, cirrhosis develops without an apparent intermediate stage of florid alcoholic hepatitis (Karasawa et al., 1980; Popper and Lieber, 1980). As noted above, histologic alcoholic hepatitis may exist in relatively asymptomatic alcoholics, and it is possible that minimal inflammation and necrosis may suffice to trigger the fibrosis. Alternatively, alcohol may have direct effects on collagen metabolism that are independent of necrosis. This latter concept is supported by studies in baboons (Nakano and Lieber, 1982) and man (Nakano et al., 1982) showing an increased number of myofibroblasts at an early fatty liver stage. Ethanol causes proliferation of myofibroblasts and this is accompanied by deposition of collagen, first in the perivenular areas, but later throughout the hepatic lobule. We can only speculate as to the factors that cause proliferation of myofibroblasts and deposition of collagen. Alcohol metabolism may be linked to collagen formation because elevated lactate (section I.A) is associated with increased peptidylproline hydroxylase activity both in vitro (Green and Goldberg, 1964) and in vivo (Lindy et al., 1971). In addition, lactate may inhibit proline oxidase (Kowaloff et al., 1977) and once again, lead to the stimulation of collagen synthesis. Both acetaldehyde and lactate also stimulated collagen synthesis in isolated myofibroblasts (Savolainen et al., 1984).

3. Treatment

Abstinence prolongs survival in patients with moderately advanced cirrhosis. Indeed, in the absence of jaundice, ascites, or hematemesis, the five-year survival rate is considerably better in abstainers (89%) than drinkers (63%) (Powell and Klatskin, 1968).

An interesting approach to the treatment of alcoholic cirrhosis is the use of colchicine. Colchicine has a number of effects on collagen metabolism, (i.e., increased collagenase activity, decreased transcellular movement of collagen). Randomized trials have been encouraging, but further study is required before its use can be recommended (Kershenobich et al., 1979).

D. Complications of Hepatic Cirrhosis

1. Ascites

The appearance of ascites in a cirrhotic individual implies a disequilibrium between hydrostatic (portal pressure) and osmotic (serum albumin) forces in the peritoneal cavity. The likelihood of ascitic accumulation is also influenced by the anatomic locus of the portal pressure increase and may be perpetuated by hyperaldosteronism. The stimulus that initiates hyperaldosteronism is not clearly understood. Increased tubular reabsorption and decreased urinary excretion of sodium appear to precede the development of ascites in dogs with dimethylnitrosamine-induced cirrhosis (Levy et al., 1977, 1979); these observations suggest that ascites formation represents an "overflow" of fluid from the intravascular compartment.

Anorexia and dyspnea may accompany large collections of ascitic fluid. A fluid wave or shifting dullness may be absent when only small amounts of fluid are present. In these cases, diagnostic sensitivity may be increased by percussion of the abdomen in the knee-chest position or by utilizing ultrasonography. When the abdominal cavity is distended with fluid, organomegaly may be difficult to evaluate, and serious, coexistent pathology may not be appreciated.

Treatment should initially be directed to the restriction of dietary sodium. A weight loss of 2 lb/day is optimal and does not exceed the maximal resorption rate of ascites from the peritoneal cavity (about 950 ml/24 hours). Weight loss in excess of 2 lb/day may result in azotemia since diuresis may occur at the expense of intravascular volume. This is especially true when peripheral edema is absent or when potent diuretics are administered. Water restriction should be reserved for patients with significant hyponatremia, and intravenous hypertonic sodium chloride is used only for severe degrees of hyponatremia (Conn, 1972).

When sodium restriction is not effective or cannot be adhered to, a spironolactone should be added to the therapeutic regimen. At a maximal dose of 400 mg/day, 75% of patients appear to respond (Conn, 1972). Spironolactone has the additional advantage of correcting total body deficiencies of potassium, a common problem in cirrhotics with ascites. Only in resistant cases should ethacrynic acid or furosemide be necessary. Although sodium excretion may be augmented, hypokalemia and azotemia (both of which augment ammonia toxicity) are frequent complications. These diuretics may be used successfully and safely when ascites is of recent onset and patients are monitored closely. Peritoneovenous shunting may be an effective surgical approach to resistant ascites, but relief is often transient due to infection, shunt clotting, or intravascular coagulopathy.

2. Variceal Hemorrhage

In general, esophageal and gastric varices are clinically silent until rupture occurs. The factors that initiate varices hemorrhage are disputed: Hemorrhage has been attributed to "explosion," "erosion," or, possibly both (Conn, 1979). However, therapeutic modalities employed to increase plasma volume in the cirrhotic (e.g., albumin infusion and ascitic reinfusion) clearly increase the risk of variceal bleeding, and the risk of variceal rupture is higher in patients with large varices than in those with small ones (Lebrec et al., 1980). When portal hypertension results from cirrhosis, variceal blood loss is poorly tolerated and frequently is followed by hepatic coma or functional renal failure. As noted before (Section I.C.1), hepatic blood flow is already precarious in the cirrhotic, and even minor reductions in blood volume may adversely affect hepatic function. Fiberoptic endoscopy is generally indicated in patients with known varices presenting with upper gastrointestinal hemorrhage: Endoscopic diagnosis is more sensitive and reliable, provides direct confirmation of variceal rupture, and excludes other potentially hemorrhagic lesions (e.g., gastritis, ulceration, and carcinoma).

Emergency management of variceal hemorrhage should begin with intravenous infusion of vasopressin at a dose of 0.4 U/minute. To avoid toxicity (myocardial, intestinal, and peripheral ischemia), the infusion should be gradually decreased over a 48-hour period. An alternative approach is to begin the vasopressin infusion at 0.3 U/min and to progressively increase the dose at 30 min intervals (to a maximum of 0.9 U/min) if hemorrhage continues (Chojkier et al., 1979). Vasopressin appears to act by decreasing portal pressure and splanchnic blood flow, but other effects on smooth muscles have been identified.

Other approaches must be instituted if vasopressin infusion fails to control bleeding within several hours. Current options include balloon tamponade, injection sclerosis, and portal-systemic anastomosis. Balloon tamponade is hazardous in the hands of physicians or nurses inexperienced in its use, but good results can be achieved with meticulous and devoted nursing (Pitcher, 1971). Injection sclerosis (using rigid endoscopes) has been reported to control bleeding in 85–90% of cases (Johnston and Rogers, 1973; Terblanche et al., 1979) but requires general anesthesia. Flexible endoscopy avoids the risks of general anesthesia and results in immediate control in 76–84% of actively bleeding patients (Lewis et al., 1980; Goodale et al., 1982). Emergency portacaval or mesocaval anastomosis effectively controls bleeding in about 50%, but is associated with a high operative mortality (Orloff et al., 1977). Other operative approaches include transesophageal ligation of varices, esophageal transection, esophagogastric devascularization (Sugiura procedure), and operative coronary vein sclerosis. Randomized, controlled studies are necessary to determine the relative value of these various modalities.

Strategies for the long-term management of patients who have survived an initial variceal bleed are also in a state of flux. Various forms of portal decompression have become less popular in light of studies that failed to show improvement in long-term survival (Resnick et al., 1974), and it remains to be shown that survival is improved by shunts that selectively decompress varices while maintaining hepatic blood flow. Other forms of therapy have been quick to fill this vacuum. In particular, promising results have been reported using pharmacologic agents (propranolol) that reduce portal flow (Lebrec et al., 1980, 1981) and employing injection sclerosis (Clark et al., 1980; Macdougall et al., 1982). The efficacy of propranolol was demonstrated over a one-year period in relatively compensated cirrhosis (absent or minimal ascites, absent or mild jaundice) and at a dose that reduced the heart rate by 25%. Routine uses of propranolol should await the results of long-term studies in a variety of cirrhotic populations (including those with advanced disease) because the drug is potentially harmful (especially in those with asthma, diabetes mellitus, or cardiac decompensation).

3. *Hepatorenal Syndrome*

In the patient with medically intractable ascites, oligura and azotemia are poor prognostic signs. Renal failure usually occurs in the context of severe hepatic decompensation, but the immediate trigger may be paracentesis, overly vigorous diuresis, or gastrointestinal hemorrhage. Other causes of renal failure in the cirrhotic must be considered, including the administration of nephrotoxic antibiotics and acute tubular necrosis. The unremarkable urinary sediment and very low urinary sodium concentrations in functional renal failure usually permit such a differentiation.

Renal blood flow is markedly reduced in the presence of both ascites and azotemia (Baldus et al., 1964), and this decline reflects increased renal vascular resistance (Baldus et al., 1964; Tristani and Cohn, 1967) rather than reduced cardiac output. A redistribution of renal blood flow away from cortical nephrons accompanies the overall decline in renal blood flow (Schroeder et al., 1967; Epstein et al., 1970; Kew et al., 1971) and these intrarenal aberrations also fail to correlate with indices of cardiac output (Epstein et al., 1977). The cause for the increase in renal vascular resistance and redistribution of blood flow is obscure, but its functional nature is underscored by the normal macroscopic and microscopic appearance of the kidneys in fatal cases and their normal performance in kidney-transplant recipients.

Management of these patients involves dietary restriction (protein and salt), and prevention of encephalopathy using neomycin or lactulose. Neomycin may be toxic in the azotemic patient, and the dose must be reduced.

4. Hepatic Encephalopathy

Encephalopathy in the alcoholic with cirrhosis may have an insidious onset. Early symptoms may be limited to changes in personal habits or sleep patterns. More obvious changes may include confusion, drowsiness, and various levels of unresponsiveness. Asterixis is characteristic of, but not specific for hepatic encephalopathy and may be found in association with constructional apraxia, hypothermia, hyperventilation, and fetor hepaticus. The diagnosis is supported by elevated arterial ammonia levels, typical EEG changes, and increased levels of ammonia, glutamine, and α-keto glutaramate in the cerebrospinal fluid.

Ammonia is thought to play a central role in the pathogenesis of hepatic encephalopathy although other toxins may also be involved. Ammonia is generated from urea in the stomach, colon, and kidney, and its systemic absorption is favored at an alkaline pH. Ammonia has been linked to encephalopathy because of its experimental effects on cerebral energy metabolism. In animals, intoxicating doses of ammonia depress levels of ATP in the brain stem, and it has been suggested that disruption of ATP-dependent metabolism may engender cerebral dysfunction (Schenker et al., 1974). Because ATP and α-ketoglutarate are consumed (and glutamine produced) in the detoxification of ammonia, the rate at which ammonia is detoxified, rather than its absolute concentration, may disrupt cerebral integrity (Bessman and Bessman, 1955).

Hepatic encephalopathy has also been related to changes in central neurotransmitters. Specifically, increases in beta-hydroxylated false neurochemical transmitters and a decrease in norepinephrine (a putative transmitter) have been found. These changes have been linked to abnormal plasma amino-acid patterns in patients with hepatic failure and encephalopathy (increased aromatic and decreased branched-chain amino acids). Favorable results have been reported in human hepatic encephalopathy when this pattern is normalized by intravenous infusion of amino acids (Fischer et al., 1976). This theory has been challenged by Ono et al. (1978) who found similar plasma amino-acid patterns in cirrhotics with and without encephalopathy. A similar negative study was carried out by Morgan et al. (1978). The latter group observed that the amino acids remained abnormal despite clinical improvement following therapy with dietary protein restriction and lactulose.

Hepatic encephalopathy is commonly precipitated by azotemia, GI blood loss, dietary protein excess, hypokalemia, infection, and constipation (Schenker et al., 1974). Protein restriction, potassium repletion, neomycin, bowel cleansing, and lactulose may all be effective in reducing the contribution of the gastrointestinal tract to ammonia production. Substitution of vegetable protein for animal protein has been proposed as an adjunctive approach to the dietary management of encephalopathy. Theoretically, the ratio of branch chain to aromatic amino acids in vegetable protein (a high ratio) should tend to correct the low ratio present in the serum of encephalopathic patients. A recent study (Uribe et al., 1982) reported the beneficial effects on encephalopathy of a 40-g vegetable protein diet (compared with 40 g of animal protein) but neglected to document the effects this dietary manipulation may have had on nitrogen balance. Moreover, in patients given lactulose, no such beneficial effect of vegetable protein was found (Shaw et al., 1983).

III. GASTROINTESTINAL COMPLICATIONS OF ALCOHOLISM

A. The Mouth

Enlargement of the parotid glands and alterations in salivary secretion are common in patients with alcoholic liver injury (Durr et al., 1975; Bode, 1980). The functional significance of these changes is unclear. The glossitis and stomatitis seen in alcoholics is probably the result of poor nutrition since they usually respond to vitamin supplementation.

B. The Esophagus

Esophageal complications of alcohol abuse include: (1) an increased incidence of esophageal cancer (Tuyns, 1970; Williams and Horn, 1977); (2) a high incidence of Barrett's epithelium (Martini and Wienbeck, 1974); and (3) functional alterations in peristaltic contraction, especially in patients with peripheral neuropathy (Winship et al., 1968).

The esophagus has also received attention in alcoholics with cirrhosis, portal hypertension, and esophageal varices. It has been proposed that reflux of gastric acid might abrade the mucosa overlying the varices and result in hemorrhage. However, LES pressures (considered an important defense against gastroesophageal reflux) were measured in cirrhotics and were not found significantly altered by the presence or absence of varices or ascites (Eckardt et al., 1976). Although LES pressures do not correlate precisely with pH probe evidence of reflux, these results fail to support the role of acid digestion in the pathogenesis of variceal hemorrhage.

C. The Stomach

Ethanol has acute and chronic effects on gastric secretion and the gastric mucosa. Acute effects include a reduction of gastric mucus, disruption of the mucosal "barrier" (with insorption of H^+ and exorption of Na^+) and a net decrease in gastric acid secretion (Cooke, 1972). Long-term consumption of alcohol decreases basal and maximal acid output (Chey et al., 1968) and appears to cause a chronic antral gastritis (Parl et al., 1979). On a clinical level, acute mucosal lesions ("hemorrhagic gastritis") are a significant cause of upper gastrointestinal blood loss in the alcoholic (Katz et al., 1976; Belber, 1978; Silverstein et al., 1981). Other sources of blood loss in the alcoholic are esophageal varices (see above), peptic ulceration, Mallory-Weiss lesions, duodenitis, and esophagitis. The clinician must not assume that patients with known esophageal varices are necessarily bleeding from this site. Endoscopic studies in patients with known varices and upper gastrointestinal hemorrhage identify varices as the cause of bleeding in only 40–50% (Waldram et al., 1974; Thomas et al., 1979). While early endoscopy may not improve overall mortality and morbidity, it is necessary in patients with varices because specific therapy (Vasopressin infusion, balloon tamponade, sclerotherapy) may be indicated if varices are indeed bleeding. Management of hemorrhagic gastritis involves stabilization of the patient and correction of clotting abnormalities (vitamin K, fresh frozen plasma, and platelets if necessary). Bleeding from gastric erosions tends to subside spontaneously, and there is no evidence that antacids and/or H_2-receptor blockers (e.g., cimetidine) alter the course of alcoholic gastritis. Surgical intervention, usually in the form of a subtotal gastrectomy, is required in only a small minority of cases.

D. The Pancreas

Alcoholic pancreatitis is considered a "chronic" form of pancreatitis because it is generally associated with irreversible changes in function and structure. The label "acute" pancreatitis should generally be reserved for entities like gallstone pancreatitis where there is potential for complete functional recovery of the pancreas. Under certain conditions, this etiologic classification fails to distinguish gallstone from alcoholic pancreatitis: An early attack in the course of alcohol-induced pancreatitis may not be reflected in abnormal pancreatic secretory parameters, while repetitive insults from gallstones *may* have a lasting effect on pancreatic secretion (Bank, 1981).

The most widely accepted theory of the pathogenesis of alcoholic pancreatitis involves precipitation of protein in peripheral pancreatic ducts (Sarles, 1974). These protein "plugs" eventually become calcified and spread to obstruct larger ducts; this in turn causes atrophy and fibrosis of "upstream" pancreatic acini. Increased concentration of protein and intraductal activation of zymogens are factors that have been implicated in protein deposition. The weakness of this theory is the absence of convincing evidence that protein precipitates are the cause and not the result of metabolic derangements in the pancreas. In addition, as demonstrated by ERCP, dilatation of the pancreatic duct may exist in the absence of calcified plugs.

Alcoholic pancreatitis generally develops after 10 to 15 years of heavy drinking. Binges in alcoholics often precipitate relapses of pancreatitis, but intermittent excesses by nonalcoholics (e.g., students) rarely provokes the disorder (Strum and Spiro, 1971).

Abdominal pain and vomiting are common during the relapse. In general, the pain is poorly localized to the upper abdomen, radiates to the back, and is relieved by bending forward. There may be a paucity of physical findings in mild episodes. In severe or complicated cases, hypoactive bowel sounds (ileus), high fever (pancreatic abscess), abdominal mass (pseudocyst), and shifting dullness (pancreatic ascites) may be encountered.

The diagnosis of alcoholic pancreatitis is based on the association of compatible clinical features, a history of alcoholism, and certain laboratory findings. Helpful diagnostic measures include the KUB (plain film of the abdomen), the serum amylase, and ultrasonography. The KUB may reveal pancreatic calcification (Figure 3), localized areas of small bowel ileus ("sentinel loops"), and various colonic gas patterns. A high serum amylase is compatible with the diagnosis of pancreatitis but is not entirely specific or sensitive. For example, the serum amylase may be within the normal range in patients with long-standing, fibrotic disease. Likewise, other intraabdominal processes (biliary tract disease, intestinal infarction, perforated ulcer), pelvic emergencies (especially ruptured ectopic pregnancy), and severe diabetic ketoacidosis may increase the serum amylase

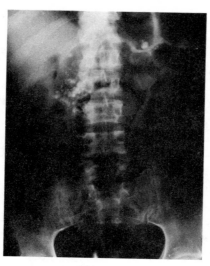

Figure 3
Plain film (KUB) of the abdomen demonstrating calcification in head and tail of the pancreas.

and cause diagnostic confusion. Ultrasonography yields information on coexistent gallstones, pancreatic size (swelling or atrophy), and such complications as pseudocyst formation and common bile duct obstruction. In obscure or confused clinical situations, pancreatic function may have to be evaluated.

Direct visualization of the pancreatic duct (endoscopic retrograde cholangiography) may also be useful in defining ductal anatomy in patients with atypical presentations and in the preoperative assessment of those who fail to resolve with medical management.

The relapse is managed with analgesia and parenteral nutrition. As pain subsides, oral feeding is cautiously reintroduced. Questions have arisen regarding the therapeutic role of nasogastric suction (Levant et al., 1974). Although this modality is clearly not beneficial in mild cases, it would be premature to abandon its use entirely. Nasogastric suction often dramatically relieves pain in patients with pancreatitis, if only by relieving gaseous distention and ileus. Short-term survival is high, but long-term outlook depends upon abstinence and the severity of sequelae such as pancreatic insufficiency, glucose intolerance, pseudocysts, and ascites.

1. Pancreatic Insufficiency

Characteristic symptoms of pancreatic insufficiency include weight loss and steatorrhea. The diagnosis is based on estimation of the amount of fat in a 72-hour stool collection, examination of stool for fat globules (Sudan stain), and various pancreatic stimulation tests. These latter examinations require duodenal intubation; they are time-consuming but very sensitive measures of insufficiency. Recent innovations in the diagnostic armamentarium include the triolein breath (Newcomer et al., 1979) and PABA tests (Arvanitakis and Greenberger, 1976). In the former test, ^{14}C-triolein is administered as part of a fatty meal and $^{14}CO_2$ is measured in expired breath at hourly intervals. The appearance of label in CO_2 depends on lipolysis, intestinal absorption of free fatty acids, hepatic oxidation, and, finally, pulmonary excretion. If subnormal $^{14}CO_2$ excretion is corrected by pancreatic extract, pancreatic insufficiency is probably present. In the latter test, PABA (para-amino-benzoic acid) is measured in the urine after oral administration of N-benzoyl-L-tyrosyl-p-aminobenzoic acid. PABA excretion depends upon the level of chymotrypsin activity in pancreatic secretion and correlates well with fecal fat determinations. Of course, other forms of steatorrhea (e.g., sprue) occur in the alcoholic and must be differentiated from pancreatic steatorrhea (small bowel biopsy and D-xylose absorption may be needed to diagnose such disorders).

Pancreatic steatorrhea is treated by giving pancreatic extract with or without measures to reduce acid inactivation (e.g., antacids and H_2-receptor antagonists). If this fails to correct steatorrhea, reduction in dietary lipid or substitution of medium chain triglycerides for long-chain triglycerides may help.

2. Glucose Intolerance

Hyperglycemia is common in patients with pancreatic insufficiency and may require more than dietary limitations for adequate control. Oral hypoglycemic drugs should be used whenever possible since even small doses of insulin may induce hypoglycemic shock. The brittle nature of the diabetes has been attributed to relative failure of glucagon secretion, but continued alcohol intake may also play a role. For example, by inhibiting gluconeogenesis and depleting glycogen stores in the liver, alcohol may potentiate the hypoglycemic actions of insulin.

3. Pancreatic Pseudocysts

Pseudocysts (cystic structures without true epithelial lining) should be suspected in patients with alcoholic pancreatitis having persistent elevations of serum amylase or evidence of a mass (on physical examination, by ultrasonography, or on CAT scan). Since many cysts will resolve spontaneously, initial management is medical (Bradley et al., 1976). However, surgical intervention must not be delayed if the cyst enlarges. Rup-

:yst, intracystic hemorrhage, and abscess formation are seri-
.ications requiring immediate laparotomy. In patients too
or surgery, ultrasonically guided percutaneous aspiration of the
.bscess is feasible. In most cases, however, decompression is
trans. t and definitive surgery (internal drainage) is still required.

4. Pancreatic Ascites

The clinical features of pancreatic ascites are relatively nonspecific
(increased abdominal girth); if a pancreatic origin is suspected, the amylase concentration should be determined in a sample of fluid obtained
during paracentesis. A high level of amylase confirms the diagnosis and
indicates the need for definitive therapy of the underlying pancreatic process. Although pancreatic ascites may resolve with therapeutic paracentesis and parenteral nutrition, surgical intervention is often necessary.

E. The Intestine

Malabsorption and diarrhea are common in alcoholics and result
from a number of interactive factors (Figure 4) which include direct toxicity of ethanol on the intestine, malnutrition, and organ (liver, pancreas)
injury.

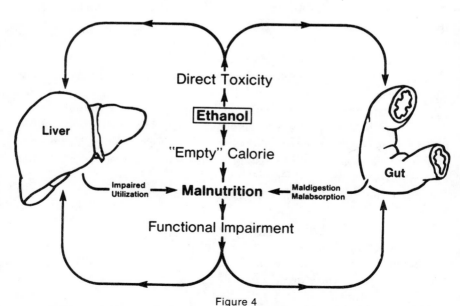

Figure 4
**Interaction of direct toxicity of ethanol on liver and gut with malnutrition
secondary to dietary deficiencies, maldigestion, and malabsorption. (From
Lieber, 1982.)**

1. Direct Toxicity

A number of toxic effects of ethanol have been identified. These actions may be caused by the high alcohol concentrations attained in the upper small intestine. Among the direct effects that have been reported are the following: (1) alterations in intestinal motility (decreased impeding waves in the jejunum) (Robles et al., 1974); (2) structural changes in the upper gastrointestinal tract (erosions, decreased villus height) (Baraona et al., 1974); and (3) impaired transport of glucose (Fox, et al., 1978), amino acids (Israel et al., 1969), electrolytes (Mekhjian and May, 1977), thiamine (Wilson and Hoyumpa, 1979), vitamin B_{12} (Lindenbaum and Lieber, 1969), and calcium (Krawitt, 1975).

2. Malnutrition

Malabsorption in alcoholics is often associated with a history of poor nutrition. Because absorptive function improves with ingestion of a normal diet (despite the continued intake of ethanol), malnutrition per se appears to be an important factor in the pathogenesis of malabsorption in alcoholics (Mezey, 1975). For example, folic acid deficiency alters intestinal morphology (Hermos et al., 1972), and these changes may augment the abnormalities in sodium and water transport produced by ethanol (Mekhjian and May, 1974). Likewise, protein malnutrition impairs intestinal function (Mayoral et al., 1967) and results in reversible pancreatic insufficiency (Mezey, 1976).

3. Organ Injury

As already discussed, pancreatic insufficiency is a cause of maldigestion in the alcoholic and may exacerbate the effects of poor dietary intake. Liver injury may also impair the luminal phase of digestion and alter the absorptive function of the intestine. Lipid uptake may be particularly sensitive to this factor since fatty acids require bile salts (micelles) for solubilization. Bile pool size is markedly depressed in patients with alcoholic cirrhosis. This factor may impair micelle formation and produce steatorrhea (Vlahcevic et al., 1971; Badley et al., 1970).

IV. NUTRITIONAL COMPLICATIONS OF ALCOHOLISM

Alcohol and nutritional status are fundamentally interrelated. At the most basic level, alcoholic beverages displace other forms of food from the diet. This is important because apart from the caloric content of ethanol and small amounts of B vitamins, alcoholic beverages have little nutritional value. At another level, alcohol affects nutrition by its effects on organ systems involved in the digestion and absorption of nutrients. This was particularly evident in the sections of this chapter dealing with the effects of alcohol on the pancreas and small intestine. Finally, ethanol may alter the activation and/or inactivation of nutrients and thereby affect nutritional status. The metabolism of pyridoxine demonstrates this latter aspect. Ethanol decreases the net synthesis of pyridoxal phosphate from pyridoxine (Veitch et al., 1975). These effects have been linked to the oxidation of ethanol and may involve the displacement (and subsequent degradation) of pyridoxal-5-phosphate from its cytosol-binding protein by acetaldehyde (Veitch et al., 1974). This facilitates hydrolysis by pyridoxal phosphatase and results in a net decrease in activation. The nutritional complications of alcoholism are of more than academic interest. Illnesses due to malnutrition are a major cause of hospitalization among alcoholics (Iber, 1971), and alcoholism remains one of the few causes of overt nutritional deficiency in Western society.

A. Folic Acid Deficiency

Megaloblastic anemia is common in malnourished alcoholics (Herbert et al., 1963) and is usually due to folate deficiency. Thrombocytopenia and granulocytopenia may accompany the megaloblastosis, especially if the deficiency of folate is severe. The hematologic manifestations of folate deficiency are rapidly reversible despite persistently low serum levels (Herbert et al., 1963). Folate deficiency per se results in small bowel mucosal changes that may contribute to malabsorption of other nutrients (Hermos et al., 1972). The pathogenesis of folate deficiency is reviewed in greater detail below (Section VI.A).

B. Pyridoxine Deficiency

Pyridoxine deficiency has been implicated in the development of sideroblastic anemias in the alcoholic. The sideroblastic changes induced by ethanol and a diet low in pyridoxine can be reversed by pyridoxine despite continued alcohol intake (Hines and Cowan, 1970).

C. Thiamine Deficiency

Thiamine deficiency in the alcoholic may result from malabsorption (Tomasulo et al., 1968) and, perhaps, defective activation (Cole et al.,

1969) of thiamine. Thiamine deficiency has been implicated in the etiology of Wernicke-Korsakoff syndrome. To be sure, even latent thiamine deficiency is common in the alcoholic, and the administration of parenteral glucose without thiamine may precipitate Wernicke's encephalopathy in such patients.

D. Iron

Iron deficiency is uncommon in the alcoholic unless such factors as GI bleeding and infection are present (Eichner et al., 1972). On the contrary, the alcoholic is much more at risk from iron overload because alcohol per se (Charlton et al., 1964) and pancreatic insufficiency may increase iron absorption and anemias in the alcoholic may be incorrectly treated with iron preparations.

E. Zinc Deficiency

Zinc deficiency has been incriminated in the pathogenesis of night blindness seen in alcoholics, possibly because of its role as a cofactor of vitamin A dehydrogenase (needed for conversion of retinol to retinal) (Russell et al., 1978). A similar importance of zinc in vitamin A metabolism in the gonad has been suggested but remains to be established in man.

F. Fat-Soluble Vitamin Deficiency

1. *Vitamin A*

Vitamin A deficiency in the alcoholic may develop as a result of decreased uptake (steatorrhea), impaired storage, increased degradation, and diminished activation.

Chronic consumption of ethanol decreases hepatic vitamin A levels, as has been demonstrated in both animal and human studies (Sato and Lieber, 1981; Leo and Lieber, 1982). Although a variety of mechanisms are probably involved, it has recently been suggested that vitamin A depletion may be a consequence of accelerated vitamin A catabolism by microsomal pathways (Sato and Lieber, 1982). On a clinical level, deficiency of this vitamin has been linked to abnormal dark adaptation and hypogonadism. Vitamin A (and zinc) repletion may reverse these conditions but must be done cautiously because chronic consumption of alcohol increases the hepatotoxicity of even moderate doses of vitamin A (Leo et al., 1982; Leo and Lieber, 1983).

2. Vitamin D

Vitamin D deficiency may result from decreased dietary intake, decreased absorption, and altered metabolism. Vitamin D depletion and impairment of calcium transport may account for the decreased bone density (Saville, 1965), increased susceptibility to fractures (Nilsson, 1970), and increased frequency of aseptic necrosis (Solomon, 1973) observed in alcoholics. Ethanol may also have direct toxic effects on bone; chronic alcohol feeding decreases trabecular bone in rats despite normal levels of 25-OH D, calcium, phosphorus, and testosterone (Baran et al., 1980).

3. Vitamin K

Steatorrhea, decreased intake, and altered colonic micronora may combine to produce vitamin K deficiency. In patients with liver injury, such deficiency may depress already marginal synthesis of clotting factors and result in significant coagulopathy (Roberts and Cederbaum, 1972). Failure of vitamin K (10 mg/day for 3 days) to correct a prolonged prothrombin time indicates severe hepatic injury.

G. Practical Considerations

Dietary management of the alcoholics should be directed at the correction of specific deficiencies. There may be increased requirements for folate, thiamine, and pyridoxine in active alcoholics, but caution must be exercised with respect to supplementation with iron and fat-soluble vitamins.

Alcoholics with liver injury present unique problems. Protein should be given in quantities that maximize nitrogen balance but do not precipitate hepatic encephalopathy (56 g/day for a 70-kg man seems optimal in this respect). Patients with ascites require additional restrictions in terms of dietary sodium.

V. ENDOCRINOLOGICAL COMPLICATIONS

Alcohol interacts with the endocrine system at a number of possible loci, including the hypothalamus, the pituitary and various target organs. In addition, liver injury may disturb peripheral metabolism of hormones by affecting hepatic blood flow, protein binding, enzymes, cofactors, or receptors.

A. Adrenocortical Function

Chronic ethanol abuse increases plasma cortisol (Mendelson et al., 1966, 1971) and is occasionally associated with physical and biochemical changes resembling those seen in Cushing's syndrome. Patients with alcohol-induced pseudo-Cushing's syndrome may exhibit increased plasma cortisol levels, an abnormal response to dexamethasone, and evidence of pituitary dysfunction. Experimental studies indicate that alcohol activates the hypothalamic-pituitary-adrenal axis resulting in ACTH release and cortisol secretion.

While liver disease (cirrhosis) per se does not consistently alter plasma cortisol levels, plasma aldosterone levels are generally increased (Wolff et al., 1962). The secondary aldosteronism that occurs in liver disease is believed to play a role in the pathogenesis of ascites (Section II.D.1.).

B. Adrenomedullary Function

Considerable evidence in man indicates that alcohol stimulates adrenal medullary secretion of catecholamines. In addition, the peripheral metabolism of the released catecholamine is altered by alcohol (Davis et al., 1967). Peripheral metabolism of catecholamines shifts from an oxidative (3-methoxy-4-hydroxymandelic acid) to a reductive pathway (3-methoxy-4-hydroxyphenylglycol), a change which may reflect changes in the NADH/NAD ratio or acetaldehyde production (Smith and Gitlow, 1967). The effects of alcohol on adrenomedullary secretion must clearly be considered when evaluating the alcoholic for the presence of a pheochromocytoma.

C. Thyroid Function

Alcohol and alcoholic liver injury have effects on thyroid function. Acute administration of ethanol increases the liver to plasma ratio of thyroid hormone (Bleeker et al., 1969; Israel et al., 1973), a finding that may explain some of the metabolic effects of alcohol. In particular, it has been proposed that chronic use of alcohol leads to a hepatic "hypermetabolic" state. In this scheme, hepatic "hyperthyroidism" leads to increased oxygen consumption, local anoxia, and, possibly liver injury (Bernstein et al., 1975; Israel et al., 1973). Propylthiouracil has been used to protect against alcohol-induced liver injury on these grounds. Two recent clinical trials on this question have yielded discrepant findings

(Orrego et al., 1979; Halle et al., 1982), and it would be premature to use PTU in other than controlled studies.

D. Gonadal Function

Alcohol use decreases plasma testosterone (Mendelson and Mello, 1974; Mendelson et al., 1977; Gordon et al., 1978), an effect that reflects both a decrease in production and increased metabolic clearance of the hormone. Depletion of NAD as a result of the metabolism of alcohol, or acetaldehyde, or both may lead to decreased conversion of pregnenolone to testosterone (Gordon et al., 1980) and, in part, account for decreases in plasma testosterone. In addition, alcohol or its oxidation may affect the levels of lutenizing hormone (LH) as well as the receptor for LH in the Leydig cell (Bhalla et al., 1979).

Alcoholic cirrhosis has long been known to affect gonadal function; indeed, hypogonadism and feminization are considered hallmarks of cirrhosis. Clinically, loss of sexual hair and libido are common in males, menstrual disorders are common in females, and vascular spiders are common in both. These clinical manifestations may reflect the following alterations in estrogen metabolism: elevated levels of estradiol and estrone (Chopra et al., 1973) and increased conversion of testosterone and androstenedione to estrogen (Gordon et al., 1975).

E. Pituitary Function

This subject has been extensively reviewed (Lieber, 1982) and is beyond the scope of the present chapter. The highly variable results in this area seen to reflect the complex interrelationship between alcohol, malnutrition, and liver injury. However, at least in terms of the gonadotropins, the hypothalamic-pituitary axis appears defective since gonadotropin levels are in the normal range despite low levels of testosterone (Kent et al., 1973). In addition, the diuretic actions of alcohol are clearly an effect on the posterior pituitary (i.e., a transient suppression of antidiuretic hormone) (Linkola et al., 1978).

F. Other Metabolic Complications

Alcoholic hypoglycemia develops after prolonged fasting or in severely malnourished individuals who ingest a large amount of ethanol. Patients may be comatose and experience convulsions. Trismus is common as are conjugate deviation of the eyes, extensor rigidity of the extremities, and flexor Babinski responses. The distinction between alcohol-induced hypoglycemia and coma due to alcoholic intoxication may be difficult; the former is suggested by the combination of trismus and coma (DeMoura et al., 1967). After drawing baseline blood samples for blood glucose determination, a diagnostic infusion of glucose (25 gm) is indicated. Plasma insulin is invariably low at the time of attack, which may be useful, in retrospect, to help eliminate a diagnosis of hypoglycemia caused by insulinoma. Alcoholic hypoglycemia is due mainly to inhibition by alcohol of hepatic gluconeogenesis (Freinkel et al., 1963), but failure of growth hormone or glucocorticoid secretion (Arky and Freinkel, 1964) may contribute.

Alcoholic ketosis usually occurs 48 hours or more after the last intake of alcohol and following a period of anorexia and hyperemesis. Decreased, normal, or moderately increased blood glucose levels contrasts with the severe ketosis (Cooperman et al., 1974). Levels of β-hydroxybutyrate are typically higher than that of acetoacetate and may be overlooked if blood ketone levels are assessed by the nitroprusside reaction (Acetest, Ketostix) which is insensitive to β-hydroxybutyrate. Malnutrition is not a prerequisite for the development of ketosis since chronic administration of ethanol, in association with a calorically adequate fat containing diet, induces marked hyperketonemia (Lefevre et al., 1970).

Alcoholic hyperuricemia is due, at least in part, to the effects of excess blood lactate on renal excretion of uric acid (Lieber et al., 1962). Oxidation of ethanol to acetaldehyde generates NADH, which reduces pyruvate to lactate. The resulting rise in blood lactate blocks renal tubular clearance of uric acid, which leads to an increase in serum uric acid concentration. An additional factor contributing to hyperuricemia is increased urate synthesis, possibly as a result of ethanol-induced turnover of ATP (Faller and Fox, 1982). These mechanisms may account for the higher prevalence of gout among alcoholics (Pell and D'Alongo, 1968) and the aggravating effect of alcohol on individuals with primary gout.

VI. HEMATOLOGIC COMPLICATIONS

A. Red Cells

Megaloblastic anemia resulting from folate deficiency is a common cause of anemia in the alcoholic. Folate deficiency usually results from decreased dietary intake, but ethanol ingestion also plays an important role. Ethanol interferes with folate metabolism in a number of ways: (1) ethanol exacerbates folate malabsorption in patients on folate-poor diets (Halsted et al., 1973); and (2) ethanol may block the delivery of storage methylfolate from the liver into the circulation or interrupt the enterophepatic circulation of folic acid (Eichner and Hillman, 1973). Megaloblastic anemia due to folate deficiency is characterized by macrocytes and hypersegmented neutrophils. The MCV (mean corpuscular volume) is typically increased but may be normal when iron deficiency coexists. Severe folate deficiency may cause thrombocytopenia and granulocytopenia as well. The diagnosis should be confirmed by measuring red cell folate levels (rather than serum folate levels). Red cell folate is a better reflection of tissue stores; serum folate responds rapidly to dietary intake of folate, falls early in the course of dietary folate deprivation, and may correlate poorly with hematologic evidence of folate deficiency. B_{12} levels must be measured in all patients with megaloblastic anemia to rule out the possibility of pernicious anemia.

Sideroblastic changes are also a common abnormality affecting red cells. Sideroblasts are red cell precursors that have increased numbers of cytoplasmic granules (possibly containing hemosiderin or ferritin). When the granules form a ring around the nucleus, the cells are termed "ring sideroblasts." Megaloblastic changes coexist with ring sideroblasts in a large percentage of patients, making it difficult to estimate the role of sideroblasts in causing anemia.

Sideroblastic changes are usually encountered in malnourished alcoholics, and a number of studies have implicated pyridoxine deficiency in its pathogenesis. Pyridoxal phosphate is required as a coenzyme in the formation of d-aminolevulinic acid; deficiency of this coenzyme would be predicted to result in the accumulation of non-heme iron in the mitochondria of developing red cells. Ethanol may also have direct inhibitory effects on heme synthesis (Freedman and Rosman, 1976) and, as such, play a role in the formation of sideroblasts.

Alcoholic liver injury may itself result in a number of red cell abnormalities. Target cells and acanthocytosis (spur cell anemia) are frequently noted in patients with severe liver disease and have been attributed to alterations in membrane lipids (Cooper et al., 1972; Cooper, 1977). For possibly similar reasons, hemolytic anemia may occur in patients with fatty liver and hyperlipemia (Zieve's syndrome), but the validity of this syndrome has been questioned (Eichner, 1973). Unusual red cells with a central slit or mouth-like zone of palor (stomatocytes) are occasionally observed in alcoholics with fatty liver (Douglass and Twomey, 1970). Neither the pathogenesis nor the significance of these erythrocyte variants has been elucidated.

B. White Cells

Quantitative and qualitative abnormalities in white cells have been noted in alcoholics. In part, white cell dysfunction may account for the alcoholic's decreased resistance to infection. Granulocytopenia in the alcoholic may be due to direct toxic effects of ethanol on the bone marrow, effects of severe folate deficiency, or sequestration of white cells in the spleen (hypersplenism). Ethanol-mediated abnormalities in the function of white cells include: (1) impaired adherence (MacGregor et al., 1974), (2) inhibited chemotaxis (MacGregor et al., 1978), (3) depressed delayed hypersensitivity of lymphocyte (Tennenbaum et al., 1969), and possibly, (4) altered phagocytosis (Atkinson et al., 1977). The net result of these various defects is that the alcoholic is liable to infections, particularly pneumonia (sometimes due to gram-negative organisms) and has a greater mortality rate when infected (Lyons and Saltzman, 1974).

C. Platelets

Alcoholic thrombocytopenia is probably the most common cause of thrombocytopenia in the United States (Cowan and Hines, 1974). Platelets recover rapidly after alcohol withdrawal, and there may even be a rebound thrombocytosis (Lindenbaum and Hargrove, 1968). Despite wide swings in the platelet count, hemorrhagic and thrombotic complications are usually absent. Thrombocytopenia appears to be a direct effect of ethanol because it can be induced in well-nourished volunteers receiving alcohol and vitamin (including folate) supplementation (Lindenbaum and Lieber, 1969). Multiple mechanisms have been invoked to explain the effect of alcohol on platelets, including ineffective platelet production and shortening of platelet survival.

VII. CARDIAC COMPLICATIONS

Alcoholic cardiomyopathy is generally found in patients who have been drinking heavily for at least 10 years. It is manifest by breathlessness, easy fatigability, palpitations, anorexia, and dependent edema. Although absence of angina pectoris is typical (Evans, 1961), ischemic-type chest pain may be a complaint in some patients (Friedman et al., 1982). The physical findings are similar to those found in other forms of dilated cardiomyopathy: lateral displacement of the apical impulse, an S-3 (and S-4) heart sound, systolic murmurs (a reflection of papillary muscle dysfunction), elevated venous pressure, hepatomegaly, and edema. The ECG findings are also not pathognomonic, occurring in a variety of diffuse myocardial diseases. Atrial and ventricular arrhythmias, intraventricular conduction abnormalities, pathologic "Q" waves, and decreased QRS voltage are common, nonspecific electrocardiographic features. The chest X-ray generally shows symmetric cardiomegaly; cardiac catheterization reveals reduced cardiac output, high diastolic pressures, and pulmonary hypertension. The histopathologic features are varied and nonspecific. Myocardial fiber hypertrophy and fibrosis are commonly found, as are lipid or glycogen vacuolization.

Treatment involves total avoidance of alcohol (Demakis et al., 1974) and anticoagulation (Fuster et al., 1981). Other standard approaches (diuretics, venodilators, and arteriolar vasodilators) are helpful, but patients with alcoholic cardiomyopathy may have increased sensitivity to digitalis toxicity (Friedman et al., 1982).

The alcoholic may suffer transmural myocardial infarction in the absence of significant coronary disease (Regan, 1974). Pathogenetic possibilities include coronary artery spasm and myocardial ischemia secondary to perivascular fibrosis. Alcoholic binges may also result in cardiac arrhythmias (generally supraventricular), a phenomenon that has been linked to ethanol-induced prolongation of His-Purkinje conduction time and shortening of corrected sinus recovery time (Greenspon et al., 1981).

The relationship of ethanol to atherosclerosis has attracted considerable attention. Moderate use of alcohol (up to 60 ml per day) appears to be associated with a lower rate of nonfatal myocardial infarction (Klatsky et al., 1974; Stason et al., 1976; Hennekens et al., 1979). This protective effect of alcohol has been attributed to elevations of HDL-cholesterol levels (Yano et al., 1977). However, it has been shown recently that moderate drinking increases HDL_3, whereas HDL_2 is associated with protection (Lieber, 1984). Alcohol abuse, on the other hand, increases the risk for developing coronary disease (Dyer et al., 1977), possibly by contributing to hypertension.

VIII. ALCOHOL WITHDRAWAL SYNDROMES

The physically dependent alcoholic is likely to experience a number of unpleasant syndromes upon withdrawal of alcohol. The severity of these syndromes varies from mild to life-threatening.

A. Tremulousness

This syndrome is the most common manifestation of withdrawal and is noted about 8 hours after the last drink. Indeed, overnight abstinence may be sufficient to produce these so-called "shakes." If abstinence persists, more marked tremors, insomnia, and hallucinations may ensue after approximately 24 hours. The *hallucinations* ("horrors") are usually visual and rarely last more than three days.

B. Withdrawal Seizures

These seizures develop 12 to 48 hours after alcohol withdrawal. They are usually grand mal, but status epilepticus is rare. Patients with such "rum fits" have normal EEG during seizure-free intervals as opposed to true epileptics.

C. Delirium Tremens

"DTs" has a longer latency than the other syndromes (three to five days) and is characterized by tachycardia, profuse perspiration, dilated pupils, and fever. The episode usually lasts about three days and is accompanied by considerable mortality (about 7%) (Thompson et al., 1975). Patients with aspiration pneumonia, severe liver injury, hyperthermia greater than 104°C, or pancreatitis have a relatively poorer prognosis (as high as 45% mortality) (Tavel et al., 1961).

D. Treatment

Mild withdrawal syndromes (tremulousness) can often be managed on an outpatient basis using small doses of chlordiazepoxide (25 mg q.i.d.). Hospitalization is required when alcohol withdrawal is more severe because such patients require general supportive measures and more intensive sedative therapy. Electrolytes should be monitored (especially Mg^{++} and phosphate) and abnormalities corrected if necessary. Vitamin repletion should be given parenterally (at least initially) because the alcoholic may have absorptive defects (vide supra IV.A and C). If intravenous glucose is required because of persistent vomiting, thiamine (50–100 mg IM) should be administered in advance. The benzodiazepines are usually used for sedation and have a wide margin of safety, even in the presence of liver disease. The dose should be titrated until modest sedation is achieved (Schenker, 1982).

Other agents such as phenothiazines and paraldehyde are no longer used extensively because of their undesirable side effects (phenothiazines cause postural hypotension and cholestatic jaundice while paraldehyde may result in local inflammation and nerve damage).

Withdrawal seizures are usually self-limited but may require intravenous diazepam if prolonged. Anticonvulsant therapy can be discontinued after the withdrawal period in patients with unremarkable EEG pathology.

IX. SUMMARY

We have reviewed the clinical features and pathogenesis of many medical complications of alcoholism. In terms of morbidity and mortality, the collective impact of these disorders is immense and growing. Alcoholism has been considered "the great imitator" because its complications mimic so many other diseases; it can also be considered "the great scourge" because it causes such extensive suffering and pain.

REFERENCES

Arky, R. A., and Freinkel, N., 1964, The response of plasma human growth hormone to insulin and ethanol-induced hypoglycemia in two patients with "isolated adrenocorticotropic defect," *Metabolism*, 13:347–350.

Arvanitakis, C., and Greenberger, N. J., 1976, Diagnosis of pancreatic disease by a synthetic peptide. A new test of exocrine pancreatic function. *Lancet*, 1:663–666.

Atkinson, J. P., Sullivan, T. J., Kelly, J. P., and Parker, C. W., 1977, Stimulation by alcohols of cyclic AMP metabolism in human leukocytes. Possible role of cyclic AMP in the anti-inflammatory effects of ethanol. *J. Clin. Invest.*, 60:284–294.

Badley, B. W. D., Murphy, G. M., Bouchier, I. A. D., and Sherlock, S., 1970, Diminished micellar phase lipid in patients with chronic nonalcoholic liver disease and steatorrhea, *Gastroenterology*, 58:781–789.

Baldus, W. P., Feichter, R. N., Summerskill, W. H. J., Hunt, J. C., and Wakim, K. G., 1964, The kidney in cirrhosis. II. Disorders of renal function, *Ann. Intern. Med.*, 60:366–377.

Bank, S., 1981, Acute and chronic pancreatitis, in *Pancreatic Disease: Diagnosis and Therapy* (T. L. Dent, ed.), pp. 167–188, Grune & Stratton, Inc., New York.

Baran, D. T., Teitelbaum, S. L., Berfeld, M. A., Parker, G., Cruvant, E. M., and Avoli, L. V., 1980, Effect of alcohol ingestion on bone and mineral metabolism in rats, *Am. J. Physiol.*, 238:507–510.

Baraona, E., and Lindenbaum, J., 1977, Metabolic effects of alcohol on the intestine, in *Metabolic Aspects of Alcoholism* (C. S. Lieber, ed.), pp. 81–116, University Park Press, Baltimore.

Baraona, E., Pirola, R. C., and Lieber, C. S., 1974, Small intesinal damage and changes in cell population produced by ethanol ingestion in the rat, *Gastroenterology*, 66:226–234.

Belber, J. P., 1978, Gastroscopy and duodenoscopy, in *Gastrointestinal Disease* (M. H. Sleisenger and J. S. Fordran, eds.), pp. 691–713, W. B. Saunders Company, Philadelphia.

Bernstein, J., Videla, L., and Israel, Y., 1975, Hormonal influences in the development of the hypermetabolic state of the liver produced by chronic administration of ethanol, *J. Pharmacol. Exper. Therap.*, 192:583–591.

Bessman, S. P., and Bessman, A. N., 1955, The cerebral and peripheral uptake of ammonia in liver disease with an hypothesis for the mechanism of hepatic coma, *J. Clin. Invest.*, 34:622–628.

Bhalla, V. K., Chen, C. J., and Gnanprakasam, M. S., 1979, Effect of in vivo administration of human chorionic gonadotropin and ethanol on the process of testicular receptor depletion and replenishment, *Life Sci.*, 24:1315–1324.

Bjorkhem, I., 1972, On the role of alcohol dehydrogenase in oxidation of fatty acids, *Europ. J. Biochem.*, 30:441–445.

Bleecker, M., Ford, D. H., and Rhines, R. K., 1969, A comparison of ^{131}I-triiodothyronine accumulation and degradation in ethanol-treated and control rats, *Life Sci.*, 8:267–275.

Bode, J. Ch., 1980, Alcohol hepatitis und Alkohoizirrhose-Klinik, Begleiterkrankungen und Therapie, in *Leberversagen* (J. Ch. Bode, P. Eckert, M. Fischer, and O. Zelder, eds.), Thieme, Stuttgart.

Borowsky, S. A., and Lieber, C. S., 1978, Interaction of methadone and ethanol metabolism, *J. Pharmacol. Exp. Ther.*, 207:123–129.

Bradley, E. L., Gonzalez, A. C., and Clements, J. L., Jr., 1976, Acute pancreatic pseudocysts: Incidence and implications, *Ann. Surg.*, 184:734–737.

Burnett, D. G., and Felder, M. R., 1980, Ethanol metabolism in peromyscus genetically deficient in alcohol dehydrogenase, *Biochem. Pharmacol.*, 28:108.

Cederbaum, A. I., Dicker, E., and Rubin, E., 1977, Transfer and reoxidation in reducing equivalents as the rate-limiting steps in the oxidation of ethanol by liver cells isolated from fed and fasted rats, *Arch. Biochem. Biophys.*, 183:638–646.

Cederbaum, A. I., Dicker, E., Lieber, C. S., and Rubin, E., 1977, Factors contributing to the adaptive increase in ethanol metabolism due to chronic consumption of ethanol, *Alcoholism: Clin. Exp. Res.*, 1:2371.

Cederbaum, A. I., Lieber, C. S., Toth, A., Beatty, D. S., and Rubin, E., 1973, Effects of ethanol and fat on the transport of reducing equivalents into rat liver mitochondria, *J. Biol. Chem.*, 248:4977–4986.

Charlton, R. W., Jacobs, P., Seftel, H., and Bothwell, T. H., 1964, Effect of alcohol on iron absorption, *Br. Med. J.*, 2:1427–1429.

Chey, W. Y., Kusakcioglu, O., Dinoso, V., and Lorber, S. H., 1968, Gastric secretion in patients with chronic pancreatitis and in chronic alcoholics, *Arch. Intern. Med.*, 122:399–403.

Chojkier, M., Groszmann, R. J., Atterbury, C. E., et al., 1979, A controlled comparison of continuous intraarterial and intravenous infusions of vasopressin in hemorrhage from esophageal varices, *Gastroenterology*, 77:540–546.

Chopra, I. J., Tulchinsky, D., and Greenway, F., 1973, Estrogen-androgen imbalance in hepatic cirrhosis, *Ann. Int. Med.*, 79:198–203.

Clark, A. W., Macdougall, B. R. D., Westaby, D., Mitchell, K. J., Silk, D. B. A., Strunin, L., Dawson, J. I., and Williams, R., 1980, Prospective controlled trial of injection sclerotherapy in patients with cirrhosis and recent variceal hemorrhage, *Lancet*, 2:552–554.

Cochrane, A. M. G., Moussouros, A., Portman, B., et al., 1977, Lymphocyte cytotoxicity for isolated hepatocytes in alcoholic liver disease, *Gastroenterology*, 72:918–923.

Cohen, J. A., and Kaplan, M. M., 1979, The SGOT/SGPT ratio—an indicator of alcoholic liver disease, *Dig. Dis. Sci.*, 24:835–838.

Cooke, A. R., 1972, Ethanol and gastric function, *Gastroenterology*, 62:501–502.

Cooper, R. A., 1977, Abnormalities of cell-membrane fluidity in the pathogenesis of disease, *New Eng. J. Med.*, 297:371–377.

Cooper, R. A., Diloy-Puray, M., Lando, P., and Greenberg, M. S., 1972, An analysis of lipoproteins, bile acids, and red cell membranes associated with target cells and spur cells in patients with liver disease, *J. Clin. Invest.*, 51:3182–3192.

Cooperman, M. T., Davidoff, F., Spark, R., and Pallotta, J., 1974, Clinical studies of alcoholic ketoacidosis, *Diabetes*, 23:433–439.

Conn, H. O., 1972, The rational management of ascites, in *Progress in Liver Diseases*, vol. 4 (H. Popper and F. Schaffner, eds.), Grune & Stratton, Inc., New York and London.

Conn, H. O., 1979, Portal hypertension and its consequences, in *Current Gastroenterology and Hepatology* (G. L. Gitnick, ed.), pp. 338–402, Houghton Mifflin Company, Boston.

Cowan, D. H., and Hines, J. D., 1971, Thrombocytopenia of severe alcoholism, *Ann. Intern. Med.*, 74:37–43.

Davis, V. E., Brown, H., Huff, J. A., and Cashaw, J. L., 1967, Ethanol-induced alterations of norepinephrine metabolism in man, *J. Lab. Clin. Med.*, 69:787–799.

Demakis, J. G., Proskey, A., Rahimtoola, S. H., Jamil, M., Sutton, G. C., Rosen, K. M., Gunnar, R. M., and Tobin, J. R., Jr., 1974, The natural course of alcoholic cardiomyopathy, *Ann. Int. Med.*, 80:293–297.

Depew, W., Boyer, T., Omata, M., Redeker, A., and Reynolds, T., 1980, Double-blind controlled trial of prednisolone therapy in patients with severe acute alcoholic hepatitis and spontaneous encephalopathy, *Gastroenterology*, 78:524–529.

DeRitis, F., Coltorti, M., and Giusti, G., 1972, Serum-transaminase activities in liver disease, *Lancet*, 1:685–687.

Devenyi, P., Rutherdale, J., Sereny, G., and Olin, J. S., 1970, Clinical diagnosis of alcoholic fatty liver, *Am. J. Gastroenterol.*, 54:579–602.

Domschke, A., Domschke, W., and Lieber, C. S., 1974, Hepatic redox state: Attenuation of the acute effects of ethanol induced by chronic ethanol consumption, *Life Sci.*, 15:132–134.

Douglass, C. C., and Twomey, J. J., 1970, Transient stomatocytosis with hemolysis: A previously unrecognized complication of alcoholism, *Ann. Intern. Med.*, 72:159–164.

Durr, H. K., Bode, J. Ch., Gieseking, R., Haase, R., v. Arnim, I., and Beckman, B., 1975, Anderungen der exokrinen Funktion der Glandula parotis und des Patienten mit Leberzirrhose und chronischem Alkoholismus, *Verh. Dtsch. Ges. Inn. Med.*, 81:1322.

Dyer, A. R., Stamler, J., Paul, O., Berkson, D. M., Lepper, N. H., McKean, H., Shekelle, R. B., Lindberg, H. A., and Garside, D., 1977, Alcohol consumption, cardiovascular risk factors and mortality in two Chicago epidemiologic studies, *Circulation*, 56:1067–1074.

Eckardt, F. F., Grace, N. D., and Kantrowitz, P. A., 1976, Does lower esophageal sphincter incompetency contribute to esophageal variceal bleeding? *Gastroenterology*, 71:185–189.

Eichner, E. R., Buchanan, B., Smith, J. W., and Hillman, R. S., 1972, Variations in the hematologic and medical status of alcoholics, *Am. J. Med.*,263:35–42.

Eichner, E. R., and Hillman, R. S., 1973, Effect of alcohol on serum folate level, *J. Clin. Invest.*, 52:584–591.

Epstein, M., Berk, D. P., Hollenberg, M. K., Adams, D. F., Chalmers, T. C.,

Abrams, H. L., and Merrill, J. P., 1970, Renal failure in the patient with cirrhosis. The role of active vasoconstriction, *Am. J. Med.*, 49:175–185.

Epstein, M., Schneider, N., and Befeler, B., 1977, Relationship of systemic and intrarenal hemodynamics in cirrhosis, *J. Lab. Clin. Med.*, 89:1175–1187.

Evans, W., 1961, Alcoholic cardiomyopathy, *Am. Heart J.*, 61:556–567.

Facchini, A., Stefanini, G. F., Bernardi, M., et al., 1978, Lymphocytotoxicity test against rabbit hepatocytes in chronic liver diseases, *Gut*, 19:189–193.

Faller, J., and Fox, I. H., 1982, Ethanol-induced hyperuricemia: Evidence for increased urate production by activation of adenine nucleotide turnover, *New Eng. J. Med.*, 307:1598–1602.

Feinman, L., Baraona, E., Matsuzaki, S., Korsen, M. A., and Lieber, C. S., 1978, Concentration dependence of ethanol metabolism in vivo in rats and man, *Alcoholism: Clin. Exp. Res.*, 2:381–385.

Fenster, L. F., 1966, The nonefficacy of short-term anabolic steroid therapy in alcoholic liver disease, *Ann. Intern. Med.*, 65:738–744.

Feytmans, E., and Leighton, F., 1973, Effects of pyravole and 3-amino-1,2,4-triazole on methanol and ethanol metabolism by the rat, *Biochem. Pharmacol.*, 22:349–360.

Fischer, J. E., Rosen, H. M., Ebeid, A. M., James, J. H., Keane, J. M., and Soeters, P. B., 1976, The effect of normalization of plasma amino acids on hepatic encephalopathy in man, *Surgery*, 80:77–91.

Fox, J. E., Bourdages, R., and Beck, I. T., 1978, Effect of ethanol on glucose and water absorption in hamster jejunum in vivo, *Am. J. Dig. Dis.*, 23:193–200.

Freedman, M. L., and Rosman, J., 1976, A rabbit reticulocyte model for the role of hemin-controlled repressor in hypochromic anemias, *J. Clin. Invest.*, 57:594–603.

Freinkel, N., Singer, D. L., Arky, R. A., et al., 1963, Alcohol hypoglycemia. I. Carbohydrate metabolism in patients with clinical alcohol hypoglycemia and the experimental reproduction of the syndrome with pure ethanol, *J. Clin. Invest.*, 42:1112–1133.

French, S. W., Reubner, B. H., Mezey, E., Tamura, T., and Halsted, C. H., 1983, Effect of chronic ethanol feeding on hepatic mitochondria in the monkey, *Hepatology*, 3:34–40.

Friedman, H. S., Geller, S. A., and Lieber, C. S., 1982, The effect of alcohol on the heart, skeletal and smooth muscles, in *Medical Disorders of Alcoholism—Pathogenesis and Treatment* (C. S. Lieber, ed.), pp. 436–479, W. B. Saunders Company, Philadelphia.

Fuster, V., Gersh, B. J., Giulaina, E. R., Tajik, A. J., Brandenburg, R. O., and Frye, R. L., 1981, The natural history of idiopathic dilated cardiomyopathy, *Am. J. Cardiol.*, 47:525–531.

Galambos, J. T., 1972, Natural history of alcoholic hepatitis. III. Histological changes, *Gastroenterology*, 63:1026–1035.

———, 1974, Alcoholic hepatitis, in *The Liver and Its Diseases* (F. Schaffner, S. Sherlock, and C. M. Leevy, eds.), pp. 255–267, Intercontinental Medical Book, New York.

Goodale, R. L., Silvis, S. E., O'Leary, J. F., Gebhard, R., Mjollness, L., Johnson, M., and Fryd, D., 1982, Early survival after sclerotherapy for bleeding esophageal varices, *Surg. Gynecol. Obstet.*, 155:523–528.

Gordon, E. R., 1977, ATP metabolism in an ethanol-induced fatty liver, *Alcoholism: Clin. Exp. Res.*, 1:21–25.

Gordon, G. G., Olivo, J., Rafi, F., and Southren, A. L., 1975, Conversion of androgens to estrogens in cirrhosis of the liver, *J. Clin. Endocr. Metab.*, 40:1018–1026.

Gordon, G. G., Southren, A. L., and Lieber, C. S., 1978, The effects of alcoholic liver disease and alcohol ingestion on sex hormone levels, *Alcoholism: Clin. Exp. Res.*, 2:259–263.

Green, H., and Goldberg, B., 1964, Collagen and cell protein synthesis by an established mammalian fibroblast line, *Nature*, 204:347–349.

Grunnet, N., Quistroff, B., and Thieden, H. I. D., 1973, Rate-limiting factors in ethanol concentration, fructose, pyruvate and pyravole, *Europ. J. Biochem.*, 40:275–282.

Halli, P., Pari, P., Kapstein, E., Kanel, G., Redeker, A. G., and Reynolds, T. B., 1982, Double-blind, controlled trial of propylthiouracil in patients with severe acute alcoholic hepatitis, *Gastroenterology*, 82:925–931.

Halsted, C. H., Robles, E. A., and Mezey, E., 1973, Intestinal malabsorption in folate-deficient alcoholics, *Gastroenterology*, 64:526–532.

Harinasuta, U., and Zimmerman, H. J., 1971, Alcoholic steatonecrosis. I. Relationship between severity of hepatic disease and presence of Mallory bodies in the liver, *Gastroenterology*, 60:1036–1046.

Hennekens, C. H., Willett, W., Rosner, B., Cole, D. S., and Mayrent, S. L., 1979, Effects of beer, wine, and liquor in coronary deaths, *JAMA*, 242:1973–1974.

Herbert, V., Zalusky, R., and Davidson, C. S., 1963, Correlation of folate deficiency with alcoholism and associated macrocytosis, anemia and liver disease, *Ann. Intern. Med.*, 58:977–988.

Hermos, J. A., Adams, W. H., Liu, Y. K., Sullivan, L. W., and Trier, J. S., 1972, Mucosa of the small intestine in folate-deficient alcoholics, *Ann. Intern. Med.* 76:957–965.

Hines, J. D., and Cowan, D. H., 1970, Studies on the pathogenesis of alcohol-induced sideroblastic bone-marrow abnormalities, *New Eng. J. Med.*, 283:441–446.

Iseri, O. A., Lieber, C. S., and Gottlieb, L. S., 1966, The ultrastructure of fatty liver induced by prolonged ethanol ingestion, *Am. J. Pthol.*, 48:535–555.

Israel, Y., Salazar, I., and Rosenmann, E., 1968, Inhibitory effects of alcohol on intestinal amino acid transport in vivo and in vitro, *J. Nutr.*, 96:499–504.

Israel, Y., Videla, L., Macdonald, A., and Bernstein, J., 1973, Metabolic alterations produced in the liver by chronic ethanol administration. Comparison between the effects produced by ethanol and by thyroid hormones. *Biochem. J.*, 134:523–529.

Israel, Y., Videla, L., and Bernstein, J., 1975, Liver hypermetabolic state after chronic ethanol consumption: Hormonal interrelations and pathogenic implications, *Fed. Proc.*, 34:2052–2059.

Israel, Y., Videla, L., Fernandes-Videla, V., and Bernstein, J., 1975, Effects of chronic ethanol treatment and thyroxine administration on ethanol metabolism and liver oxidative capacity, *J. Pharmacol. Exp. Ther.*, 192:565–574.

Jauhonen, P., Baraona, E., Miyakawa, H., and Lieber, C. S., 1982, Mechanism for selective perivenular hepatotoxicity of ethanol, *Alcoholism: Clin. Exp. Res.*, 6:350–357.

Johnson, O., 1974, Influences of the blood ethanol concentration on the acute ethanol-induced liver triglyceride accumulation in rats, *Scand. J. Gastroenterol.*, 2:207.

Johnston, G. W., and Rogers, H. W., 1973, A review of 15 years' experience in the use of sclerotherapy in the control of acute haemorrhage from esophageal varices, *Br. J. Surg.*, 60:797–800.

Joly, J-G., Villeneuve, J-P., and Mavier, P., 1977, Chronic ethanol administration induces a form of cytochrome P-450 with specific spectral and catalytic properties, *Alcoholism: Clin. Exp. Res.*, 1:17–20.

Karasawa, T., Kushida, T., Shitake, T., and Kaneda, H., 1980, Morphologic spectrum of liver diseases among chronic alcoholics, *Acta Pathol. Jpn.*, 30:505–514.

Kater, R. M. H., Carulli, N., and Iber, F. L., 1969, Differences in the rate of ethanol metabolism in recently drinking alcoholic and nondrinking subjects, *Am. J. Clin. Nutr.*, 22:1608–1617.

Katz, D., Pitchumoni, C. S., Thomas, E., and Antonelle, M., 1976, The endoscopic diagnosis of upper-gastrointestinal hemorrhage, *Dig. Dis.*, 21:182–189.

Kent, J. R., Scaramuzzi, R. J., Lauwers, W., et al., 1973, Plasma testosterone, estradiol and gonadotropins in hepatic insufficiency, *Gastroenterology*, 64:111–115.

Kershenobich, D., Uribe, M., Suarez, G. I., et al., 1979, Treatment of cirrhosis with colchicine. A double-blind randomized trial, *Gastroenterology*, 77:532–536.

Kew, M. C., Brunt, P. W., Varma, R. R., Hourigan, K. J., Williams, H. S., and Sherlock, S., 1971, Renal and intrarenal blood-flow in cirrhosis of the liver, *Lancet*, 2:504–509.

Klatsky, A. L., Friedman, G. D., and Siegelaub, A. B., 1974, Alcohol consumption before myocardial infarction: Results from Kaiser-Permanente Epidemiologic study of myocardial infarction, *Ann. Int. Med.*, 81:294–301.

Koop, D. R., Morgan, E. T., Tarr, G. E., and Coon, M. J., 1982, Purification and characterization of a unique isozyme of cytochrome P-450 from liver microsomes of ethanol-treated rabbits, *J. Biol. Chem.*, 257:8472–8480.

Kostelnik, M. E., and Iber, F. L., 1973, Correlation of alcohol and tolbutamide blood clearance rates with microsomal enzyme activity, *Am. J. Clin. Nutr.*, 26:161–164.

Kowaloff, E. M., Phang, J. M., Granger, A. S., et al., 1977, Regulation of proline oxidase activity by lactate, *Proc. Natl. Acad. Sci. USA*, 74:5368–5371.

Krawitt, E. L., 1975, Effect of ethanol ingestion on duodenal calcium transport, *J. Lab. Clin. Med.*, 85:665–671.

Lane, B. P., and Lieber, C. S., 1966, Ultrastructural alterations in human hepatocytes following ingestion of ethanol with adequate diets, *Am. J. Path.*, 49:593–603.

Lebrec, D., DeFleury, P., Rueff, B., Nakum, H., and Benhamou, J. P., 1980, Portal hypertension, size of esophageal varices, and risk of gastrointestinal bleeding in alcoholic cirrhosis, *Gastroenterology*, 79:1139–1144.

Lebrec, W. K., Poynard, T., Hillon, P., and Benhamou, J.-P., 1981, Propranolol for prevention of recurrent gastrointestinal bleeding in patients with cirrhosis, *New Eng. J. Med.*, 305:1371–1374.

Lefevre, A., Adler, H., and Lieber, C. S., 1970, Effect of ethanol on ketone metabolism, *J. Clin. Invest.*, 49:1775–1782.

Lelbach, W. K., 1975, Cirrhosis in the alcoholic and its relation to the volume of alcohol abuse, *Ann. N.Y. Acad. Sci.*, 252:85–105.

Leo, M. A., Arai, M., Sato, M., and Lieber, C. S., 1982, Hepatotoxicity of moderate vitamin A supplementation in the rat, *Gastroenterology*, 82:194–205.

Leo, M. A., and Lieber, C. S., 1982, Hepatic vitamin A depletion in alcoholic liver injury, *New Eng. J. Med.*, 307:597–601.

Leo, M. A., and Lieber, C. S., 1983, Hepatic fibrosis after long-term administration of ethanol and moderate vitamin A supplementation in the rat, *Hepatology*, 2:1–11.

Levant, J. A., Secrist, D. M., Resein, H., Sturdevant, R. A. L., and Guth, P. H., 1974, Nasogastric suction in the treatment of alcoholic pancreatitis. A controlled study, *JAMA*, 229:51–53.

Levy, M., 1977, Sodium retention and ascites formation in dogs with experimental portal cirrhosis, *Am. J. Physiol.*, 233F:572–585.

Levy, M., Wexler, M. J., and McCaffrey, C., 1979, Sodium retention in dogs with experimental cirrhosis following removal of ascites by continuous peritoneovenous shunting, *J. Lab. Clin. Med.*, 94:933–946.

Lewis, J., Chung, R. S., and Allison, J., 1980, Sclerotherapy of esophageal varices, *Arch. Surg.*, 115:476–480.

Lieber, C. S., 1982, *Medical Disorders of Alcoholism: Pathogenesis and Treatment*, W. B. Saunders Company, Philadelphia.

———, 1984, To drink (moderately) or not to drink? *New Eng. J. Med.*, 310:846–848.

Lieber, C. S., and DeCarli, L. M., 1970, Hepatic microsomal ethanol-oxidizing system: In vitro characteristics and adaptive properties in vivo, *J. Biol. Chem*, 245:2505–2512.

———, 1972, The role of the hepatic microsomal ethanol oxidizing system (MEOS) for ethanol metabolism in vivo, *J. Pharmacol. Exp. Ther.*, 181:279–287.

———, 1974, An experimental model of alcohol feeding and liver injury in the baboon, *J. Med. Primatol.*, 3:153–163.

Lieber, C. S., Jones, D. P., and Losowsky, M. S., 1962, Interrelation of uric acid and ethanol metabolism in man, *J. Clin. Invest.*, 41:1863–1870.

Lieber, C. S., Jones, D. P., Mendelson, J., and DeCarli, L. M., 1963, Fatty liver, hyperlipemia and hyperuricemia produced by prolonged alcohol consumption, despite dietary intake, *Trans. Assoc. Am. Phy.*, 76:289–300.

Lieber, C. S., Jones, D. P., and DeCarli, L. M., 1965, Effects of prolonged ethanol intake: Production of fatty liver despite adequate diets, *J. Clin. Invest.*, 44:1009–1021.

Lieber, C. S., DeCarli, L. M., and Rubin, E., 1975, Sequential production of fatty liver, hepatitis, and cirrhosis in sub-human primates fed ethanol with adequate diets, *Proc. Nat. Acad. Sci. USA*, 72:437–441.

Lieber, C. S., Leo, M. A., Mak, K. M., DeCarli, L. M., and Sato, S., 1984, Choline fails to prevent liver fibrosis in alcohol-fed baboons but causes toxicity, *Hepatology* (in press).

Lieberman, F. L., and Reynolds, T. B., 1967, Plasma volume in cirrhosis of the liver: Its relation to portal hypertension, ascites, and renal failure, *J. Clin. Invest.*, 46:1297–1308.

Lieberman, F. L., Ito, S., and Reynolds, T. B., 1969, Effective plasma volume in cirrhosis with ascites. Evidence that a decreased value does not account for renal sodium retention, a spontaneous reduction in glomerular filtration rate (GFR), and a fall in GFR during drug-induced diuresis, *J. Clin. Invest.* 48:975–981.

Lindenbaum, J., and Hargrove, R. L., 1968, Thrombocytopenia in alcoholics, *Ann. Intern. Med.*, 68:526–532.

Lindenbaum, J., and Lieber, C. S., 1969, Alcohol-induced malabsorption of vitamin B_{12} in man, *Nature (London)*, 224:806.

——, 1969, Hematologic effects of alcohol in man in the absence of nutritional deficiency, *New Eng. J. Med.*, 281:333–338.

Lindy, S., Pedersen, F. B., Turto, H., et al., 1971, Lactate, lactate dehydrogenase and protocollagen proline dydroxylase in rat skin autograft, Hoppe-Seylers' *Z. Physiol. Chem.*, 352:1113–1118.

Linkola, J., Ylikhari, R., Fyhrquist, F., and Wallenius, M., 1978, Plasma vasopressin in ethanol intoxication and hangover, *Acta Physiol. Scand.*, 104:180–187.

Lue, S. L., Paronetto, F., and Lieber, C. S., 1979, Cytotoxicity of lymphocytes in alcoholic fatty liver: Respective role of lymphocytes and target cells, *Gastroenterology*, 76:1290.

Lyons, H. A., and Saltzman, A., 1974, Diseases of the respiratory tract in alcoholics, in *The Biology of Alcoholism*, vol. 3, *Clinical Pathology* (B. Kissin and H. Begleiter, eds.), pp. 403–434, Plenum Press, New York.

Macdougall, B. R. D., Theodossi, A., Westaby, D., Dawson, J. L., and Williams R., 1982, Increased long-term survival in variceal hemorrhage using injection sclerotherapy. Results of a controlled trial, *Lancet* 1:124–127.

MacGregor, R. R., Spagnuolo, P. J., and Lentnek, A. L., Inhibition of granulocyte adherence by ethanol, prednisone, and aspirin, measured with an assay system, *New Eng. J. Med.*, 291:642–646.

Martini, G. A., and Wienbeck, M., 1974, Begunstigt Alkohol die Entstehung eines Barrett-Syndroms (Endobrachyosophagus), *Dtsch. Med. Wochenschr.* 99:434.

Matloff, D. S., Selinger, M. J., and Kaplan, M., 1980, Hepatic transaminase activity in alcoholic liver disease, *Gastroenterology*, 78:1389–1392.

Matsuzaki, S., and Lieber, C. S., 1975, ADH-independent ethanol oxidation in the liver and its increase by chronic ethanol consumption, *Gastroenterology*, 69:845.

Mayoral, L. G, Tripathy, K., Garcia, F. T., Klahr, S., Bolano, S. O., and Ghitis, J., 1967, Malabsorption in the tropics: A second look, *Am. J. Clin. Nutr.*, 20:866.

Mekhijan, H. S., and May, E. S., 1977, Acute and chronic effects of ethanol on fluid transport in the human small intestine, *Gastroenterology*, 72:1280–1286.

Mendelson, J. H., and Stein, S., 1966, Serum cortisol levels in alcoholic and nonalcoholic subjects during experimentally induced alcohol intoxication, *Psychosomatic Med.*, 28:616–626.

Mendelson, J. H., Ogata, M., and Mello, N. K., 1971, Adrenal function and alcoholism. I. Serum cortisol, *Psychomatic Med.*, 33:145–157.

Mendelson, J. H., and Mello, N. K., 1974, Alcohol aggression and androgens, in *Aggression* (S. H. Frazier, ed.), pp. 225–247, The Williams & Wilkins Company, Baltimore.

Mendelson, J. H., Ellingboe, J., Mello, N. K., and Kuehnle, J., 1978, Effects of alcohol on plasma testosterone and luteinizing hormone levels, *Alcoholism: Clin. Exp. Res.*, 2:255–258.

Mezey, E., 1975, Intestinal function in chronic alcoholism, *Ann. N.Y. Acad. Sci.*, 252:215–227.

Mezey, E., Jow, E., Slavin, R. E., and Tobon, F., 1970, Pancreatic function and intestinal absorption in chronic alcoholism, *Gastroenterology*, 59:657–664.

Mezey, E., and Tobon, F., 1971, Rates of ethanol clearance and activities of the ethanol-oxidizing enzymes in chronic alcoholic patients, *Gastroenterology*, 61:707–715.

Mezey, E., and Potter, J. J., 1976, Changes in exocrine pancreatic function produced by altered dietary protein intake in drinking alcoholics, *Johns Hopkins Med. J.*, 138:7–12.

Mezey, E., Potter, J. J., French, S. W., Tamura, T., and Halsted, C. H., 1983, Effect of chronic ethanol feeding on hepatic collagen in the monkey, *Hepatology*, 3:41–44.

Mikkelsen, W. P., Turrill, F. L., and Kern, W. H., 1968, Acute hyaline necrosis of the liver: A surgical trap, *Am. J. Surg.*, 116:266–272.

Morgan, M. Y., Milsom, J. P., and Sherlock, S., 1978, Plasma ratio of valine, leucine and isoleucine to phenylalanine and tyrosine in liver disease, *Gut*, 19:1068–1073.

Nakano, M., and Lieber, C. S., 1982, Ultrastructure of initial stages of perivenular fibrosis in alcohol fed baboons, *Am. J. Path.*, 106:145–155.

Nakano, M., Worner, T. M., and Lieber, C. S., 1982, Perivenular fibrosis in alcoholic liver injury: Ultrastructure of histologic progression, *Gastroenterology*, 83:777–785.

Nasrallah, S. M., Nassar, V. H., and Galambos, J. T., 1980, Importance of terminal hepatic venule thickening, *Arch. Pathol. Lab. Med.*, 104:84–86.

Newcomer, A. D., Hofmann, A. F., DiMagno, E. P., Thomas, P. J., and Carlson, G. L., 1979, Triolein breath test—A sensitive and specific test for fat malabsorption, *Gastroenterology*, 76:6–13.

Okuda, K., and Takigawa, N., 1970, Rat liver 5-cholestane-3, 7, 12, 26-tetroldehydrogenase as a liver alcohol dehydrogenase, *Biochem. Biophys. Acta*, 22:141–148.

Ono, J., Hutson, D. G., Dombro, R. S., et al., 1978, Tryptophan and hepatic coma, *Gastroenterology*, 74:196–200.

Orloff, M. J., Duguary, L. R., and Kosta, L. D., 1977, Criteria for selection of patients for emergency portacaval shunt, *Am. J. Surg.*, 134:146–152.

Orrego, H., Kalant, H., Israel, Y., et al., 1979, Effect of short-term therapy with propylthiouracil in patients with alcoholic liver disease, *Gastroenterology*, 76:105–115.

Papenberg, J., vonWartburg, J. P., and Aebi, H., 1970, Metabolism of ethanol and fructose in the perfused rat liver, *Enzymol. Biol. Clin.*, 11:235–250.

Paronetto, F., and Lieber, C. S., 1976, Cytotoxicity of lymphocytes in experimental alcoholic liver injury in the baboon, *Proc. Soc. Exp. Biol. Med.*, 153:495–497.

Parl, F. F., Lev, R., Thomas, E., and Pitchumoni, C. S., 1979, Histologic and morphometric study of chronic gastritis in alcohol patients, *Human Pathol.,* 10:45–56.

Pell, S., and D'Alonzo, C. S., The prevalence of chronic disease among problem drinkers, *Arch. Environ. Health,* 16:679–684.

Pikkarainen, P. H., and Lieber, C. S., 1980, Concentration dependency of ethanol elimination rates in baboons: Effect of chronic alcohol consumption, *Alcoholism: Clin. Exp. Res.,* 4:40–43.

Pitcher, J. L., 1971, Safety and effectiveness of the modified Sengstaken-Blakemore tube: A prospective study, *Gastroenterology,* 61:291–298.

Popper, H., and Lieber, C. S., 1980, Histogenesis of alcoholic fibrosis and cirrhosis in the baboon, *Am. J. Path.,* 98:695–716.

Powell, W. J., and Klatskin, G., 1968, Duration of survival in patients with Laennec's cirrhosis. Influence of alcohol withdrawal and possible effects of recent changes in general management of the disease, *Am. J. Med.,* 44:406–420.

Ratnoff, O. D., and Patek, A. J., Jr., 1942, Natural history of Laennec's cirrhosis of the liver. An analysis of 386 cases. *Medicine (Baltimore),* 21:207–268.

Regan, T. J., Wu, C. F., Weisse, A. B., Haider, B., Ahmed, S. S., Oldewurtel, H. A., and Lyson, M. M., 1974, Acute myocardial infarction in toxic cardiomyopathy without coronary obstruction, *Circulation,* 51:453–461.

Resnick, R. H., Iber, E., Ishihara, A. M., Chalmers, T. C., and Zimmerman, H., 1974, A controlled study of the therapeutic portacaval shunt, *Gastroenterology,* 67:843–857.

Roach, M. K., Khan, M., Knapp, M., and Reese, W. N., 1972, Ethanol metabolism in vivo and the role of hepatic microsomal ethanol oxidation, *Q. J. Stud. Alc.,* 33:751–755.

Robles, E. A., Mezey, E., Halsted, C. H., and Schuster, M. M., 1974, Effect of ethanol on motility of the small intestine, *Johns Hopkins Med. J.,* 135:17–24.

Rogers, A. E., Fox, J. G., and Gottlieb, L. S., 1981, Effects of ethanol and malnutrition on non-human primate liver, in *Frontiers in Liver Disease* (P. D. Berk and T. C. Chalmers, eds.), pp. 167–175, Thieme-Stratton, Inc., N.Y., N.Y.

Rubin, E., and Lieber, C. S., 1968, Alcohol-induced hepatic injury in nonalcoholic volunteers, *New Eng. J. Med.,* 278:869–876.

Russell, R. M., Morrison, S. A., Smith, F. R., Oaks, E. V., and Carney, E., 1978, Vitamin A reversal of abnormal dark adaptation in cirrhosis, *Ann. Intern. Med.,* 88:622–626.

Sabesin, S. M., Hawkins, H. L., Kuiken, L., and Ragland, J. B., 1977, Abnormal plasma lipoproteins and lecithin-cholesterol acyltransferase deficiency in alcoholic liver disease, *Gastroenterology,* 72:501–518.

Salaspuro, M. P., Lindros, K. O., and Pikkarainen, P., 1975, Ethanol and galactose metabolism as influenced by 4-methylpyrazole in alcoholics with and without nutritional deficiencies. Preliminary report of a new approach to pathogenesis and treatment in alcoholic liver disease, *Ann. Clin. Res.,* 7:26–72.

Salaspuro, M., and Lieber, C. S., 1977, Non-ADH pathway of alcohol metabolism: Its increase in activity at high ethanol concentrations and after chronic ethanol consumption, *Gastroenterology,* 73:1245.

Salaspuro, M. P., Shaw, S., Jayatilleke, E., Ross, W. A., and Lieber, C. S., 1981,

Attenuation of ethanol-induced hepatic redox change after chronic alcohol consumption: Mechanism and metabolic consequences, *Hepatology*, 1:33–38.

Sargent, W. Q., Simpson, J. R., and Beard, J. D., 1974, The effects of acute and chronic ethanol administration in divalent cation excretion, *J. Pharm. Exp. Therap.*, 190:507–514.

Sarles, H., 1974, Chronic calcifying pancreatitis—Chronic alcohol pancreatitis, *Gastroenterology*, 66:604–616.

Sato, C., Matsuda, Y., and Lieber, C. S., 1981, Increased hepatotoxicity of acetaminophen after chronic ethanol consumption in the rat, *Gastroenterology*, 80:140–148.

Sato, M., and Lieber, C. S., 1981, Hepatic vitamin A depletion after chronic ethanol consumption in baboons and rats, *J. Nutr.*, 111:2015–2023.

———, 1982, Increased metabolism of retinoic acid after chronic ethanol consumption in rat liver microsomes, *Arch. Biochem. Biophys.*, 213:557–564.

Savolainen, E-R., Leo, M. A., Timpl, R., and Lieber, C. S., 1984, Acetaldehyde and lactate stimulate collagen synthesis of cultured baboon liver myofibroblasts, *Gastroenterology*, 87:777–787.

Schenker, S., Breen, K. J., and Hoyumpa, A. M., 1974, Hepatic encephalopathy: Current status, *Gastroenterology*, 66:121–151.

Schenker, S., 1982, Effects of alcohol on the brain: Clinical features, pathogenesis, in *Medical Disorders of Alcoholism—Pathogenesis and Treatment* (C. S. Lieber, ed.), pp. 480–525, W. B. Saunders Company, Philadelphia.

Schroeder, E. T., Shear, L., Sancetta, S. M., and Gabuzda, G. J., 1967, Renal failure in patients with cirrhosis of the liver. III. Evaluation of intrarenal blood flow by para-aminohippurate extraction and response antiotensin, *Am. J. Med.*, 43:887–896.

Shaw, S., Heller, E. A., Friedman, H. S., Baraona, E., and Lieber, C. S., 1977, Increased hepatic oxygenation following ethanol administration in the baboon, *Proc. Soc. Exp. Biol. Med.*, 156:509–513.

Shaw, S., Worner, T. M., and Lieber, C. S., 38:59–63, 1983, Comparison of animal and vegetable protein sources in the dietary management of hepatic encephalopathy, *Am. J. Clin. Nutr.*

Shigeta, Y., Nomura, F., Iida, S., Leo, M. A., Felder, M. R., and Lieber, C. S., 1983, Ethanol metabolism in vivo by the microsomal ethanol oxidizing system in deermice lacking alcohol dehydrogenase (ADH), *Biochem. Pharmacol.*, 33:807–814.

Silverstein, F. E., Gilbert, D. A., Tedesco, F. J., Buenger, N. K., and Pershing, J., 1981, The national ASGE survey on upper gastrointestinal bleeding, *Gastrointes. Endoscopy*, 27:73–102.

Smith, M., Hopkinson, D. A., and Harris, H., 1973, Studies on the subunit structure and molecular size of the human alcohol dehydrogenase isozymes determined by the different loci ADH_1, ADH_2 and ADH_3, *Ann. Human Genet.*, 36:401–414.

Stamatoyannopoulos, G., Chen, S., and Fukui, M., 1975, Liver alcohol-dehydrogenase in Japanese: High population frequency of atypical form and its possible role in alcohol sensitivity, *Am. J. Human Gen.*, 27:789–796.

Stason, W. B., Neff, R. K., Miettinen, I. S., and Jick, H., 1976, Alcohol consumption and nonfatal infarction, *Am. J. Epidemiol.,* 104:603–608.

Strum, W. B., and Spiro, H. M., 1971, Chronic pancreatitis, *Ann. Int. Med.,* 74:264–277.

Summary of Vital Statistics of the City of New York, 1979, Department of Health, The City of New York, Bureau of Health Statistics and Analysis, New York.

Tavel, M. E., Davidson, W., and Betterton, T. D., 1961, A critical analysis of mortality associated with delirium tremens: A review of 39 fatalities in a nine-year period, *Am. J. Med. Sci.,* 242:18–29.

Tennenbaum, J. I., Ruppert, R. D., St. Pierre, R. L., and Greenberger, N. J., 1969, The effect of chronic alcohol administration on the immune responsiveness of rats, *J. Allergy,* 44:272–281.

Terblanche, J., Northover, J. M. A., Bornman, P., Kahn, D., Bargezat, G. O., Sellars, S., Campbell, J. A. H., and Saunders, S. J., 1979, A prospective evaluation of injection sclerotherapy in the treatment of acute bleeding from esophageal varices, *Surgery,* 85:239–245.

Theorell, H., and Chance, B., 1951, Studies on liver alcohol dehydrogenase. II. The kinetics of the compounds of forse liver alcohol dehydrogenase and reduced idphosph pyridine nucleotide, *Acta Chem. Scand.,* 5:1127–1144.

Thieden, H. I. D., 1971, The effect of ethanol concentration on ethanol oxidation in rat liver slices, *Acta Chem. Scand.,* 25:3421–3427.

Thomas, E., Rosenthal, W. S., Rymer, W., and Katz, D., 1979, Upper gastrointestinal hemorrhage in patients with alcoholic liver disease and esophageal varices, *Am. J. Gastroenterology,* 72:623–629.

Thompson, W. L., Johnson, A. D. and Maddrey, W. L., 1975, Diazepam and paraldehyde for treatment of severe delirium tremens, *Ann. Intern. Med.,* 82:175–180.

Thurman, R. G., McKenna, W. R., and McCaffrey, T. B., 1976, Pathways responsible for the adaptive increase in ethanol utilization following chronic treatment with ethanol: Inhibitor studies with the hemoglobin-free perfused rat liver, *Molecular Pharmacol.,* 12:156–166.

Tomasulo, P. A., Kater, R. M. H., and Iber, F. L., 1968, Impairment of thiamine absorption in alcoholism, *Am. J. Clin. Nutr.,* 21:1340–1344.

Tristani, F. E., and Cohn, J. N., 1967, Systemic and renal hemodynamics in oliguric hepatic failure: Effect of volume expansion, *J. Clin. Invest.,* 46:1894–1906.

Tuyns, A. J., 1970, Cancer of the oesophagus: Further evidence of the relation to drinking habits in France, *Int. J. Cancer,* 5:151–162.

Ugarte, G., Pino, M. E., and Insunza, I., 1967, Hepatic alcohol dehydrogenase in alcoholic addicts with and without hepatic damage, *Am. J. Dig. Dis.,* 12:589–592.

Ugarte, G., Pereda, I., Pino, M. E., and Iturriaga, H., 1972, Influence of alcohol intake, length of abstinence and meprobamate on the rate of ethanol metabolism in man, *Q. J. Stud. Alc.,* 33:698–705.

Uribe, M., Marquez, M. A., Ramos, G. G., Ramos-Uribe, M. H., Vargas, F., Villalobos, A., and Ramos, C., 1982, Treatment of chronic portal-systemic encephalopathy with vegetable and animal protein diets: A controlled crossover study, *Dig. Dis. Sci.,* 27:1109–1116.

VanWaes, L., and Lieber, C. S., 1977a, Early perivenular sclerosis in alcoholic fatty liver, an index of progressive liver injury, *Gastroenterology,* 73:646–650.

———, 1977b, Glutamate dehydrogenase, a reliable marker of liver cell necrosis in the alcoholic, *Br. J. Med.,* 2:1508–1510.

Veich, R. L., Guynn, R., and Veloso, D., 1972, The time-course of the effects of ethanol on the redox and phosphorylation states of rat liver, *Biochem. J.,* 127:387–397.

Veitch, R. L., Lumeng, L., and Li, T. K., 1974, The effect of ethanol and acetaldehyde on vitamin B_6 metabolism in liver, *Gastroenterology* 66:868.

———, 1975, Vitamin B_6 metabolism in chronic alcohol abuse: The effect of ethanol oxidation on hepatic pyridoxal 5′-phosphate metabolism, *J. Clin. Invest.,* 55:1026–1032.

Vlahcevic, Z. R., Buhac, I., Farrar, J. T., Bell, C. C., and Swell, L., 1971, Bile acid metabolism of cholic acid metabolism. I. Kinetic aspects of cholic acid metabolism, *Gastroenterology,* 60:491–498.

vonWartburg, J. P., Papenberg, J., and Aebi, H., 1965, A atypical human alcohol dehydrogenase, *Can. J. Biochem.,* 43:889–898.

Waldram, R., Davis, M., Nunnerley, H., and Williams, R., 1974, Emergency endoscopy after gastrointestinal hemorrhage in fifty patients with portal hypertension, *Br. Med. J.,* 4:94–96.

Williams, R. R., and Horn, J. W., 1977, Association of cancer sites with tobacco and alcohol consumption and socioeconomic status of patients: Interview study from the third national cancer survey, *J. Nat. Cancer Inst.,* 58:547.

Wilson, F. A., and Hoyumpa, A. M., 1979, Ethanol and small intestinal transport, *Gastroenterology,* 76:388–403.

Winship, D. H., Carlton, R. C., Zaboralskie, F. F., and Hogan, W. J., 1968, Deterioration of esophageal peristalsis in patients with alcoholic neuropathy, *Gastroenterology,* 55:173–178.

Witte, M. H., Dumont, A. E., Cole, W. R., Witte, C. L., and Kintner, K., 1969, Lymph circulation in hepatic cirrhosis: Effect of portacaval shunt, *Ann. Intern. Med.,* 70:303–310.

Wolff, H. P., Lommer, D., and Torbica, M., 1962, Studies in plasma aldosterone metabolism in some heart, liver and kidney disease, *Schweiz. Med. Wschr.,* 95:387–395.

Yano, K., Phoads, G. G., and Kagan, A., 1977, Coffee, alcohol and risk of coronary heart disease among Japanese men living in Hawaii, *New Eng. J. Med.,* 297:405–409.

CHAPTER 3

Genetic Determinants of Alcoholism

Donald W. Goodwin, M.D.
Professor of Psychiatry, Chairman of the Department
University of Kansas Medical Center
Kansas City, Kansas

I. ALCOHOLISM: A FAMILY DISEASE

A. Historical Background

The idea that alcoholism runs in families dates back to antiquity. Aristotle declared that drunken women "bring forth children like themselves." Plutarch said, "One drunkard begets another" (Burton, 1906). During the "gin epidemic" in eighteenth-century England, the notion that alcoholism was not only familial but hereditary was strong, with many tracts denouncing consumption of spirits on the grounds that it produced alcoholism in the offspring (Warner and Rosett, 1975). In the early nineteenth century Benjamin Rush, holding similar views, warned against prescribing alcohol to pregnant women (Rush, 1787), and throughout the nineteenth century there are numerous references in medical and religious works referring to the transmission of alcoholism from generation to generation. Fournier (1877) believed, as did many of his generation, that not only did alcoholism promote alcoholism in subsequent generations but also other forms of "depravity," most conspicuously mental retardation. He wrote: "It is common to witness the son of a drunkard becoming addicted to excess in drinking at an early age but the principle of transmission does not confine manifestations to a reiteration of the same form of derangement but other phenomena of disordered nerve elements are legitimately traced in children through many generations back to a drunken progenitor." While it was agreed that alcoholism ran in families, however, not everyone agreed that alcoholism was associated with other illnesses. As noted later, this controversy persists to the present time.

B. Systematic Studies

Late in the nineteenth century for the first time investigators began systematic studies of the families of alcoholics. Previously the evidence had been entirely anecdotal. One of the first systematic studies was conducted by Long (1879) when he questioned 200 Michigan doctors about the offspring of alcoholics. They attributed about 21% of "inherited disease" to alcohol, without specifying the disease. Shuttleworth and Beach (1900) found alcoholic parentage in 19% of the idiots at a paupers' home and in 13% at a charitable institution. MacNicholl (1905) surveyed the schoolchildren of New York City in one of the largest studies ever attempted of alcohol as a cause of mental retardation. He found that of 6624 children of drinking parents, 53% were retarded, whereas among 13,000 children of abstainers, only 10% were retarded.

In 1909 Crothers reported that of 4400 inebriates he treated over 35 years in practice, 70% had predecessors who drank moderately or excessively. In the first two decades of the century several other investigators reported similar findings, with only one exception: Elderton and Pearson (1910) reported that children of alcoholics were as normal as children of nonalcoholics. As Warner and Rosett (1975) commented in their excellent review, this led to heated controversy. Opponents criticized the investigators for using moderate drinkers rather than abstainers as a control group and for failing to determine whether the parent's drinking began before or after the birth of the children studied. Even John Maynard Keynes criticized the study on statistical grounds.

With this one exception, every family study of alcoholism, irrespective of country of origin, has shown much higher rates of alcoholism among the relatives of alcoholics than in the general population. The lifetime expectancy rate for alcoholism among males appears to be about 3% to 5%; the rate for females ranges from 0.1% to 1% (Goodwin, 1971). These studies include the following:

Boss (1929), examining the siblings and parents of 909 male and 166 female alcoholics, found that alcoholism occurred in 53% of the fathers, 6% of the mothers, 30% of the brothers, and 3% of the sisters. Pohlisch (1933) compared the siblings and parents of chronic alcoholics with the siblings and parents of opiate addicts with respect to alcoholism and morphinism. Alcoholism was found in 22% of the brothers of alcoholics and 6% of the brothers of opiate addicts. Alcoholism occurred in 47% of the fathers of alcoholics and 6% of the fathers of opiate addicts. Conversely, among the parents and siblings of opiate addicts, opiate addiction occurred more frequently than did alcoholism. Studying a large sample of alcoholics and their families, Brugger (1934) found that about 25% of the fathers were alcoholic. Other authors reporting similar figures are Amark (1953), Gregory (1960), and Winokur and Clayton (1968). Viewing the situation from another aspect, Dahlberg and Stenberg (1934) reported that 25% of hospitalized alcoholics come from families where one of the parents abused alcohol. About half of hospitalized alcoholics today come from alcoholic families.

A more recent study by Winokur et al. (1970) showed a particularly high prevalence of alcoholism among the full siblings of alcoholics. Among the full siblings of male alcoholics there was a lifetime expectancy of excessive drinking in 46% of the brothers and 5% of the sisters; the lifetime expectancy of alcoholism among the full siblings of female alcoholics was 50% in the brothers and 8% in the sisters. These expectancy rates are higher than those reported in most other studies, possibly because the investigators studied family members rather than relying solely on information from alcoholic probands. A study by Rimmer and Chambers (1969) has shown that "family studies" in which family members are interviewed show higher rates of alcoholism than occur in "family history studies" where only alcoholic probands are interviewed.

Aware that "familial" does not necessarily mean "hereditary," several of these authors have attempted to analyze their data in such a way as to control for environmental factors. Dahlberg and Stenberg (1934) established that one of the parents of their alcoholics was an alcoholic in 25% of the cases and that both parents were abstainers in 12% of the cases. The severity of alcoholism in the subjects was the same if their parents were alcoholics or abstainers. The authors interpreted this finding as indicating a hereditary influence in alcoholism. Amark (1953) reported that "periodic" and "compulsive" alcoholics more frequently had alcoholic children than did alcoholics whose illnesses presumably were less severe. Home environments were found to be equally "good" or "bad" in both groups, again suggesting that alcoholism had a hereditary component. Utilizing a pedigree approach to an investigation of a single large family, Kroon (1924) concluded that alcoholism was influenced by a sex-linked hereditary trait—a subject that comes up again in the section on genetic markers.

Alcoholism also has been studied with regard to its possible association with other psychiatric illnesses. On the basis of studies by Brugger (1934), Amark (1953), Winokur et al. (1970), Bleuler (1932), and Guze et al. (1967), it appears there is an excess of depression, criminality, sociopathy, and "abnormal personality" in the families of alcoholics.

Typically, depression occurs most often in the female relatives and alcoholism or sociopathy in the male relatives. In these studies, relatives of alcoholics were no more often schizophrenic, mentally defective, manic, or epileptic than were relatives of nonalcoholics.

II. PROPOSED EXPLANATIONS FOR GENETIC TRANSMISSION

A. Pre-Darwinian Explanations

From biblical times until the theories of Darwin were accepted in the late nineteenth century, two explanations were offered for children of alcoholics either being alcoholic or suffering from some other "degenerative" disease or "depravity." One was theological, reflecting the biblical notion that the "sins of the father are visited upon the sons," and the other naturalistic.

The naturalistic view, held by writers of antiquity such as Plato and Aristotle, as well as many subsequent generations of physicians through Benjamin Rush and other nineteenth-century writers, was based on the theory, espoused by Lamarck among others, of the inheritance of acquired characteristics. The children of alcoholics became alcoholic or suffered other disorders because either one or both of their parents drank alcohol at time of conception, or because the mother drank alcohol during pregnancy. Drinking during pregnancy has been discouraged by many societies, including Carthage and Sparta which had laws prohibiting use of alcohol by newly married couples. The Bible also warned against imbibing during pregnancy: recall, for example, the angel who informed Samson's mother that she was pregnant and that she should not drink wine during her pregnancy (Warner and Rosett, 1975).

With the advent of modern medicine in the seventeenth and eighteenth centuries, leading physicians frequently expressed this belief in the deleterious effects of alcohol on the "germ cell," or fetus. Morel (Warner and Rosett, 1975) stated that parental drunkenness produced depravity, alcohol excess, and degradation in the first generation of offspring, with progressively more severe symptoms in their children until the fourth generation produced sterility, heralding extinction of the line. Bezzola (1901) proposed that alcohol caused damage to the germ cell, resulting in idiot children. Studying birth records in Switzerland, he found an increase in the birth of idiots nine months after wine festivals, with a corresponding drop in normal births.

Rarely, if ever, was a nonbiological explanation given for the alcoholism "taint" running through families. Even theologians tended to ascribe the transmission of alcoholism from generation to generation to a toxic effect of alcohol on the fetus. It is difficult to find an environmental explanation for alcoholism until the second or third decade of the twentieth century, when emphasis shifted to social factors in mental illness and Lamarckian genetics virtually disappeared (except in Russia).

B. Environmental Explanations

Biological explanations for mental illness waned coincident with the rise of social work, sociology, child-rearing systems, and psychological theorists such as Freud and the behaviorists. By 1940 these influences had become so strong that such distinguished students of alcoholism as E. M. Jellinek, having reviewed the evidence for a genetic factor in alcoholism, categorically stated there was none (Jellinek and Jolliffe, 1940). With rare exceptions, interest in identifying biological factors in alcoholism was in eclipse roughly from 1930 through the 1960s.

Environmental explanations for alcoholism were numerous and varied. Here are only three: (1) The parents are "bad" parents. They frustrate the child, making him or her feel anxious in later life. The person drinks to feel less anxious. (2) The family "teaches" the child to drink. A boy sees his father drink and follows his example. He learns from observation that certain problems can be solved by drinking: fatigue, depression, shyness. (3) The values of the family are transmitted to the child, and these values promote drinking. For example, young men who cannot cry because of the machismo they learned from their fathers may find that alcohol provides consolation for occasions when crying would be consoling. The evidence supporting these theories ranges from a little to none at all (Goodwin, 1976).

Today it is fashionable to blame alcoholism on multiple factors: biological, sociological, psychological. In some ways this is clearly true. Genes give us enzymes to metabolize alcohol; society gives us alcohol to metabolize; and our psyches respond in specific ways to these combined factors. Nevertheless, beyond this obvious level, the evidence for multiple causes of alcoholism is no better or worse than the evidence for a single cause. The cause of alcoholism, in truth, is unknown. But it *does* run in families and this is a starting point.

C. Genetic Explanations

"Familial," of course, is not synonymous with "hereditary." Speaking French may also be familial but presumably it has no genetic basis.

Nevertheless, in studying familial disorders, it is important to determine whether the illness is influenced by heredity. Unless the illness follows a precise Mendelian mode of inheritance, as Huntington's chorea does, separating "nature" from "nurture" is difficult. The temptation, however, to attempt to disentangle the two is apparently strong. Nature-nurture studies are still popular, despite widespread skepticism about their feasibility.

The main problem in assessing the relative importance of heredity and environment is that early in life both are usually provided by an individual's progenitors. Through the years, a number of strategies have been developed to circumvent this problem with regard to alcoholism. In general, these can be grouped into three types: (1) twin studies, (2) genetic marker studies, and (3) adoption studies.

1. Twin Studies

One method for evaluating whether genetic factors may predispose individuals to a particular disease is to compare identical with fraternal twins where at least one member of each pair has the illness.

Originally proposed by Galton, this approach assumes that monozygotic and dizygotic twins differ only with respect to genetic makeup and that environment is as similar for members of a monozygotic pair as for a dizygotic pair. Given these assumptions, the prediction is that genetic disorders will be concordant more often among identical twins than among fraternal twins.

The twin approach has been applied to alcoholism in two large-scale studies, one Swedish, the other Finnish. In the former study, Kaij (1960) located 174 male twin pairs where at least one partner was registered at a temperance board because of a conviction for drunkenness or other indication of alcohol abuse. He personally interviewed 90% of the subjects and established zygosity by anthropometric measurements and blood type. The concordance rate for alcohol abuse in the monozygotic group was 54%; in the dizygotic group it was 28%, a statistically significant difference. Moreover, by dividing alcohol abusers into subgroups based on severity, the largest contrast occurred when individuals with most extensive use of alcohol were considered.

Kaij also found that social and intellectual "deterioration" was more correlated with zygosity than with extent of drinking—i.e., a "deteriorated" heavy-drinking monozygotic twin was more likely to have a light-drinking partner showing signs of deterioration than was true of dizygotic twins where one partner was deteriorated. He interpreted this as indicating that "alcoholic deterioration" occurred more or less independently of alcohol consumption and may be a genetically determined contributor to the illness rather than a consequence.

In the Finnish study Partanen et al. (1966a) found more equivocal evidence of a genetic predisposition to alcoholism. They studied 902 male twins, 28 to 37 years of age, a substantial proportion of all such twins born in Finland between 1920 and 1929. Zygosity diagnosis was based on anthropometric measures and serological analysis. The authors also studied a sample of brothers of the same age as the twins. Little difference in within-pair variation was found between dizygotic twins and the non-twin brothers. Subjects were personally interviewed and evaluated by personality and intelligence tests.

In contrast to Kaij, Partanen et al. found no difference between monozygotic and dizygotic twins with regard to consequences of drinking (perhaps the most widely accepted criterion today for diagnosing alcoholism). More or less normal patterns of drinking, however, did appear to reflect genetic factors. Frequency and amount of drinking were significantly more concordant among monozygotic twins than among dizygotic twins. Abstinence also was more concordant among identical twins. The authors found no signs of heritability for the presence of "additive" symptoms, arrests for drunkenness, or various social complications of drinking, but loss of control was subject to genetic influence in younger twins: Heritability was -0.07 for older pairs, but 0.54 for younger twins.

A third twin study utilizing questionnaire data was conducted in the United States. Leohlin (1977) studied 850 pairs of like-sex twins chosen from a group of some 600,000 high school juniors who took the National Merit Scholarship Questionnaire Test. Included in the questionnaire were 13 items related to attitudes toward alcohol and drinking practices. Also included were items permitting a rough approximation of zygosity. Leohlin found that putative monozygotic twins were more concordant for "heavy drinking" than were putative dizygotic twins. Drinking customs and attitudes toward drinking appeared to be uninfluenced by zygosity. Leohlin conceded that his data were "somewhat fragile" but suggestive.

Cederlof et al. (1977) examined 13,000 twin pairs and reported that normal drinking was not subject to hereditary influence, but MZ/DZ ratios were increased for excessive drinking, particularly in women. Perry (1973) investigated attitudes toward various drugs and reported heritabilities of 0.51 for alcohol, and 0.19 and 0.12 for coffee and cigarettes, respectively.

Jonsson and Nilsson (1968) reported findings based on questionnaire data obtained from 7500 twin pairs in Sweden. Zygosity diagnoses were known for about 1500 pairs. Monozygotic twins were significantly more concordant with regard to quantity of alcohol consumed than were dizygotic twins. Social-environmental factors, on the other hand, seemed to explain much of the variation in consequences from drinking, a result corresponding closely to that reported in the Partanen et al. study (1966a).

Vesell et al. (1971) studied the elimination rates of alcohol in 14 pairs of twins. The subjects were given 1 ml/kg of 95% ethanol solution orally, and the ethanol elimination rate was followed by taking blood samples over a four-hour period. They found that the heritability value for the ethanol elimination rate was 0.98. In short, the rate was almost totally controlled by genetic factors.

Forsander and Ericksson (1974) compared six monozygotic and eight dizygotic male twin pairs in Finland. A heritability value of 80% was found for ethanol elimination rates and a heritability value of 60–80% for acetaldehyde in venous blood.

On the basis of these two studies, it would appear that the alcohol elimination rate is under a high degree of genetic control, although further studies with larger samples are necessary to confirm this.

Like all approaches to the nature-nurture problem, twin studies have a number of weaknesses. For example, the assumption that identical and fraternal twins have equally similar environments is open to question. In Partanen's study, identical twins differed from fraternal twins in that they lived longer together, were more concordant with respect to marital status, and were more equal in "social, intellectual, and physical dominance relationships." Even in rare instances where monozygotic twins are reared apart, zygosity may influence environmental effects, e.g., a person's appearance influences people's behavior toward him or her—individuals who look alike may be treated alike. In this and other ways, the interaction between physical characteristics and the environment may tend to reduce intrapair differences in identical twins and increase differences in fraternal twins.

Further, twins represent a genetically selected population (Partanen et al., 1966b). They have higher infant mortality, lower birth weight, slightly lower intelligence, and their mothers are older.

Separated twins provide an opportunity to answer the criticism that MZ twins may have been raised in a more similar fashion than DZ twins. Six pairs of reared-apart MZ twins with an alcoholic proband are known: three from Kaij's study (1960) and three from the twin registry at the Maudsley Hospital (Murray and Gurling, 1980). In five of the six pairs the co-twin also abused alcohol.

2. Genetic Marker Studies

An association of alcoholism with known inherited characteristics would afford support for a biological factor in the etiology of alcoholism. Studies exploring this possibility include the following:

Nine studies have compared ABO blood types in alcoholics versus nonalcoholics (Swinson, 1983). Two found that blood Group A predominated in alcoholics and cirrhotics. Seven studies failed to confirm the association. Other serological markers (e.g., proteins) have also been studied, with conflicting results (Swinson, 1983).

In three studies, alcoholics were compared to controls with regard to secretion of ABH blood group substances in saliva (Swinson and Madden, 1973). All three found a remarkable increase in nonsecretors among alcoholics, but *only* in those with blood Group A. This is the most consistent finding in the genetic market literature, and it warrants further study. Although the high rate of nonsecretors may represent an acquired change rather than genetic marker, it is difficult to understand why this only occurs in Group A alcoholics.

One investigator (Peeples, 1962) reported an increased percentage of nontasters of phenylthiocarbamide (PTC) among alcoholics (PTC taste response being inherited as an autosomal dominant trait), but others (Swinson, 1983) failed to find the difference, and loss of taste sensitivity in alcoholics may explain the original finding.

At least nine studies (Cruz-Coke, 1964; Swinson, 1983) report an association between color-blindness and alcoholism. Usually the color-blindness disappears after the acute alcohol symptoms subside, suggesting a toxic or nutritional rather than a genetic etiology. A pedigree study, however, suggests the issue is not closed (Cruz-Coke and Varela, 1966). Color vision was studied in relatives of alcoholics, and it was found that male nonalcoholic relatives did not differ from male controls, but that female relatives differed significantly, indicating transmission by sex-linked recessive genes.

Varela et al. (1969) concluded that the inconsistent findings may be attributable to variable sensitivity of color-blindness tests and repeated their original study, using a more sensitive test (the Fansworth-Munsell 100-Hue test). They also studied color vision in the nonalcoholic first-degree relatives of alcoholics and in a group of control subjects. The visual defect, they found, mainly involved the Tritan and Tetartan axis. More importantly, they discovered that male nonalcoholic relatives of alcoholics did not differ significantly from male controls, but that female relatives did differ significantly from control females in the Tritan and Tetartan axis, indicating that sex-linked recessive genes affecting blue-yellow discrimination ability were associated with alcoholism.

Hill et al. (1975) reported that the homozygous SS (of the MNSs system) was more frequently found (P < 0.01) in nonalcoholic family members than in their alcoholic relatives. They postulated the possibility that the SS condition constituted a "protective factor against alcohol-

ism.'' In analyzing the blood samples for the third component of complement, C3, the same authors found that all of the alcoholics and their
nonalcoholic relatives had an SS phenotype, whereas from available
population data only 54% should have had this phenotype (P < 0.01). In a
subsequent study Winokur et al. (1976) found no evidence of an association between alcoholism and specific markers, including those reported
by Hill et al.

In a group of male alcoholics, Kojic et al. (1977) studied palmar and
fingerprint characteristics as well as the ABO, MN, SS, Kell, Duffy,
Lewis, and P blood groups, Rh and Hp phenotypes, HLA and Au antigens, immunoglobulins, blood sugar, cholesterol, SGOT, SGPT, and
karyotypes. In comparison with the normal population, the alcoholics
showed increased occurrence of whorls and arches on the fingers, decrease in the total finger ridge count, sharpening of the atd angle, and
separation of the lower from the upper transverse line. Genetic markers in
the blood of alcoholics showed greater frequencies of A, Lewis ab +,
Lewis a − b, Duffy a −, Duffy a +, SS, and M blood groups, CcD − ee,
Hp1 − 1, Hp2 − 1 phenotypes, and HLA − 5, HLA − 7, w10, w16, and w5
antigens.

Results of a comparative analysis of serum haptoglobin levels in
alcoholic and nonalcoholic human subjects revealed that levels of haptoglobin were significantly higher in the alcoholic group, but genetic typing
revealed no differences in the frequency of the HP2 allele in either group
(De Torok et al., 1976). Thus, it was speculated that the presence of a
regulator gene may be present prior to the onset of heavy drinking, and
that the elevated haptoglobin levels in the alcoholic sera may help explain
the atypical iron overload in alcoholics.

The genetic marker studies are intriguing, however inconsistent their
findings. One reason for the inconsistency undoubtedly arises from the
still primitive state of population genetics. Genetic factors influencing
taste, color vision, blood factors, and so forth vary so widely from population to population that deciding what is ''normal'' becomes highly arbitrary. Phenotype, moreover, is constantly influenced by environment, so
that in the case of color-blindness, for example, it is virtually impossible
to distinguish a sex-linked genetic defect from an acquired impairment
unless color-blindness is studied in family members. In their latest study,
Varela et al. (1969) did study family members of color-blind alcoholics
and found a familial pattern of color-blindness consistent with sex-linked
recessive transmission. The study needs replication; if confirmed by other
investigators, it would provide the strongest evidence available to date
that at least certain types of alcoholism are associated with a genetic
factor.

As of now, however, the sex-linked hypothesis appears improbable on clinical grounds. As Winokur (1967) has pointed out, if the hypothesis were true, 50% of the brothers of alcoholic probands should be affected because the mother would distribute her X-linked recessive alcoholism gene and normal gene equally to her sons. If fathers of some of the alcoholic probands also had alcoholism, 50% of the sisters of these probands would also be affected with alcoholism because this number of sisters would have received a recessive gene for alcoholism from both their fathers and heterozygous mothers. Clinical data are consistent with neither of these expectations. Family studies of alcoholics are unanimous in showing a high prevalence of alcoholism among the fathers of alcoholics but not among sisters.

Kaij and Dock (1975) directly tested the hypothesis of a sex-linked factor influencing the occurrence of alcoholism by comparing alcohol abuse rates in 136 sons of the sons versus 134 sons of the daughters of 75 alcoholics. No substantial difference between the groups of grandsons was found in frequency of alcoholism, suggesting that a sex-linked factor was not involved. The total sample was also used to calculate the risk of registration for alcohol abuse among the grandsons; the rate of registration by the grandsons' fifth decade of life was 43%, approximately three times that of the general male population. This result is incompatible with an assumption of a recessive gene being involved in the occurrence of alcoholism, although it fits with the assumption of a dominant gene.

As mentioned above, the finding by three groups of investigators of a statistically significant increase in Group A nonsecretors also warrants further investigation. To be sure, the finding, if replicated in other studies, may represent an acquired change rather than constitute a genetic marker. However, it is difficult to see why the excessive intake of alcohol should affect the secretion of ABH substance in the saliva only of Group A alcoholics. To rule out the possibility that nonsecretion of ABH substances by alcoholics is an acquired change, sibship studies would be helpful or, alternatively, a prospective study of people of known blood groups and secretor status before they become alcoholics.

Pharmacogenetic markers have drawn attention recently. The pharmacokinetics and metabolism of many drugs, including alcohol, appear to be under a high degree of genetic control. The best evidence for this comes from twin studies where it has been shown repeatedly that identical twins metabolize specific drugs at a similar rate and fraternal twins metabolize specific drugs at different rates.

In the case of alcoholism, an interesting pharmacogenetic finding was reported by Schuckit and Rayses (1979), who found higher levels of acetaldehyde in the blood of moderate-drinking sons of alcoholics than in sons of nonalcoholics after an alcohol challenge. If replicated, this finding would not only help identify individuals at high risk for alcoholism, it would also have theoretical implications for the addictive process itself. Replication has been difficult, partly because of technical problems in measuring blood acetaldehyde. However, a recent study by Thomas et al. (1982) suggests the observation may be valid.

Thomas et al. found that in alcoholic patients with fatty liver the activity of cytosolic acetaldehyde dehydrogenase was lower than in controls. Sequential studies in abstaining alcoholics showed that the cytosol acetaldehyde dehydrogenase activity remained low, although the previously low activity of alcohol dehydrogenase returned to normal values. It was suggested that reduced cytosolic acetaldehyde dehydrogenase activity may represent a primary defect in alcoholism and even contribute to the addiction process. There was no evidence of a missing or abnormal enzyme in the alcoholic group.

Family members of alcoholics do *not* differ from family members of nonalcoholics in the rate of ethanol elimination (Schuckit and Rayses, 1979; Utne et al., 1977). There exists, however, the possibility of an "atypical" isoenzyme of alcohol dehydrogenase producing a more rapid buildup of acetaldehyde, and/or differences in aldehyde dehydrogenase activity in families of alcoholics. Neither possibility has been studied as of this writing.

Another type of "marker" study involves platelet monoamine oxidase activity (believed to correspond closely to MAO activity in brain synaptosomes). In two studies of the relatives of alcoholic individuals (Major and Murphy, 1978; Sullivan et al., 1978), highly consistent results were obtained. Both investigations involved a large number of subjects and demonstrated higher incidences of alcoholism in the relatives of low-MAO alcoholics compared to high-MAO alcoholics. There is a large, albeit inconsistent, literature relating variations in central monamine metabolism with alcoholism; the MAO studies are important and deserve replication. Based on twin studies, platelet MAO activity also is under a high degree of genetic control.

Twin studies have also shown that electroencephalographic patterns are highly influenced by genetic factors and that EEG responses to alcohol are also in large part genetically controlled (Propping, 1978). Several studies report that alcoholics have a smaller percentage of alpha activity on their EEG record than do nonalcoholics, although this could be attributable to effects of chronic drinking on the brain. However, a recent study by the author and associates (unpublished) indicates that nonalcoholic sons of alcoholics also have a decreased percentage of alpha. On receiving alcohol, they show an *increase* of alpha, so their

EEGs resemble those of sons of nonalcoholics receiving the same amount of alcohol. In short, alcohol appears to have a "normalizing" effect on the EEG of sons of alcoholics—a provocative finding, if reproducible. It suggests that low alpha may predict future alcoholism in young people and may even relate to etiology.

Genetic marker studies have also been conducted in a search for predictors of cirrhosis in alcoholics. Although epidemiological data suggest that the development of cirrhosis in alcohol abusers is related to the duration and amount of ethanol intake, the fact that only a small percentage of alcohol abusers develop cirrhosis remains unexplained and suggests a possible predisposing genetic factor. Several previous studies have reported an association between various human leucocyte antigens (HLA) and alcoholic cirrhosis (Rada et al., 1981). In the most recent study, HLA antigen frequencies were determined in cirrhotic and noncirrhotic alcoholics and in a control group of nonalcoholic patients without liver disease. No statistically significant differences in HLA frequencies among the groups were found. Since HLA is only one class of marker, it is possible other markers will be found that will help predict which alcoholics are most likely to get cirrhosis (a very useful predictor to have, and one worth searching for).

3. Adoption Studies

Another approach to separating "nature" from "nurture" is to study individuals separated from their biological relatives soon after birth and raised by nonrelative adoptive parents.

Beginning in 1970, the author and colleagues from Washington University in St. Louis and Denmark started a series of adoption studies in Denmark to investigate the possibility that alcoholism in part has genetic origins (Goodwin, 1979). The studies involved interviewing four groups of subjects, all children of alcoholics. The first group consisted of sons of alcoholics (average age, 30 years) raised by nonalcoholic foster parents. The second group consisted of sons of alcoholics (average age, 33 years) raised by their alcoholic biological parents. The third and fourth groups consisted, respectively, of daughters of alcoholics (average age, 37 years) raised by nonalcoholic foster parents, and daughters of alcoholics (average age, 32 years) raised by their alcoholic biological parents. Paired with each group was a control group matched for age and, in the adopted samples, circumstances of adoption. All adoptees were separated from their biological parents in the first few weeks of life and adopted by nonrelatives. The interviews were conducted by Danish psychiatrists "blind" to the overall purpose of the study and the identity of the interviewees, whether they were children of alcoholics or controls. The results were as follows:

1. Sons of alcoholics were about four times more likely to be alcoholic than were sons of nonalcoholics, *whether raised by nonalcoholic foster parents or raised by their own biological parents.* They were no more likely to be "heavy" drinkers or have other psychiatric or personality disorders.

2. Of the adopted daughters of alcoholics, 2% were alcoholic and 2% more had serious problems from drinking. In the adopted control group, 4% were alcoholic. Of the nonadopted daughters, 3% were alcoholic and 2% were problem drinkers. None of the nonadopted control women was alcoholic. Thus, both in the proband and control female groups, a higher-than-expected prevalence of alcoholism was found. Nothing was known about the biological parents of the controls other than they did not have a hospital diagnosis of alcoholism (the alcoholic parents of the probands were identified because they had been hospitalized with this diagnosis). Possibly some of the biological parents of the alcoholic controls were alcoholics. However, this could not be demonstrated one way or the other, and the findings from the daughter-adoption study are inconclusive.

In both the adopted and nonadopted daughter groups there were low rates of heavy drinking. About 8% of the subjects were heavy drinkers, as compared to nearly 40% of the male subjects. Therefore, of women who met the criteria for heavy drinking, a substantial number developed serious problems from drinking that required treatment.

As with the male adoptees, the adopted-out daughters of alcoholics and controls did not differ with regard to other variables such as depression or drug abuse. There has been speculation, based on family studies, that female relatives of alcoholics are prone to be depressed, while male relatives are subject to alcoholism (Winokur and Clayton, 1968). Indeed, 30% of daughters *raised* by alcoholics had been treated for depression by age 32, compared to about 5% of the controls. Apparently, growing up with an alcoholic parent increases the risk of depression in women but not in men, a susceptibility that does not exist if daughters are raised by nonalcoholic foster parents. This does not deny the possibility of a genetic predisposition to depression in female relatives of alcoholics; many genetic disorders require an environmental "trigger" to become clinically apparent.

Summarizing the results of the Danish studies:

1. Children of alcoholics are particularly vulnerable to alcoholism, whether raised by their alcoholic parents or by nonalcoholic foster parents.

2. The vulnerability is specific for alcoholism and does not involve increased risk for other psychopathology, including abuse of other substances.
3. Alcoholism is not on a continuum with "heavy drinking," or even with "problem drinking" (defined as heavy drinking that results in problems but does not justify the term "alcoholism" as defined in these studies).
4. More definitive conclusions could be drawn from studies of the sons of alcoholics than of the daughters because the female control adoptees also had a higher rate of alcoholism than would be anticipated from the estimated prevalence in the general population.
5. The men in the study were relatively young to be diagnosed as alcoholic. Where they met the criteria for alcoholism, they had almost always received treatment, suggesting they had a severe form of alcoholism. The women alcoholics also had a severe form of alcoholism, requiring treatment, but were somewhat older.

Four other adoption studies have been conducted, two subsequent to the Danish studies.

In the early 1940s, Roe (1944) obtained information about 49 foster children in the 20- to 40-year age group, 22 of normal parentage and 27 with a biological parent described as a "heavy drinker." Neither group had adult drinking problems. Roe concluded there was no evidence of hereditary influences on drinking.

This conclusion can be questioned on several grounds. First, the sample was small. There were only 21 men of "alcoholic" parentage and 11 of normal parentage. Second, the biological parents of the probands were described as "heavy drinkers," but it is not clear how many were alcoholic. Most had a history of antisocial behavior; none had been treated. All of the biological parents of the proband group in the Danish study received a hospital diagnosis of alcoholism at a time when this diagnosis was rarely employed in Denmark.

In the early 1970s, Schuckit et al. (1972) also studied a group of individuals reared apart from their biological parents who had either a biological parent or a "surrogate" parent with a drinking problem. (This was technically a "half-sibling" study rather than an adoption study, but the principle was the same.) The subjects were significantly more likely to have a drinking problem if their biological parent was considered alcoholic than if their surrogate parent was alcoholic.

Bohman (1978) studied 2000 adoptees born between 1930 and 1949 by inspecting official registers in Sweden for notations about alcohol abuse and criminal offenses in the adoptees and their biological and adoptive parents. There was a significant correlation between registrations for abuse of alcohol among biological parents and their adopted sons. Registered criminality in the biological parents did not predict criminality or alcoholism in the adopted sons.

Further analyzing the Swedish cohort, Cloninger and Bohman (Cloninger et al., 1981; Bohman et al., 1981) identified two distinct patterns of alcohol abuse with different modes of inheritance. They described "Type 1" alcoholism as the more common, occurring in individuals who began drinking in their mid-20s to 30s and did not develop problems until middle age. The type was marked by a high risk of liver disorder and hospitalization, but little antisocial behavior and relatively low risk of social and occupational problems. Natural children of parents who had Type 1 alcoholism had a twofold greater risk of developing alcoholism themselves.

However, sons who were genetically susceptible were placed at even greater risk for developing severe disability if they were raised in adoptive homes of low social status, had fathers in unskilled occupations, and required extensive hospital care early in childhood. In Type 1 alcoholism, both congenital and environmental predisposition factors were necessary for a person to have an increased risk.

Type 2 alcoholism was associated with prominent social problems, but few medical problems. In families with Type 2 alcoholism, it was found that alcoholism increases ninefold in adopted sons, regardless of their postnatal environment, but not with daughters. The heritability of predisposition to Type 2 alcoholism was about 90% in men.

Confirmation of the "two-type" hypothesis requires further extensive study.

In the most recent adoption study, Cadoret and Gath (1978) investigated 84 adult adoptees separated at birth from their biological relatives and having no further contact with them. Alcoholism occurred more frequently in adoptees whose biological background included alcoholism than it did in other adoptees. Alcoholism was not correlated with other biological parental diagnosis.

In general, the studies just summarized produced results similar to those found in the Danish adoption studies: Alcoholism in the biological parents predicted alcoholism in their male offspring raised by unrelated adoptive parents, but it did not predict other psychiatric illness.

III. FAMILIAL ALCOHOLISM

In 1940, Jellinek (Jellinek and Jolliffe, 1940) proposed a diagnostic category called "familial alcoholism," which was characterized by early age of onset and a particularly severe course. Neglected for nearly 40 years, the concept of familial alcoholism has recently awakened new interest. The impetus for the revival has been the twin and adoption studies indicating a possible genetic predisposition to alcoholism.

Two kinds of research have evolved from these studies: (1) comparisons of familial and nonfamilial alcoholics, and (2) comparisons of children of alcoholics with children of nonalcoholics (high-risk studies). A number of centers are pursuing these lines of research, with the findings just beginning to appear in the literature. Here is a review of some early findings:

A. Familial versus Nonfamilial Alcoholics

Separating alcoholics into familial and nonfamilial types, studies indicate that familial alcoholism includes at least the first three of the following four features:

1. A Family History of Alcoholism

If an alcoholic reports having one close relative who is alcoholic, he or she often reports having two or more (Jones, 1972).

2. Early Onset of Alcoholism

The sons of alcoholics in the Danish study (Goodwin, 1979) were alcoholic by their late 20s. Usually male alcoholics are in their mid- or late-30s before they are identified as alcoholics. In the Kaij (1960) and Partenan et al. (1966) studies, younger identical twins were concordant for alcoholism more often than older twins. In five separate reports (Jones, 1972; McKenna and Pickens, 1981; Penick et al., 1978; Powell et al., 1982; Schuckit et al., 1970), younger alcoholics more often have alcoholic relatives than do older alcoholics, or there is other evidence that familial alcoholism has a relatively early age of onset.

3. Severe Symptoms, Requiring Treatment at an Early Age

The alcoholic biological parents in the Danish studies had been identified because they had received the diagnosis in a Danish hospital. It is customary in many Danish hospitals to avoid the diagnosis of alcoholism when another diagnosis is available, e.g., a personality disorder. Therefore, it can safely be assumed that the alcoholic parents were severely alcoholic, and this may explain why their offspring were so clearly alcoholic at a young age. In the twin study of Kaij (1960) the concordance rate for alcoholism in identical twins rose as a function of the severity of the alcoholism. Another study (Knight, 1937) reported that "essential" alcoholism is associated with a family history of alcoholism more often than is "reactive" alcoholism, "essential" being defined as alcoholism apparently unrelated to external events (as "endogenous" depression is often contrasted with "reactive" depression) as well as connoting severity and lack of other psychopathology. Amark (1953) noted that periodic (severe) alcoholics had a family history of alcoholism more often than did less severe alcoholics.

In five recent studies (Frances et al., 1980; Fitzgerald & Mulford, 1981; Ohayon, 1981; Templer et al., 1974; McKenna and Pickens, 1981), familial alcoholics had a more severe illness than nonfamilial alcoholics. In two studies (Knight, 1973; Frances et al., 1980) they had a worse prognosis following treatment.

4. Absence of Other Conspicuous Psychopathology

This was found in both the Danish son and daughter adoption studies (Goodwin, 1979) and the subsequent two adoption studies (Bohman, 1978; Cadoret and Gath, 1978). However, three groups (Cadoret and Gath, 1978; Frances et al., 1980; Tarter, 1981) report that familial alcoholics more often have a childhood history of hyperactivity and conduct disorder; two groups (Schuckit et al., 1970; Frances et al., 1980) report more antisocial behavior; and two studies (McKenna and Pickens, 1981; Penick et al., 1978) found that multiple psychiatric syndromes characterized familial alcoholism. The issue of psychopathology associated with alcoholism is clearly unresolved.

Finally, a study by Begleiter et al., (1982) compared familial and nonfamilial alcoholics (matched for age, education, and drinking history) and found greater structural and functional abnormalities in the family-history-positive group as measured by computerized tomography and evoked brain potentials. Both groups had been abstinent for at least a month and off medication for at least three weeks. The study suggested the possibility of an anatomical substrate for the hyperactivity and conduct disorders associated with alcoholism in other studies.

The issue of general psychopathology associated with alcoholism remains unclear, but the early-onset and severity association is highly consistent across studies.

B. High-Risk Studies

Family and adoption studies suggest that between 20% and 25% of sons of alcoholics will themselves become alcoholic. Children of alcoholics therefore can be considered a "high-risk" group with regard to the future development of alcoholism. A number of high-risk studies of alcoholism are now in progress and have yielded the following results:

After drinking alcohol, college-age sons of alcoholics show greater tolerance for alcohol than do matched controls. The tolerance is reflected in superior performance on the pursuit rotor task and less subjective intoxication. At the same time, they show greater muscle relaxation. Schuckit et al., who reported these findings (Schuckit, 1980a; Schuckit, 1980b), also found that sons of alcoholics had higher blood levels of acetaldehyde after alcohol ingestion than did sons of nonalcoholics (Schuckit and Rayses, 1979). As noted, attempts to replicate this finding have not always been successful. None of the subjects was alcoholic, and all were matched for drinking history.

In another study, Lipscomb et al. (1979) found that sons of alcoholics showed increased body sway after drinking when compared to controls.

High-risk studies conducted in Denmark found that sons of alcoholics generated more alpha rhythm on the EEG after drinking alcohol than did controls and also had poorer scores on the categories test of the Halstead Battery (unpublished data). Alcoholics fairly consistently do poorly on the categories test, usually attributed to the deleterious effects of alcohol. Since the Danish study suggests that their nonalcoholic sons also do poorly on the categories test, the interpretation of the previous studies may need revision.

Supporting a possible link between childhood hyperactivity and later alcoholism, one group (Lund and Landesman-Dwyer, 1979) reported that sons of alcoholics more often give a history of hyperactivity than do controls. As noted earlier, hyperactivity and conduct disorders appear more common in familial alcoholics than in nonfamilial alcoholics.

Investigating the possibility that sons of alcoholics metabolize alcohol abnormally, Utne and co-workers (1977) compared the disappearance rate of blood alcohol in two groups of adoptees, 10 with an alcoholic parent and 10 without. As noted earlier, there was no difference.

High-risk studies are based on the assumption that one-fifth or one-quarter of the sons of alcoholics will become alcoholic. Long-term follow-up will be required to discover which of the sons become alcoholic. The rationale for high-risk studies ultimately depends on this follow-up information, permitting correlations with a broad range of premorbid variables.

In any case, group differences between children of alcoholics and nonalcoholics are consistently being found. This, together with twin and adoption data and variables correlated with familial alcoholism, tends to suggest that familial alcoholism represents a separate diagnostic entity.

REFERENCES

Amark, C., 1953, A study in alcoholism: Clinical, social-psychiatric and genetic investigations, *Acta Psychiat. Neurol. Scand.*, suppl. 70.

Begleiter, H., Porjesz, B., and Kissin, B., 1982, Brain dysfunction in alcoholics with and without a family history of alcoholism, *Alcoholism: Clin. Exp. Res.*, 6:136.

Bezzola, D., 1901, A statistical investigation into the role of alcohol in the origin of innate imbecility, *Quart. J. Inebr.*, 23:346–354.

Bleuler, M., 1932, Psychotische Belastung von Korperlich Kranken, Z., *Gesamte Neurol. Psychiat.*, 142:780–782.

Bohman, M., 1978, Genetic aspects of alcoholism and criminality, *Arch. Gen. Psychiat.*, 35:269–276.

Bohman, M., Sigvardsson, S., and Cloninger, C. R., 1981, Maternal inheritance of alcohol abuse, *Arch. Gen. Psychiat.*, 38:965–969.

Boss, M., 1929, Zur Frage der erbbiologischen Bedeutung des Alkohols, *Mschr. Psychiat. Neurol.*, 72:264–268.

Brugger, C., 1934, Familienuntersuchungen bei Alkoholdeliranten, Z., *Gesamte Neurol. Psychiat.*, 151:740–741.

Burton, R., ("Democritus Junior"), 1906 (orig. 1621), *The Anatomy of Melancholy*, vol. 1, part I, section 2: Causes of melancholy. William Tegg, London.

Cadoret, R., and Gath, A., 1978, Inheritance of alcoholism in adoptees, *Br. J. Psychiat.*, 132:252–258.

Cederlof, R., Friberg, L., and Lundman, T., 1977, The interactions of smoking, environment and heredity and their implications for disease aetiology, *Acta Med. Scand.* 202 (Suppl. 612):1–128.

Cloninger, C. R., Bohman, M., and Sigvardsson, S., 1981, Inheritance of alcohol abuse, *Arch. Gen. Psychiat.*, 38:861–868.

Crothers, T. D., 1909, Heredity in the causation of inebriety, *Brit. Med. J.*, 2:659–661.

Cruz-Coke, R., 1964, Colour blindness and cirrhosis of the liver, *Lancet*, 2:1064–1065.

Cruz-Coke, R., and Varela, A., 1966, Inheritance of alcoholism: Its association with colour blindness, *Lancet*, 2:1282–1284.

Dahlberg, G. and Stenberg, S., 1934, *Alkoholismen som Samhallsproblem*, Oskar Eklunds, Stockholm.

DeTorok, D. and Johnson-Decrow, C. A., 1976, Quantitative and qualitative plasma protein studies on alcoholics versus non-alcoholics, *Annals of the New York Academy of Sciences*, 273:167–174.

Elderton, E. and Pearson, K., 1910, *A first study of the influence of parents' alcoholism on the physique and ability of the offspring* (Eugeni Laboratory Memoir X), Cambridge University Press, London.

Fitzgerald, J., and Mulford, H., 1981, Alcoholics in the family? *Int. J. Addic.*, 16:349–357.

Forsander, O. and Eriksson, K., 1974, Forekommer det etnologiska skillnader i alkoholens amnesomsattningen (in Swedish), *Alkoholpolitik*, 37:315.

Fournier, E. H., 1877, Annual oration, *Trans. Med. Ass. Ala.*, 30:94–117.

Frances, R., Timm, S., and Bucky, S., 1980, Studies of familial and nonfamilial alcoholism. I. Demographic studies, *Arch. Gen. Psychiat.*, 37:564–566.

Goodwin, D. W., 1971, Is alcoholism hereditary? A review and critique, *Arch. Gen. Psychiat.*, 25:545–549.

————, 1976, *Is Alcoholism Hereditary?* Oxford University Press, New York.

————, 1979, Alcoholism and heredity, *Arch. Gen. Psychiatr.*, 36:57–61.

Goodwin, D. W., Schulsinger, F., Hermansen, L., Guze, S. B., and Winokur, G., 1973, Alcohol problems in adoptees raised apart from alcoholic biological parents, *Arch. Gen. Psychiat.*, 28:238–243.

————, 1975, Alcoholism and the hyperactive child syndrome, *J. Nerv. Ment. Dis.*, 160:349–353.

Goodwin, D. W., Schulsinger, F., Moller, N., Hermansen, L., Winokur, G., and Guze, S. B., 1974, Drinking problems in adopted and nonadopted sons of alcoholics, *Arch. Gen. Psychiat.*, 31:164–169.

Goodwin, D. W., Schulsinger, F., Knop, J., Mednick S., Guze, S. G., 1977, Alcoholism and depression in adopted-out daughters of alcoholics, *Arch. Gen. Psychiat.*, 34:751–755.

Gregory, I., 1960, Family data concerning the hypothesis of hereditary predisposition toward alcoholism, *J. Ment. Sci.*, 106:1068.

Guze, S., Wolfgram, E., and McKinney, J., 1967, Psychiatric illness in the families of convicted criminals: A study of 519 first degree relatives, *Dis. Nerv. Syst.*, 28:651.

Hill, S. Y., Goodwin, D. W., Cadoret, R., Osterland, C. K., and Doner, S. M., 1975, Association and linkage between alcoholism and eleven serological markers, *Q. J. Stud. Alc.*, 36:981–993.

Jellinek, E. M. and Jolliffe, N., 1940, Effect of alcohol on the individual; review of the literature of 1939, *Q. J. Stu. Alc.*, 1:110–181.

Jones, R. W., 1972, Alcoholism among relatives of alcoholic patients, *Q. J. Stud. Alc.*, 33:810–813.

Jonsson, E. and Nilsson, T., 1968, Alkoholkonsumption ho s monozygota och dizygota tvillingar (in Swedish), *Nord. Hyg. Tidskr.*, 49:21.

Kaij, L., and Dock, J., 1975, Grandsons of alcoholics, *Arch. Gen. Psychiat.*, 32:1379–1381.

Kaij, J., 1960, Studies on the Etiology and Sequels of Abuse of Alcohol, Department of Psychiatry, University of Lund, Lund.

Knight, R. P., 1937, Dynamics and treatment of chronic alcoholism, *Bull. Menninger Clin.*, 1:233–250.

Kojic, T. Stojanovic, O. Dojcinova, A. and Jakulic, S. 1977, "Possible Genetic Predisposition for Alcohol Addiction." Unpublished communication.

Kroon, H. M., 1924, Die Erblichkeit der Trunksucht in der Familie X, *Genetica*, 6:319.

Leohlin, J. C., 1977, An analysis of alcohol-related questionnaire items from the National Merit twin study, in Nature and nurture in alcoholism, *Annals of the New York Academy of Science* (F. A. Seixas, G. S. Omenn, E. D. Burk, and S. Eggleston, eds.), 197:117–120.

Lipscomb, R., Carpenter, J., and Nathan, P., 1979, Static ataxia: A predictor of alcoholism, *Br. Jour. Addic.*, 74:289–294.

Long, J. F., 1879, Use and abuse of alcohol, *Trans. Med. Soc. N.C.*, 26:87–100.

Lund, C., and Landesman-Dwyer, S., 1979, Pre-delinquent and disturbed adolescents: The role of parental alcoholism in *Currents in Alcoholism* (M. Galanter, ed.), Grune & Stratton, Inc., New York.

MacNicholl, T. A., 1905, A study of the effects of alcohol on school children, *Quart. J. Inebr.*, 27:113–117.

Major, L. F., and Murphy, D. L., 1978, Platelet and plasma amine oxidase activity in alcoholic individuals, *Br. J. Psychiat.*, 132:548–554.

McKenna, T., and Pickens, R., 1981, Alcoholic children of alcoholics, *J. Stud. Alc.*, 42:1021–1029.

Murray, R. M., and Gurling, H., 1980, Genetic contributions to normal and abnormal drinking, in *Psychopharmacology of Alcohol* (M. Sandler, ed.), Raven Press, New York.

Ohayon, J., 1981, Familial and nonfamilial alcoholics, University of Pittsburgh, Ph.D. thesis.

Partanen, J., Bruun, K., and Markkanen, T., 1966a, *Inheritance of drinking behavior*, Rutgers University Center of Alcohol Studies, New Brunswick, New Jersey.

————, 1966b, Inheritance of drinking behavior. A study on intelligence, personality, and use of alcohol of adult twins, *Finnish Foundation for Alcohol Studies*, 14:159.

Peeples, E. E., 1962, "Taste sensitivity to penylthiocarbamide in alcoholics." Master's thesis, Stetson University, Deland, Florida.

Penick, E., Read, M., Crowley, P., and Powell, B., 1978, Differentiation of alcoholics by family history, *J. Stud. Alc.*, 39:1944–1948.

Perry, A., 1973, The effect of heredity on attitudes toward alcohol, cigarettes and coffee, *J. Appl. Psychol.*, 58:275–277.

Pohlisch, K., 1933, Soziale und personliche Bedingungen des chronischen Alcoholismus, in *Sammlung psychiatrischer und neurologischer Einzeldarstellungen*, (G. Thieme, ed.) Verlag, Leipzig, Germany.

Powell, B. J., Penick, E., Othmer, E., Bingham, S. F., and Rice, A. S., 1982, Prevalence of additional psychiatric syndromes among male alcoholics, *J. Clin. Psych.*, 43:404–408.

Propping, P., 1978, Alcohol and alcoholism, *Human Genetics*, Suppl. 1:91–99.

Rada, R. T., Knodell, R. G., Troup, G. M., Kellner, R., Hermanson, S., and Richards, M., 1981, HLA antigen frequencies in cirrhotic and non-cirrhotic male alcoholics: A controlled study, *Alcoholism: Clin. Exp. Res.*, 5:118–191.

Rimmer, J. and Chambers, D. S. 1969, Alcoholism: Methodological considerations in the study of family illness, *Amer. J. Orthopsychiat.* 39:760.

Roe, A., 1944, The adult adjustment of children of alcoholic parents raised in foster homes, *Q. J. Stud. Alc.*, 5:378–393.

Rush, B., 1787, An enquiry into the effects of spirituous liquors upon the human body and their influence upon the happiness of society. Thomas Dobson, Philadelphia.

Schuckit, M., 1980a, Biological markers: Metabolism and acute reactions to alcohol in sons of alcoholics, *Pharma. Biochem. Behavior*, 13:9–16.

————, 1980b, Self-rating of alcohol intoxication by young men with and without family histories of alcoholism, *J. Stud. Alc.*, 41:242–249.

Schuckit, M. A., Goodwin, D. W., and Winokur, G., 1972, A half-sibling study of alcoholism, *Am. J. Psychiat.*, 128:1132–1136.

Schuckit, M., Rimmer, J., Reich, T., and Winokur, G., 1970, Alcoholism: Antisocial traits in male alcoholics, *Am. J. Psychiat.*, 117:575–576.

Schuckit, M., and Rayses, V., 1979, Ethanol ingestion: Differences in acetaldehyde concentrations in relatives of alcoholics and controls, *Science*, 203:54–55.

Shuttleworth, G. E. and Beach, F., 1900, Idiocy and imbecility, in *A system of Medicine by Many Writers*, Allbutt, T. C., ed., Macmillan, New York.

Sullivan, J. L., Stanfield, C. N., Schanberg, S., and Cavenar, J. O., Jr., 1978,

Platelet monoamine oxidase and serum dopamine-b-hydroxylase activity in chronic alcoholics, *Arch. Gen. Psychiat.,* 35:1209–1212.

Swinson, R. P., and Madden, J. S., 1973, ABO blood groups and ABH substance secretion in alcoholics, *Q. J. Stud. Alc.,* 34:64–70.

Swinson, R. P., 1983, Genetic markers and alcoholism, in *Recent Developments in Alcoholism* (M. Galanter, ed.), Plenum Press, New York.

Tarter, R., 1981, Minimal brain dysfunction as an etiological predisposition to alcoholism, in *Evaluation of the Alcoholic: Implications for Research, Theory and Practice* (R. Meyer et al., eds.), pp. 167–191, U.S. Department of Health and Human Services, Rockville, Md.

Templer, D., Ruff, C., and Ayres, J., 1974, Essential alcoholism and family history of alcoholism, *Q. J. Stud. Alc.,* 35:655–657.

Thomas, M., Halsall, S., and Peters, T. J., 1982, Role of hepatic acetaldehyde dehydrogenase in alcoholism, *Lancet,* Nov. 13:1057–1059.

Utne, H. E., Hansen, F. V., Winkler, K., and Schulsinger, F., 1977, Ethanol elimination rate in adoptees with and without parental disposition towards alcoholism, *J. Stud. Alc.,* 38:1219–1223.

Varela, A., Rivera, L., Mardones, J., and Cruz-Coke, R., 1969, Color vision defects in non-alcoholic relatives of alcoholic parents, *Brit. J. Addict.,* 64:67.

Vesell, E. S., Page, J. G., and Passananti, G. T., 1971, Genetic and environmental factors affecting ethanol metabolism in man, *Clin. Pharmacol. Ther.,* 12:192.

Warner, R. H. and Rosett, H. L., 1975, The effects of drinking on offspring. An historical survey of the American and British literature, *J. Stud. Alc.,* 36:(11) 1395–1420.

Winokur, G., 1967, X-borne recessive genes in alcoholism, Letters to the editor, *Lancet,* 2:466.

Winokur, G. and Clayton, P. J., 1968, Family history studies, IV. Comparison of male and female alcoholics, *Q. J. Stud. Alc.,* 29:885.

Winokur, G., Reich, T., Rimmer, J., and Pitts, F., 1970, Alcoholism, III. Diagnosis and familial psychiatric illness in 259 alcoholic probands, *Arch. Gen. Psychiat.,* 23:104.

Winokur, G., Tanna, V., Elston, R., and Go, R., 1976, Lack of association of genetic traits with alcoholism; C3, Ss and ABO system, *J. Stud. Alc.,* 37:9; 1313–1315.

CHAPTER 4

Alcohol Problems in Special Populations

Barbara W. Lex, Ph.D., M.P.H.
Associate in Psychiatry (Anthropology), Harvard Medical School
Assistant Research Anthropologist, Alcohol and Drug Abuse Research Center
McLean Hospital
Belmont, Massachusetts

INTRODUCTION

Although fermentation is an ubiquitous natural process, there has been no single pattern of alcoholic beverage use common to all societies. The ways in which alcoholic beverages are used and abused are influenced by a series of interdependent factors including personality and psychopathology, availability, and socioculturally prescribed patterns of acceptable drinking and abstinence. Such factors interact to shape individual behaviors and promote or inhibit development of drinking problems. In societies that proscribe alcohol use, only a small percentage are likely to drink, but these people generally tend to be the most deviant individuals, as well as those most likely to exhibit a relatively high incidence of pathological drinking. Conversely, in societies where drinking is an integral component of the culture, the percentage of drinkers who experience difficulties with alcohol is likely to be relatively small (Marshall, 1979). Moreover, socioculturally distinctive groups have different beliefs and expectations about behavior associated with alcohol use, which in turn influence individual responses (MacAndrew and Edgarton, 1969). In addi-

NOTE: This chapter is an expanded revision of material originally prepared by Peter Bourne, M.D., and Enid Light, M.A., "Alcohol Problems in Blacks and Women," which appeared in the first edition of *The Diagnosis and Treatment of Alcoholism*.

tion, patterns in societies that indigenously used alcohol tend to differ from those where it has recently been introduced.

Perspectives on alcohol problems and alcoholism in America were formerly based on clinical impressions or observations limited to adult white males. It is now recognized that a society as heterogeneous as the United States is best viewed as an aggregation of numerous subgroups. There is considerable variation in patterns of alcohol use and alcohol problems in distinctive subgroups who share common racial or ethnic backgrounds—such as blacks, Hispanics, and American Indians. Persons who share demographic characteristics of sex or age—such as women, youth, and the elderly—similarly constitute discernible subgroups whose alcohol-use patterns and problems also have implications for diagnosis and treatment.

For lack of a better term, we will refer to these various subgroups as *special populations*—special in terms of their uniformity on some dimensions and their differences from more typical societal patterns and problems. Persons in these special populations are exposed to unique sets of influences on beliefs and behaviors which depart from those affecting persons involved in the major sociocultural patterns of American society. Examination of alcohol problems among subgroups distinguished by disparate identifying criteria may involve unwarranted assumptions of homogeneity and some inappropriate comparisons, but it is nonetheless important to acknowledge that information about membership in special populations may facilitate the diagnosis and treatment of alcoholism.

I. ALCOHOLISM AND WOMEN

A. Introduction

Perceptions of women and their problems have been altered by the changing sociopolitical climate in the United States over the past 15 years. The women's liberation movement exposed a wide range of social issues pertinent to women and focused both public and professional attention on the legitimacy of research and treatment for women as a "special population." Changing attitudes about women have stimulated questioning of traditional assumptions that held that problem drinking, alcoholism, and related medical sequelae are identical for men and women; that women are constitutionally or socially protected from alcohol problems; and that the prognosis for alcoholic women is different from that for alcoholic men. In the public arena, a number of prominent women have acknowledged their alcohol problems and thereby lessened the stigma for others. And, in terms of resource allocations, there has been a gradual shift toward the funding of research projects and treatment programs especially designed for the alcohol problems of women.

A neglect of women in alcohol research appears to have been associated with a popular notion that women are far less likely than men to develop alcohol problems (cf. Mello, 1980) and that studies of male alcoholics present fewer logistical problems (Hyman, 1976). In addition, certain lines of investigation have had to await development of research techniques capable of measuring neuroendocrine hormones in females (cf. Cicero, 1980). However, events of the recent past have by no means closed the gap in knowledge about factors promoting or perpetuating alcohol problems in women. Instead, this review discusses current findings and points to a number of unanswered questions.

B. Differences between Male and Female Alcoholics

There are numerous reviews of the psychological and social differences between male and female alcoholics (Lolli, 1953; Lisansky, 1957; Wanberg and Knapp, 1970; Curlee, 1970; Beckman, 1976; Schuckit and Morrissey, 1976; Waller and Lorch, 1978; Blume, 1980; Braiker, 1982). In summary, the most frequently cited differences are as follows:

1. Women typically consume less alcohol than men. They are less likely to drink daily, to drink continuously, or to engage in binges, and they usually prefer spirits or wine to beer.
2. Women usually begin both drinking and problem drinking at a later age than men.
3. Women progress more rapidly from the onset of drinking through the later stages of alcoholism than do men—a phenomenon known as "telescoping."
4. Women, more frequently than men, attribute onset of problem drinking to a specific life stress or traumatic event. These landmark events are usually associated with female physiological functioning or life crises peculiar to women.
5. More stigma attaches to the female alcoholic, even to the extent that skid-row women maintain more solitary drinking patterns than their male counterparts and remain more sensitive to social disapproval of public drinking (Garrett and Barr, 1973).
6. Female alcoholics are more likely to have affective disorders, and male alcoholics are more likely to be sociopathic.
7. The pattern of consequences stemming from alcohol abuse for men is different from that affecting women. Men feel the consequences of alcohol abuse more frequently in their jobs or career

paths, while for women disruptions are more likely to occur in family life. In comparison with alcoholic men, a higher percentage of alcoholic women are separated or divorced.

8. Alcoholic women are more likely than alcoholic men to have had an alcoholic role-model in their nuclear families. The frequency of drinking problems among the husbands of alcoholic women is considerably greater than that found for either the general population or for the wives of alcoholic men.

9. There appear to be different medical sequellae of alcohol abuse for each sex.

10. Alcoholic women are more frequently characterized as feeling guilty, anxious, or depressed than alcoholic men.

There is less than consensus regarding significant differences between men and women in the development, expression, and consequences of alcoholism. Differential distribution of other variables, such as age, socioeconomic status, ethnicity, or psychopathology may account for reported differences (Schuckit and Morrissey, 1976; Schuckit, 1978). Furthermore, once data for alcoholics of each sex have been controlled for confounding factors such as underlying psychiatric disorder, socioeconomic status, and occupational status, the most appropriate comparisons are made with males and females in the *general population*. Thus Schuckit and Morrissey (1976) suggested that the association between drinking practices and socioeconomic status is much more dramatic for women than for men. Lower socioeconomic status women, they assert, have drinking histories similar to those generally reported for male alcoholics, while those reported for women of higher socioeconomic status more closely resemble the stereotypic alcoholic female.

C. Prevalence

1. Male and Female Rates of Alcohol Consumption and Alcohol Problems

Recent estimates of the number of female alcoholics range from 1 million (Braiker, 1982) to 2 million (Hill, 1982), depending on case definition in the absence of medical diagnoses. A 1979 national survey examined consumption patterns, adverse social consequences of drinking, and symptoms of alcohol dependence or loss of control of drinking in a sample of 762 men and 1010 women over age 18 (Clark and Midanik, 1982).

Fifty-four percent of both men and women reported consumption of between 1 and 60 alcoholic drinks per month, while consumption of more than 60 drinks per month was reported by 21% of men versus 5% of women. Adverse social consequences of drinking were reported by 7% of men and 3% of women, while symptoms of alcohol dependence or loss of control of drinking were reported by 15% of men and 6% of women (Clark and Midanik, 1982).

Although middle-aged persons typically predominate in clinical populations, survey results showed drinking problems to be more prevalent in men under age 40 and women under age 50. The number of men who reported consumption of more than 60 drinks per month, adverse social consequences of drinking, or symptoms of alcohol dependence diminished more or less linearly with age. Consumption of more than 60 drinks per month was highest (36%) for men aged 21 to 25 and, with minor fluctuations, decreased to 8% for ages 61 to 70, then rose again to 13% for men aged 70 and over. Alcohol problems showed a consistent linear decrease with age. Fifteen percent of men aged 18 to 20, but 4% aged 70 and over, reported adverse social consequences of drinking. Similarly, 35% of males aged 18 to 20, but only 2% of males aged 70 and over, reported symptoms of alcohol dependence. Abstinence also showed linear increase with age. Only 5% of males aged 18 to 20 reported abstinence, versus 41% of men aged 70 and over (Clark and Midanik, 1982). Among men, then, it appears that highest rates of both alcohol consumption and alcohol-related problems are concentrated in younger age groups. At least some portion of the decline with age may be attributable to abstinence.

The picture of drinking patterns and drinking problems in women was more complex. Rates of consumption of more than 60 drinks per month, adverse social consequences of drinking, and symptoms of alcohol dependence appear to be less influenced by age and did not show consistently parallel trends. Consumption of more than 60 drinks per month was most frequent in women aged 31 to 40 (9%) and 41 to 50 (10%). Younger women (aged 18 to 20 and 21 to 25) reported lower percentages of consumption of more than 60 drinks per month (5% and 6%, respectively). Symptoms of alcohol dependence for women of ages 18 to 20 and 21 to 25 were much higher (16% and 13%, respectively) than for women aged 31 to 40 and 41 to 50 (4% and 5%, respectively). Percentages reporting adverse social consequences of drinking were more similar among the four age groups in this comparison, and ranged from 3% to 6%. Moreover, among all women, large increases in the numbers of abstainers did not appear until after age 41. With the exception of the 21-to-25-year-old group (15% abstainers), the number of abstainers in groups under age 40 averaged 30% (Clark and Midanik, 1982). Consequently, factors influencing abstinence among women may be different from those influencing abstinence among men.

Marital status also appears to affect male and female drinking patterns differentially. Rates for consumption of more than 60 drinks per month, adverse social consequences of drinking, and symptoms of alcohol dependence were highest among men who had never married or who were divorced or separated (averaging 30%, 13%, and 25%, respectively). Lowest rates were reported by married men (17%, 4%, and 10%, respectively), while widowers were intermediate (reporting rates of 11%, 17%, and 19%, respectively). Numbers of men reporting abstinence ranged from 13% of never-married men to 35% of widowers (Clark and Midanik, 1982).

Among women, rates for consumption of more than 60 drinks per month, adverse social consequences of drinking, and symptoms of alcohol dependence were highest among women who had never married (8%, 16%, and 15%, respectively). Lowest rates of consumption of more than 60 drinks per month were reported by widows, and no widows reported experiencing any alcohol-related problems. Married women and divorced or separated women reported almost equal percentages of consumption of more than 60 drinks per month (5% and 6%, respectively) and adverse social consequences of drinking (2% and 3%, respectively), but more divorced or separated women (8%) than married women (5%) reported symptoms of alcohol dependence. Rates of abstinence ranged from 65% for widows to 26% among divorced or separated women (Clark and Midanik, 1982).

In summary, drinking problems were least frequent among widowed women and married men, and most frequent among women who had never married and among men who either had never married or who were divorced or separated. Drinking practices of divorced or separated women appear to most closely resemble those of married women, while drinking practices of divorced or separated men appear to most closely resemble those of men who never married. The affect of age on drinking practices of both widowed women and women who had never married could not be discerned from available data, but that may explain at least some portion of the differences between these two groups.

Marital status is experienced differently by men and women, and the contribution of age must also be examined. More precise analysis of drinking patterns and drinking-problems frequencies grouped according to sex, age, and marital status appears especially necessary for appropriate comparisons between men and women, as well as for more complete elucidation of female drinking practices.

2. Trends in Male and Female Rates of Alcohol Consumption and Alcohol Problems

Some observers feel that the extent of drinking problems among women has increased and will continue to increase (Fraser, 1973;

Gunther, 1975; Korcok, 1978), while others feel that no real change has occurred in the recent past (Schuckit and Morrissey, 1976; Ferrence, 1980). Ferrence (1980) reviewed studies of the prevalence of problem drinking among women. She devoted special attention to examining the validity of evidence that supports the alleged convergence between rates of problem drinking for males and for females and the alleged existence of numerous "hidden" female alcoholics awaiting case-finding among middle-class housewives. Partially at issue is the willingness of women to report their drinking patterns accurately. Ferrence (1980) found no evidence of female underreporting for consumption data obtained via self-report or cross-sectional survey. Instead, studies of reliability of both youthful and adult respondents reveal that women at all levels of consumption were more reliable than men and more accessible to interviewers.

Among high-school students, sex ratios of drinking rates derived from cross-sectional survey data indicate that females are almost as likely as males to drink at least occasionally and to become intoxicated once in a while. This consumption pattern showed a convergence trend two decades ago, and subsequently the proportion of male to female drinkers (sex ratio) has gradually approached unity (expressed as "100"). However, sharp increases in sex ratios occur as drinking frequency increases. Male rates of reported daily drinking were two to three times higher than female rates, and males reported frequent heavy drinking (5 or more drinks on 10 occasions within two weeks) more than four times as often as females (Johnston et al., 1979; Ferrence, 1980). In adults, over the past four decades prevalence of at least occasional use of alcohol has gradually increased for *both* sexes. In the United States, a little more than three-fourths of all males and slightly less than two-thirds of all females drink an alcoholic beverage in the course of a year (in Canada, sex ratios for most recent cross-sectional surveys are even lower, 114, with slightly higher proportions of men and women reporting some amount of annual alcohol use). Yet since men are still 20% more likely to drink alcoholic beverages than are women, convergence in sex ratios will occur during the next decade only if the slow rate of increase in alcohol use prevalence among women surpasses the slight but continuing increment in prevalence among men.

Ten percent to 17% of men consume alcohol daily, compared to between 2% to 5% of women, yielding male to female ratios ranging from 250 to more than 400. Among heavy drinkers, sex ratios exceed 200, and male heavy drinkers are four times more prevalent than females. Rates of heavy drinking range from 15% to 22% for males and from 3% to 6% for females (Ferrence, 1980).

The number of persons of each sex reporting drinking problems is smaller. Johnson et al. (1977) proposed a range of rates for "serious problem drinking" among adults that lies between 10% and 15% for males, and 3% and 5% for females. If survey data for heavy drinking are controlled for sex differences in body weight and composition as well as for consumption at hazardous levels (10 cl and over of absolute alcohol per day, consumed in one drinking episode) (cf. Blume, 1980), the sex ratio is 264 (that is, 2.64 males for every female) (Ferrence, 1980). This is the best available conservative estimate of sex differences in problem drinking as surveyed in the general population. All sex ratios are crude ratios; they are not adjusted for age, socioeconomic status, or geographic region.

Lack of convergence in sex ratios is also revealed by careful analysis of mortality data, especially that for liver cirrhosis. Ferrence (1980) found no evidence for convergence in sex ratios among Canadians in rates of liver cirrhosis or other alcohol-related mortality data, nor were there any indications of underreporting of alcohol-related deaths among women. Morbidity data, for treatment of alcohol-related disorders (liver cirrhosis, alcoholism, or alcoholic psychosis), alcoholism treatment, and alcohol-related offenses in Canada do not provide conclusive evidence of convergence in sex ratios.

3. *Women in Treatment Populations*

It also has been alleged that many women with alcohol problems remain untreated. This view appears likely to be based on clinical impressions—or actual sex ratios of clients treated in public alcoholism-treatment facilities. Patterns of service utilization indicate that, in general, more women than men seek help for emotional or medical problems (Weissman and Klerman, 1977), and that female alcoholics are more likely to seek help from a psychiatrist (Woodruff et al., 1973). Thus alcoholic women may be underrepresented in programs that deliver care to alcoholics—such as detoxification units or half-way houses—but nonetheless may receive treatment in other sectors of the health-care delivery system.

Most information about alcoholism has been obtained from impoverished individuals treated in government-supported treatment facilities (Polich et al., 1980). A study of 3411 middle income persons who were first admissions for alcohol treatment in nine proprietary hospitals found 23% to be female (Mendelson et al., 1982). Age distributions for men and women were similar. At admission, the majority were between 35 and 59 years of age, with the average age of 47. Significantly more women than men were widowed or divorced, but the majority were employed at the time of admission.

The stereotype of the typical "hidden" female alcoholic as a middle-aged suburban housewife does not bear scrutiny. The highest rates of problem drinking are found among younger, lower-class women, both employed and unemployed, who are single, divorced, or separated (Knupfer, 1967; Cahalan and Cisin, 1976a; Johnson et al., 1977; Liban and Smart, 1980). Heavy drinking is less likely to occur among women who are not in the labor force (Johnson et al., 1977; Ferrence, 1980), and alcoholism is less likely among married women (Mulford, 1977). The "hidden" alcoholic housewife seems to be the female counterpart of the skid-row bum among male alcoholics (Mulford, 1977), i.e., deviant, remarkable, and, perhaps, shocking. This image appears bound up in the stigma attached to female alcoholism, but the purported effects of such social stigma remain to be investigated (Ferrence, 1980). Contrary to the notion that alcoholic women are likely to be protected, in treatment populations female alcoholics are found more likely to be married to heavy drinkers—and thus perhaps insulated from spousal criticism of drinking but definitely more exposed to heavy alcohol use patterns—or divorced, lacking the protection that a spouse is purported to provide (Ferrence, 1980).

4. Future Trends

Increased consumption of alcohol is associated with increased affluence and integration of drinking patterns (Brenner, 1975; Bruun et al., 1975). Hence, it might be assumed that convergence in sex ratios will occur as more women enter the labor force, control more disposable income, and experience greater exposure to the patterns of heavy drinking associated with the workplace.

Yet working women may not drink like men. Participation in the labor force does not necessarily provide as much disposable income for women as for men. Women's jobs are more closely supervised, and women are less likely to be employed in jobs conferring high risks for alcohol problems, such as bartending. Women are more likely to share personal problems with intimates as well as to seek professional help, and they also lack male traditions of heavy drinking in groups. Women also have been shown to use more psychoactive drugs other than alcohol to cope with stress (Ferrence, 1980; Ferrence and Whitehead, 1980). For women in their childbearing years, widespread concern about fetal alcohol syndrome may discourage even moderate social drinking. Similarly, broad public appeal of the ecology movement has raised awareness of the limits of clinical health care and focused increasing attention on lifestyle behaviors, including alcohol consumption (Beauchamp, 1981). Moreover, convergence of male and female drinking rates contradicts the generalization demonstrated cross-culturally (Bacon et al., 1965; Barry, 1968; Bacon, 1976; Marshall, 1979) that alcoholic beverages are most usually used by young males, rather than by females, preadolescents, or older persons.

D. Biomedical Consequences of Alcoholism in Women

Pathophysiological sequellae of alcohol abuse or alcoholism affect virtually every organ system. However, the vast majority of information about the consequences of excessive alcohol intake has been obtained from studies of male problem drinkers or alcoholics. Studies of alcohol-related pathophysiology in animal models also have largely excluded female research animals (Cicero, 1980; Mello, 1980). Nevertheless, there is now growing evidence that not only are different health-risk factors associated with alcohol usage for men and for women but also certain alcohol-related health problems are unique to women. In addition to psychiatric disorders, some information is available concerning sex differences in overall mortality and morbidity, gynecological disorders, liver disorders, cardiovascular disorders, neoplasms, smoking disorders, and disorders of the central nervous system (Wilkinson, 1980).

In comparison to male alcoholics, some investigators have observed accelerated development of physical morbidity in female alcoholics. Ashley et al. (1977) conducted a comparative study of disease profiles of 736 male and 135 female alcoholics voluntarily admitted to the inpatient treatment unit of the Addiction Research Foundation. Although the women had shorter heavy drinking histories (mean 14.1 years versus 20.2 for men), at admission both males and females had similar prevalence rates for most diseases. Fatty liver and chronic obstructive pulmonary disease were found to be more prevalent among men, and anemia, especially folate deficiency, was more prevalent among women. In addition, women reported significantly shorter average duration of excessive drinking before the onset of fatty liver, hypertension, obesity, anemia, malnutrition, gastrointestinal hemorrhage, and ulcers requiring surgery.

Findings from a number of studies suggest that women are at greater risk for the development of physical morbidity related to alcohol abuse than men. Barchha et al. (1968) found that peptic ulcer, cirrhosis of the liver, and pancreatitis occurred in 39% of alcoholic women but only 25% of patients in general hospital wards. Studies of Swedish public health insurance societies indicate that female alcoholics begin to experience moderate increases in morbidity five to six years prior to treatment for alcoholism but exceed men and women in the general population, as well as male alcoholics, in their amount of disability rates, sick periods, and duration of illness both before and after treatment (Medhus, 1974; Dahlgren and Idestrom, 1979).

Spain (1945), Summerskill et al. (1960), and Wilkinson et al. (1969a; 1969b) reported women were more susceptible to the development of alcoholic liver disease than men. Among women, increased prevalence of both alcoholic hepatitis and liver cirrhosis has been found despite shorter duration of excessive alcohol intake (Wilkinson et al., 1969a; Krasner et al., 1977; Pequignot et al., 1974). Menopause appears to increase the risk for cirrhosis of the liver in alcoholic women. Wilkinson et al. (1969a) found a dramatic increase in prevalence of liver cirrhosis in women aged 40 to 60, but only a slight increase for men in that age range.

Female mortality rates for alcoholic cirrhosis (Spain, 1945; Tokuhata et al., 1971) and alcoholic hepatitis (MJA, 1976; Krasner et al., 1977) have been reported to be higher than those for men. Tokuhata et al. (1971) reported that the mean age at death of women dying of alcoholic cirrhosis was approximately five years younger (51.8 years) than for men (56.7) dying of the same disease—a trend contrary to that expected for the general population. The median age at death for nonwhite (predominantly black) alcoholic women dying of liver cirrhosis was especially low (45.8). Analysis of death certificates by Kramer et al. (1968) indicated a 260% increase in liver cirrhosis mortality among black women in the years 1957 to 1966. Liver cirrhosis in women is associated with steady drinking (Pequignot et al., 1974; Krasner et al., 1977) and a shorter duration of excessive drinking (Wilkinson et al., 1969a; Lelbach et al., 1974; Galambos et al., 1972). Although the exact mechanisms are unknown, Galambos et al. (1972) implicated estrogen effects on liver dysfunction, and Krasner et al. (1977) reported an association of alcoholic cirrhosis with immune destruction of hepatocytes in the pathogenesis of alcoholic liver disease in women.

In addition to comparisons of morbidity and mortality rates between male and female alcoholics, the morbidity and mortality rates for female alcoholics must also be calculated against age-specific risk tables for females in the general population. As anticipated, the ratio of observed to expected morbidity or mortality is higher for female alcoholics. Higher mortality rates have been reported for accidents (Schmidt and de Lint, 1972; Medhus, 1975) and for suicides (Medhus, 1975). Schmidt and de Lint (1972) reported significant excess mortality for cirrhosis of the liver, arteriosclerotic and degenerative heart diseases, vascular lesions of the central nervous system, and pneumonia. However, reported ratios have varied, especially because different populations have been studied.

Data from the Third National Cancer Survey (Cutler and Young, 1975) show an association between alcohol and cancers of the breast, thyroid, and malignant melanoma in analyses that controlled for age, race, and smoking status. The relationship between breast cancer and alcohol consumption seems to be supported by other studies (Breslow and Enstrom, 1974; Lyon et al., 1976). Williams (1976) has hypothesized that alcohol stimulated the anterior pituitary secretion of prolactin and under stimulation of this hormone, breast tissues exhibit increased mitotic activity and are therefore more susceptible to the development of a malignancy. In females, greater use of alcohol is associated with higher rates of cancer of the lip, tongue, pharnyx, and esophagus, while in males higher rates are found for oral, pharyngeal, and laryngeal cancers. Although exposure to both tobacco smoking and alcohol intake interacts synergistically, cancers of the mouth and esophagus in both males and females are more strongly related to drinking (Hill, 1982).

Comparison of mortality causes in 110 male and 100 female alcoholics in a Swedish study found four times the rate of cancer in males (Dahlgren and Myrhed, 1977). However, among cancer patients heavy drinking appears to increase the risk for multiple primary cancers. In a prospective study of male and female multiple primary cancer patients, Schottenfeld et al. (1974) found less exposure to alcohol and tobacco and better survival among women. Heavy drinking—defined as consumption of seven or more alcoholic drinks per day—was found to increase the risk of cancer of the upper digestive system, larynx, and lung. Heavy drinking was reported by 38% of men and 14% of women with single primary cancers, and by 62% of men and 43% of women with multiple primary cancers.

Klatsky et al. (1977b), in an extensive study of blood pressure and drinking behavior, reported that men and women who were heavy drinkers were equally at risk for developing hypertension and that heavy drinkers had a significantly higher prevalence of hypertension than those who drank less. A shorter history of heavy drinking prior to the onset of hypertension for women has been reported (Ashley et al., 1977). It should be noted that since the prevalence of hypertension is higher among blacks than whites, alcoholic or heavy-drinking black women are at high risk for development of this disease.

Mortality ratios calculated for deaths from cardiovascular disorders show alcoholic women to have at least the same risk as alcoholic men, but few studies comparing morbidity rates of cardiovascular disorders in male and female alcoholics have been conducted (Hill, 1982). A comparison of 22 male and 14 female alcoholics, matched for drinking histories and absence of physical morbidity, found women to be less vulnerable to the effects of alcohol on the myocardium (Wu et al., 1976). Among cirrhosis patients, myocardial infarction and atherosclerosis are less prevalent (Ruebner et al., 1961; Hirst et al., 1965; Vanecek, 1976). Studies of risk factors in cardiovascular disease have shown a positive protective effect of low levels of alcohol use (Kannel, 1976). A case-control study of 513 female myocardial infarction patients and 918 female hospital controls found current moderate alcohol consumption reduced the relative risk of myocardial infarction to .7 (Rosenberg et al., 1981). In a study of risk factors for coronary artery occlusion (Anderson et al., 1977) it was observed that male patients used more alcohol than female patients, and that greater alcohol consumption was associated with protection from coronary artery occlusion.

Regarding CNS disorders, few data are available for women (Hill, 1982). Both Wernicke-Korsakoff syndrome (Victor et al., 1971) and alcoholic dementia (Horvath, 1975) are more prevalent among alcoholic women than alcoholic men. One study comparing neuropsychological function in both alcoholic and nonalcoholic women (Hatcher et al., 1977) found alcoholic women to have deficits in both spatial and verbal abstraction. Earlier studies of male alcoholics reported deficits only in spatial abstraction (Hill, 1982).

In the general population, more women than men attempt suicide (Bratfos, 1971), but more men than women complete suicidal acts (Gibbs et al., 1966). Overall, suicide rates for alcoholics exceed those for the general population by six- to twenty-fold (Goodwin, 1973). In studies of clinic populations, rates of suicide attempts range from 7 per 100 to 37 per 100 for women, and 0 per 100 to 15 per 100 for men (Curlee, 1970; Rathod and Thompson, 1971; Rimmer et al., 1971; Dalgren and Myrhed, 1977). Study of mortality in 139 male and 118 female alcoholics treated in a Stockholm hospital showed a higher number of excess suicide deaths in female alcoholics. For female alcoholics, the ratio of observed to expected suicide deaths was 17.5, versus 5 for male alcoholics (Lindelius et al., 1974).

E. Subgroups of Alcoholic Women

Although an inclination to draw a profile of "the typical alcoholic woman" still exists, it is generally agreed that female alcoholics comprise a heterogeneous group (Beckman, 1976; Schuckit and Morrissey, 1976; Gomberg, 1976a; Sandmaier, 1980a; Hill, 1982). Like male alcoholics, female alcoholics differ from one another on a variety of important dimensions including age, race, ethnicity, religion, psychopathology, occupational status, education, and socioeconomic status. Consequently, numerous subgroup classifications have appeared in recent years.

Kinsey (1966) distinguished three subgroups based on age of onset in a study of female state hospital patients. Types included those with early onset and rapid development of alcoholism, those with early onset and later development of alcoholism, and those with later onset and rapid development of alcoholism. Gomberg (1976a) suggested that age of onset might be an important variable, especially insofar as prognosis might be predicted. It also appears reasonable to expect factors that promote or perpetuate alcohol abuse to differ across life-cycle stages.

Schuckit and Morrissey (1976) argued that socioeconomic factors significantly differentiate the development and expression of alcoholism in different populations of alcoholic women. Alcoholic women treated in a private hospital serving middle- and upper-class patients were found to differ from those treated in a public facility serving a lower-class, indigent population. Alcoholic women of higher social status closely resembled "typical" alcoholic women as profiled in published reports, while lower status alcoholic women more closely resembled the published descriptions of alcoholic men that usually were obtained from studies of lower status individuals.

Several efforts have been made to distinguish subgroups of female alcoholics on the basis of psychopathology (Schuckit et al., 1969; Rimmer et al., 1972; Schuckit, 1972). Schuckit and Morrissey (1976) suggested that all alcoholics can be subtyped on the basis of prior diagnosis of psychological disorders. They suggest two major categories: primary alcoholics (individuals having no major preexisting psychiatric disorder) and secondary alcoholics (those who evidence alcoholism intercurrent with other psychiatric problems). Within the category of "secondary alcoholic," Schuckit and Morrissey (1976) further identified "affective disorder alcoholics" (women with primary affective disorders and secondary alcoholism) and "sociopathic alcoholics" (women with histories of serious antisocial life-styles antedating their alcohol abuse). Other investigators have also distinguished between female alcoholics with discernible disorders preceding the onset of problem drinking or disorders developed during long periods of abstinence, and those "primary" female alcoholics who do not evidence disorders (Rimmer et al., 1972; Beckman, 1976).

Numerous investigators have attempted classifications of alcoholics based on personality types (Morey and Blashfield, 1981). Using the MMPI, Mogar et al. (1970) subtyped male and female alcoholics. They differentiated among five distinct MMPI types of female alcoholic— normal, depressive, hysterical, psychopathic, and passive-aggressive— and four types of male alcoholic—passive-aggressive, depressive-compulsive, schizoid prepsychotic, and passive dependent. Eshbaugh et al. (1980) compared MMPI scores of female alcoholic patients with those for male alcoholic patients. The mean profiles for both men and women were almost identical, manifesting elevated scores on the depression and psychopathic deviance (social maladjustment) scales. Cluster analysis of this sample of female alcoholics revealed five significantly different groups, namely "delinquent," "schizoid," "narcissistic, passive-aggressive," "hysterical," and "depressive with obsessive-compulsive features." The five types were further collapsed into two groups, one including character disturbances and the other including "neurotic" disturbances. Eshbaugh et al. (1980) argued that the etiology of excessive drinking may stem from poor behavior control in character-disordered women, while neurotic women may consume excessive amounts of alcohol to self-medicate anxiety and depression. However, the most useful product of a classification system for alcoholics is referral to appropriate treatment. To date the promising activity of cluster-analytic strategies has not achieved this goal (Morey and Blashfield, 1981). Since only a subset of "neurotic" or "character-disordered" women become alcoholics, it appears more useful to employ diagnostic criteria, such as DSM-III criteria (American Psychiatric Association, 1980) or RDC Criteria (Spitzer, Endicott, and Robins, 1978), to distinguish primary from secondary alcoholics.

Other delineations have been suggested. For example, Beckman (1976) concluded that distinctions should be made between female alcohol abusers who are "polydrug" abusers and those who abuse only alcohol. In general, more women than men are seen by physicians, report more anxiety and depression, and thus are more likely to receive prescriptions for psychoactive drugs (James, 1975; Dahlgren and Myrhed, 1977; Schuckit and Morrissey, 1979), despite their proven lack of efficacy in the treatment of alcoholism.

The disproportionate rate of alcoholism among black women may warrant their inclusion in a separate category, especially if different sociocultural factors contribute to their development and expression of alcohol problems. A study of 32 black and 118 white women entering alcoholism treatment (Corrigan and Anderson, 1982) found no significant differences in the age of onset of drinking (mean 21.4 versus 20.5 years), age of onset of problem drinking (mean 37 versus 34 years), duration of drinking before entering treatment (mean 6.3 versus 5.7 years), number of drinks per day (mean 11.81 versus 11.03), or type of preferred beverage (distilled spirits). In contrast to alcoholic white women, however, alcoholic black women were significantly less likely to drink alone (59% versus 75%) or to drink in bars or restaurants (28% versus 74%) but were more likely to have heavy-drinking female friends (47% versus 21%). Black women also were less likely to hide their drinking (53% versus 69%) or to conceal the amount that they drank (47% versus 70%). In addition, black women were less likely to be concerned about their emotional health (22% versus 50%), and their husbands were less likely to criticize their drinking behavior (9% versus 30%). Although this sample was small, these findings suggest that the social context of drinking among black alcoholic women differs from that among white alcoholic women, and that peer and family factors may be important in maintaining abusive drinking patterns.

Others have suggested that sexual orientation appears to influence women's drinking patterns (Saghir and Robins, 1973; Lewis, Saghir, and Robins, 1982). In their descriptive study of 10 alcoholic lesbians, Diamond and Wilsnack (1978) identified strong dependency needs, low self-esteem, and a high prevalence of depression as strongly associated with excessive drinking, but this study used no standardized diagnostic criteria. In a case-control study of 57 homosexual women and 43 heterosexual female controls, the lifetime prevalence of heavy and problem drinking was significantly higher in the homosexual sample (Lewis, Saghir, and Robins, 1982). Using criteria established by Guze et al. (1963) and Feighner et al. (1972), 28% of lesbian women versus 5% of control women were diagnosed as alcoholic. Heavy drinking or possible alcoholism was identified in 33% of the lesbian sample, but in only 7% of the controls. Personality traits, psychiatric diagnosis, gender identity, frequency of visits to gay bars, and family history of alcoholism all failed to explain pathogenic drinking by lesbian women. Since rates for excessive and problem drinking are comparable among heterosexual men, homosexual men, and homosexual women (Saghir and Robins, 1973), Lewis, Saghir, and Robins (1982) suggested that certain environmental factors selectively act to protect heterosexual women from engaging in heavy and problem drinking.

F. Factors That Contribute to Problem Drinking among Women

Most authorities in the field of alcohol studies believe that the development of alcohol problems is a complex process for which no single factor has been shown to explain or predict why some people develop alcohol problems and others do not (Mello and Mendelson, 1978). It is generally believed that alcoholism in women, or in men, is the result of a combination of behavioral, biological, and sociocultural variables (Mello, 1980). These factors are so interwoven that it has proven difficult to unravel possible etiological factors from the direct effects of alcoholism.

A number of psychosocial theories have been proposed to explain alcohol problems in men. These have incorporated fundamentally untestable speculations about the role of alcohol in reduction of anxiety, attainment of power, or satisfaction of needs for dependency (e.g., Horton,

1943; White, 1948; McCord et al., 1960; Blane, 1968; McClelland et al., 1972). For women, although the two concepts are usually not carefully distinguished, psychological conflicts in either female gender identity (individual perception of one's sex status) or in performance of the female "sex role" (specific expectations of behavior associated with one's sex status) (Leland, 1980b) have been alleged to somehow precipitate alcohol problems (e.g., Parker, 1972; Beckman, 1975, 1976; Scida and Vannicelli, 1979). However, the specific content of traditional or contemporary sex roles as well as the ways in which these behaviors might be linked to alcohol abuse have not been elicited (Knupfer, 1982). Nor is there any obvious link between known male-female differences in biological capacity, such as strength, information processing, or reproductive capacity, and the development of alcohol problems (Leland, 1980b). Instead, it has been only intuitively assumed that mutually exclusive expectations and behavioral norms are inherent in self-evidently different male and female "sex roles," and that for some women these ill-defined polar differences somehow promote or perpetuate excessive use of alcohol.

1. Psychological Factors and Psychiatric Disorders

Attempts to delineate a unique female alcoholic personality syndrome have been disappointing (Beckman, 1975; Hill, 1982). Studies comparing the scores of male and female alcoholics in MMPI profiles or other personality scales have been inconclusive (Beckman, 1975, 1976). Small sample sizes and social class bias in the few available longitudinal studies of male and female drinking patterns and drinking problems (Jones, 1968, 1971; Fillmore, 1974, 1975) preclude study of youthful characteristics that might predict alcohol abuse later in adult life. Differences among alcoholic women, alcoholic men, and women experiencing other types of emotional or psychological disturbance have also remained obscure (Beckman, 1976).

Alcohol abuse has many manifestations and is no longer regarded as merely symptomatic of underlying psychological disorder (Mello, 1980). History of affective illness or intercurrent clinical depression frequently has been found in association with alcohol problems. However, the extent to which other psychiatric disorders contribute to alcohol problems has been systematically explored via epidemiological study only within the last decade (Weissman and Myers, 1980). In a prospective study of 184 men first studied in college, Vaillant (1980) identified 5 men with affective disorder consequent to alcohol abuse among 26 problem drinkers. However, there are no comparable prospective studies of women. Both treated prevalence studies and community surveys indicate that women are more likely than men to become depressed (Weissman and Klerman,

1977). It has been observed that among women, affective disorders and alcoholism often appear to be related illnesses, close relatives are more likely to be diagnosed as affective disorder alcoholics, and primary depression is more likely to occur antecedent to alcohol problems (Pitts and Winokur, 1966; Winokur and Clayton, 1968; Schuckit, 1973).

2. Biological Factors

Differences in age, drinking patterns, and symptoms of alcohol dependence distinguish alcoholic women from alcoholic men (Saunders, 1980). The onset of problem drinking in women occurs four to eight years later than in men (Lisansky, 1957; Horn and Wanberg, 1969; Rathod and Thompson, 1971; Rimmer et al., 1971; Beckman, 1976), but alcoholic women have shorter drinking histories before coming to treatment (Lisansky, 1957; Sclare, 1970; Curlee, 1970; Beckman, 1976; Dahlgren, 1978). Overall, alcoholic women consume less alcohol, and drink less frequently than alcoholic men (Horn and Wanberg, 1969; Rimmer et al., 1971; Schuckit and Morrissey, 1976), report fewer binges and continuous drinking (Wanberg and Horn, 1970; Rimmer et al., 1971; Schuckit and Morrissey, 1976), and report fewer blackouts, morning drinking episodes, and episodes of delirium tremens (Rimmer et al., 1971; Tamerin et al., 1976). The extent to which these differences derive from biological factors requires careful investigation.

Genetic and familial factors appear to be important in the development of alcoholism (Schuckit et al., 1972; Goodwin et al., 1973, 1974). Danish male adoptees separated from their alcoholic biological parents soon after birth and raised by nonrelatives were compared with control adoptees (Goodwin et al., 1973). Nearly four times the rate of alcoholism was found in the group of adoptees separated from alcoholic biological parents. However, in a similar study of female adoptees (Goodwin et al., 1977) the relative infrequence of alcoholism in Danish women hampered investigation of the importance of genetic variables in females. Forty-nine adopted women with alcoholic biological parents were compared with 47 adopted daughters of nonalcoholics. In each group, 4% had alcoholism or serious drinking problems. Since the estimated prevalence of alcoholism among Danish women lies between 0.1% and 1%, it was suggested that alcoholism may have a partial genetic basis in women. However, the small sample size precluded definite conclusions.

Beckman (1976) reviewed the literature on family background in female alcoholics and concluded that alcoholic women are more likely than alcoholic men to have an alcoholic parent, especially the father. The estimates of prevalence of alcoholism in fathers of female alcoholics have been reported to be as high as 59% (Wood and Duffy, 1966; Rathod and

Thompson, 1971). In comparison to alcoholic men in the same treatment populations, alcoholic women have a higher rate of alcoholism than their parents, siblings, or spouses (Sherfey, 1955; Lisansky, 1957). There also appears to be a concordance between alcoholism and affective disorders in the same family. It has been reported that as high as 50% of the mothers and sisters of alcoholic women have diagnosable affective disorders (Winokur et al., 1970). Reports that alcoholic women experience a high incidence of disruptive emotional behavior and emotional deprivation as children (Lisansky, 1957; Kinsey, 1968; Rathod and Thompson, 1971) and frequently perceive themselves to have had cold, severe, domineering mothers and warmer, gentler, but often alcoholic fathers (Wood and Duffy, 1966; Kinsey, 1968; Driscoll and Bar, 1972) may be the result of familial genetic propensities. Whether factors such as temperament, psychological disturbance, or psychosocial variables are implicated remains unknown (cf. Mello, 1983).

3. Alcohol and Sexuality

Few studies have investigated acute or chronic alcohol effects on female sexuality (Wilson, 1981). Although Lemere and Smith (1973) found little evidence of sexual dysfunction in female alcoholics via examination of medical records, there have been a number of recurring reports that alcoholic women are characterized by promiscuity (Wall, 1937) or frigidity (Levine, 1955; Curran, 1957; Kinsey, 1966). Schuckit (1972) reconciled these seemingly antithetical viewpoints by observing that alcoholic women are diagnostically heterogeneous. Diagnosis of 103 alcoholic women in a Washington University sample (Winokur et al., 1970) identified 61% as primary alcoholics, 25% as having affective disorder, less than 5% as sociopathic alcoholics, and about 5% as hysteric. Case analysis indicated that marked impulsiveness and promiscuity are associated with sociopathic alcoholism, while marked sexual aversion and exaggerated somatic complaints are associated with hysteric alcoholics. Alcoholic women in other diagnostic categories manifested less extreme disruptions in interpersonal, marital, and sexual adjustment.

Some evidence indicates that alcohol may enhance feelings of sexuality in certain women. High proportions of women, not known to be either alcoholic or experiencing sexual dysfunction, sampled in several studies (Jones and Jones, 1976b; Wilson and Lawson, 1976) reported that alcohol increased their perceived sensation of sexual excitation. Women interviewed by Jones and Jones (1976b) reported feelings of sexual excitement occurring at the 0.04 BAL on the ascending limb—this feeling was described as "one of clitoral tingling or itching with a warm sensation that spreads throughout the groin area" (p. 132).

However, subjective feelings of enhanced sexual response were at variance with objective physiological measures (vaginal pressure pulse using a vaginal photoplethysmograph) of sexual arousal (Wilson and Lawson, 1976). Such discrepancy between subjectively perceived and objectively measured sensations of sexual excitation may be, in part, reflective of expectation within a cultural milieu which overtly emphasizes a positive relationship between alcohol and sexual activity. Wilson and Lawson (1976) suggested that perceived association between increasing levels of alcohol intoxication and sexual arousal may be instrumental in the development or maintenance of moderate or excessive drinking patterns. However, in evaluating this conclusion, it is necessary to consider experimental effects on laboratory subjects as well as to acknowledge absence of subjective and behavioral assessments of sexual arousal and functioning (Wilson, 1981).

4. Gynecological Aspects of Alcoholism in Women

It has been suggested that possible changes in mood associated with female physiological functioning may have an important modulating influence on temporal parameters of drinking patterns (Mello, 1983). Alterations in patterns of alcohol use in women may be related to specific changes in sex hormonal balances—such as those which occur periodically during the menstrual cycle, following childbirth, and in relation to menopause—and particularly to the feelings of dysphoria and anxiety which are frequently associated with these physical events (cf. Mello, 1980). There is clinical evidence that alcoholic women frequently report a relationship between the onset of their problem drinking and hormonally disruptive events such as childbirth, hysterectomy, or the menopause. Cyclical increases in drinking during the premenstruum as a method to alleviate the symptoms of premenstrual tension also have been reported (Podolsky, 1963; Belfer and Shader, 1976; Belfer et al., 1971; Jones and Jones, 1976a, 1976b).

Podolsky (1963) reported clinical observations of self-medication of dysphoria during the premenstruum associated with increased alcohol use in seven female alcoholics. Belfer et al. (1971) found that 67% of the menstruating women and 46% of the nonmenstruating women in their study related their drinking behavior to their menstrual cycles. Driscoll and Barr (1972), however, found no simple, direct relationship between the menstrual cycle and alcohol abuse. Nonetheless, after equivalent alcohol doses, it has been suggested that blood alcohol concentrations differ across menstrual cycle phases. Jones and Jones (1976a, 1976b) reported that significantly higher peak blood alcohol levels and absorption rates occur during the premenstruum.

As Mello (1980) has observed, many alcoholic individuals report that their excessive drinking occurs in attempts to relieve anxiety and depression. Because cyclic patterns of increased anxiety and depression are often associated with certain menstrual cycle phases, especially the premenstruum, menstruum, and ovulation (Dalton, 1964, 1969; Moos, 1969; Smith, 1975; Steiner and Carroll, 1977), it is logical to speculate that menstrual cycle phases may be associated with alcohol use patterns in some women (Mello, 1980). Nevertheless, to date there has been only one published study of alcohol use in alcoholic women (Tracey and Nathan, 1976), and no reports of menstrual cycle status were incorporated in those findings. At this writing, rigorous studies of alcohol use across menstrual cycle phases remain to be conducted (see also Mello, 1980; 1983).

Alcoholic women frequently attribute the onset of their drinking problems to female physiological dysfunctions other than premenstrual tension, such as menopause and various gynecological problems (dysmenorrhea, infertility, frequent miscarriages, and hysterectomy) (Lindbeck, 1972; Kinsey, 1966; Belfer and Shader, 1976; Curlee, 1970; Hoffman and Noem, 1979; Gomberg, 1980). Studies of stress and alcohol problems have investigated factors in the lives of middle-class alcoholic women (Curlee, 1969; Lisansky, 1957; Fort and Porterfield, 1961; Wood and Duffy, 1966). In contrast, Morrissey and Schuckit (1978) studied the temporal relationship of life stresses to the onset of alcohol abuse in 293 women of all social classes treated at a detoxification facility. Although 262 (89.4%) experienced a stressful gynecological event, only 8% reported temporal concordance with alcohol abuse. Fewer than one-fourth of the sample reported temporal concordance for any type of life stress, including death of a family member, separation or divorce, depression, or suicide attempt, in addition to stressful gynecological events. The closest association between stressful life events and the onset of alcohol abuse was found in the lowest social class, with the smallest association found for women in the higher social classes.

It has been suggested that a woman's emotional perception and acceptance of physiological functions, rather than the physiological functions per se, are critical to the development of alcohol problems (Lisansky, 1957; Podolsky, 1963). Gomberg (1980) argued that the onset of alcoholic drinking in most women occurs long before menopause might act as a precipitant. For women already drinking heavily, however, the hormonal changes that take place at menopause may promote liver cirrhosis (Spain, 1945; Wilkinson et al., 1971; Rankin et al., 1975; Morgan and Sherlock, 1977; Schmidt and Popham, 1980).

Prevalence of problem drinking and alcoholism is highest in women in the 35- to 64-year age category. The "middle years" are alleged to be particularly stressful for many women. Curlee (1969) found that 21% of women treated in a private alcoholism facility attributed their alcoholism to the middle-age identity crisis that has been called the "empty-nest syndrome." Each of these women reported sudden onset of problem drinking that was related to marked changes associated with attaining middle age. Curlee reported that these women exhibited unusual dependency upon other nuclear family members for their identity. When the roles fundamental to these relationships changed, the women rapidly progressed from early heavy drinking to symptoms characteristic of the later stages of alcoholism—often within a year or two, and sometimes in a matter of months.

5. Social and Cultural Factors

Relationships have been established between a number of sociodemographic factors and various patterns of alcohol consumption. National drinking practices surveys have demonstrated statistical correlations between extent of drinking and age, sex, socioeconomic status, ethnic background, education, occupation, and degree of urbanization (Cahalan et al., 1969; Cahalan, 1970; Cahalan and Room, 1972). In general, national surveys indicate that the percentage of drinkers increases as social status increases. However, rates of heavy drinking, heavy escape drinking, and problem drinking are highest in lowest status groups. Lower-status women report higher rates of abstinence than upper-status women, but when they drink, they are more likely to drink heavily. This pattern is particularly characteristic of black women, and it has also been described for some American Indian women and an increasing number of Hispanic women.

Relative to black men, black women are at higher risk for developing alcoholism (Bailey et al., 1965) than are white women in comparison to white men (Roebuck and Kessler, 1972). Several interpretations of this phenomenon have been offered. Bailey et al. (1965) attributed alcoholism in black women to a combination of stresses associated with dual social roles and permissive cultural norms. Knupfer et al. (1963) suggested that the extent to which women have economic independence from men delimits other behaviors, including drinking patterns. Thus, purported greater economic independence is thought to permit black women to drink like black men. Study of sex differences in the use of psychoactive drugs (Ferrence and Whitehead, 1980) provides further illumination. Although this analysis omitted alcohol use, for licit and illicit psychoactive drugs, males generally control production and distribution, influence drug availability, and determine context of use. Access, however, is also affected by legal status of a drug, so that alcohol is more like tobacco, i.e., legal and widely available, than it is like cocaine or heroin, i.e., illegal and obtained only via highly restricted distribution channels. Legal drugs are also far less expensive than illegal drugs, so that the legal status of alcohol contributes to its relatively small cost and wide availability. Higher rates of heavy drinking by black women cannot be explained by greater availability of disposable income, for blacks earn less than whites. Exposure to heavy-drinking males, proportionately more numerous among blacks, as well as to other heavy-drinking women, may account for some portion of the heavy drinking rate among black women, as may differences in values regarding expenditures.

Black women also have been shown to have poorer treatment outcomes than white women (Corrigan and Anderson, 1982; Idelburg, 1982). A one-year follow-up study of black and white women treated for alcoholism (Corrigan and Anderson, 1982), found that only 13% of black women (versus 41% of the combined sample) abstained, and 9% (versus 12% of the combined sample) drank on rare occasions. No difference was found in the likelihood of remaining in treatment. However, two-thirds of the black women were of lower socioeconomic status, while the white women were distributed across several socioeconomic strata. Black women scored a mean of 9.3 on a psychiatric impairment scale, versus a mean of 4.9 for white women; and on a case-by-case basis, black women also were found to have fewer social and emotional supports and greater exposure to heavy-drinking mates and friends. In a 12-year follow-up study of 24 black and 24 white female alcoholics matched for age and hospitalization (Idleburg, 1982), 69% of black women were found to be uncontrolled drinkers, while 78% of the white women had become abstinent. Mortality among black women (10 deaths) was double the rate for white women (5 deaths). No significant differences were found between black and white women for religious affiliation, educational level, marital status, age at index admission, number of alcohol dependence symptoms at index admission, or site of hospitalization.

Societal norms for drinking patterns and tolerance of drunkenness traditionally have been different for each sex. Strong disapproval of female drinking and intoxication has been attributed to fears of compromise in the reproductive and nurturing roles of wife and mother (Knupfer et al., 1963; Child et al., 1965). Intolerance of female drunkenness persists despite technological advances diminishing requirements of division of labor by sex and the accompanying "sexual revolution" (Gomberg, 1976a). A number of recent changes in American society accentuate fears that vulnerable women will abuse alcohol (cf. Whitehead and Ferrence, 1976; Wechsler, 1979). These changes include: (1) decrease in the number of women who abstain, thus increasing the pool of drinkers who might become alcoholic; (2) increase in the number of teen-age girls who use alcohol, raising concerns that no age-specific decreases in consumption will occur in their lifetimes; (3) increases, however slight, in the amount of disposable income controlled by women as they increasingly participate in the labor force; (4) increased exposure to alcohol use as more women attend college and enter the workplace; (5) increased numbers of women "challenging" traditional female norms and life-styles; (6) changes in the form and content of "sex roles"; and (7) increased exposure to alcoholic beverage advertising specifically targeted at the "women's" market.

G. Alcohol and Reproduction

1. Alcohol Use and Pregnancy

For some women the occurrence of pregnancy itself seems to contribute to a reduction in their alcohol intake, but the psychological or physical factors that contribute to this change are unknown. Little et al. (1976) reported that in a sample of predominantly white, middle-class obstetrical patients at a health maintenance organization in Seattle, Washington, approximately two-thirds of the women reported drinking less during early pregnancy than before pregnancy. The percentage of women whose average daily intake exceeded 1.0 oz of absolute alcohol prior to pregnancy dropped from 7% to 2% during pregnancy, and for women drinking from 0.51 to 1.0 oz of absolute alcohol prior to pregnancy, the percentage dropped from 18% to 4% during pregnancy. These findings were corroborated in an epidemiological study of mothers of diverse socioeconomic and cultural backgrounds in Southern California: approximately 17% of a sample of 6864 women delivering infants at participating hospitals indicated that they stopped drinking during pregnancy. Self-reported reasons for diminished use of alcoholic beverages included adverse physiological effects (nausea, stomach irritation, headache, diuresis); other physical reasons (unpalatable taste, unpleasant smell, or simple lack of appeal), and increased health concerns for themselves and their unborn babies. Heavy (more than 0.5 oz) drinkers were more likely to report changed physiological reactions or loss of appeal of alcoholic beverages, while lighter drinkers (less than 0.5 oz) attributed their diminished intake to health concerns for their unborn children. According to Little (1976), the stigma of alcohol use extends to the physician-patient relationship, for women were more likely to underreport alcohol use during prenatal visits than they were to underreport their smoking behavior. In contrast, pregnant women are alleged to be more likely to report their alcohol use to research investigators accurately and to be willing to participate in scientific studies.

2. Effect of Alcohol on Offspring

Although for several hundred years alcohol consumption was popularly associated with high rates of fetal and infant mortality, morbidity, and physical and mental abnormalities, this association was clinically ignored during much of the twentieth century. The systematic study of adverse effects of alcohol on the fetus and infant only began about 15 years ago (for historical review, see Warner and Rosett, 1975; Rosett, 1980). Current research on this topic was stimulated by the independent reports of Jones and Smith (1973) and Jones et al. (1973, 1974) in the United States, and Lemoine et al. (1968) in France, which described a common pattern of abnormal development that occurred in some children of alcoholic mothers who drank heavily during pregnancy. This pattern of altered growth, morphogeneses, and behavioral impairment has been called the fetal alcohol syndrome (FAS).

According to Rosett (1980), the effects of few other teratogens have been investigated as thoroughly as that of alcohol and its metabolites. The effects of alcohol on the fetus are complex, with multiple biochemical pathways and pathophysiological alterations potentially involved in embryonic and fetal growth and development at different stages of gestation. Clinical descriptions of FAS include: growth and performance abnormalities (pre- and postnatal growth deficiency, microencephaly, fine motor dysfunction); characteristic craniofacial defects (short palpebral fissures, epicanthal folds, maxillary hypoplasia, cleft-palate, micrographia); and limb abnormalities (joint anomalies, altered palmar crease pattern). Various other abnormalities such as cardiac defects, anomalies of external genitalia, small hemangiomas, and deformed ears have also been observed (Clarren and Smith, 1978). Once seen and described, this syndrome is easily recognized by nursery room staff, general practitioners, and therapists (Streissguth, 1976a). Indeed, initial publication of reports by Jones and by Lemoine prompted numerous others (Ferrier et al., 1973; Hall and Ornstein, 1974; Saule, 1974; Palmer et al., 1975; Tenbrinck and Buchin, 1975; Barry and O'Nuallain, 1975; Root et al., 1975; Christoffel and Salafsky, 1975; Manzke and Grosse, 1975; Reinhold et al., 1975; Loiodice et al., 1975; Mulvihill et al., 1976; Mulvihill and Yeager, 1976; Bierich et al., 1976; Ijaiya et al., 1976; Majewski et al., 1976; Hanson et al., 1976; and Noonan, 1976) to identify infants and children exhibiting partial or full FAS. All cases were offspring of severely alcoholic mothers who drank heavily during pregnancy.

By 1980, 245 clinical cases of fetal alcohol syndrome had been retrospectively identified world wide. Prospective studies, however, have identified only a few infants manifesting FAS. It appears likely that FAS occurs when a high maternal blood alcohol level coincides with a critical stage in embryonic development. Rosett (1980) has suggested that average alcohol consumption is less important than the effects of alcohol binges during critical development periods.

A number of studies which compare the outcome of pregnancy between heavy drinking or alcoholic women and moderate or light drinkers have reported that alcohol consumption appears related to increases in rates of miscarriage (Kinsey, 1966; Wilsnack, 1973; Sokol et al., 1980; Harlap and Shiono, 1980), prenatal mortality (Jones et al., 1974), stillbirths (Sokol et al., 1980), growth retardation in length (Ouellette and Rosett, 1976), birthweight (Kaminski et al., 1976; Russell, 1977), head circumference (Ouellette and Rosett, 1976), and functional abnormalities, i.e., jitteriness and tremulousness (Rosett et al., 1976).

Streissguth (1976a, 1976b) reported that the most disabling aspect of FAS is mental impairment, ranging from borderline intellectual functioning to moderately severe impairment. In all cases the severity of intellectual deficit was positively correlated with the severity of dysmorphogenesis. The prognosis for mental retardation in FAS children is poor, with only limited response to environmental intervention (Streissguth, 1978).

Sander et al. (1977) investigated the 24-hour sleep-awake state distributions in newborns exposed throughout pregnancy to high maternal alcohol intake. These infants were compared to newborns whose mothers began pregnancy as heavy drinkers but who significantly reduced their intake or abstained from alcohol following their prenatal clinic contact, as well as to a control group of infants whose mothers were classified as abstinent or rare drinkers. The group of infants whose mothers drank heavily throughout pregnancy showed grossly abnormal patterns in sleep substages. These infants had a different quality of sleep from the control group: their respiratory amplitude was poorly stabilized, they exhibited more frequent startles and more extended body movements, and they evidenced respiratory rate irregularities. Significantly, infants whose mothers reduced or were able to abstain from alcohol intake during the third trimester of pregnancy exhibited less severe abnormalities than did those infants whose mothers continued to drink through their entire pregnancies.

Women who are not considered or known to be alcoholic by their physicians, but who consume critical amounts of alcohol during critical gestational periods may have infants who exhibit subtle functional disturbances such as hyperactivity, jitteriness, and poor food intake (Rosett et al., 1976). These subtle disturbances may interfere with the establishment of the infant-mother bond, promote inadequate care-giving, and diminish sense of maternal adequacy regarding the nurturing role (Sander et al.,

1977). Since alcoholic or problem-drinking women may be vulnerable regarding personal adequacy, as well as experiencing other problems, detection and provision of care-giving support may be necessary to prevent a postnatal environment that is further detrimental to infants already impaired at birth. Intervention may be necessary to minimize the impact of learning disabilities and behavioral disturbances.

That alcohol, rather than some other factor such as deficient maternal nutrition, smoking, emotional stress, or caffeine, is the teratogenic agent implicated in FAS and many milder functional abnormalities in infants and children has received some empirical support from clinical and animal studies (Randall et al., 1977; Chernoff, 1975). However, it is likely that multiple stressors such as smoking, environmental or emotional stress, or poor nutrition interact synergistically in affecting the fetus (Rosett, 1980).

Social class also appears to play an important role in FAS. Not only are the majority of children diagnosed as having FAS of lower socioeconomic status, the most profoundly retarded and physically malformed FAS children are also found in lower socioeconomic groups (Streissguth, 1976a). It is unclear whether differences among FAS children reflect selection bias, variation in genetic background, greater resources available to mothers in higher socioeconomic strata, or a combination of factors. A recent case-control study (Boone, 1982) of very low birthweight (VLBW) (less than or equal to 1500 g) infants delivered to impoverished black women in a Washington, D.C., public hospital, however, indicated that alcohol abuse was only one of at least ten interactive factors that profiled high risk mothers. At highest risk for VLBW infants were mothers who were underweight, abusers of alcohol and nicotine, ineffective contraceptors, frequently pregnant, rural migrants, chronically ill, depressed and lacking social supports, victims of psychological or physical violence, with histories of poor pregnancy outcome. According to Boone, "nicotine and alcohol addictions, poor nutrition, and social and psychological adjustment problems exacerbate one another" and generated an intolerable burden for socioeconomically disadvantaged women when added to ineffective contraception and inadequately spaced pregnancies. For VLBW infants, then, alcohol abuse only contributes a portion of the risk. Accordingly, a carefully executed case-control study of mothers of FAS children appears necessary in order to identify the combination of risk factors operating in FAS (see Rosett, 1980).

H. Treatment of Alcoholic Women

Alcoholism treatment programs traditionally have been geared to the needs of males—their most numerous clients (cf. Henderson and Anderson, 1982). Yet although in recent years advocates of the needs of alcoholic women have argued for sexually segregated facilities to provide emotionally and socially sensitive treatment, this position may be viewed as overdrawn as well as unsupported by any empirical evidence (Braiker, 1982). Since outcome data for treatment programs for women are lacking (Blume, 1980; Braiker, 1982), considerations of investigators have often served as guidelines.

Gomberg (1976a) suggested that six aspects of the social support systems of female alcoholics require improvement. These included awareness of greater social stigma and related reluctance to seek treatment, as well as greater need for health care and enhancement of personal appearance, vocational training and employment counseling, conjoint therapy with significant others, coping and life-skills training for single women, assistance with specific parental responsibilities, and, especially because alcoholic women are more likely to be separated or divorced, greater need for child-care services affiliated with treatment programs (cf. Blume, 1980; Henderson and Anderson, 1982; Sandmaier, 1980b). However, a study of structural factors in treatment utilization of 53 alcoholism treatment facilities in two California counties (Beckman and Kocel, 1982) found women more likely to choose agencies with higher percentages of professional staff, aftercare services, and treatment programs for children. Neither provider attitudes toward female alcoholics nor the type of agency (public or private) was associated with women's utilization rates, and support services, such as transportation, vocational counseling, or legal aid, were found to be of lesser importance to women than child-related services. Thus, the alcoholic women studied appear to have chosen treatment for themselves and their children that addressed the central impact of alcohol problems, while social support requirements were of lesser importance.

Schuckit (1978) asserted that any hypothesized sex differences in treatment needs are actually based on common sense appreciation of alcoholic women's economic and occupational positions, reproductive capacity, and intercurrent psychological disorders, as well as the fact that most alcoholism counselors are male. Recognition that 25% of female alcoholics have primary affective disorder (Schuckit and Morrissey, 1976; Schuckit, 1978) argues for careful history-taking, precise psychiatric diagnosis, and appropriate referral to psychiatric treatment.

It has been suggested (Little et al., 1976) that a pregnant woman's receptivity to alcohol treatment is enhanced by the normal crises associated with pregnancy along with her general increased concern for her own health and that of her unborn baby. For certain women, concern may be further increased by aversion to drinking. Some authors have advocated therapeutic abortions of fetuses exposed to alcohol (Jones et al., 1974; Hanson et al., 1976). In the intervention model proposed by Rosett (1980) the treatment goal is reduction or elimination of alcohol use, especially during the third trimester of pregnancy. Heavy-drinking women seen in a prenatal clinic are referred to psychiatric treatment and treated by a team consisting of a psychiatrist and a female counselor. Abstinence is praised and criticism of drinking avoided, education about alcohol and pregnancy imparted, and psychological support and practical help obtained for disadvantaged women.

The first step toward assisting alcoholics or problem drinkers whose children may be at risk is to identify them. Because the etiology of FAS is largely known, recognition of this syndrome by physicians, therapists, or social workers should lead to counseling mothers about current or future pregnancies. Such women should be informed of the likelihood of impairment in future offspring. Physicians and others also should be alerted to elicit drinking histories in prenatal clinics.

II. ALCOHOL PROBLEMS AMONG YOUTH

A. Introduction

Because drinking is such a common adult social behavior in the United States, learning to use alcoholic beverages appears to have become one of the rites of passage among American adolescents. Recent epidemiological studies of all age groups in the general population indicate that young adults are the most frequent users and largest consumers of alcohol (Room, 1972; Alcohol and Health, 1975; Harford and Mills, 1978; Polich, 1979). In national surveys, experimentation with alcohol has been reported by one-half of 7th-grade students and by almost 90% of 12th-grade students (Jessor and Jessor, 1975; Donovan and Jessor, 1978). A recent national survey of 12- to 17-year-olds in households (Abelson et al., 1977) and a recent survey of high school seniors (Johnston et al., 1979) found that alcohol was used more frequently than any other licit or illicit drug. Since alcohol is clearly the drug most widely used by young people, some authors consider alcohol abuse to be the primary drug problem among contemporary American youth (Rachal et al., 1975; Robins, 1980). Yet chronic physiological or psychological dependence on alcohol in youth is rare (Smart and Finley, 1976; Blane, 1979; Smart, 1979a; Chauncey, 1980). Instead, episodic or frequent heavy use of alcohol is associated with a variety of problems experienced by between 10% to 20% of all adolescents (Braucht, 1982).

B. Prevalence

Youthful drinking practices are most usually studied via surveys of convenient "captive" populations of high-school students. However, estimates derived from these surveys cannot be confidently generalized to all youth. It has been estimated that 20% of high-school students will be absent on any given day and that problem drinkers are likely to be more numerous among absentees (Rachal et al., 1982). Moreover, alcohol problems may be strongly associated with other characteristics of high-school "drop-outs" (Globetti, 1972, 1977), such as psychopathology, race, or ethnicity. Thus it is likely that school-based surveys underestimate problem drinking prevalence in the school-aged population. In addition, because of legal, economic, and social constraints on their behavior, frequent heavy drinking is less prevalent among high-school youth than among post-high-school youth.

1. Drinking Patterns

Frequency of alcohol consumption is the most commonly investigated variable in prevalence studies of adolescent drinking practices (Braucht, 1982). The amount of alcohol consumed by adolescents increased in the decade 1965 to 1975 (Rachal et al., 1982) and then leveled off. Prevalence of adolescent drinking, frequency of consumption, and quantities consumed reported in a national survey of 10th- to 12th-grade students in 1975 were very similar to findings for the same assessments conducted among 10th- to 12th-grade students in 1978 (Harford and Spiegler, 1982).

The large majority of youth rarely drink. A 1978 study of 4918 10th- to 12th-grade students revealed that 87% reported alcohol use at least once during their lifetime, while 81% reported alcohol use at least once during the year prior to the survey (Rachal et al., 1982). Slightly less than 2% reported drinking daily, 8% reported drinking three or four times per week, and over 20% reported drinking once or twice per week. In assessments of the amount of alcohol consumed per month, one-fourth were classified as abstainers or negligible drinkers, 7.6% as infrequent drinkers, 18.8% as light drinkers, 16.6% as moderate drinkers, and 17.3% as moderate-to-heavy drinkers. Heavy drinkers, who consumed five or more drinks at least once each week, constituted 14.8% of the sample (Rachal et al., 1982).

Although sex differences in drinking patterns have become less marked in recent years (Wechsler and McFadden, 1976), a national survey in 1978 found heavy drinking more characteristic of young male drinkers. Heavy drinking was reported by 9% of the adolescent females and 20% of the adolescent males. Roughly two-thirds of adolescent females abstained or drank lightly to moderately, but only one-half of the adolescent males consumed alcohol at those lower rates (Alcohol and Health, 1981).

Surveys also have examined drinking practices of racial or ethnic group members formally enrolled in high school. Among 10th- to 12th-grade students, blacks were more likely to abstain (36.1%) than whites (21.1%) or Hispanics (21.1%) in 1978. Black students also had a lower rate of heavier drinking (3.9%) than whites (12.2%) or Hispanics (4.2%) (Alcohol and Health, 1981). However, variables that affect remaining in school, such as socioeconomic status, are complex and experienced differently by white, black, and Hispanic youths, and are likely to preclude valid comparisons across these three groups. In addition, Padilla et al. (1979) found that among Hispanic youths ages 12 to 17 residing in public housing projects in East Los Angeles, weekly prevalence of alcohol use was less than monthly prevalence of alcohol use generally reported for national household samples of the same age groups. This observation supports findings indicating lower alcohol consumption frequency among Hispanics, but Hispanics also used 14 times the weekly rate of inhalants and twice the weekly amount of marijuana generally reported for national samples. Consequently, direct comparisons of rates of drinking or of heavy drinking across ethnic or racial groups must be considered in the context of other substance use and polydrug abuse.

2. Drinking Problems

Estimates of the extent of adolescent drinking problems typically have been derived from consumption data. More precise estimates of the frequencies of specific alcohol-related problems have been less systematic. Variations in definitions of drinking "problems" also affect these estimates. Acute consequences of adolescent drinking are usually identified as drunkenness, serious or fatal traffic accidents, trouble with law enforcement officials, difficulties with teachers or school authorities or impaired school work, and conflict with dates, friends, or family members (Rachal et al., 1976; Donovan and Jessor, 1978; Rachal et al., 1982).

A national survey of 13,122 junior- and senior-high-school students conducted in 1974 (Rachal et al., 1976) provides a major source of estimates of the extent of adolescent drinking problems. Problem drinkers were defined as either those who reported drunkenness at least four times during the previous year or those who reported experiencing adverse consequences in two life areas during the same interval. Accordingly, 27.8% of the sample were identified as problem drinkers. Donovan and Jessor (1978) used stricter criteria for problem drinking to reanalyze these survey data. In their analysis, 9.4% of the sample reported having been drunk at least twice per month during the previous year, and 8.9% reported adverse consequences of drinking twice in one life area and one in another during the year prior to the survey.

Drinking may have variable effects on young people (cf. Blane, 1979). In a 1978 survey, 10th to 12th graders were queried about problems associated with drinking that had occurred during the previous year. In that study, 10% reported criticism from dates, 17% reported conflict with friends, and 23% reported driving while intoxicated. However, only 1% acknowledged that drinking had caused them serious problems (Rachal et al., 1982). Thus, although it has been estimated that 3.3 million youths are problem drinkers (Alcohol and Health, 1981), these estimates must be cautiously interpreted.

3. Frequent Heavy Drinking among Young Adults

Blane (1979) has argued that there are two subpopulations within the general population that have alcohol-related problems: alcoholics and frequent heavy drinkers. Studies of "problem drinkers" have consistently failed to reveal a coherent syndrome analogous to that manifested by alcoholics (Cahalan, Cisin, and Crossley, 1969; Cahalan, 1970; Cahalan and Room, 1974). Instead events labeled as the outcome of "problem drinking" (belligerence, problems with spouse, friends, or neighbors, and problems with job, finances, police, or health) are highly variable and disconnected. Usually these events can be retrospectively attributed to episodes of acute alcohol intoxication associated with frequent heavy drinking (Polich, 1979). However, only a portion of the high-risk group of frequent heavy drinkers experience alcohol-related problems.

In a national drinking problems survey (Cahalan and Cisin, 1976b), the highest rates of alcohol-related problems were found in the 21- to 24-year-old group. To confirm stability of frequent heavy-drinking patterns and associated drinking problems, Polich (1979) reanalyzed data from four sample surveys of drinking patterns and drinking problems in the household population of the United States. Daily alcohol consumption levels were used to determine percentages of frequent heavy drinkers in each age and sex group. Frequent heavy drinking (consumption of five or more alcoholic drinks per day) was reported by 13% of males ages 18 to 24, versus 7% of males in older age groups and much smaller percentages (< 3.5%) of females in all age groups. Males ages 18 to 24 comprised only 9% of the total sample, but comprised 30% of all persons reporting consumption of five or more alcoholic drinks per day. During a three-year period, 19% of males ages 18 to 24 experienced adverse consequences of drinking, but there was little patterning or clustering among alcohol-related problems.

However, household surveys are likely to be biased toward stable populations. Young males not residing in households are not represented and may have greater prevalence of frequent heavy drinking and more alcohol-related problems. Further, even those young males residing in households may be underrepresented in a household survey sample because they are less likely to be at home to be interviewed and their absence may be related to alcohol use. For the 18-to-24 age group, highest rates of frequent heavy drinking are found among military personnel, who tend to be young, less well-educated, and geographically distant from family ties (Polich, 1979), and lowest rates are found among individuals residing with their parents while attending college or working (Blane, 1979).

In the general population, problems directly attributable to alcohol can be differentiated by age as well as sex. Age- and sex-specific rates of selected alcohol-related problems among 18- to 24-year-old men and women were compared with rates for older groups of men and women for the year 1976 (Blane, 1979). Acute problems, such as drunken driver mortality and driving while intoxicated, were more prevalent in the younger age group. The rate for drunken driver mortality in 18- to 24-year-old men (37 per 100,000 licensed drivers) was 42% greater than the rate for 35- to 54-year-old men (26 per 100,000 licensed drivers). No comparable data were available for women. The rate for driving while intoxicated for 18- to 24-year-old men (1728 per 100,000 licensed drivers) was 35% greater than the rate for 35- to 54-year-old men (1276 per 100,000 licensed drivers). The rate for 18- to 24-year-old women (123 per 100,000 licensed drivers) was 34% greater than the rate for 35- to 54-year-old women (92 per 100,000 licensed drivers). In contrast, chronic problems, as measured by rates of liver cirrhosis and of psychiatric treatment for alcohol abuse, were more marked in older age groups. Liver cirrhosis rates were less than 1 per 100,000 for men and for women ages 18 to 24 versus 36 per 100,000 for men, and 18 per 100,000 for women, ages 35 to 54. Rates of psychiatric treatment for alcohol abuse for 24- to 44-year-old men were 4.4 times the rates for 18- to 24-year-old men, and for 25- to 44-year-old women, 7.3 times the rates for 18- to 24-year-old women.

Twelve problems indirectly attributable to alcohol (disorderly conduct, vandalism, serious crimes against persons, other assaults, rape, sex offenses, prostitution and commercialized vice, offenses against family and children, divorce, accident mortality, motor vehicle fatalities, and suicide) also showed higher rates among young adults, but the contribution of alcohol to these events has been inadequately documented and investigated (Blane, 1979). Contributions of other variables, such as socioeconomic status, are complex. Decline of these problems with increased age may simply reflect an increased capacity to behave in more socially acceptable ways (Blane, 1979).

C. Consequences of Problem Drinking among Youth

1. Mortality

Traffic accidents are the major cause of mortality among youth (Weiss, 1976; Holinger, 1979). In 1978, automobile drivers under age 20 were involved in 11,500 of 43,500 crashes resulting in one or more fatalities (National Safety Council, 1979; Alcohol and Health, 1981). Investigations of traffic fatalities involving younger drivers consistently reveal that between 45% and 60% are alcohol related (Douglass, 1982). The typical profile of young drivers involved in severe automobile crashes is that of the beer-drinking male in a single vehicle accident while driving at an excessive speed during nighttime hours (Waller, 1970). Associated characteristics include personal and social problems, limited education, unemployment, and prior traffic accidents and violation convictions (Douglass, 1982).

The consistent finding that blood alcohol levels higher than 0.20% are less frequent in younger drivers involved in traffic accidents may indicate that increased risk results from inexperience in both drinking and driving (Hyman, 1968; Smart, 1979a; Alcohol and Health, 1981). This association has prompted some to advocate increases in legal ages for alcoholic beverage purchase (Moore and Gerstein, 1981), and others to mount programs to reduce the number of alcohol-related traffic casualties. Safety campaigns targeted at youth are mainly fielded via public-school driver education or health education classes, and are based on the assumption that knowledge of drinking and driving consequences will reduce incidence. Yet formal education programs are unlikely to reach the population at highest risk (Smart, 1979a), and perhaps instead unnecessarily increase the absolute number of youthful drivers as well as increase exposure to driving at younger ages (Robertson and Zader, 1977). In addition, actual contribution of alcohol to traffic accidents can be documented only in a minority (28%) of cases (Shinar et al., 1978; Roizen, 1982).

2. Interpersonal Relationships

In general, disturbed relationships with family and friends are interrelated with problem drinking. Problem drinking, especially among adolescent boys, has been found to be strongly associated with antisocial attitudes that include rejection of social obligations (Wilsnack and Wilsnack, 1979). Mayer and Filstead (1980) argued that adolescent use of alcohol as a palliative in stressful social relationships presages later social dysfunction by retarding development of mature sociability and intimacy. However, whether alcohol abuse is a cause or an effect of strains on adolescent sociability is difficult to discern from available data (Wilsnack and Wilsnack, 1979).

Sociocultural expectations of youthful drinking behaviors may act to shape the intimate and social behaviors of young people in ways that may be considered specifically appropriate for their age group. An ethnographic account of excessive drinking by a group of young white working-class males (Burns, 1980) disclosed the complex interplay of contextual factors in protracted drinking episodes. Marked increase in "rowdy" behavior appeared to be associated both with increased geographic distance from the community and with increased social distance from scrutiny by significant others, as well as with increased intoxication. Transgressions of conventional social norms (e.g., driving an automobile at excessive speed, fighting, altercations with bartenders and bar patrons, and an encounter with the police) occurred among strangers outside the community. The young men interpreted these events as appropriate expressions of group identity rather than as deliberately antisocial acts. Individual behaviors potentially dangerous to persons or to their reputations, however, were curbed by other group members. Thus "rowdy" drinking appeared to be part of the social behavior expected of young men, but it also was anticipated that attainment of more socially responsible roles (husband, father, and breadwinner) would foster more restrained drinking behavior. Accordingly, the social consequences of problem drinking appear to be the most severe when excessive drinking occurs in improper contexts or when it exceeds the boundaries of behavior set by peer groups.

D. Relationships between Problem Drinking and Alcoholism

There is no direct linear relationship between youthful problem drinking and subsequent development of alcoholism. Not only do alcohol consumption rates decline with age, many middle-aged alcoholics also report abstinence or moderate intake during youth. Women tend to have drinking patterns different from men; both drinking frequency and consumption rates increase over time, but the absolute levels are consistently lower.

According to Blane (1979), age-related trends are inadequately explained by conventional notions, such as "burning out" or "settling down," that insufficiently account for specific factors and processes.

Aversive consequences of drinking or shifts in peer associations appear likely sources of change in drinking practices. Studies of problem drinking conducted over three-year intervals (Cahalan and Cisin, 1976a) have shown that for many individuals problem drinking is a brief, self-limiting condition. In the longitudinal study reported by Vaillant (1982), 49% of 110 men diagnosed at some point as alcohol abusers became abstinent for at least one year by age 47. No single factor was associated with abstinence, and some men reported influence of multiple factors. These included substitute dependencies (53%), confrontation with medical complications (49%), participation in Alcoholics Anonymous (37%), new intimate relationships (32%), supervision by employers or courts (24%), and religious participation (12%). The contribution of alcohol treatment to abstinence was minimal.

E. Factors that Contribute to Adolescent Problem Drinking

Adolescent problem drinkers are not a homogeneous group (Braucht, 1974; Braucht, 1982), and personal and environmental factors that influence development of problem drinking do not derive from a single source. Zucker (1976, 1979) has argued that multiple factors operate at four levels of influence: sociocultural and community background; family of origin; peer group, spouse, and children; and intrapersonal cognitive, personality, and genetic factors. The relative influence of each group of factors changes with age (Zucker, 1979). However, this model only appears to have utility in retrospective study of developmental factors leading to alcohol-related problems.

Results of prospective studies of problem drinking youths vary according to characteristics of groups selected for study. A three-year follow-up study of risk factors associated with alcohol abuse among 841 Swiss Army conscripts (Sieber, 1979) found heavy alcohol consumption most strongly associated with lack of social integration, negative relationships with parents, frequent peer group interactions, low paternal social status, and heavy consumption of both tobacco and marijuana, but parental drinking appeared unimportant. However, other follow-up studies have found children of alcoholics at higher risk for problem drinking or alcoholism as well as hyperactivity and juvenile delinquency (Goodwin et al., 1974, 1977). Contributions of hereditary or environmental factors are difficult to determine because exactly which intergenerational factors are conferred—and the mechanisms for their transmission—remain to be specified (Mello, 1983). Some investigators attribute causality to disruption in emotional bonds between parent and child (Barry, 1974; Wolin et al., 1980), but as yet there is no satisfactory familial explanation that accounts for the absence of problem drinking or alcoholism in some off-spring of alcoholics.

The effects of parental, peer group, and environmental factors that contribute to initiation and perpetuation of adolescent problem drinking have been reviewed for cross-sectional studies (Braucht, 1982; Harford and Spiegler, 1982). Compared to nonproblem drinkers, problem drinkers are more likely to be precocious drinkers. Peer factors in adolescent problem drinking include disproportionate peer influence as well as numerous peer models of problem drinking and other deviant behaviors. Parental factors in adolescent problem drinking include heavy drinking parents, lack of parental involvement in life activities, emotionally remote or negative parents, and relative absence of parental disapproval and control of drinking (Braucht, 1982; Harford and Spiegler, 1982).

In addition, cross-sectional studies have shown a cluster of personality characteristics associated with problem drinking by adolescents. These characteristics include tolerance of deviance, relative disinterest in religion, positive valuation of the effects of drinking, lowered valuation of education and expectations of personal educational success, and heightened values favoring self-determination and autonomy from parents. Some investigators have alleged the existence of a greater number of personal problems and "alienation" among problem drinking adolescents (Jessor and Jessor, 1977; Horman, 1979).

In follow-up studies, adolescent problem drinking has been associated with school failure and related school problems such as truancy and dropping out, use of marijuana and other illicit drugs, precocious sexual activity, and delinquent behavior (Robins, 1980). This constellation of characteristics overlaps with criteria established for Antisocial Personality Disorder, and about 20% of youths with alcohol-related problems meet this diagnosis (Schuckit, 1979).

F. Intervention and Treatment for Adolescent Problem Drinkers

Only a small minority of young people who experience alcohol-related problems are alcoholic. According to Smart (1979a, 1979b) there is no substance to the assertion that lack of social supports and early histories of alcoholic drinking combine to increase difficulties in treating younger alcoholics. Instead, outcomes are equally good for both groups. In addition, no different types of treatment are required.

Offspring of alcoholics may benefit from early intervention. Health, emotional, interactional, economic, and social problems are likely to occur within the context of their families (Deutsch, 1982; Hewitt, 1982).

Accordingly, careful and comprehensive assessments and treatment plans are necessary.

For other youth, effective efforts to prevent problem drinking appear to rely on adequate identification of factors that predispose young people to misuse alcohol (Donovan and Jessor, 1978). General alcohol prevention education programs using "scare" techniques are thought to have encouraged experimentation rather than to have deterred abusive drinking. Approximately one-half of drinking problems among youth are time-limited and associated with youthful drinking practices rather than lifelong behavior styles (Blane, 1979). Some drop-outs or potential drop-outs, delinquent or predelinquent youth, and minority youth are high-risk groups (Hewitt, 1982).

Typical interventions for high-risk groups include community-based, culturally sensitive programs offering alcohol education as well as realistic alternatives to adolescent drinking activities. Suggested behavioral approaches to disruptions in peer and family relationships associated with problem drinking include the teaching of social skills, values clarification, decision analysis, relaxation and meditation techniques, assertiveness skills, and alternative activities, including physical exercise or creative work (Hewitt, 1982). However, lack of program evaluation and outcome studies precludes any cogent assessment of effectiveness as well as any general recommendation for selection of programs (Green, 1979; Douglass, 1982).

III. ALCOHOLISM AND PROBLEM DRINKING IN THE ELDERLY

A. Introduction

There was relatively little interest in research on elderly persons prior to the 1970s. An increase in both the absolute number of elderly persons and their proportion in the general population has focused more attention on their problems. In the United States between 1970 and 1977, the size of the population aged 60 and over increased by 15%, while the size of the general population only increased by 6% (Administration on Aging, 1978). By 1980, the number of persons aged 60 and over was estimated to be 36.3 million, comprising 16.7% of the entire population of the nation (Statistical Abstracts, 1981). Although elderly persons typically are thought to drink less than younger persons (Cahalan, Cisin, and Crossley, 1969; Clark and Midanik, 1982), a variety of studies investigating alcohol problems or alcoholism in elderly persons have reported prevalence estimates ranging from 2% to 10% (Bailey et al., 1965; Siassi et al., 1973; Schuckit, 1980; Barnes, 1982; Atkinson and Schuckit, 1983). Thus the prevalence of alcohol problems and alcoholism among elderly persons is at least as great as it is among other age groups (Atkinson and Schuckit, 1983). In a sample of 3411 male and female first admissions to nine proprietary hospitals, 7.2% reported onset of excessive drinking after age 55 (Mendelson et al., 1982).

Numerous factors combine to create adversities for elderly persons who are too often ill-prepared for unexpected longevity. In general, elderly persons are at high risk for poor health and disability, are more likely to have mental and emotional difficulties, and are more likely to require long-term and institutional care (Kramer et al., 1973; Kovar, 1977). Elderly persons also are more likely to experience social isolation and the loss of primary social supports and usual social roles as well as to be unemployed and dependent on public sources of support (Kovar, 1977; Chown, 1977; Pfeiffer, 1977). Adding alcohol-related problems to this list may place an almost intolerable burden on vulnerable individuals and on society.

B. Prevalence

Study of alcohol problems and alcoholism in the elderly is complicated by difficulties in identifying cases (Atkinson and Schuckit, 1983) as well as by lack of consistency in definitions of groups to be investigated (Gomberg, 1982a). Transition to "elder" status at age 65 was a common social definition, arbitrarily imposed by the age eligibility criterion for Old Age Survivors Insurance and, later, for Medicare (Eisdorfer and Basen, 1979). In recent years, recognition of increased longevity has prompted a legal redefinition of retirement age to 70 years or the complete elimination of any retirement ceiling. Neugarten (1975) proposed subdividing the elderly population into at least two empirical subgroups: the "young-old," including persons between ages 55 and 75, and the "old-old," including persons over age 75. However, no consistent set of age cut-off points has been used in studies of drinking practices, problem drinking, or alcoholism.

Alcohol consumption typically declines with age. In a community survey of drinking practices among 447 elderly men and women in the Washington, D.C., area (Guttman, 1977), negligible use or total abstinence was reported by 56.2%. Daily alcohol use was reported by 18.6%, and alcohol use a few times per week to a few times per month, by 24.6%. Comparison of alcohol consumption patterns for middle-aged and elderly persons reported in a recent national survey (Clark and Midanik, 1982) indicated a marked increase in the percentage of abstainers after age 50. The percentage of abstainers increased by 16% among men and 18% among women over age 51. The proportion of heavy drinkers among women was highest at ages 41 to 50 (10%), then declined to 4% for ages 51 to 60, and to 1% for ages 61 to 70. In contrast, the proportion among men aged 51 to 60 (17%) dropped by more than one-half to 8% for ages 61 to 70, then rose again to 13% for ages 70 and over (after Gomberg, 1982a).

Social characteristics of the elderly impede accurate estimates of alcoholism prevalence. According to Schuckit and Pastor (1978, 1979), older persons residing in the community are more likely to be widowed and retired or unemployed; they are therefore less likely to experience marital or job problems that might bring them to the attention of the police or prompt referral alcohol treatment. Community-based surveys estimate rates of alcoholism at between 2% and 10% of elderly persons (Bailey et al., 1965; Siassi et al., 1973; Barnes, 1982). Those elderly persons associated with highest rates of problem drinking or alcoholism show a typical social profile of being widowed, divorced, or single men who have experienced difficulty with the police and who live in impoverished areas (Bailey et al. 1965).

Estimates of alcoholism among institutionalized elderly people are higher. Alcoholism rates have been estimated at 15% for elderly persons residing in nursing homes (Graux, 1969). Pascarelli and Fisher (1974) reported a 12% rate of alcoholism for persons age 60 and older living in a single-occupancy hotel. Rates of alcoholism for elderly persons hospitalized for medical diagnostic procedures range from 15% to 30% (Barchha et al., 1968; Moore, 1971), and for elderly medical outpatients, rates of alcoholism range from 5% to 15% (Atkinson and Schuckit, 1983). Estimates for elderly psychiatric patients range from 5% to 50% (Atkinson and Schuckit, 1983). Estimates for elderly patients treated in alcohol treatment settings range from 3% for persons 65 and above treated in NIAAA-funded agencies (Alcohol and Health, 1981) to 10% for all persons aged 60 and over coming to treatment (Atkinson and Schuckit, 1983).

Sex ratios for male and female problem drinkers or alcoholics range from 2 or 3 to 1 (Schuckit et al., 1977) to 5 to 1 (Rathbone-McCuan et al., 1976). Given the longer life expectancy of women, these ratios are striking (Gomberg, 1982a).

Nonwhite rates for admission to an emergency alcohol-health-care system (Westie and McBride, 1979), to public mental hospitals (Gorwitz et al., 1970), and for alcoholic psychoses (Locke et al., 1960) are all higher than those for whites in younger age groups, but they decline with age. A similar pattern was observed for arrests for public intoxication (Zax et al.,

1974), and for participation in skid row life-styles (Bahr and Caplow, 1973).

C. Consequences of Alcohol Abuse in the Elderly

1. *Medical Sequelae of Alcohol Abuse and Alcoholism in the Elderly*
Diminished tolerance to alcohol generally occurs with advancing age (Rosin and Glatt, 1971). Constant amounts of alcohol administered to individuals of various ages typically produce higher blood alcohol levels in elderly individuals (Vestal et al., 1977). The aging process promotes higher body adipose content, shifts in metabolism, and cell loss in target organs, especially the central nervous system. Absorption may decrease, but the sensitivity of target organs may also increase (Frolkis, 1977). Consequently, even the smaller amount of alcohol more typically consumed by elderly persons may be augmented by the aging process to have extensive effects (Vestal et al., 1977). Even small amounts of alcohol decrease cardiac output and coronary artery circulation in individuals with heart disease (Gould et al., 1971; Smith, 1977), decrease respiration in individuals with lung disease (Schuckit and Pastor, 1978), increase neurological deficits (Parsons and Farr, 1981), and exacerbate diabetes (Schuckit, 1980).

Elderly alcoholics have decreased physical reserve and are at higher risk for intercurrent medical illnesses (Schuckit and Pastor, 1979). Among 113 general hospital patients over age 65 studied on acute medical and surgical wards, Schuckit and Miller (1976) found elderly alcoholic men to have higher rates of chronic obstructive pulmonary disease (25%) than nonalcoholic controls (15%). This finding closely paralleled prevalence of smoking one or more packs of tobacco cigarettes per day (25% versus 10%), but rates for pneumonia were similar for each group (about 13%). Twenty-five percent of the alcoholics also manifested organic brain syndrome. In a sample of 100 consecutive admissions of patients over age 60 to a county psychiatric screening ward, 44% were found to be alcoholic, and 61% of the alcoholics were diagnosed as brain-damaged (Gaitz and Baer, 1971). Liver cirrhosis, peptic ulcer, and nutritional deficiencies also are likely to occur in elderly alcoholics (Neville et al., 1968; Gaitz and Baer, 1971; Schuckit and Miller, 1976; Zimberg, 1978). However, alcohol abstinence syndrome is less likely to occur in elderly alcoholics (Zimberg, 1978).

2. *Interaction of Alcohol with Medication in the Elderly*
It has been estimated that elderly people use 25% of all prescription drugs (Basen, 1977). Alcohol may have adverse interactions with a vari-

ety of drugs, including salicylates, antidiabetic agents, anticonvulsants, nitroglycerin, antibiotics, and digoxin (Charalampous and McCaul, 1977), CNS depressants and other psychoactive drugs (Charalampous and McCaul, 1977; Seixas, 1979). Alcohol can produce confusional states often misdiagnosed as organic brain syndromes when used in combination with commonly used over-the-counter sleeping preparations (Atkinson and Schuckit, 1983).

Two studies illustrate the frequency of alcohol interactions with prescription drugs. Pascarelli and Fisher (1974) investigated drug dependence in 86 impoverished men and women aged 60 and over living in a single occupancy hotel. Each person had a mean number of two prescription medications, and 65% of the 172 prescription medications used by this sample were psychoactive drugs, especially propoxyphene and chlordiazepoxide. Alcoholism was diagnosed in 12% of the sample. Guttman (1977) found that more than half of a sample of 447 elderly women in the Washington, D.C., area combined licit prescription medications (mainly cardiovascular medications or psychoactive drugs) with alcohol and/or over-the-counter medications. More men than women combined alcohol with prescription medications (Guttman, 1977). The findings have many disturbing implications. In addition to toxic drug-alcohol interactions, alcohol can mask signs of other physical disorders, such as pain, and thereby delay diagnosis and treatment (Horowitz, 1975). Moreover, the contribution of alcohol to acute drug reactions treated in hospital emergency rooms has been inadequately investigated for elderly persons (Atkinson and Schuckit, 1983).

3. *Social and Psychological Sequelae of Alcohol Abuse in the Elderly*

Increased rates of suicide are associated with problem drinking in the elderly (Schuckit and Miller, 1976), especially in persons with primary affective disorder (Atkinson and Schuckit, 1983). In a study of 113 general hospital patients over age 65, alcoholics reported more suicide attempts (5%) than nonalcoholic controls (1%) (Schuckit and Pastor, 1979).

Disruptive behavior by elderly alcoholics may elicit neglect or violence from family members or care-takers (Rathbone-McCuan, 1980). Among elderly patients with organic brain syndrome, alcoholics received less tolerance and attention from family members than nonalcoholics (Gaitz and Baer, 1971).

Elderly problem drinkers and alcoholics are more susceptible to falls, self-neglect, confusion, and querulous behaviors (Rosin and Glatt, 1971), loneliness, social isolation, and loss of income (Rathbone-McCuan et al., 1976; Gomberg, 1982a). It has been asserted that elderly alcoholic women are especially stigmatized—for their combined age, gender, and alcoholism—and that historically the highest rates of arrests among elderly men were for public drunkenness (Gomberg, 1982a).

D. Types of Elderly Problem Drinkers and Alcoholics

Attempts to differentiate among subgroups of elderly alcoholics have used criteria such as age of onset of problem drinking, duration of problem drinking, and patterns of drinking (Carruth et al., 1973; Mayfield, 1974). One group, called "early onset alcoholics," or "survivors," is comprised of persons over age 60 characterized by long and relatively continuous histories of heavy drinking that began before age 40 (cf. Atkinson and Schuckit, 1983). Having survived the risks of early mortality associated with high alcohol intake, they nonetheless manifest alcohol-related morbidity, especially liver cirrhosis, brain damage, and clinical depression. A second group, called "late onset alcoholics," or "reactors," develops alcoholism after age 40 (cf. Atkinson and Schuckit, 1983). As a group, they are less likely to manifest alcohol-related morbidity and exhibit fewer behavioral disturbances. Yet a third group, the "intermittents," is characterized by a history of abstinence or moderate drinking punctuated by periodic relapse to binge drinking (Gomberg, 1982a).

Estimates of the proportions of each group among elderly problem drinkers or alcoholics vary. Gomberg (1982a) has suggested that the "intermittent" category comprises a "sizeable" but unspecified proportion. However, it is difficult to discern whether this group is physically dependent on alcohol, largely because discussion of "intermittents" has been generally omitted from studies investigating types of elderly problem drinkers in clinical samples. This may mean that their numbers are not as great as has been suggested, or that persons in this category remain undetected and untreated.

Atkinson and Schuckit (1983) discussed two subtypes of elderly alcoholics: those with early onset and those with late onset of drinking problems. Earlier onset alcoholics usually had alcohol-related problems prior to age 40, became abstinent during their late 50s, and survived beyond age 65. In contrast, late onset alcoholics developed alcohol problems after age 40 and continued to drink past age 65. Schuckit and Miller (1976) found that about half of the alcoholics diagnosed in a general hospital sample were late onset alcoholics. Gaitz and Baer (1971) found 5% of alcoholics in a psychiatric hospital sample over age 60 began drinking after age 55. Thus, the distribution of early and late onset alcoholics is affected by age criteria as well as the source of the sample (Atkinson and Schuckit, 1983). Validation of these empirical categories across community and institutional samples, exploration of their relationship to affective disorders, and more accurate estimates of their distribution is warranted for accurate planning and delivery of appropriate health care services.

E. Factors That Contribute to Problem Drinking in Elderly Persons

1. Limitations of Existing Data

There has been little study of factors associated with the onset of problem drinking in the elderly. Discussion of precipitating factors is hampered for several reasons. Definitions and criteria used to study problem drinking in younger populations often do not apply to the elderly, no longitudinal studies are available, and no comparative studies exist that specifically contrast older and younger problem drinkers (Mishara and Kastenbaum, 1980). It is unlikely that any universally valid precipitating factors promote or perpetuate alcohol abuse among elderly persons.

In contemporary American society, infirmities incurred as aging progresses combine with increased need for economic and social support to channel large numbers of elderly persons into the care of health and social welfare agencies. In such contexts, certain problems, such as alcohol abuse, become more visible and compelling. Consequently, available data are largely drawn from various institutional settings or from surveys of social service or health care personnel. These data necessarily reflect the eligibility criteria and the missions of specific institutions and are unlikely to be generalizable across the entire elderly population. Furthermore, Gomberg (1982a) has argued that the characteristics of some institutions, especially nursing homes and domiciliary settings, may promote or perpetuate problem drinking or alcoholism.

2. Current Knowledge

Given these limitations, existing data are relatively silent on specific factors and processes promoting or perpetuating problem drinking in the elderly. According to Gomberg (1982a), mere association of problem drinking with "stresses" of aging is an overly simplistic interpretation. Instead, the different subgroups of elderly problem drinkers or alcoholics are likely to be differentially affected by various antecedents. The "survivor" group of early onset drinkers is more likely to manifest longstanding personality disturbances (Rosin and Glatt, 1971). For this group, the factors precipitating abusive drinking are so temporally remote that they are likely to have little relevance to problems of aging. Intermittent drinkers are purported to relapse to excessive drinking in response to psychosocial stressors (Gomberg, 1982a). Since only certain elderly individuals exhibit this response to stress, underlying mood or affective disorders may be involved. Reactive (late onset) drinkers are alleged to drink abusively more or less continuously as a response to some experience of loss, especially bereavement, retirement, or declining physical health (Rosin and Glatt, 1971). Some portion of this group also may develop alcoholism secondary to primary affective disorder. Schuckit and Miller (1976) found fewer severe problems and more stable life-styles in late onset drinkers.

Some sort of stress associated with aging inevitably affects all elderly persons. Clearly, research is needed to illuminate the differences among abstainers, elderly nonproblem drinkers, and elderly problem drinkers and alcoholics. Some (Gomberg, 1982a) have suggested that conservative values gained by living through the era of National Prohibition serves as a protection against abusive drinking. Although abstinence does increase with age, in all likelihood the experience of Prohibition across any given age cohort was shaped by numerous intervening variables, including the availability of bootleg beverages. Other arguments (Gomberg, 1982a) suggest that low income, vulnerability to medical, physiological, and behavioral affects of alcohol, or life-cycle differences, promote abstinence or diminished consumption, but again, these factors fail to distinguish between elderly persons who abuse alcohol and those who do not. This topic invites careful investigation.

F. Treatment of Alcohol Problems in the Elderly

According to Mishara and Kastenbaum (1980), elderly persons with alcohol problems comprise only a small number of patients or clients receiving care from health or social welfare providers. Since they are likely to be unrecognized, their problems are likely to be misdiagnosed and treated ineffectively. For younger alcoholics, treatment referrals frequently stem from prompting by co-workers or family members, but older persons out of the labor force and lacking social supports are not likely to experience similar pressures. Moreover, many elderly persons with intact family ties may be protected by relatives who fear the stigma commonly associated with alcohol abuse. Lack of information about resources or money to pay for care also may be deterrents (Dobbie, 1978).

Elderly persons are most likely to receive medical care in hospitals (Mishara and Kastenbaum, 1980). Recommendations for alternative settings for elderly alcohol abusers include community-based noninstitutional care or social welfare agencies specifically serving older people (Zimberg, 1978; Mishara and Kastenbaum, 1980). However, it appears logical to deliver services in frequently used settings in which careful medical, psychiatric, and drinking histories can be taken and appropriate diagnoses made. Such settings include community hospitals as well as nursing homes. Depending on diagnoses, Atkinson and Schuckit (1983) recommended brief hospitalization, modified according to the special needs of the elderly. Such needs include nutritional assessment and supplementation, and social casework. Appropriate education and information for personnel in facilities serving the elderly appears necessary to facilitate referrals and implementation of treatment plans.

Schuckit (1980) observed that long-term facilities for care of mentally or physically deteriorated elderly alcoholics are inadequate. Placement of such individuals in nursing homes has been resisted by staff because of expected behavior stereotypes (Atkinson and Schuckit, 1983). Expanded provision of long-term care may be especially feasible within the Veterans Administration medical system (Farber, 1978).

Elderly persons generally receive care via highly fragmented services, such as meal delivery programs, homemaker service programs, and outpatient clinics. Atkinson and Schuckit (1983) endorsed a coordinated treatment-team approach to provide thorough medical and psychiatric evaluation, general supportive care, detoxification when necessary, and rehabilitation. The importance of combating social isolation and boredom by rebuilding social networks and by participation in self-help groups in any treatment program for elderly alcoholics has been generally recognized (Glasscock, 1979; Snyder and Way, 1979).

IV. ALCOHOL ABUSE AND ALCOHOLISM AMONG BLACK AMERICANS

A. Introduction

Black Americans constitute the largest ethnic minority in the United States. Approximately 26.5 million black Americans, comprising 11.7% of the total population, were enumerated in 1980 (Statistical Abstracts, 1981). Yet despite the relative size of this special population, comparatively little information specifically documents black drinking patterns, drinking practices, drinking problems, or alcoholism (Clark and Midanik, 1982), or illuminates ways in which differentiation among black subgroups may shape these behaviors (cf. Lewis, 1955; Sterne, 1967; Harper, 1976; Gomberg, 1982b).

Neglect of research on black drinking problems and alcoholism appears to have been a by-product of changing trends in the American political climate over the past two decades. Most of the numerous sociological or ethnographic studies of black Americans (e.g., Liebow, 1967; Hannerz, 1969; Rainwater, 1970; Ladner, 1971; Stack, 1974) were stimulated by the civil rights movement and the subsequent "War on

Poverty'' of the 1960s. These works mainly focused on portrayals of the life-styles of black Americans in the lowest socioeconomic strata, and interpretations of their findings largely implicated exogenous social and economic conditions. The extent to which certain behaviors of disadvantaged groups that were traditionally considered to be merely deviant (such as a high rate of illegitimate births) should be reinterpreted and labeled as predictable outcomes of disadvantaged social status became an issue for heated debate. Furthermore, during this interval only limited information was available about the prevalence of alcohol problems in the general population, and prevailing ideas about factors shaping origins, expressions, and consequences of alcohol abuse also lacked conceptual refinement.

For these reasons, observations of drinking practices as well as of abusive drinking patterns were only coincidentally included in narratives generally depicting lower-class black life-styles. Consequently, although alcohol use has been alleged to be an especially important factor in the social, health, and mental health problems of blacks (King et al., 1969; Bourne, 1973; Harper, 1976; Bourne and Light, 1979), only a few investigations have directly and systematically undertaken to explore the implications of this assumption (King, 1982). Most available studies are either descriptive or drawn from institutionalized samples or small-scale community surveys (Harper, 1978). Persistent inadequacies in studies of alcohol use and abuse among blacks include inconsistent reporting of data by sex, predominant focus on urban males, general paucity of studies of females, and scant attention to rural populations of either sex (Benjamin, 1976; Harper, 1976; Inge, 1976; Lopez-Lee, 1979). As a result, generalizability of these findings is necessarily limited.

B. Prevalence

1. Drinking Patterns

Historically, high rates of drinking problems were reported for black populations. For example, a community prevalence study (Bailey et al., 1965) found higher rates of heavy drinking and alcoholism for black males (37 per 1000) and females (20 per 1000) than for white males (31 per 1000) and females (5 per 1000), and in the 25-year follow-up study of drinking problems in 235 black men aged 30 to 36 who had attended St. Louis elementary schools (Robins and Guze, 1971), almost half of the sample (48%) experienced alcohol-related problems. Among the men studied by Robins and Guze, family members had expressed concern about excessive alcohol use for 35%, 20% had been arrested for behaviors associated with alcohol use, 6% reported job problems related to alcohol use, and 6%

reported physical fights while intoxicated. Adverse health consequences included 9% hospitalized for alcohol abuse, 3% diagnosed as alcoholic, and 3% reporting liver damage.

Until recently, the 9% black subsample of the drinking practices surveys of the 1960s (Cahalan and Cisin, 1969) provided the most widely cited source of information about black drinking patterns. In comparison with whites of both sexes, higher rates of abstinence were found among blacks, and higher rates of heavy drinking were found among black women. Among black men, 38% were abstainers, versus 31% of white men; among black women, 51% were abstainers, in comparison with 39% of white women. Similar rates for heavy drinking were reported by black men (19%) and white men (21%), but almost three times more black women (11%) than white women (4%) reported heavy drinking. Similar alcohol consumption patterns among blacks were reported for a 1979 national household survey of adult drinking practices (Clark and Midanik, 1982).

Less markedly different alcohol consumption patterns were revealed by health examination data routinely collected for 12,731 black men and women and 88,528 white men and women ages 15 to 17 in Oakland and San Francisco (California) health maintenance organizations from 1964 to 1968 (Klatsky et al., 1977a). In that sample, abstinence from alcohol use was reported by 23.0% of black men and 41.7% of black women, versus 15.5% of white men and 25% of white women. Consumption of two or less alcoholic drinks per day was modal, and reported by 49.8% of black men and 40.3% of black women, versus 62.2% of white men and 59.7% of white women. Consumption of three or more alcoholic drinks per day was reported by 14.7% of black men and 4.3% of black women versus 16.6% of white men and 5.8% of white women. However, these findings may underrepresent persons omitted from the population seeking routine health examinations in a health maintenance organization, and persons undergoing such examinations may underreport alcohol consumption, especially if their intake is at higher quantities and frequencies. Since regional drinking practices also depart from those reported for national samples (Cahalan and Room, 1972; Clark and Midanik, 1982), it appears that more appropriate comparisons might be made with findings from other studies conducted in California.

A community survey of drinking practices among 322 black adults (aged 18 to 59) in two predominantly black San Francisco neighborhoods during 1979 and 1980 (Department of Alcohol and Drug Programs, 1981), found 37% of men and 63% of women to be abstainers or infrequent drinkers who reported no alcohol consumption during the previous month. Seventeen percent of men and 8% of women were frequent drinkers (reported alcohol consumption on 17 or more days during the previous month), and 14% of men and 3% of women were heavy drinkers (reported alcohol consumption on 17 or more days during the previous month and intake of at least 4 drinks on 11 of those occasions). Among an additional 94 men and women over age 60 who were surveyed, 55% of the men and 90% of the women abstained or drank alcohol less than once per month, while 14% of the men, but none of the women, were heavy drinkers.

2. *Drinking Problems*

Surveys of blacks in two San Francisco neighborhoods have shown that among persons aged 18 to 59, marital problems (26%), job problems (23%), family problems (21%), being the victim of a crime (17%), and police problems (8%) were significantly associated with alcohol consumption on 17 or more days during the previous month, while among persons over age 60, health problems were significantly associated with abstinence or absence of alcohol consumption during the previous month (Lipscomb and Trochi, 1981). However, apart from a tendency of usual amounts of alcohol consumed to diminish in quantity with age, no statistically significant differences in sociodemographic characteristics differentiated among levels of alcohol consumption and no linear trends were observed (Lipscomb and Trochi, 1981). Nonetheless, about 8% identified themselves as having experienced alcohol problems, and these "problem" drinkers could be distinguished from others in the sample by the amount of alcohol consumed during the most recent episode of heavy consumption (mean 12.1 versus 5.1 drinks) as well as by scores on a drinking consequences scale (mean 2.9 versus 0.6) and the mean number of friends reported to have alcohol problems (1.2 versus 0.6). However, only 38% of the "problem" drinkers had ever obtained any form of treatment for alcohol abuse, and all but three persons in this group denied current alcohol problems. Thus it appears that excessive alcohol consumption occurs across age, sex, and marital status groups, and that among heavy drinkers, episodes of consumption more than double the typical amount are associated with emergence of alcohol problems. However, factors permitting or promoting episodes of excessive intake—as well as denial of alcohol problems—among blacks remain to be identified.

Two recent studies provide information about blacks treated for alcohol problems. Blacks constituted 5.2% (77) of 1484 male first admissions for alcoholism treatment in nine proprietary hospitals in 1977 and 1978 (Babor et al., 1981). In comparison with men in seven other ethnoreligious groups (Irish, German, Scandinavian, French, Hispanic, and

Mormon), blacks were youngest at admission (mean age 41.6 years), began drinking earliest (mean age 16.8), began excessive drinking at the youngest age (mean 30.7 years), and reported "out of control" drinking at an average age of 40.8 years (only 0.9 years older than the average age of the youngest group, Hispanics). Blacks were the group most likely to be laborers (83.6%), and the least likely to be married (50.6%). Of all groups, blacks were most likely to be referred to treatment via television advertisements (54.5%), and at admission, lack of social and economic resources for black patients was reflected in their rating by the treatment staff as having the smallest percentage of patients with good treatment prognosis (71%). Further, at discharge blacks were most likely to be referred to outpatient medical services (24.4%), social service agencies (24.1%), and psychological counseling (21.3%). Blacks also reported the greatest number of symptoms of alcohol dependence (mean 5.1) and the highest percentages of decreased ability to perform usual duties (83.6%), criticism of drinking by friends (83.1%), and alcohol-related job loss (30.3%). In 1979, 18% of all clients receiving alcohol treatment in NIAAA-funded programs were black (NIAAA, 1981a). Black clients entered treatment at the same rate as non-black clients (41%), similar proportions of black and non-black clients were male (80%), and educational levels were comparable (10 or 11 years of education). In comparison with non-black clients, however, black clients were slightly older (mean age 40, versus 37 years), more likely to be unemployed (54% versus 45%), and to earn an average of $2000 less per year. Black clients reported one or two more years of heavy drinking, higher average daily alcohol consumption (9.1 to 7.1 ounces of absolute alcohol per day versus 5.6 ounces), and received more emergency care (16% versus 7%) and less social setting detoxification (31% versus 42%). Black outpatients were slightly more likely to require medical referrals (11% versus 8%), social or vocational therapy (10% versus 5%), social service (15% versus 12%), and follow-up or aftercare services (23% versus 19%). Black outpatients also averaged more treatment visits (16.1 versus 9.9) and had lengthier contacts (20.1 versus 11.6 contact hours per client).

Thus, in comparison with other groups receiving treatment, the consequences of problem drinking and alcoholism appear more severe for blacks, especially in light of their relatively more circumscribed social and economic resources. For blacks, earlier exposure to alcohol use combined with more marginal social and economic status appears to foster conditions which permit or promote greater or more frequent alcohol intake that, in turn, generates more serious social and economic—and health—problems.

C. Consequences of Alcohol Abuse among Black Americans

1. Mortality

Blacks are at higher risk for certain alcohol-related causes of mortality and morbidity. Liver cirrhosis rates are especially high. King (1982) reported a 352% increase in the rate of liver cirrhosis among United States blacks between 1940 and 1974, from 5.8 per 100,000 to 20.4 per 100,000. In postmortem findings for all deaths at the Los Angeles County-University of Southern California Medical Center between 1970 and 1975 (Lopez-Lee, 1979), liver cirrhosis was attributed as the cause of death in 20% of all male and 10% of all female cases. Among men, liver cirrhosis was reported for 17.7% of black, 19.9% of white, and 26.3% of Mexican-American deaths. Johnson (1975) disputed the representativeness of those percentages, arguing that black males resist treatment and are thus underrepresented in municipal and county hospitals. Among California blacks during the interval between 1979 and 1981, two-thirds of all cirrhotic deaths were found to be attributable to alcohol, versus 56% of cirrhotic deaths among all California non-blacks (Department of Alcohol and Drug Programs, 1982b). Although blacks comprised approximately 7.7% of the total California population in 1980, over one three-year period they accounted for 9% of all deaths from liver cirrhosis in that state. A recent survey of liver cirrhosis mortality data for seven metropolitan areas (Baltimore, Chicago, Detroit, Los Angeles, New York, Philadelphia, and Washington, D.C.) found the rate for blacks to be 44% higher than the rate for whites. Among males aged 25 to 34, rates for blacks were 10 times higher than for whites (Malin et al., 1982).

2. Morbidity

Medical and psychiatric consequences of alcohol abuse and alcoholism appear more severe for blacks than for whites. Johnson (1975) asserted that the sickest patients in general hospitals are black males, black females, white males, and white females, in that order. In comparison with the general population, an urban community prevalance study (Bailey et al., 1965) found black alcoholics to experience more chronic illness. A study of alcoholism prevalence in general hospital patients (Barchha et al., 1968) found the rate for black males (38%) to be double that for white males (19%) of similar socioeconomic status, although no racial differences were observed for women.

Alcohol abuse appears to increase morbidity and decrease life expectancy in blacks. Study of a sample of patients admitted for treatment of pneumonia at the Johns Hopkins Hospital revealed intercurrent alcoholism in 38% (Moore et al., 1977). Health examination data showed higher rates of systolic or diastolic hypertension among blacks consuming six or more alcoholic drinks per day (15.14% of men and 24.18% of women) than among those who abstained (10.18% of men and 14.71% of women) (Klatsky et al., 1977b). Alcoholism also has been found to increase milk intolerance in blacks. Decreased intestinal disaccharidase activities lower than 1 U/g were found in all adequately nourished black alcoholics studied, but in only 50% of nonalcoholic black controls (Perlow et al., 1977). Keller (1978) studied factors associated with cancer and liver cirrhosis in black and white Veterans Administration hospital patients. Blacks with liver cirrhosis were significantly younger than those hospitalized for cancer. Black cirrhotics were 3 times more likely to have cancer of the esophagus, and 28 times more likely to have cancers of the liver and gall bladder. Black and white patients reported consuming similar quantities of alcohol daily, but black patients were significantly more likely to drink whisky. Among blacks, increased rates of fetal alcohol syndrome (Russell, 1977; Streissguth, 1978) and very low birthweight infants associated with prenatal alcohol abuse (Boone, 1982) have been observed.

Rimmer et al. (1971) compared alcoholic white and black men and women in both a public and private psychiatric hospital in St. Louis. More blacks (52%) than whites (11%) exhibited medical complications. Blacks experienced almost triple rates of alcoholic hallucinosis (47% versus 16%), and double rates of delirium tremens (54% versus 26%). Black women reported more hospitalizations and more binge drinking than white women. Rosenblatt et al. (1971) found greater prevalence of alcoholic psychoses and other mental disorders in low socioeconomic status blacks treated for alcohol dependence syndrome. However, Locke et al. (1960) reported that high rates of first admissions to public mental health hospitals in Ohio for treatment of alcoholic psychoses were related to both the effects of poor nutrition on physical and mental health and the lack of appropriate treatment facilities in impoverished communities. Vitols (1968) compared treated black and white alcoholics in a North Carolina state psychiatric hospital. Despite earlier onset of heavy alcohol use, black alcoholics were less likely to be referred to treatment and more likely to be incarcerated or ignored. Rushing (1969) found black alcoholics less likely than white alcoholics to commit suicide. However, study of depressive symptoms in 103 black men seeking treatment for alcoholism found 65% to experience mild to severe symptoms as measured by the Beck Depression Inventory (Fine and Steer, 1977). Since most studies of psychiatric problems and alcohol abuse among blacks were conducted one or two decades ago, investigation of the extent of these problems in contemporary populations appears necessary. In addition to detailed study of intercurrent psychiatric disorders in treated populations, community prevalence studies using standardized assessment instruments also seem warranted.

3. Social Consequences

According to Harper (1976, 1978), high rates of problem drinking and alcoholism in high density urban black communities have been exacerbated by concurrent social and health problems. Assaults, homicides, accidents, trouble with the law, and family problems are consequences most typically associated with alcohol abuse by blacks.

Historically, rates of arrest for public intoxication were several times higher for black males than for white males (Zax et al., 1964), and black males were disproportionately represented in arrests for drunken driving, liquor-law violations, vagrancy, and disorderly conduct (Sterne, 1967). A study of automobile drivers by Hyman (1968) found black men more likely than white men to have blood alcohol levels above 0.10%. More recently, although 7.7% of the population of California in 1980 was black, in 1981 the rates for driving under the influence of alcohol by California blacks was 8.3%, and for public drunkenness arrests, 11.6% (Department of Alcohol and Drug Programs, 1982b).

A number of studies have reported an association between alcohol abuse and crime in black populations. Robins and Guze (1971) found that 20% of their sample of 235 black males in St. Louis aged 30 to 36 reported arrests resulting from excessive drinking. A follow-up study of 51 black felons in Missouri found those diagnosed as alcoholic in discharge or parole records were more likely to be reincarcerated or convicted of another felony. Harper (1976) studied blood alcohol levels of black homicide victims in four cities (Atlanta, Cleveland, Miami, and Washington, D.C.) for 1974. Percentages of positive findings ranged from 49% to 63%. However, Roizen (1982) found little evidence to support the contention that crimes by lower socioeconomic status blacks are causally associated with alcohol use. For nonoffenders, drinking practices and patterns were similar across racial groups of comparable socioeconomic status. Criminal offenders were found to consume more alcohol and to have more alcohol-related problems than the general population. However, black offenders were less likely than white offenders to consume alcohol before a criminal event. According to Roizen, drinking styles and drinking environments appear to increase the negative consequences of drinking for blacks. Blacks were typically found to concentrate heavy drinking on weekends and in public places. Ethnographic study showed local taverns frequented by lower socioeconomic status blacks to be shelters for transients as well as bases for planning and coordinating criminal activities. Hence, the role of alcohol in crimes committed by blacks appears to be less central than was previously assumed.

Alcohol also appears to be a less important factor for black participation in skid row life-styles. Comparisons of black and white inhabitants of skid row (Blumberg et al, 1973) found blacks less likely to be alcoholic (44%) than whites (74%). Blacks were younger, less likely to be homeless, and more likely to drink on weekends. Blacks also were more likely to maintain social relationships with persons outside of the skid row area, but were less likely than whites to obtain employment.

D. Drinking Styles among Black Americans

Bourne (1973) and Harper (1976, 1978) summarized ways in which drinking patterns described for blacks differ markedly from those considered to be characteristic of whites. Blacks have been reported either to abstain or to drink heavily, to begin drinking at earlier ages, to purchase larger containers of more expensive beverages, to concentrate drinking on weekends, and to share alcoholic beverages among groups of relatives or friends. Individuals engaged in manual labor are reported to drink on the job, thus extending weekend drinking and promoting alcoholic dependence. Black alcoholics tend to be younger than white alcoholics. Although black alcoholics are found in various socioeconomic strata, problem drinking among blacks usually has been found in association with health and social problems in impoverished urban communities. Blacks are more likely to lack factual information about deleterious effects of alcohol abuse, less likely to perceive alcoholism as a disease requiring treatment, and less likely to seek treatment or to be admitted to alcoholism treatment facilities.

The extent to which these generalizations actually characterize black drinking practices and patterns is not known. The sparse and uneven qualities of most available studies seriously restricts evaluation of popular assumptions and stereotypes. Also unknown is the way in which socioeconomic status affects drinking practices and patterns. For example, sharing beverages appears more likely to be currently associated with lack of disposable income than with historical patterns of reciprocity or conditions imposed by slavery. The younger age of black alcoholics may be related to earlier exposure to alcoholic beverages, but whether this occurs in the home, in the community among peers, or as a result of more numerous heavy drinking role models among blacks cannot be determined.

One study of black drinking practices among 416 persons over age 18 was conducted in two San Francisco neighborhoods during 1979 and 1980 (Department of Alcohol and Drug Programs, 1981; Lipscomb and Trochi, 1981). Heaviest consumption, averaging 3.4 drinks per occasion, was most usually of liquor (63%), and most frequently occurred in friends' homes or in bars (48%), at parties or celebrations (52%), and in mixed company (41%). More than one-half of the persons surveyed reported having their most recent drink on a Friday or Saturday. Ethnographic study of persons in these neighborhoods found that alcohol was widely used as a "party food," and also believed to have "warming" or pain-killing medicinal properties. Purchase by brand name was associated with esteemed social status, and habitual drinking or uncontrolled intoxicated behavior was considered to be socially unacceptable, especially by women. "Problem" drinking was interpreted as transitory and a legitimate means for coping with socioeconomic and discriminatory stressors, "alcoholism" defined as constant use and psychological dependence on alcohol, and "addiction" considered to be the result of a defect in will power. Thus alcohol consumption appeared positively associated with palliative effects, and the possible contribution of alcohol to personal problems was overlooked. Recognition of physiological aspects of alcohol dependence also appears absent from popular black beliefs. The applicability of these findings to blacks in other locales and of differing socioeconomic status is not known, and the generalizability of these and other assertions about black drinking practices remain to be tested.

E. Factors That Contribute to Alcohol Abuse among Black Americans

Several authors have reviewed the role of alcohol in the history of blacks in the United States (Larkins, 1965; Sterne, 1967; Bourne, 1973; Davis, 1974; Harper, 1976; 1978; Bourne and Light, 1979). These works emphasize the importance of historical factors in shaping contemporary drinking practices. Antecedent factors mentioned include former slave status, discriminatory prohibition, racial prejudice, poverty, inferior education, segregation, unemployment, and unstable family life. Two factors have been considered especially important in promoting and maintaining alcohol abuse among blacks (Bourne, 1973). It has been alleged that for blacks, prescribed alcohol use became associated with unbridled celebration as a reward for hard work. Further, no restrictions were placed on behaviors consequent to drinking, so that drunkenness became normative for any drinking occasion. In addition, abstinence among blacks has been reported to be strongly associated with participation in religious groups eschewing alcohol use (Sterne, 1967; Harper, 1976). As a consequence, blacks are reputed to lack models for moderate alcohol consumption.

Testing of these assumptions via ethnographic study of blacks in different socioeconomic strata appears warranted.

The retrospective follow-up study of black men conducted by Robins and Guze (1971) found that early life experiences predicted alcohol problems in adult life. Despite the popular belief that residence in impoverished black urban communities promotes alcohol abuse, this association was not demonstrated. Instead, stable family background, good school performance, absence of juvenile arrests, and lack of drug experimentation were associated with absence of alcohol problems in black male adults. More recently, Dembo et al. (1978) reported adolescent alcohol use, irrespective of ethnic background, to be most closely associated with perceptions of high rates of violence and drug use in neighborhoods, peer involvement, proportion of time spent in "street" leisure activities, and membership in disrupted families. Review of these and other studies of alcohol problems among blacks leads to the unavoidable conclusion that their presence or absence results from a multifactorial process. Additional follow-up studies, as well as prospective studies, are needed to determine the proportionate contribution of each of several factors to this process.

V. ALCOHOL ABUSE AND ALCOHOLISM AMONG HISPANIC AMERICANS

A. Introduction

Persons of Spanish origin comprise the second largest minority group in the United States. The 1980 census officially enumerated the number of persons of Mexican-American, Puerto Rican, Cuban, and other Hispanic descent at 14.6 million, or 6.5% of the total population (Statistical Abstracts, 1981). However, because of a variety of historical factors, there may be more people in this category than disclosed by census data. Problems in precise enumeration arise from reconciling social definitions of group membership with official enumeration criteria. In addition, illegal immigration status may have promoted undercounting.

Hispanic Americans are of heterogeneous backgrounds, and intergroup tensions prevail among them (Abad et al., 1974). Close to 60% report Mexican origin, approximately 15% report Puerto Rican origin, and a little under 6% report Cuban origin. The remainder are divided among 7% reporting Central (mainly Dominican Republic) or South (mainly Columbian or Chilean) American origin, or are classified as other Hispanic origin (U.S. Bureau of the Census, 1979). The majority of Mexican-Americans live in the Southwest (California, New Mexico, Texas,

Arizona, and Colorado), territories annexed from Mexico in 1848. The majority of Puerto Ricans reside in New York, reflecting migration that began after World War II. Cubans began to migrate to the United States after 1959 and located primarily in Florida. Persons of Central American or South American origin migrated northward in recent decades, and mainly reside in East Coast cities.

Persons in various Hispanic groups vary considerably in educational, occupational, and income levels, health status, and degree of acculturation, especially bilingualism (Trevino, 1975; Simpson and Simpson, 1976; Hall et al., 1977, Technical Systems Institute, 1980; Gomberg, 1982b). Most research on Hispanic alcohol use and abuse is drawn from studies of Mexican-Americans (Alocer, 1982), who tend to be younger and to have less education and lower incomes than the general population (Gomberg, 1982b). Little information is available about alcohol problems among Cuban-Americans, who are more likely to be older and of middle-class origin (Gomberg, 1982b). In comparison to the general population, alcohol use and abuse have been consistently found to be higher for males in all Hispanic groups except Cuban-Americans (Alcohol and Health, 1981; Alocer, 1982; Gomberg, 1982b).

B. Prevalence

1. Drinking Patterns

Hispanic Americans are at high risk for alcohol abuse and alcoholism. National drinking practices surveys (Cahalan et al., 1969; Cahalan and Room, 1972; Cahalan, 1974; Cahalan and Cisin, 1976a; Cahalan and Treiman, 1976; Cahalan et al., 1976) found rates of heavy drinking and problem drinking to be higher among Mexican-American and Puerto Rican men than among men in the overall population. In addition, studies of skid row inhabitants in 10 American cities (Siegal et al., 1975) found an overrepresentation of Mexican-Americans.

In the national drinking practices study (Cahalan et al., 1969) comparisons revealed that 30% of all Hispanics who drank, drank heavily versus 17% of all whites who drank and 17% of the entire subsample of drinkers. In a later study of problem drinking men (Cahalan and Room, 1972), 43% of Hispanics surveyed reported problems associated with heavy drinking versus 11% of whites and 14% of the entire sample.

Community surveys also have revealed high rates of heavy drinking among Hispanic Americans. A community survey of whites, Spanish-Americans, and Indians in a small Colorado town (Graves, 1967; Jessor et al., 1968) found 10% of Spanish-Americans to be heavy drinkers, versus 3% of whites and 25% of Indians. Haberman and Sheinberg (1967) studied indirect indicators of problem drinking in a sample of residents of the five boroughs of New York City. The highest rates of implicative drinking, 212 per 1000, were found among Puerto Rican men.

Hispanic women are more likely to abstain from alcohol than are women in other groups (Technical Systems Institute, 1977, 1980; Lopez-Lee, 1979). Study of drinking patterns among 402 Spanish-speaking men and women in three California areas found rates of heavy drinking ranging from 8% to 43% for men and 2% to 10% for women, and rates of abstinence ranging from 11% to 39% for men and 37% to 68% for women (Technical Systems Institute, 1977). Paine (1977) studied 138 Mexican-American families in Houston, Texas. Fifty-three percent of the conjugal pairs consisted of a husband who used alcohol and a wife who abstained, 33% were comprised of a pair who both abstained, and 12% consisted of a husband and a wife who both used alcohol. Haberman and Sheinberg (1967) reported a 1 to 4.6 ratio of male to female abstainers among New York City Puerto Ricans.

Studies comparing Hispanic and white youths reveal Hispanic youths to have lower overall alcohol consumption rates and to be more likely to abstain (Levy, 1973; Guinn and Hurley, 1976; Sanchez-Dirks, 1978). However, Hispanic youths are more likely to use inhalants or marijuana (Padilla et al., 1979). Factors promoting change from abstinence or poly-drug use to high rates of heavy alcohol consumption and alcohol problems among Hispanic adults are unknown (cf. Gomberg, 1982b).

2. Drinking Problems

Three studies provide information about characteristics of Hispanic problem drinkers or alcoholics. Study of drinking practices and alcohol-related problems among 402 Spanish-speaking men and women in three California locales (Technical Systems Institute, 1977) found the percentage of current problem drinkers or alcoholics among men to range from 3.1% to 8.0%, and the percentage of former problem drinkers or alcoholics among men to range from 1.5% to 3.4%. No women reported current drinking problems or alcoholism, and only in one community (East Los Angeles) did any women report former drinking problems or alcoholism (1.5%).

In 1977, 9% of all clients (27,000 persons) receiving outpatient alcohol treatment in 500 NIAAA-funded programs were of Spanish origin (NIAAA, 1978). Spanish-origin clients were reported to enter treatment at higher rates (46%) than non-Spanish-origin clients (41%), and higher percentages of admissions of Spanish-origin clients were male (89% to 95%) than were non-Spanish-origin clients (83% to 88%). In comparison to non-Spanish clients, at admission Spanish-origin clients were one to four years younger (ages 33 to 38), had been heavy drinkers from one to two more years (duration of heavy drinking ranged from 8.9 to 12.1 years), consumed less absolute alcohol per day (2.6 to 5.6 ounces), and had fewer prior treatment experiences. Spanish-origin clients were also more likely to be married, to have one to two years less education, and to earn lower household incomes (about $1750 less per year) than non-Spanish-origin clients. Spanish-origin clients were more likely to have been referred to treatment via the criminal justice system, and to require detoxification at admission.

Study of 1484 male first admissions for hospital treatment of alcoholism (classified as Irish, German, French, Scandinavian, black, or Mormon) in nine proprietary hospitals during 1977 and 1978 found that 6.76% (n = 183) identified themselves as Hispanic (Babor et al., 1981). Their average age at admission was 43.5 years, and the average age at which drinking began was 17.4 years. Excessive drinking occurred at an average age of 31.8 years, and "out-of-control" drinking was reported by a mean age of 39.7 years. Only blacks reported these events as occurring at younger ages. In general, Hispanics tended to be laborers (82.6%), married (58%), and employed (54.9%). Among all of the ethnoreligious groups, Hispanics had the highest rates of three or more citations (23%) or convictions (16%) for driving under the influence of alcohol, arrests for drunk and disorderly behavior (37.2%), suicide attempts (16.4%), psychiatric referrals (18.8%) and referrals to Alcoholics Anonymous (43.6%) at discharge, and highest prevalence of alcohol problems or heavy drinking among their grandparents (33.6%), brothers (51.5%), and sisters (24.8%). The major source of referral to treatment for Hispanics was via television advertisement (50.8%), and only blacks reported more referrals from this source. In the general population, referrals to treatment most frequently come from family members or co-workers (Atkinson and Schuckit, 1983), so the extent to which minority persons were referred via an impersonal source is striking (cf. McCusker et al., 1971).

C. Consequences of Alcohol Abuse among Hispanic Americans

1. Biomedical Consequences

The major consequence of alcohol abuse reported for Hispanic Americans is liver cirrhosis. A mortality study by Edmundson (Alcohol and Health, 1981) analyzed results for all autopsies conducted for 1970 at the University of California Medical Center in Los Angeles County. This facility mainly serves low-income populations. Liver cirrhosis accounted for 52% of the deaths of Mexican-American men, in comparison with 24% of white men and 22% of black men, and 20% of Mexican-American women, in comparison with 23% of white women and 22% of black women. Confirmation of excess liver cirrhosis mortality rates in post-mortem studies conducted for Mexican-Americans in San Antonio, Texas, and for Puerto Ricans was provided by Alocer (1982). For New York City, Alers (1978) found that liver cirrhosis was the third-ranked cause of mortality among Puerto Ricans, but the fifth-ranked cause of mortality for the general population.

Study of alcohol-related causes of mortality (alcohol dependence, alcoholic psychoses, and cirrhosis of the liver attributable to alcohol) in California between 1970 and 1974 found the percentage of Spanish-surname persons among the deceased to be only slightly higher than the percentage of Spanish-surnamed residents of the state. However, among the Spanish-surname population the alcohol-related deaths occurred at younger ages. For persons under age 44, 31% of alcohol-related deaths were among Spanish-surname individuals, versus 19% of the general population (Hall et al., 1977). These findings appear concordant with the younger ages, shorter drinking histories, and greater need for detoxification indicated by the characteristics of Spanish-origin clients in NIAAA-funded alcohol treatment programs (NIAAA, 1978).

2. Social Consequences

In a study of drinking behavior of California residents in 1974 (Cahalan, 1976), 13.1% of the Mexican-Americans surveyed reported adverse social consequences of drinking, versus 9.5% of the total sample. A study of 138 Mexican-American families in Houston, Texas, found 13% to have experienced legal problems associated with drinking, primarily driving while intoxicated, and 8% to have experienced family problems, largely marital conflict. In almost every case, family conflict over alcohol use predicted legal problems associated with alcohol use. In addition, 6% experienced economic problems associated with drinking (Paine, 1977).

Legal infractions, especially motor vehicle and drunkenness offenses, appear to be the major adverse social consequences reported in association with excessive alcohol use by Hispanic Americans. Although some of the disproportionate number of arrests of Hispanic Americans have been attributed to increased police vigilance of minority persons (Morales, 1972), studies have consistently shown that, in comparison with the general population, Hispanic Americans have higher than average rates of driving while intoxicated, and for public drunkenness (Hyman, 1968; Hyman et al., 1972; Hall et al., 1977; Alocer, 1982). Study of persons arrested by the Los Angeles police department for traffic accidents involving injuries or fatalities in 1975 showed that a greater proportion resided in predominantly Spanish-speaking areas (Hall et al., 1977). Mexican-Americans comprised 16% of the California population during 1974 and 1975, but account for 23% of arrests for traffic fatalities or injuries in 1974, and 21% of such arrests in 1975 (Hall et al., 1977). Similarly, Hispanics comprised 19% of the California population in 1980, but accounted for 29% for all arrests for driving under the influence of alcohol and 32.5% of all arrests for public intoxication in 1981 (Department of Alcohol and Drug Programs, 1982b).

D. Drinking Styles among Hispanic Americans

The extent to which any reported observations of Hispanic drinking practices, beliefs, values, or behaviors may be generalized to all persons of Hispanic origin is limited. Heterogeneity in Hispanic American drinking patterns is well-illustrated in the work of Gordon (1978, 1981) and of the Technical Systems Institute (1977, 1980). Gordon investigated drinking patterns among 7700 Dominicans, 3300 Puerto Ricans, and 1000 Guatemalans who were recent migrants to an economically depressed northeast coastal city. Dominicans were found to drink less than before migration, Guatemalans to drink more, and Puerto Ricans to retain their premigration drinking rates. Dominicans typically sipped scotch, and drank heavily on Saturday nights but moderately on Fridays and Sundays. Dominicans were more likely to have family responsibilities and to value tranquil social relationships as well as to seek upward social mobility and economic advancement. Guatemalans gulped beer and drank heavily during extended weekends. Guatemalan men were more likely to be single wage-workers, geographically distant from family ties, for whom barroom life filled a social void. Among Puerto Rican men, patterns were variable. About 10% of young Puerto Rican males manifested daily intercurrent abusive alcohol and drug consumption, mixing inhalants, barbiturates, cocaine, marijuana, or methadone with alcohol in order to become narcotized. This pattern was associated with unemployment and support by public assistance, loss of legitimate family roles, family conflict, and violence. Observation in three California communities (Technical Systems Institute, 1977) found a variety of drinking patterns and drinking contexts associated with distinctive Mexican-American subgroups. The typical pattern for migrant farm workers, largely male, included almost continuous access to beer on the job, in buses or trucks transporting laborers between worksites, and after work in bars in lieu of other recreation. Among men who had been born in the United States, laborers and industrial workers appeared to drink steadily in a controlled fashion in neighborhood bars after work, while the younger males who patronized bars and clubs with sexually oriented entertainment exhibited boisterous behavior. In contrast, among recent migrants, both men and women drank moderately in restaurants featuring traditional music and dancing. Persons in higher social strata patronized ethnically mixed bars and clubs, and their behavior was indistinguishable from patrons of other ethnic backgrounds. From these findings it can only be concluded that sex, age, birthplace, recency of migration, participation in family and domestic life, employment opportunities, alcohol availability, drug availability, and social welfare institutions are some of the major factors shaping drinking practices and drinking problems among Hispanic Americans.

E. Factors That Contribute to Alcohol Abuse among Hispanic Americans

Factors contributing to alcohol abuse among Hispanic Americans have been poorly defined and incompletely identified. Alocer (1982) reviewed studies of drinking practices and drinking problems in other Hispanic groups in the Americas. He observed that for both native Indian and *mestizo* (mixed) populations, the practice of heavy drinking was reported, often in ritual or convivial settings. High rates of drinking problems also were observed in contemporary Latin American nations, in Mexico, and in Puerto Rico. However, rates prevailing in other nations or on the island of Puerto Rico do not necessarily explain rates for the continental United States. Other intervening variables must be examined.

One popular explanation of Hispanic drinking practices lies in misperception of the concept of *machismo*, i.e., appropriate manly behavior. This concept, however, was traditionally associated with personal autonomy, strength, dignity, honor (and the absence of shame), respect, and responsibility, and conveyed no explicit demand for excessive alcohol consumption or manifestation of alcohol-related problems (cf. Technical Systems Institute, 1977). Instead, among Mexican-Americans in California and Texas (Madsen, 1964; Johnson and Matre, 1978) both undignified drunken comportment and refusal to drink were found to violate the norms of *machismo*. Ethnographic study of Spanish-speaking men and women in three California locales (Technical Systems Institute, 1977) indicated that both popularization and distortion of this concept have occurred. Accordingly, it has been suggested that for some the meaning of *machismo* has shifted to symbolize assertion of masculine entitlement, sexual potency, and "toughness," including the "right" to drink, especially as an earned reward for acting as breadwinner in a social milieu offering only limited occupational opportunities to Hispanic men.

Several differences in drinking norms, beliefs, and values may distinguish Hispanic Americans. Johnson and Matre (1978) found Mexican Americans in Texas to have a greater tolerance for both drinking behavior and for drinking problems. De Rios and Feldman (1977) reported that Mexican-Americans in Southern California generally attributed addictive drinking to a loss of free will rather than to immorality or a disease process. The ethnographic study of Spanish-speaking persons in three California communities (Technical Systems Institute, 1977) found excessive drinkers to evoke censorship only after they embarrassed persons associated with the drinker, generated marital strife, or committed visibly antisocial acts. Problem drinking or alcoholism was considered to be a failure to act responsibly, but not an illness. A majority of persons failed to perceive alcoholism as a specific problem requiring treatment. Instead, excessive drinking was believed to be merely more visible among Hispanics than among whites, while disproportionately high arrest rates were attributed to social discrimination and increased police vigilance of minority persons. Reluctance to seek help for alcohol problems was observed to stem from concerns about shame or loss of autonomy, apprehension about contacting white bureaucracies, and, for some, fear of discovery of illegal immigration status.

Minority group status, immigrant status, low income status, low social status, acculturation, and culture shock all have been cited as causal factors in Hispanic American drinking (Madsen, 1964; Graves, 1967; Abad and Suarez, 1974; de Rios and Feldman, 1977; Paine, 1977; Dobkin-de-Rios, 1979; Alocer, 1982). While these factors may contribute stressors, their impact does not inevitably lead to alcohol abuse. Guinn (1978) found no association between alcohol use or abuse and socioeconomic status among Mexican-American youth in South Texas. Instead, the father's use of alcohol was a better predictor of alcohol abuse, and frequent alcohol use was associated with mistrust of major societal institutions, especially family, school, or religion. Maril and Zavaleta (1979) found no causal association between low income and drinking problems in a study of 785 impoverished Mexican-American women in Texas. Only 2% of the women and 4% of the men in that sample reported problem drinking. However, it does not appear unlikely that alcohol abuse will exacerbate problems associated with migration, limited employment opportunities, and minority group status.

VI. ALCOHOL ABUSE AND ALCOHOLISM AMONG AMERICAN INDIANS AND ALASKA NATIVES

A. Introduction

Contemporary American Indians and Alaska Natives officially number slightly more than 1.4 million persons and constitute 0.6 per cent of the total population of the United States (Statistical Abstracts, 1981), although social definitions of group membership may somewhat increase those figures. The comparatively small size of this population limits knowledge of drinking patterns and problems. No findings pertinent to Indians were provided in the results of the 1979 alcohol use and alcohol problems survey of adults in the United States (Clark and Midanik, 1982). In addition, Indians are highly heterogeneous in tribal origin, extent of preservation of traditions, and degree of urbanization. No large-scale drinking practices or drinking problem surveys or alcoholism prevalence studies have been conducted across tribes or communities, in part because many are located in widely dispersed, geographically remote locations. Consequently, the considerable individual and group variation across disparate sociocultural settings limits statement of generalizations applicable to all Indians. Nonetheless, several indirect indicators of alcohol-related problems among Indians reveal rates of alcohol abuse and alcoholism that are several times greater than those for the general population.

B. Prevalence

1. Drinking Patterns

Drinking prevalence rates among Indians vary according to the specific tribes or communities that have been studied (Westermeyer, 1974). No single pattern can be expected because tribes are so numerous: In the United States some 280 different tribes are recognized by the Bureau of Indian Affairs (Heath, 1982). In addition, Indians who have migrated to cities come from heterogeneous backgrounds. Weibel (1982) alluded to the presence of members of more than 100 tribes in the city of Los Angeles, and the numbers of tribes represented in other urban areas is largely unknown. Although roughly one-half of all Indians now live in cities, urban drinking patterns rarely have been quantified, and comparisons with drinking patterns of reservation inhabitants are almost completely lacking. However, one recent study (Beltrame and McQueen, 1979) reported 19.3% of rural Lumbee to be heavy drinkers versus 32.6% of the Lumbee who had migrated to Baltimore, and a comparison of 105 Indians of various tribal backgrounds residing in Los Angeles with 86 Indians residing in rural California (Weibel-Orlando, 1982) found that more than twice the number of urban Indians drank two or more times per day (16.% versus 5.8%).

High rates of both heavy drinking and of abstinence generally characterize Indian groups (Lemert, 1982; May, 1982). May (1982) found considerable lack of uniformity in actual alcohol consumption rates recently reported for four different "hard-drinking" tribes living on reservations.

Depending on the group surveyed, between 30% and 84% of all adults reported drinking at least once per year. In comparison to findings for national drinking practices surveys in the United States, the rates of abstinence were shown to be lower in two groups, similar in a third, and higher in a fourth.

With few exceptions (e.g., Levy and Kunitz, 1974), most studies of Indian drinking have focused on visible drinking by males, and fail to provide information about female drinking practices (May, 1977; Leland, 1978, 1980a; Lemert, 1982; Weibel, 1982). Highest alcohol consumption prevalence rates are observed in males between the ages of 25 to 44, although the number of females who drink alcohol has been reported to be increasing (Indian Health Service, 1977). Both the number of drinkers and the quantity and frequency of consumption decline after age 40 (Indian Health Service, 1977).

Several studies report high rates of alcohol use for Indian adolescents. In one study, one-third of young people surveyed were reported to have begun to use alcohol by age 11 (Goldstein et al., 1979). In national surveys of adolescent drinking practices, the 1978 survey showed that 42% of Indian males and 31% of Indian females reported problem drinking versus 34% of white males and 25% of white females (Donovan and Jessor, 1978). In the 1974 survey of adolescent drinking practices, Indian females were more likely to be heavy drinkers than white females or black males (Rachal et al, 1975). Survey data from 2080 7th- through 12th-grade students living on reservations (Oetting and Beauvais, 1982) indicated that 85.6% have used alcohol versus 92.4% of a comparison group of 2017 non-Indian urban 7th- through 12th-grade students. Among Indian students, during a two-month period at least 42.2% reported at least one episode of becoming "high" on alcohol, and 34.8% reported drunkenness (involving staggering, falling down, vomiting, or blacking out) versus 26.6% of non-Indian students who became "high," and 21.3% who were drunk. The contrast is much more marked in a comparison of 12th-grade students (213 Indians and 232 non-Indians). Among Indian students, 95.3% had used alcohol at least once, and during the previous two months 66.9% reported getting high while 46.2% reported being drunk. Although slightly fewer (90.9%) non-Indian 12th-grade students had ever used alcohol, during the previous two months 45.3% reported being high and 27.2% reported being drunk. Local surveys of Indian adolescents across tribal groups reveal consumption rates ranging from 56% to 89%, and heavy alcohol consumption rates also vary, ranging from 17% to 46% (May, 1982). However, among Indian adolescents exclusive use of alcohol may be exceptional. In the study conducted by Oetting and Beauvais (1982), only 0.5% of Indian 7th- through 12th-graders reported "heavy" alcohol use, and 5.2% reported "light" alcohol use, while 36.5% reported combined alcohol and marijuana use. About one-half of the students who combined alcohol with marijuana became high or drunk during a two-month period. However, no comparable data are available for adolescents who did not attend school, or for adults, limiting the application of these findings.

2. Drinking Problems

Admission rates for alcohol treatment also reveal high prevalence of alcohol problems among Native Americans. In Alaska, Native Alaskans constituted 65% of all client admissions to state-funded alcoholism programs in 1977 (Mala, 1979). In 1980, an estimated 13,465 Indian clients received treatment in 460 NIAAA-funded programs (NIAAA, 1981b). The mean age at admission was four years younger than that of non-Indian clients (32 years versus 36 years), and almost 28% were women, in comparison with 18% in other NIAAA-funded programs. In comparison to non-Indian clients, Indian clients were more likely to have never married (43% versus 34%) and to be unemployed (70% versus 50%), and their gross annual income was 26% less. Indian clients reported shorter histories of heavy drinking (mean 9.5 versus 11.0 years), but consumed similar amounts of absolute alcohol per day (5.8 versus 6.0 ounces), and had similar patterns of prior treatment experiences. Indian clients were most likely to be either self-referred or referred by law enforcement agencies. One-third received some type of inpatient care, 37% were referred to Alcoholics Anonymous, 23% were referred to social assistance services, and 13% referred for detoxification. In 1974, alcohol "misuse" accounted specifically for 8% of outpatient visits to Indian Health Service Mental Health clinics by boys, and 4% of similar visits by girls (Beiser and Attneave, 1978).

C. Consequences of Alcohol Abuse among American Indians

1. Mortality

According to the Indian Health Service (Andre, 1979), recent studies reported five of the ten most frequent causes of death among Indians to be alcohol-related. The five categories include accidents, liver cirrhosis, alcoholism, suicide, and homicide. Together these causes are believed to account for 35% of all Indian deaths.

According to Roizen (1982), the precise contribution of alcohol to events such as accidents and suicide (as well as crimes) is difficult to determine. Because findings may be variously interpreted by different vested interests, range estimates are preferable to point estimates. Stratton et al. (1978) reported a range of 6 per 100,000 to 294 per 100,000 for alcohol-related deaths (classified as due to alcoholic cirrhosis, alcoholism, delirium tremens, or alcohol poisoning) across eleven tribal areas in Oklahoma. In most reports, however, range estimates across tribal groups are lacking, and rates published by the Indian Health Service are summarized by state.

Among American Indians, accidental deaths have been designated the major cause of mortality, accounting for 21% of all deaths. The Indian Health Service has estimated that 75% of those events were alcohol-related (Andre, 1979). Liver cirrhosis was reported as the fourth-ranking cause of death, accounting for almost 6% of Indian deaths. This rate was more than 3½ times as great as the overall national cirrhosis mortality rate. Liver cirrhosis mortality rates were found to be higher at every age level among Indians than among whites or blacks. In 1975, one-fourth of the deaths among Indian women aged 35 to 44 were attributable to cirrhosis. In 1976, age-adjusted liver cirrhosis mortality rates for Indians were 59.75 per 100,000 for men, and 49.84 per 100,000 for women (Johnson, 1980). For the years 1977 through 1979, the age-adjusted Indian and Alaska Native 3-year average alcoholism mortality rates (for alcoholic psychoses, alcoholism, and cirrhosis of the liver with mention of alcohol) for ages 25 to 34, 35 to 44, and 45 to 54 years were respectively 25, 11, and 7 times national levels, and for 10-year age groups between ages 25 and 84, rates ranged from 2.1 to 6.7 times as large as those calculated for the nonwhite population of the United States (Indian Health Service, 1982). The age-adjusted rate of alcoholism deaths for Indians and Alaska Natives in reservation states was 57.3 per 100,000 versus 7.4 per 100,000 for the overall population of the United States, yielding a ratio of 7.7.

Suicide accounted for 2.0% of all Indian deaths. This rate was twice the overall national suicide mortality rate. The Indian Health Service has estimated that about 80% of all Indian deaths by suicide are alcohol-related. According to Westermeyer (1974), however, historically some groups had high rates of suicide that have only recently appeared to be associated with alcohol use. Moreover, Leland (1980a) found wide ranges in suicide rates reported for specific tribes or groups, from 8 per 100,000 to over 120 per 100,000. Homicide accounted for 2% of all Indian deaths. It was estimated that in 90% of all homicides in Indian communities either the victim or the assailant had consumed alcohol (Andre, 1979). Although few sex ratios have been calculated, Leland (1980a) found that young Indian males were most typically reported to commit suicide or homicide.

High rates of alcohol-related mortality also occur among Alaska Natives. Mala (1979) observed that although Alaska Natives comprise only 17% of the state population, they accounted for 60% of all deaths due to alcoholism and for 25% of all deaths due to liver cirrhosis in 1977. Alcohol-related death rates among Alaska Natives also reveal wide ranges across specific ethnic groups (Kraus and Buffler, 1979).

2. Morbidity

Alcohol abuse also disproportionately affects American Indian morbidity. A study conducted in 1965 found 773 person-days lost for alcohol-related illnesses and injuries treated at a reservation clinic serving 908 adults in Utah (Slater and Albrecht, 1972). Miller et al. (1975) reported that 76% of Alaska Natives admitted to 12 hospitals in 1974 for alcohol-related problems also received treatment for alcohol-related medical complications. The Indian Health Service provides health care to approximately one-half million Indians and Alaska Natives (Beiser and Attneave, 1978). The rate of alcohol-related discharges (with alcoholic psychosis, alcoholism, cirrhosis of the liver—alcoholic, acute pancreatitis, chronic pancreatitis, or toxic effect of ethyl alcohol mentioned as first-, second-, or third-listed diagnosis) reported for Indian Health Service and contract general hospitals for 1979 was 8018 per 100,000 discharges (Indian Health Service, 1980). The comparison rates for general population patients was 2573 per 100,000, and for other-than-white patients, 4099 per 100,000. The ratio of male to female patients was approximately 2.5 to 1. Rates were highest for ages 45 to 64, with one out of four discharges of males being alcohol-related. One-half of the 4892 discharges with alcohol-related primary diagnosis reported no alcohol-related secondary diagnoses, but the most frequently mentioned secondary diagnoses were injuries, accidents, poisoning, or violence. Thirty percent of alcohol-related secondary diagnoses were associated with injuries, and 16% with diseases of the digestive system.

Intercurrent illnesses associated with alcohol abuse that have been observed among American Indians include alcoholic pancreatitis, heart disease, malnutrition, peptic ulcer, and trauma (Westermeyer, 1972a; Shore et al., 1973; Nelson, 1977; Cohen, 1982). A study of rates of fetal alcohol syndrome (FAS) and fetal alcohol effects (FAE) infants among American Indians in the Southwest (May et al., in press), found lowest rates (4.59 and 5.34 per 1000 women of childbearing age) for Pueblos and Navajos, and a much higher rate (30.49 per 1000 women of childbearing age) for women of the Plains tribes. Rates for Pueblo and Navajo births were comparable to those for the United States, France, and Sweden. The higher rates for Plains Indian women were also associated with multiple FAS or FAE births.

Alcohol-related morbidity data for Indians off the reservation are relatively sparse. Lang (1979) reported that Indians in Minneapolis were shown to experience more alcohol-related health problems than non-

Indians. Poor nutrition may be especially severe among Indian alcoholics. Westermeyer (1972a) studied nutritional status in hospitalized Chippewa and non-Chippewa alcoholics. Mean protein levels for Chippewa alcoholics were 6.7 mg/100 ml, versus 7.2/100 ml in non-Chippewa alcoholics. Additional abnormal tests reported for Chippewa alcoholics included decreased carotene (73%), serum iron (58%), vitamin C (58%), and hemoglobin (34%) levels. In contrast to non-Chippewa alcoholics, the poor nutritional status of Chippewa alcoholics combined with their tendency to postpone treatment to contribute to greater severity of abstinence symptoms.

3. Social Consequences

Westermeyer (1976) argued that the multiple manifestations of chronic alcohol abuse are best studied in terms of alcohol-associated events, rather than via definition and identification of individual cases. Accordingly, he used a social indicator strategy to estimate the prevalence of alcohol-related events involving Indians in Minnesota. Disproportionately high prevalence rates were found in populations served by morgues, jails and prisons, welfare agencies, and foster homes, but almost no Indians directly received treatment for alcohol problems in clinics or hospitals.

Alcohol abuse is a major disrupting factor in Indian family life (Leon, 1968; Ablon, 1971; Brody, 1977; Leland, 1978; Beiser and Attneave, 1982; Weibel, 1982). Ablon (1971) found that Indians relocated in San Francisco experienced marital conflict, unemployment, and problems with the law as a result of alcohol use. Brody (1977) reported increased wife-beating, child neglect, and conflict with neighbors and friends by binge-drinking Inuit Eskimos. Leland (1978) found 35% of women in a reservation population in Nevada were directly affected by male alcohol abuse. Foulks (1982) studied consequences of problem drinking in 88 Inuit Eskimos. Over 50% reported problems with family and spouse, and 62% reported physical fights associated with alcohol consumption.

Almost two decades ago Stewart (1964) observed that arrest rates for Indians were 40 times higher than those for the overall United States population, with 71% of those arrests for "drunkenness." However, Heath (1982) noted that historically the majority of arrests of Indians were associated with illegal possession of alcoholic beverages on "dry" reservations or with increased police vigilance of public drinking in off-reservation jurisdictions. Similar findings were reported by Jessor et al. (1968) and Levy and Kunitz (1974). More recently, arrest rates for Indians driving while intoxicated in Los Angeles County were found to be seven times greater than the proportion of Indian drivers in the county population (Alcohol and Health, 1981), and for the state of California, in 1981 the arrest rates for public drunkenness were 5.5 times greater than the proportion of Indians in the state population (Department of Alcohol and Drug Programs, 1982b).

D. Drinking Styles among American Indians

There is no single style or pattern of drinking manifested by all Indians. Patterns typically observed include abstinence, moderate drinking, more-or-less continuous heavy addictive drinking, and binge drinking. According to May (1977), most research has focused on noticeably flamboyant binge drinking that is erroneously perceived to be both peculiar to and widespread among American Indians.

Two major types of American Indian problem drinkers are typically identified, and these appear to have influenced numerous works on Indian drinking practices. Ferguson (1968) called these types "recreational" and "anxiety" drinkers. Recreational drinkers are typically young males (ages 15 to 35) who sporadically participate in groups that consume large amounts of alcohol over prolonged time periods at social events, such as all-night dances or day-long rodeos (cf. Lemert, 1982). For recreational drinkers, intoxication is valued, encouraged, expected by peers, and used to facilitate interaction between the sexes. However, these episodes may occur weeks or months apart (Ferguson, 1968; Levy and Kunitz, 1974; Goldstein et al., 1979). In contrast, anxiety drinkers are solitary continuous drinkers, psychologically and physiologically dependent on alcohol. They are downwardly mobile and tend to cluster in areas (such as vacant lots or alleys), often in towns and cities convenient to "dry" reservations (Lemert, 1982). Among their own people they are generally identified by a term akin to "alcoholic," and they are stigmatized or ostracized (Ferguson, 1968; Westermeyer, 1981).

Moderate drinking patterns appear more typical of acculturated Indians. Moderate drinkers are more likely to drink at home, or if in public places, to follow patterns typifying the reference group with which they identify (Westermeyer, 1972b; Levy and Kunitz, 1974; Weibel-Orlando et al., 1982; May, 1982). Abstinence also warrants attention. Thomas (1981) observed that numerous reform religious movements which have emerged among Indians have incorporated strong social and religious sanctions against alcoholic beverages into their beliefs.

Ethnographic study of urban and rural Indian drinking patterns (Department of Alcohol and Drug Programs, 1980), found heavy drinking most strongly associated with lengthy private secular outdoor events attended only by Indians, especially in rural areas. Limits on drinking behaviors and quantities consumed were conferred by increased age, female gender, higher social status, non-Plains tribal affiliation, strong commitment to Indian traditions, and absence of more flamboyant expressions of Indian identity, such as ornate clothing or distinctive hair styles. Analysis of life histories of urban and rural Indians (Weibel-Orlando et al., 1982) indicated that for daily drinkers, abusive drinking patterns existed prior to migration to Los Angeles. In rural areas, economic factors limit alcohol availability. Urban areas, however, provide social services that support and perpetuate daily alcohol consumption, and such areas may attract chronic heavy drinkers. Social networks of heavy-drinking urban men were found to include greater numbers of heavy-drinking friends, indicating the importance of peer factors in drinking behavior. These data suggest that younger males of Plains Indian heritage, with low social status but considerable preoccupation with Indian identity, are the most vulnerable to alcohol abuse, and, if they migrate to cities, the absence of economic constraints combines with participation in heavy-drinking peer groups to permit and promote more frequent consumption of large quantities of alcohol. Although some (e.g., Levy and Kunitz, 1974) have observed that members of Plains tribes may somehow be attracted to alcohol intoxication by their familiarity with alteration of consciousness obtained via religious or magical practices, this interpretation fails to acknowledge basic differences between conditions attained with the use of exogenous agents and those that are attained by means of physiological manipulations.

E. Factors That Contribute to Alcohol Abuse among American Indians

1. Possible Sociocultural Factors

Biases and misconceptions abound in the study of American Indian alcohol use and abuse (cf. Honigmann, 1980). Leland (1980a) listed social and cultural factors usually asserted to be deprivations that "cause" Indian drinking problems (cf. Baker, 1977). These include political oppression, war, forced migration, loss of traditional culture, discriminatory prohibition, unemployment, low income, inferior education, institutionalization in boarding schools, discrimination, substandard housing, inadequate recreational substitutes, poor adjustment to urban life, social disorganization, social isolation, and tolerance of deviance, as well as poor health and inadequate diet. The existence of many social ills in Indian lives is indisputable. However, several factors that have been much discussed cannot be operationalized and tested. According to Leland (1980a), economic factors have the strongest demonstrated association with American Indian alcohol problems.

Beltrame and McQueen (1979) compared drinking patterns among

223 rural and 215 urban male Lumbee Indians. In both communities, unemployment or low occupational status was associated with high rates of heavy drinking. Ferguson (1968) found higher treatment success rates for Navajos attaining steady employment or community involvement. Stratton et al. (1978) reported a strong association between Indian unemployment rates and rates of alcohol-related deaths and arrests. In 1975, the highest rates of Indian alcohol-related arrests and deaths in Oklahoma were found in an area where the Indian unemployment rate was 22 times the overall state unemployment rate, and the lowest rates were found in areas where Indian unemployment rates ranged from 1.5 to 6 times the overall unemployment rate. Comparison of 70 American Indian alcoholic inpatients with 48 black, 78 white, and 75 Hispanic alcoholic inpatients in a mental health center found Indians had the greatest unemployment, lowest income, least education, fewest family and social supports, and greatest social role disruptions (Wanberg et al., 1978). Westermeyer (1972a) found Chippewa alcoholics less likely than non-Chippewa alcoholics to be employed or living with a spouse. He argued that for minority persons, marital instability stems from job insecurity, and that marital instability diminishes restraints on alcohol consumption (cf. Liebow, 1967). A 10-year follow-up of 45 alcoholic Indians in Minnesota (Westermeyer and Peake, 1983) found 16% improved, 16% unchanged, 7% missing, and 62% doing worse or deceased. Good outcome was positively associated with employment and stable family supports, as well as participation in helping others with alcohol-related problems. Thus it appears that participation in family, work, and community social roles promotes improvement of alcohol-related problems.

2. Explanatory Models

At least two explanatory models of cultural factors have been used to account for high rates of alcohol abuse among American Indians. One model incorporates factors associated with traditional culture and social structure; the other involves factors associated with cultural aspects of "modern" society (May, 1982). In the traditional-factors model, Indians at high risk for alcohol problems are reputed to be those whose ancestors were nomadic hunting-and-gathering peoples who formerly lived in small, loose-knit groups that valued individualistic behavior, personal prowess, and magical power derived from alterations of consciousness. Examples are people indigenous to the Plains, Great Basin, and Alaska. At much lower risk are descendants of sedentary agriculturalists or fisherman who lived in large, formally organized communities and valued strict social controls. These Indians are believed to be less likely to produce or to tolerate deviance. Examples include groups east of the Mississippi, Pueblo peoples, and inhabitants of the Northwest Coast.

The modern-factors model attributes alcohol abuse patterns to social and cultural change, culture conflict, and social disorganization. Accordingly, groups that retain traditions are predicted to show lower rates of deviant behavior, including alcohol abuse, while those that experience rapid change are expected to have fewer means of restricting deviant behavior.

Stratton et al. (1978) found that the regions of Oklahoma occupied by groups having hunting-and-gathering traditions, loose-knit social organization, and beliefs in personal magical power had the highest rates of alcohol-related deaths and arrests, while the regions of Oklahoma occupied by groups having sedentary origins, communal values, and strict social controls had the lowest rates (cf. Thomas, 1981). Because unemployment rates also—but more strongly—predicted the distribution of these alcohol-related problems in Oklahoma, it is difficult to disentangle the effects of the "traditional" and "modern" factors in these findings. To complicate this picture further, Oklahoma tribal groups with sedentary origins also have longer histories of contact with Euroamerican culture, including adherence to Protestant religious faiths strongly espousing prohibition of alcohol use (Department of Alcohol and Drug Programs, 1982a). It thus appears that certain "modern" factors, such as specific religions, may confer protection against alcohol abuse that outweighs risks conferred by loss of traditional behaviors, although it also might be argued that these faiths were adopted by those groups as a prophylaxis for their vulnerability. May (1982) argued for a combination of the two models, with focus on individuals and on families. He predicted that individuals having no role in either traditional or modern contexts would be more likely to manifest alcohol abuse. It appears that any testing of these models of the distribution of alcohol abuse among various Indian groups needs to proceed systematically across tribal groups, and that the utility of any model will lie in its ability to predict alcohol abuse rates in ways that are useful for prevention and treatment.

3. Issues of Biological Susceptibility

Since the early 1970s, numerous investigators (Fenna et al., 1971; Lieber, 1972; Wolff, 1972; 1973; Ewing et al., 1974; Bennion and Li, 1976; Hanna, 1976; Reed et al., 1976; Farris and Jones, 1977; Seixas, 1978; Zeiner et al., 1976, 1979) have studied hypothesized differences in sensitivity to alcohol and in metabolism of alcohol in various racial and ethnic groups. These studies and their findings were carefully reviewed by Mello (1983). A major premise of such studies is that biological differences in alcohol sensitivity and metabolism may in some way affect vulnerability to alcohol use in certain groups (Leland, 1976, 1980a; Mello, 1983; Schaefer, 1982).

One viewpoint expects increased consumption in persons with increased rates of alcohol metabolism associated with rapidly decreasing intoxication, and decreased consumption in persons with decreased alcohol metabolism generating more persistent intoxication. However, a series of alcohol metabolism studies in different racial and ethnic groups have yielded equivocal findings (Leland, 1980a; Mello, 1983; Schaefer, 1982). Fenna et al. (1971) reported slower rates of alcohol metabolism in Canadian Indians and Inuits than in Caucasian controls. Caucasians manifested a significantly faster disappearance rate than the other two groups. There were no differences in the amounts of alcohol required to produce peak blood levels. However, Reed et al. (1976) found faster rates of alcohol metabolism in Ojibwa Indians than in Chinese and Caucasian subjects. No differences in alcohol metabolism were found in a study comparing American Indians and Caucasians (Bennion and Li, 1976).

Alcohol sensitivity studies have been conducted to test the general hypothesis that sensitivity to alcohol or intolerance to alcohol may somehow confer protection from alcohol abuse (Mello, 1983). Increased sensitivity to alcohol is manifested by facial and body "flushing" (peripheral vasodilation), increased heart rate, decreased blood pressure, diaphoresis, nausea, headaches, diarrhea, general dysphoria, rapid absorption and elimination of alcohol, and rapid increase in acetaldehyde levels (Ewing et al., 1980; Mello, 1983). The signs and symptoms of increased alcohol sensitivity are primarily exaggerations of the peripheral and internal changes usually produced by alcohol (cf. Mello, 1983). Increased sensitivity to alcohol has been established in Oriental infants and adults (Wolff, 1972; Ewing et al., 1974).

In contrast, evidence for increased alcohol sensitivity in American Indians is equivocal. Hanna (1978) found lesser levels of increased alcohol sensitivity in subjects from populations related to Asiatic gene pools, namely Eskimos, American Indians, Hawaiians, Indochinese, and persons of mixed Asian ancestry. Wolff (1973) found increased facial flushing in Cree Indians, but Zeiner et al. (1976) found decreased facial flushing in Tarahumara Indians.

Further studies of alcohol sensitivity in American Indians and Alaska Natives appear to require rigorous elicitation of pedigrees in order to establish genetic composition of experimental groups as well as to diminish possible effects of individual differences (cf. Leland, 1980a; Schaefer, 1982). Rigorous selection and matching of subjects and controls also is necessary, especially for differences in body structure, composition, and weight, as well as nutritional status and drinking patterns (Mello, 1983). According to Leland (1980a), the primary social benefit of identification of increased alcohol sensitivity among American Indians would be provision of a scientific basis for prevention programs.

VII. TREATMENT OF ALCOHOL PROBLEMS IN ETHNIC AND RACIAL MINORITIES

Numerous reviewers have discussed problems associated with language and cultural barriers to treatment of alcohol problems in different racial and ethnic groups (cf. Leland, 1980a; Westermeyer, 1981; Alocer, 1982; King, 1982; Weibel, 1982). Westermeyer (1981) summarized recommended treatment approaches. He observed that drinking patterns typical of certain ethnic groups may influence occurrence of alcohol-related problems. Accordingly, episodic drinkers are more likely to manifest acute problems associated with binge drinking, while controlled heavy drinkers more typically exhibit problems associated with chronic alcohol use. However, needs for biomedical treatment transcend sociocultural boundaries. Biomedical treatment of alcohol abuse problems is consistent across ethnic or racial groups, and includes detoxification (when necessary), elicitation of medical, psychiatric, and drinking histories, evaluation of current nutritional and health status, and diagnosis and treatment of intercurrent medical and psychiatric illnesses.

Assessment of resources, including need for vocational rehabilitation, family and peer support, and community involvement is also necessary. According to Westermeyer (1981), application of psychotherapies and sociotherapies is also remarkably similar across ethnic or racial groups, and includes individual psychotherapy, marital or family counseling, group therapy, behavioral conditioning, residential treatment, partial residential treatment, and vocational rehabilitation as appropriate to the needs of the patient. However, outcome and evaluation studies of these interventions are almost completely lacking. Indigenous therapies using variants of traditional healing ceremonies or religious movements eschewing alcohol use also have been adapted for intervention in alcohol use problems (e.g., Dozier, 1966; Albaugh and Anderson, 1974; Jilek, 1976; Trotter and Chavira, 1978), but they remain unevaluated (Westermeyer, 1981; Iber, 1982).

Efficacy of nonmedical treatment modalities for alcohol abuse appears to derive from their intervention in the social isolation experienced by alcohol abusers, regardless of ethnic or racial background. Gradual erosion of traditional values, attitudes, and behaviors accompanies progression of drinking problems (Favazza, 1981; Westermeyer, 1981). According to Westermeyer (1981), alcohol becomes a central focus of existence, displacing traditional loyalties; future needs of a group are sacrificed in favor of short-term goals associated with alcohol use; family, friends, and other members of a group may be exploited in order to obtain alcohol; and the "usefulness" of other people is gauged by their participation in alcohol-centered activities. Irrespective of racial or ethnic origin, a "subculture" of alcohol abusers is likely to form, one in which relationships are brittle and derived from mutual focus on alcohol. Thus ethnic values are functionally suspended (cf. Favazza, 1981). In contrast, treatment disaffiliates alcohol abusers from an alcohol-centered milieu, involves personal and social reorientation, and usually includes resurgence of ethnic identity (Westermeyer, 1981).

Some (cf. Harper, 1976; Leland, 1980a; Alocer, 1982; Blume, 1982; Lewis, et al. 1982) report arguments that indigenous treatments and personnel are necessary in treatment settings serving special populations. However, Westermeyer (1981) has argued that although indigenous health workers may aid in attracting alcohol abusers to treatment and increase acceptance and compliance, social and cultural restoration occurs irrespective of treatment staff backgrounds. The syndrome of problem drinking is sufficiently uniform across racial and ethnic groups that cultural factors per se appear to have less than a central role in treatment processes. Furthermore, Iber (1982) has cogently identified several additional factors that diminish the attractiveness of special treatment programs. These include reverse stereotyping and imposition of exclusionary criteria, perpetuation of segregation, absence of cultural objectivity, and limited cost-effectiveness.

Nonetheless, removal of language barriers as well as knowledge of social and cultural factors appears essential for recognition and referral. Lack of information about consequences of alcohol abuse may be greater among ethnic and racial minorities (cf. Harper, 1976; Leland, 1980a; Alocer, 1982). Recognition of alcohol-related problems may be masked by ethnic, racial, linguistic, or socioeconomic differences. Appropriate education and information for personnel in facilities serving ethnic and racial minorities appears especially necessary because the additional stresses of alcohol abuse on persons already made vulnerable to health risks by their minority status adds an intolerable burden to the lives of individuals, their families, and their communities, as well as for the larger society.

REFERENCES

Abad, V., and Suarez, J., 1974, Cross-cultural aspects of alcoholism among Puerto Ricans, in *Proceedings of the Fourth Annual Alcoholism Conference of the National Institute on Alcohol Abuse and Alcoholism,* pp. 282–294, National Institute on Alcohol Abuse and Alcoholism, Rockville, Md.

NOTE: Bibliographic assistance for this chapter was provided by A. M. Cooper, D. B. Heath, and Lois Lowe.

Abad, V., Ramos, T., and Bryce, E., 1974, A model for delivery of mental health service to Spanish-speaking minorities, *Am. J. Orthopsychiat.*, 44:584–595.

Abelson, H. I., Fishburne, P. M., and Cisin, I. H., 1977, *National Survey of Drug Abuse: 1977, A Nationwide Study—Youth, Young Adults, and Older People*, National Institute on Drug Abuse, Rockville, Md.

Ablon, J., 1971, Culture conflict in urban Indians, *Ment. Hyg.*, 55:199–205.

Administration on Aging, 1978, *Statistical Notes*, 2:1–16.

Albaugh, B., and Anderson, P., 1974, Peyote in treatment of alcoholism among American Indians, *Am. J. Psychiat.*, 131:1247–1250.

Alcohol and Health, 1975, Second special report to the U.S. Congress, U.S. Government Printing Office, Washington, D.C.

——, 1981, Fourth special report to the U.S. Congress, U.S. Government Printing Office, Washington, D.C.

Alers, J. V., 1982, *Puerto Ricans and Health—Findings from New York City*, Hispanic Research Center, Monograph No. 1, Fordham University, New York.

Alocer, A. M., 1982, Alcohol use and abuse among the Hispanic American population, in *Special Population Issues, Alcohol and Health Monograph No. 4*, pp. 361–382, National Institute on Alcohol Abuse and Alcoholism, Rockville, Md.

American Psychiatric Association, 1980, *Diagnostic and Statistical Manual*, Third Edition, American Psychiatric Association, Washington, D.C.

Anderson, A. J., Barboriak, J. J., and Rimm, A. A., 1977, Risk factors and angiographically determined coronary occlusion, *Am. J. Epidemiol.*, 107:8–14.

Andre, J. M., 1979, *The epidemiology of alcoholism among American Indians and Alaska Natives*, Indian Health Service, Albuquerque, N.M.

Ashley, M. J., Olin, J. S., le Riche, W. H., Kornaczewski, A., Schmidt, W., and Rankin, J. G., 1977, Morbidity in alcoholics, *Arch. Intern. Med.*, 137:883–887.

Atkinson, J. H., Jr., and Schuckit, M. A., 1983, Geriatric alcohol and drug abuse, in *Advances in Substance Abuse* (N. K. Mello, ed.), JAI Press, Greenwich, Conn.

Babor, T. F., Miller, K. D., and Mendelson, J. H., 1981, *Ethnic-religious differences in the manifestation and treatment of alcoholism*, paper presented to the Epidemiology Section, Twenty-Seventh International Institute on the Prevention and Treatment of Alcoholism, Vienna.

Bacon, M. K., 1976, Cross-cultural studies of drinking: Integrated drinking and sex differences in the use of alcoholic beverages, in *Cross-Cultural Approaches to the Study of Alcohol* (M. W. Everett, J. O. Waddell, and D. B. Heath, eds.), pp. 23–39, Mouton, The Hague.

Bacon, M. K., Barry, H., III, and Child, I. L., 1965, A cross-cultural study of drinking: II. Relations to other features of culture, *Q. J. Stud. Alc.*, Suppl. 3:29–48.

Bahr, H. M., and Caplow, T., 1973, *Old Men Drunk and Sober*, New York University Press, New York.

Bailey, M. B., Haberman, P. W., and Alksne, H., 1965, The epidemiology of alcoholism in an urban residential area, *Q. J. Stud. Alc.*, 26:19–40.

Baker, J. M., 1977, Alcoholism and the American Indian, in *Alcoholism: Development, Consequences, and Interventions* (N. J. Estes and M. E. Heinemann, eds.), pp. 194–203, C. V. Mosby Company, St. Louis.

Barchha, R., Stewart, M. A., and Guze, S. B., 1968, The prevalence of alcoholism among general hospital ward patients, *Am. J. Psychiat.,* 125:681–684.

Barnes, G. M., 1982, Patterns of alcohol use and abuse among older persons in a household population, in *Alcoholism and Aging: Advances in Research* (W. G. Wood and M. F. Elias, eds.), pp. 3–15, CRC Press, Inc., Boca Raton, Fla.

Barry, H., 1968, Sociocultural aspects of alcohol addiction, *Addictive States,* 46:455–471.

———, 1974, Psychological factors in alcoholism, in *The Biology of Alcoholism,* vol. 3, *Clinical Pathology* (B. Kissin and H. Begleiter, eds.), pp. 53–107, Plenum Press, New York.

Barry, R. G. G., and O'Nuallain, S., 1975, Foetal alcoholism, *Ir. J. Med. Sci.,* 144:286–288.

Basen, M. M., 1977, The elderly and drugs—problem overview and program strategy, *Public Health Rep.,* 92:43–48.

Beauchamp, D. E., 1981, The paradox of alcohol policy: The case of the 1969 alcohol act in Finland, in *Alcohol and Public Policy: Beyond the Shadow of Prohibition* (M. H. Moore and D. R. Gerstein, eds.), pp. 225–254, National Academy Press, Washington, D.C..

Beckman, L. J., 1975, Women alcoholics: A review of social and psychological studies, *J. Stud. Alc.,* 36:799–823.

———, 1976, Alcoholism problems and women: An overview, in *Alcoholism Problems in Women and Children* (M. Greenblatt and M. A. Schuckit, eds.), pp. 65–96, Grune & Stratton, Inc., New York.

Beckman, L. J., and Kocel, K. M., 1982, The treatment-delivery system and alcohol abuse in women: Social policy implications, *J. of Social Issues,* 38:139–151.

Beiser, M., and Attneave, C. L., 1978, Mental health services for American Indians: Neither feast nor famine, *White Cloud Journal,* 1:3–10.

———, 1982, Mental disorders among Native American children: Rates and risk periods for entering treatment, *Am. J. Psychiat.,* 139:193–198.

Belfer, M. L., Shader, R. I., Carroll, M., and Harmatz, J. S., 1971, Alcoholism in women, *Arch. Gen. Psychiat.,* 25:540–544.

Belfer, M. L., and Shader, R. I., 1976, Premenstrual factors as determinants of alcoholism in women, in *Alcoholism Problems in Women and Children* (M. Greenblatt and M. A. Schuckit, eds.), pp. 97–102, Grune & Stratton, Inc., New York.

Beltrame, T., and McQueen, D. V., 1979, Urban and rural Indian drinking patterns: The special case of the Lumbee, *Int. J. Addict.,* 14:533–548.

Benjamin, R., 1976, Rural black folk and alcohol, in *Alcohol Abuse and Black America* (F. D. Harper, ed.), pp. 49–60, Douglass Publishers, Alexandria, Va.

Bennion, L. J., and Li, T. K., 1976, Alcohol metabolism in American Indians and whites: Lack of racial differences in metabolic rate and liver alcohol dehydrogenase, *New Engl. J. Med.,* 294:9–13.

Bierich, J. R., Majewski, F., Michaelis, R., and Tillner, I., 1976, Über das embryofetal Alkohosyndrom [on the embryo-fetal alcohol syndrome], *Eur. J. Pediatr.,* 121:155–177.

Blane, H. T., 1968, *The Personality of the Alcoholic: Guises of Dependency,* Harper & Row, New York.

———, 1979, Middle-aged alcoholics and young drinkers, in *Youth, Alcohol, and Public Policy* (H. T. Blane and M. E. Chafetz, eds.), pp. 5–38, Plenum Press, New York.

Blumberg, L., Shipley, T. E., Jr., and Schandler, I. W., 1973, *Skid Row and Its Alternatives; Recommendations from Philadelphia,* Temple University Press, Philadelphia.

Blume, S., 1980, Clinical research: Casefinding, diagnosis, treatment, and rehabilitation, in *Alcohol and Women,* Research Monograph no. 1., pp. 121–149, National Institute on Alcohol Abuse and Alcoholism, Rockville, Md.

———, 1982, Do special populations have special alcoholism treatment needs? Debate, National Council on Alcoholism Conference, April 5, 1982, Washington, D.C.

Boone, M. S., 1982, A socio-medical study of infant mortality among disadvantaged blacks, *Human Organization,* 41:227–236.

Bourne, P. G., 1973, Alcoholism in the urban Negro population, in *Alcoholism: Progress in Research and Treatment* (P. G. Bourne and R. Fox, eds.), pp. 211–226, Academic Press, New York.

Bourne, P. G., and Light, E., 1979, Alcohol problems in blacks and women, in *The Diagnosis and Treatment of Alcoholism* (J. H. Mendelson and N. K. Mello, eds.), pp. 84–123, McGraw-Hill Book Company, New York.

Braiker, H. B., 1982, The diagnosis and treatment of alcoholism in women, in *Special Population Issues,* Alcohol and Health Monograph No. 4, pp. 111–139, National Institute on Alcohol Abuse and Alcoholism, Rockville, Md.

Bratfos, O., 1971, Attempted suicide, *Acta Psychiatr. Scand.,* 47:38–56.

Braucht, G. N., 1974, A psychosocial typology of adolescent alcohol and drug abusers, in *Alcoholism: A Multilevel Problem* (M. E. Chafetz, ed.), U.S. Government Printing Office, Washington, D.C.

———, 1982, Problem drinking among adolescents: A review and analysis of psychosocial research, in *Special Population Issues,* Alcohol and Health Monograph No. 4, pp. 143–164, National Institute on Alcohol Abuse and Alcoholism, Rockville, Md.

Brenner, M. H., 1975, Trends in alcohol consumption and related illnesses: Some effects of economic changes, *Am. J. Pub. Health,* 65:1279–1292.

Breslow, N. E., and Enstrom, J. E., 1974, Geographic correlations between cancer mortality rates and alcohol-tobacco consumption in the United States, *J. National Cancer Institute,* 53:631–639.

Brody, H., 1977, Alcohol, change, and the industrial frontier, *Études/Inuit/ Studies,* 1:31–46.

Bruun, K., Edwards, G., Lumio, M., Mäkelä, M., Pan, L., Popham, R. E., Room, R., Schmidt, W., Skog, O.-J., Sulkunen, P., and Österberg, E., 1975, *Alcohol Control Policies in Public Health Perspective,* vol. 25, The Finnish Foundation for Alcohol Studies, Helsinki, Finland.

Burns, T. B., 1980, Getting rowdy with the boys, *J. Drug Issues,* 10:273–286.

Cahalan, D., 1970, *Problem Drinkers,* Josey-Bass, Inc., San Francisco.

———, 1976, *Ethnoreligious Group Differences, 1974 California Drinking Survey,* Social Research Group, Berkeley, Calif.

Cahalan, D., and Cisin, I. H., 1976a, Drinking behavior and drinking problems, in *The Biology of Alcoholism,* vol. 4, *Social Aspects of Alcoholism* (B. Kissin and H. Begleiter, eds.), pp. 77–116, Plenum Press, New York.

————, 1976b, Epidemiological and social factors associated with drinking problems, in *Alcoholism: Interdisciplinary Approaches to an Enduring Problem* (R. E. Tartar and A. A. Sugarman, eds.), Addison-Wesley Publishing Co., Reading, Mass.

Cahalan, D., Cisin, I. H., and Crossley, H. M., 1969, *American Drinking Practices,* Monograph No. 6, Rutgers Center of Alcohol Studies, New Brunswick, N.J.

Cahalan, D., Roizen, R., and Room, R., 1976, Alcohol problems and their prevention: Public attitudes in California, in *The Prevention of Alcohol Problems* (R. Room and S. Sheffield, eds.), pp. 354–403, California Office of Alcoholism, Sacramento, Calif.

Cahalan, D., and Room, R., 1972, *Problem Drinking among American Men,* Monograph No. 7, Rutgers Center of Alcohol Studies, New Brunswick, N.J.

————, Cahalan, D., and Treiman, B., 1976, *Drinking Behavior, Attitudes, and Problems in San Francisco,* Social Research Group, Berkeley, Calif.

Carruth, B., Williams, E. P., Mysak, P., and Boudreaux, L., 1975, Community care providers and the older problem drinker, *Grassroots,* July Suppl.:1–5.

Charalampous, K. D., and McCaul, D. S., 1977, Alcohol and sedative drugs— drug interactions, in *The Kinetics of Psychiatric Drugs* (J. C. Schoola and J. L. Claghorn, eds.), pp. 266–294, Brunner/Mazel, New York.

Chauncey, R. L., 1980, New careers for moral entrepreneurs: Teenage drinking, *J. Drug Issues,* 12:45–70.

Chernoff, G., 1975, A mouse model of fetal alcohol syndrome, *Teratology,* 11:14A.

Child, I. L., Barry, H., III, and Bacon, M. K., 1965, Sex differences in a cross-cultural study of drinking, *Q. J. Stud. Alc.,* Suppl. 3:49–61.

Chown, S. M., 1977, Morale, careers, and personal potentials, in *Handbook on Psychology of Aging* (J. E. Borren and K. Schaie, eds.) Van Nostrand, New York.

Christoffel, K. K., and Salafsky, I., 1975, Fetal alcohol syndrome in dizygotic twins, *J. Pediatr.,* 87:963–967.

Cicero, T. J., 1980, Sex differences in the effects of alcohol and other psychoactive drugs on endocrine function: Clinical and experimental evidence, in *Alcohol and Drug Problems in Women* (O. J. Kalant, ed.), pp. 545–593, Plenum Press, New York.

Clark, W., and Midanik, L., 1982, Alcohol use and alcohol problems among U.S. adults: Results of the 1979 national survey, in *Alcohol Consumption and Related Problems,* Alcohol and Health Monograph No. 1, pp. 3–52, National Institute on Alcohol Abuse and Alcoholism, Rockville, Md.

Clarren, S. K., and Smith, D. W., 1978, The fetal alcohol syndrome, *New Engl. J. Med.,* 298:1063–1067.

Cohen, S., 1982, Alcohol and the Indian, *Drug Abuse and Alcoholism Newsletter,* 11(4):1–3.

Corrigan, E. M., and Anderson, S. C., 1982, Black alcoholic women in treatment, *J. of Addictions and Health,* 3:49–58.

Curlee, J., 1969, Alcoholism and the "empty nest," *Bull. Menninger Clin.,* 33:165–171.

————, 1970, A comparison of male and female patients at an alcoholism treatment center, *J. Psychol.,* 74:239–247.

Curran, F. J., 1957, Personality studies in alcoholic women, *J. Nerv. Ment. Dis.*, 86:645–667.

Cutler, S. J., and Young, J. L., 1975, *Third National Cancer Survey: Incidence Data,* National Cancer Institute Monograph No. 41, National Cancer Institute, Washington, D.C.

Dahlgren, L., 1978, Female alcoholics. III. Development and pattern of problem drinking, *Acta Psychiatr. Scand.,* 57:325–335.

Dahlgren, L., and Idestrom, C.-M., 1979, Female alcoholics. V. Morbidity. *Acta Psychiatr. Scand.,* 60:199–213.

Dahlgren, L., and Myrhed, M., 1977, Alcoholic females. II. Causes of death with reference to sex differences, *Acta Psychiatr. Scand.,* 56:81–91.

Dalton, K., 1964, *The Premenstrual Syndrome,* Charles C Thomas, Springfield, Ill.

———, 1969, *The Menstrual Cycle,* Pantheon Books, New York.

Davis, F., 1974, Alcoholism among American blacks, *Addiction,* 3:8–16.

de Rios, M. D., and Feldman, D. F., 1977, Southern California Mexican American drinking patterns: Some preliminary observations, *J. Psychedelic Drugs,* 9:151–158.

Dembo, R. W., Burgos, W., Babst, D. V., Schmeidler, J., and La Grand, L. E., 1978, Neighborhood relationships and drug involvement among inner city junior high school youths: Implications for drug education and prevention programming, *J. Drug Education,* 8:231–252.

Department of Alcohol and Drug Programs, 1980, An executive summary of "The Ethnography of California Urban Indian Drinking Patterns in Drinking Settings," mimeographed, Sacramento, Calif.

———, 1981, An executive summary of the "Black Population Drinking Practices Research Study Report," mimeographed, Sacramento, Calif.

———, 1982a, Black Drinking Practices Study—Report of Ethnographic Research, mimeographed, Sacramento, Calif.

———, 1982b, The Black Population and Indicators of Alcohol Use/Misuse, mimeographed, Sacramento, Calif.

Deutsch, C., 1982, *Broken Bottles, Broken Dreams: Understanding and Helping the Children of Alcoholics,* Teachers College Press, New York.

Diamond, D. L., and Wilsnack, S. C., 1978, Alcohol abuse among lesbians: A descriptive study, *J. of Homosexuality,* 4:123–142.

Dobbie, J., 1978, *Substance Abuse among the Elderly,* Addiction Research Foundation, Toronto.

Dobkin-de-Rios, M. D., 1979, Mexican migrant tubercular patients' attitudes concerning alcohol, *J. Psychedelic Drugs,* 11:347–350.

Donovan, J. E., and Jessor, R., 1978, Adolescent problem drinking: Psychosocial correlates in a national sample study, *J. Stud. Alc.,* 39:1506–1524.

Douglass, R. L., 1982, Youth, alcohol, and traffic accidents, in *Special Population Issues,* Alcohol and Health Monograph No. 4, pp. 147–223, National Institute on Alcohol Abuse and Alcoholism, Rockville, Md.

Dozier, E. P., 1966, Problem drinking among American Indians: The role of sociocultural deprivation, *Q. J. Stud. Alc.,* 27:72–87.

Driscoll, G. Z., and Barr, H. L., 1972, *Comparative study of drug dependent women,* Proceedings of the twenty-third annual meeting of the Alcohol and Drug Problems Association of North America, Atlanta, Georgia.

Eisdorfer, C., and Basen, M. M., 1979, Drug misuse by the elderly, in *Handbook on Drug Abuse* (R. L. DuPont, A. Goldstein, J. O'Donnell, and B. Brown, eds.), pp. 271–276, National Institute on Drug Abuse, Rockville, Md.

Eshbaugh, D. M., Tosi, D. J., and Hayt, C. N., 1980, Women alcoholics: A typological description using the MMPI, *J. Stud. Alc.*, 41:310–317.

Ewing, J. A., Rouse, B. A., and Alderhold, R. H., 1980, Studies of the mechanism of Oriental hypersensitivity, in *Currents in Alcoholism*, vol. 5, *Biomedical Issues and Clinical Effects of Alcoholism*, Grune & Stratton, Inc., New York.

Ewing, J. A., Rouse, B. A., and Pellizzari, E. D., 1974, Alcohol sensitivity and ethnic background, *Am. J. Psychiat.*, 131:206–210.

Farber, S. J., 1978, The future role of the VA Hospital system: A national health policy dilemma, *New Engl. J. Med.*, 298:625–628.

Farris, J. J., and Jones, B. M., 1977, Ethanol metabolism in male American Indians and whites, *Alcoholism: Clin. Exp. Res.*, 2:77–81.

Favazza, A., 1981, Alcohol and special populations, *J. Stud. Alc.*, Suppl. 9:87–98.

Feighner, H. P., Robins, E., Guze, S. B., et al., 1972, Diagnostic criteria for use in psychiatric research, *Arch. Gen. Psychiat.*, 26:57–63.

Fenna, D., Mix, L., Schaefer, O., and Gilbert, J.A.L., 1971, Ethanol metabolism in various racial groups, *Can. Med. Assoc. J.*, 105:472–475.

Ferguson, F. N., 1968, Navajo drinking, some tentative hypotheses, *Human Organization*, 27:159–167.

Ferrence, R. G., 1980, Sex differences in the prevalence of problem drinking, in *Research Advances in Alcohol and Drug Problems*, vol. 5, *Alcohol and Drug Problems in Women* (O. J. Kalant, ed.), pp. 69–124, Plenum Press, New York.

Ferrence, R. G., and Whitehead, P. C., 1980, Sex differences in psychoactive drug use: Recent epidemiology, in *Research Advances in Alcohol and Drug Problems*, vol. 5, *Alcohol and Drug Problems in Women* (O. J. Kalant, ed.), pp. 125–201, Plenum Press, New York.

Ferrier, P. E., Nicod, I., and Ferrier, S., 1973, Fetal alcohol syndrome, *Lancet*, 2:1496.

Fillmore, K. M., 1974, Drinking and problem drinking in early adulthood and middle age, *Q. J. Stud. Alc.*, 35:819–840.

———, 1975, Relationships between specific drinking problems in early adulthood and middle age, *J. Stud. Alc.*, 36:882–907.

Fine, E. W., and Steer, R. A., 1977, Relationship between alcoholism and depression in Black men, in *Currents in Alcoholism*, vol. 2 (F. A. Seixas, ed.), pp. 35–43, Grune & Stratton, Inc., New York.

Fort, T., and Porterfield, A. G., 1961, Some backgrounds and types of alcoholism among women, *J. Health Hum. Behav.*, 2:283–292.

Foulks, E. S., 1982, Emerging social stratification and patterns of alcohol use in North Alaska, in *Eskimo Capitalists: Oil, Alcohol, and Politics* (S. Klausner and E. S. Foulks, eds.), Allan Held Publishers, Osmond, N.J.

Fraser, J., 1973, The female alcoholic, *Addictions*, 20:64–80.

Frolkis, V. V., 1977, Aging of the autonomic nervous system, in *Handbook of the Psychology of Aging* (J. E. Birren and K. W. Schaie, eds.), Van Nostrand, New York.

Gaitz, C. M., and Baer, P. E., 1971, Characteristics of elderly patients with alcoholism, *Arch. Gen. Psychiat.*, 24:372–378.

Galambos, J. T., Popper, H., and Schaffner, F. (eds.), 1972, Alcoholic hepatitis: Its therapy and prognosis, in *Progress in Liver Diseases*, vol. 4, pp. 567–588, Grune & Stratton, Inc., New York.

Garrett, G. R., and Bahr, H. M., 1973, Women on skid row, *Q. J. Stud. Alc.*, 34:1228–1243.

Gibbs, J. P., Merton, R. K., and Nisbet, R. A. (eds.), 1966, Suicide, in: *Contemporary Social Problems*, Second Edition, pp. 281–321, Harcourt, Brace, & World, Inc., New York.

Glassock, J. A., 1979, Rehabilitating the older alcoholic, *Aging*, 299:19–24.

Globetti, G., 1972, Problem and non-problem drinking among high school students in abstinence communities, *Int. J. Addict.*, 7:511–523.

———, 1977, Teenage drinking, in *Alcoholism: Development, Consequences, and Intervention* (N. J. Estes and M. E. Heinemann, eds.), pp. 162–173, C. V. Mosby Company, St. Louis.

Goldstein, G. S., Oetting, E. R., Edwards, R., and Garcia-Mason, V., 1979, Drug use among Native American young adults, *Int. J. Addict.*, 14:855–860.

Gomberg, E. S., 1976a, Alcoholism in women, in *The Biology of Alcoholism*, vol. 4, *Social Aspects of Alcoholism* (B. Kissin and H. Begleiter, eds.), pp. 117–166, Plenum Press, New York.

———, 1976b, The female alcoholic, in *Alcoholism: Interdisciplinary Approaches to an Enduring Problem* (R. E. Tartar and A. A. Sugarman, eds.), Addison-Wesley Publishing Co., Reading, Mass.

———, 1980, Risk factors related to alcohol problems among women: Proneness and vulnerability, in *Alcohol and Women*, Research Monograph No. 1, pp. 83–120, National Institute on Alcohol Abuse and Alcoholism, Rockville, Md.

———, 1982a, Alcohol use and alcohol problems among the elderly, in *Special Population Issues*, Alcohol and Health Monograph No. 4, pp. 263–290, National Institute on Alcohol Abuse and Alcoholism, Rockville, Md.

———, 1982b, Special populations, in *Alcohol, Science, and Society Revisited* (E. L. Gomberg, H. R. White, and J. A. Carpenter, eds.), pp. 337–354, University of Michigan Press, Ann Arbor.

Goodwin, D., 1973, Alcohol in suicide and homicide, *Q. J. Stud. Alc.*, 34:144–156.

Goodwin, D., Schulsinger, F., Hermansen, L., Guze, S. B., and Winokur, G., 1973, Alcohol problems in adoptees raised apart from alcoholic biological parents, *Arch. Gen. Psychiat.*, 238–243.

Goodwin, D. W., Schulsinger, F., Møller, N., Hermansen, L., Winokur, G., and Guze, S. B., 1974, Drinking problems in adopted and nonadopted sons of alcoholics, *Arch. Gen. Psychiat.*, 31:164–169.

Goodwin, D. W., Schulsinger, F., Knap, J., Mednick, S., and Guze, S. B., 1977, Alcoholism and depression in adopted-out daughters of alcoholics, *Arch. Gen. Psychiat.*, 34:751–755.

Gordon, A. J., 1978, Hispanic drinking after migration: The case of Dominicans, *Med. Anthro.*, 2:61–84.

———, 1981, The cultural context of drinking and indigenous therapy for alcohol problems in three migrant hispanic cultures: An ethnographic report, *J. Stud. Alc.*, Suppl. 9:217–240.

Gorwitz, K., Bahr, A., Warthen, F. J., and Cooper, M., 1970, Some epidemiological data on alcoholism in Maryland, *Q. J. Stud. Alc.*, 31:423–443.

Gould, L., Zahir, M., and Demartino, A., 1971, Cardiac effects of a cocktail, *JAMA*, 218:1799–1802.

Graux, P., 1969, Alcoholism of the elderly, *Rev. Alc.,* 15:61–63.

Graves, T. D., 1967, Acculturation, access, and alcohol in a tri-ethnic community, *Amer. Anthrop.,* 69:306–321.

Green, L. W., 1979, Toward national policy for health education, in *Alcohol, Youth, and Social Policy* (H. T. Blane and M. E. Chafetz, ed.), pp. 283–305, Plenum Press, New York.

Guinn, R., 1978, Alcohol use among Mexican-American youth, *J. School Health,* 48:90–91.

Guinn, R., and Hurley, R. S., 1976, Comparison of drug use among Houston and lower Rio Grande Valley secondary students, *Adolescence,* 11:455–459.

Gunther, M., 1975, Female alcoholism: The drinker in the pantry, *Today's Health,* 53:15–18.

Guttman, D., 1977, *A survey of drug taking behavior of the elderly,* National Institute on Drug Abuse, Rockville, Md.

Guze, S. B., Tuasen, V. B., and Stewart, M. A., 1963, The drinking history: A comparison of reports by subjects and their relatives, *Q. J. Stud. Alc.,* 24:249–260.

Haberman, P. W., and Sheinberg, J., 1967, Implicative drinking reported in a household survey: Corroborative note on subgroup differences, *Q. J. Stud. Alc.,* 28:538–543.

Hall, B. D., and Ornstein, W. A., 1974, Noonan's phenotype in an offspring of an alcoholic mother, *Lancet,* 1:680–681.

Hall, D. C., Chaikin, K., and Piland, B., 1977, A review of problem drinking behavior literature associated with the Spanish-speaking population groups, vol. III, Stanford Research Institute, Menlo Park, Calif.

Hanna, J. M., 1976, Ethnic groups, human variation, and alcohol use, in *Cross-Cultural Approaches to the Study of Alcohol* (M. W. Everett, J. O. Waddell, and D. B. Heath, eds.), pp. 235–242, Mouton, The Hague.

———, 1978, Metabolic responses of Chinese, Japanese, and Europeans to alcohol, *Alcoholism: Clin. Exp. Res.,* 2:89–92.

Hannerz, U., 1969, *Soulside: Inquiries into Ghetto Culture and Community,* Columbia University Press, New York.

Hanson, J. W., Jones, K. L., and Smith, D. W., 1976, Fetal alcohol syndrome: Experience with 41 patients, *JAMA,* 235:1458–1460.

Harford, T. C., and Mills, G. S., 1978, Age-related trends in alcohol consumption, *J. Stud. Alc.,* 39:207–210.

Harford, T. C., and Spiegler, D. L., 1982, Environmental influences in adolescent drinking, in *Special Population Issues,* Alcohol and Health Monograph No. 4, pp. 167–193, National Institute on Alcohol Abuse and Alcoholism, Rockville, Md.

Harlap, S., and Shiono, P. H., 1980, Alcohol, smoking, and the incidence of spontaneous abortion in the first and second trimester, *Lancet,* 1:173–176.

Harper, F. D. (ed.), 1976, *Alcohol abuse and black America,* Douglass Publishers, Alexandria, Va.

———, 1978, Alcohol use among North American blacks, in *Research Advances in Alcohol and Drug Problems,* vol. 4. (Y. Israel, F. B. Glaser, H. Kalant, R. E. Popham, W. Schmidt, and R. G. Smart, eds.), pp. 349–366, Plenum Press, New York.

Hatcher, E. M., Jones, M. K., and Jones, B. M., 1977, Cognitive deficits in alcoholic women, *Alcoholism: Clin. Exp. Res.,* 1:371–377.

Heath, D. B., 1982, Alcohol use among North American Indians: A cross-cultural survey of patterns and problems, in *Research Advances in Alcohol and Drug Problems* vol. 7 (Y. Israel et al., eds.), Plenum Press, New York.

Henderson, D. C., and Anderson, S. C., 1982, Treatment of alcoholic women, *J. of Addictions and Health*, 3:34–48.

Hewitt, L., 1982, Current status of alcohol education programs for youth, in *Special Population Issues*, Alcohol and Health Monograph No. 4, pp. 227–262, National Institute on Alcohol Abuse and Alcoholism, Rockville, Md.

Hill, S. Y., 1982, Biological consequences of alcoholism and alcohol-related problems among women, in *Special Population Issues*, Alcohol and Health Monograph No. 4, pp. 43–73, National Institute on Alcohol Abuse and Alcoholism, Rockville, Md.

Hirst, A. E., Hadley, G. G., and Gore, I., 1965, The effect of chronic alcoholism on atherosclerosis, *Am. J. Med. Sci.*, 249:143–149.

Hoffman, H., and Noem, A. A., 1975, Social background variables, referral sources, and life events in male and female alcoholics, *Psychol. Rep.*, 37:1087–1092.

Holinger, P. C., 1979, Violent deaths among the young: Recent trends in suicide, homicide, and accidents, *Am. J. Psychiat.*, 136:1144–1147.

Honigmann, J. J., 1980, Perspectives on alcohol behavior, in *Alcohol and Native People of the North* (J. Hamer and J. Steinbring, eds.), pp. 267–285, University Press of North America, Lanham, Md.

Horman, R. E., 1979, The impact of sociopolitical systems on teenage alcohol abuse, in *Youth, Alcohol, and Social Policy* (H. T. Blane and M. E. Chafetz, eds.), pp. 263–282, Plenum Press, New York.

Horn, J. L., and Wanberg, K. W., 1969, Symptom patterns related to excessive use of alcohol, *Q. J. Stud. Alc.*, 30:35–58.

Horowitz, L. D., 1975, Alcohol and heart disease, *JAMA*, 239:959–960.

Horton, D. J., 1943, The function of alcohol in primitive societies: A cross-cultural study, *Q. J. Stud. Alc.*, 4:199–320.

Horvath, T. B., 1975, Clinical spectrum and epidemiological features of alcoholic dementia, in *Alcohol, Drugs, and Brain Damage, Proceedings of a Symposium: Effects of Chronic Use of Alcohol and other Psychoactive Drugs on Cerebral Function* (J. G. Rankin, ed.), pp. 1–16, Addiction Research Foundation, Toronto.

Hyman, M. M., 1968, The social characteristics of persons arrested for driving while intoxicated, *Q. J. Stud. Alc.*, Suppl. 4:138–177.

———, 1976, Alcoholics 15 years later, *Ann. N.Y. Acad. Sci.*, 273:613–623.

Hyman, M. M., Helrich, A. R., and Besson, G., 1972, Ascertaining police bias in arrests for drunken driving, *Q. J. Stud. Alc.*, 33:148–159.

Iber, F. L., 1982, Do special populations have special alcoholism treatment needs? Debate, National Council on Alcoholism Conference, April 5, 1982, Washington, D.C.

Idleburg, D., 1982, *An Exploratory Study of Treatment Outcomes in a 12 Year Follow-Up of Black and of White Female Alcoholics*, unpublished Ph.D. dissertation, Washington University, St. Louis.

Ijaiya, K., Schwenck, A., and Gladtke, E., 1976, Fetales Alkoholsyndrome [fetal alcohol syndrome], *Dtsch. Med. Wochenschr.*, 101:1563–1568.

Indian Health Service, 1977, *Alcoholism: A High Priority Health Problem*, Indian Health Service, Rockville, Md.

———, 1980, *Alcohol-Related Discharges from Indian Health Service and Con-*

tract General Hospitals: Fiscal Year 1977, Indian Health Service, Rockville, Md.

————, 1982, *Age-Specific Mortality Rates per 100,000 Population for Indians and Alaska Natives in Reservation States, U.S. All Races, and U.S. Other than White,* Indian Health Service, Rockville, Md.

Inge, R., 1976, Alcoholism and blacks: A synthesis of findings, *Urban League Review,* 2:9.

James, J. E., 1975, Symptoms of alcoholism in women: A preliminary survey of AA members, *J. Stud. Alc.,* 36:1564–1569.

Jessor, R., and Jessor, S. L., 1975, Adolescent development and the onset of drinking: A longitudinal study, *J. Stud. Alc.,* 36:27–51.

————, 1977, *Problem Behavior and Psychosocial Development: A Longitudinal Study of Youth,* Academic Press, New York.

Jessor, R., Graves, T. D., Hanson, R. C., and Jessor, S. L., 1968, *Society, Personality, and Deviant Behavior: A Study of a Tri-Ethnic Community,* Holt, Rinehart and Winston, New York.

Jilek, W., 1976, "Brainwashing" as a therapeutic technique in contemporary Canadian Indian spirit dancing: A case of theory building, in *Anthropology and Mental Health,* pp. 201–213, Mouton, The Hague.

Johnson, J. J., 1975, Alcoholism: A social disease from a medical perspective in *Textbook of Black-Related Diseases* (R. A. Williams, ed.), McGraw-Hill Book Company, New York.

Johnson, L. V., and Matre, M., 1978, Anomie and alcohol use: Drinking problems in Mexican American and Anglo neighborhoods, *J. Stud. Alc.,* 39:894–902.

Johnson, P., Armor, D. J., Polich, S., and Stambul, H., 1977, *U.S. Adult Drinking Practices: Time Trends, Social Correlates, and Sex Roles,* Rand Corporation, Santa Monica, Calif.

Johnson, S., 1980, Cirrhosis mortality among American Indian women: Rates and ratios, 1975 and 1976, in *Currents in Alcoholism,* vol. 5 (M. Galanter, ed.), pp. 455–463, Grune & Stratton, Inc., New York.

Johnston, L. D., Bachman, J. G., and O'Malley, P. M., 1979, *Drugs in the Class of 1978: Behavior, Attitude, and Recent National Trends,* National Institute on Drug Abuse, Rockville, Md.

Jones, M. C., 1968, Personality correlates and antecedents of drinking patterns in adult males, *J. Consult. Clin. Psychol.,* 32:2–12.

————, 1971, Personality correlates and antecedents of drinking patterns in women, *J. Consult. Clin. Psychol.,* 36:61–69.

Jones, B. M., and Jones, M. K., 1976a, Alcohol effects in women during the menstrual cycle, *Ann. N.Y. Acad. Sci.,* 273:576–587.

————, 1976b, Women and alcohol intoxication, metabolism, and the menstrual cycle, in *Alcoholism Problems in Women and Children* (M. Greenblatt and M. A. Schuckit, eds.), pp. 103–136, Grune & Stratton, Inc., New York.

Jones, K. L., and Smith, D. W., 1973, The fetal alcohol syndrome: Recognition in early infancy and historical perspective, *Lancet,* 2:999–1001.

Jones, K. L., Smith, D. W., Ulleland, C. N., and Streissguth, A. P., 1973, Pattern of malformation in offspring of chronic alcoholic mothers, *Lancet,* 1:1269–1271.

Jones, K. L., Smith, D. W., Streissguth, A. P., and Myrianthopoulos, N. C., 1974, Outcome in the offspring of chronic alcoholic women, *Lancet,* 1:1076–1078.

Kaminski, M., Rueau-Rouquette, C., and Schwartz, D., 1976, Consumption of alcohol among pregnant women and the outcome of pregnancy, *Paris Revue d'Epidemiologie et Sante Publique,* 24:27–40.

Kannel, W. B., 1976, Some lessons in cardiovascular epidemiology from Framingham, *Am. J. Cardiol.,* 37:261–282.

Keller, A. Z., 1978, Liver cirrhosis, tobacco, alcohol, and cancer among blacks, *J. Nat. Med. Assoc.,* 70:575–580.

King, L. J., Murphy, G. E., Robins, L. N., and Darvish, H., 1969, Alcohol abuse: A crucial factor in the social problems of Negro men, *Am. J. Psychiat.,* 125:96–104.

King, L. M., 1982, Alcoholism: Studies regarding black Americans 1977–1980, in *Special Population Issues,* Research Monograph No. 4., pp. 385–407, National Institute on Alcohol Abuse and Alcoholism, Rockville, Md.

Kinsey, B. A., 1966, *The Female Alcoholic: A Social Psychological Study,* Charles C Thomas, Springfield, Ill.

————, 1968, Psychological factors in alcoholic women from a state hospital sample, *Am. J. Psychiat.,* 124:1463–1466.

Klatsky, A. L., Friedman, G. D., Siegelaub, A. B., and Gerard, M. J., 1977a, Alcohol consumption among white, black, or Oriental men and women: Kaiser-Permanente Multiphasic Health Examination data, *Am. J. Epidemiol.,* 105:311–323.

————, 1977b, Alcohol consumption and blood pressure: Kaiser-Permanente Multiphasic Health Examination data, *New Engl. J. Med.,* 296:1194–1200.

Korcok, M., 1978, Women—Alcohol and other drugs, *Focus,* 1:4.

Kovar, M. G., 1977, Health of the elderly and use of health services, *Public Health Rep.,* 92:9–19.

Knupfer, G., 1967, The epidemiology of problem drinking, *Am. J. Pub. Health,* 57:973–986.

————, 1982, Problems associated with drunkenness in women: Some research issues, in *Special Population Issues,* Alcohol and Health Monograph No. 4, pp. 3–39, National Institute on Alcohol Abuse and Alcoholism, Rockville, Md.

Knupfer, G., Fink, R., Clark, W., and Goffman, A., 1963, *Factors Related to Amount of Drinking in an Urban Community,* California Drinking Practices Study Report No. 6, California State Department of Health, Berkeley, Calif.

Kramer, K., Fuller, L., and Fisher, R., 1968, The increasing mortality attributed to cirrhosis and fatty liver in Baltimore (1957–1966), *Ann. Intern. Med.,* 69:273–282.

Kramer, M., Taube, C. A., and Redick, R. W., 1973, Patterns of use of psychiatric facilities by the aged: Past, present, and future, in *The Psychology of Adult Development and Aging,* American Psychological Association, Washington, D.C.

Krasner, N., Davis, M., Partmann, B., and Williams, R., 1977, Changing pattern of alcoholic liver disease in Great Britain: Relation to sex and signs of autoimmunity, *Br. Med. J.,* 1:1497–1550.

Kraus, R. F., and Buffler, P. A., 1979, Sociocultural stress and the American native in Alaska: An analysis of changing patterns of psychiatric illness and alcohol abuse among Alaska Natives, *Culture, Medicine, and Psychiatry,* 3:111–151.

Ladner, J., 1971, *Tomorrow's Tomorrow: The Black Woman*, Doubleday & Company, New York.

Lang, G. C., 1979, Survival strategies of Chippewa drinkers in Minneapolis, *Central Issues in Anthropology*, 1:19–40.

Larkins, J. R., 1965, *Alcohol and the Negro: Explosive Issues*, Record Publishing Co., Zebulon, N.C.

Leland, J., 1976, *Firewater Myths: North American Indian Drinking and Alcohol Addiction*, Rutgers Center of Alcohol Studies, New Brunswick, N.J.

———, 1978, Women and alcohol in an Indian settlement, *Med. Anthro.*, 2:85–119.

———, 1980a, Native American alcohol use: A review of the literature, in *From Tulapai to Tokay: A Bibliography of Alcohol Use and Abuse among Native Americans of North America* (P. D. Mail and D. R. McDonald, compilers), pp. 1–56, HRAF Press, New Haven, Conn.

———, 1980b, Sex roles, family organization, and alcohol abuse, in *Alcohol and the Family* (J. Orford and J. Harwin, eds.), Croom Helm, London.

Lelbach, W. K., Gibbons, R., Israel, Y., Kalant, H., Popham, R., Schmidt, W., and Smart, R. (eds.), 1974, Organic pathology related to volume and pattern of alcohol use, in *Research Advances in Alcohol and Drug Problems*, p. 93, John Wiley & Sons, New York.

Lemere, F., and Smith, J. W., 1973, Alcohol induced sexual impotence, *Am. J. Psychiat.*, 130:212–213.

Lemert, E., 1982, Drinking among American Indians, in *Alcohol, Science, and Society Revisited* (E. L. Gomberg, H. R. White, and J. A. Carpenter, eds.), pp. 80–95, University of Michigan Press, Ann Arbor.

Lemoine, P., Harousseau, H., Borteyru, J. P., and Menuet, J. C., 1968, Les enfants des parents alcooliques: Anomalies observees a propos/de 124 cas., *Arch. Fr. Pediatr.*, 25:830–831.

Leon, R. L., 1968, Some implications for a preventive program for American Indians, *Am. J. Psychiat.*, 125:232–236.

Levine, J., 1955, The sexual adjustment of alcoholics, *Q. J. Stud. Alc.*, 16:675–680.

Levy, J. E., and Kunitz, S. J., 1974, *Indian Drinking: Navajo Practices and Anglo-American Theories*, John Wiley & Sons, New York.

Levy, L., 1973, Drug use on campus: Prevalence and social characteristics of collegiate drug users on campuses of the University of Illinois, *Drug Forum*, 2:141–171.

Lewis, C. E., Saghir, M. T., and Robins, E., 1982, Drinking patterns in homosexual and heterosexual women, *J. Clin. Psychiatry*, 43:277–279.

Lewis, H., 1955, *Blackways of Kent*, University of North Carolina Press, Chapel Hill.

Liban, C., and Smart, R. G., 1980, Generational and other differences between males and females in problem drinking and its treatment, *Drug. Alc. Depend.*, 5:207–222.

Lieber, C. S., 1972, Metabolism of ethanol and alcoholism: Racial and acquired factors, *Ann. Intern. Med.*, 76:326–327.

Liebow, E., 1967, *Tally's Corner: A Study of Negro Streetcorner Men*, Little, Brown and Company, Boston.

Lindbeck, V., 1972, The woman alcoholic: A review of the literature, *Int. J. Addict.*, 7:567–580.

Lindelius, R., Salum, I., and Agren, G., 1974, Mortality among male and female alcoholic patients treated in a psychiatric unit, *Acta Psychiatr. Scand.*, 30:612–618.

Lipscomb, W. R., and Trochi, K., 1981, *Black Drinking Practices Study Report to the Department of Alcohol and Drug Programs*, Source, Inc., Berkeley, Calif.

Lisansky, E. S., 1957, Alcoholism in women: Social and psychological concomitants, I, social history data, *Q. J. Stud. Alc.*, 18:586–623.

Little, R. E., 1976, Alcohol consumption during pregnancy, as reported to the obstetrician and to an independent interviewer, *Ann. N.Y. Acad. Sci.*, 273:588–592.

Little, R. E., Schultz, F. A., and Mandell, W., 1976, Drinking during pregnancy, *Q. J. Stud. Alc.*, 37:375–379.

Locke, B. L., Kramer, M., and Pasamanick, B., 1960, Alcoholic psychoses among first admissions to public mental hospitals in Ohio, *Q. J. Stud. Alc.*, 21:457–474.

Loiodice, G., Fortuna, G., Guidetti, A., Ria, N., and D'Elia, R., 1975, Considerazioni cliniche intorno a due casi de malformazioni congenite in bambini nadi da madri affette da alcoholismo cronico [clinical notes on two cases of congenital deformity in children born of chronic alcoholic mothers], *Minerva Pediatr.*, 27:1891–1893.

Lolli, G., 1953, Alcoholism in women, *Council Rev. Alcohol*, 5:9–11.

Lopez-Lee, D., 1979, Alcoholism among third world women: Research and treatment, in *Women Who Drink* (V. Burtle, ed.), pp. 98–115, Charles C Thomas, Springfield, Ill.

Lyon, J. L., Klauber, M. R., Gardner, J. W., and Smart, C. R., 1976, Cancer incidence in Mormons and non-Mormons in Utah, 1966–1970, *New Engl. J. Med.*, 294:129–133.

MacAndrew, C., and Edgarton, R. B., 1969, *Drunken Comportment: A Social Explanation*. Aldine Press, Chicago.

McClelland, D. C., Davis, W. H., Kalin, R., and Wanner, E., 1972, *The Drinking Man,* The Free Press, New York.

McCord, W., McCord, J., and Gudeman, J., 1960, *Origins of Alcoholism*, Stanford University Press, Stanford, Calif.

McCusker, J., Cherubin, C. F., and Zimberg, S., 1971, The prevalence of alcoholism in a general municipal hospital population, *N.Y. State J. Med.*, 71:751–754.

Madsen, W., 1964, *Mexican-Americans of South Texas,* Holt, Rinehart and Winston, Inc., New York.

Majewski, F., Bierich, J. R., Loser, H., Michaelis, R., Leiber, B., and Bettecken, F., 1976, Zur Klinik und pathogenese der Alkoholembryopathie [Clinical aspects and pathogenesis of alcohol embryology], *Muñch. Med. Wochenschr.*, 118:1635–1642.

Mala, T. A., 1979, Status of mental health of Alaska Natives, *Alaska Med.*, 21:1–3.

Malin, H., Coakley, J., Kaelber, C., Munch, N., and Holland, W., 1982, An epidemiologic perspective on alcohol use and abuse in the United States, in *Alcohol Consumption and Related Problems*, Alcohol and Health Monograph No. 1., pp. 99–153, National Institute on Alcohol Abuse and Alcoholism, Rockville, Md.

Manzke, H., and Grosse, F. R., 1975, Inkomplettes und Komplettes des Alkohol-Syndrom: Bei drei Kindern einer Trinkerein [Incomplete and complete alcohol syndrome: Three children of an alcoholic mother], *Med. Welt.*, 26:709–712.

Maril, R. L., and Zavaleta, A. N., 1979, Drinking patterns of low-income Mexican American women, *J. Stud. Alc.*, 40:480–484.

Marshall, M., 1979, Introduction, in *Beliefs, Behaviors, and Alcoholic Beverages: A Cross-Cultural Survey* (M. Marshall, ed.), pp. 1–11, University of Michigan Press, Ann Arbor.

May, P. A., 1977, Explanations of Native American drinking, *Plains Anthro.*, 22:223–232.

————, 1982, Susceptibility to substance abuse among American Indians: Variation across sociocultural settings, in *Problems of Drug Dependence* (L. S. Harris, ed.), 1981, Research Monograph No. 41, National Institute on Drug Abuse, Rockville, Md.

May, P. A., Hymbaugh, K. J., and Aase, J. M., 1984, The epidemiology of fetal alcohol syndrome among American Indians of the Southwest, *Social Biol.*, 30.

Mayer, J. E., and Filstead, W. J., 1980, Adolescence and alcohol, in *Adolescence and Alcohol*, Ballinger Publishing Company, Cambridge, Mass.

Mayfield, D. G., 1974, Alcohol problems in the aging patient, in *Drug Issues in Geropsychiatry* (W. G. Fann and G. L. Maddox, eds.), Williams & Wilkins Company, Baltimore.

Medhus, A., 1974, Morbidity among female alcoholics, *Scand. J. Soc. Med.*, 2:5–11.

————, 1975, Mortality of female alcoholics, *Scand. J. Soc. Med.*, 3:111–115.

Medical Journal of Australia, 1976, *Comments*, Alcoholic hepatitis, Feb. 28, pp. 250–251.

Mello, N. K., 1980, Some behavioral and biological aspects of alcohol problems in women, in *Alcohol and Drug Problems in Women* (O. J. Kalant, ed.), pp. 263–298, Plenum Press, New York.

————, 1983, Etiological theories of alcoholism, in *Advances in Substance Abuse* (N. K. Mello, ed.) vol. 3, pp. 271–312, JAI Press, Greenwich, Conn.

Mello, N. K., and Mendelson, J. H., 1978, Alcohol and human behavior, in *Handbook of Psychopharmacology*, vol. 12, *Drugs of Abuse* (L. L. Iversen, S. D. Iversen, and S. H. Snyder, eds.), pp. 235–317, Plenum Press, New York.

Mendelson, J. H., Miller, K. D., Mello, N. K., Pratt, H., and Schmitz, R., 1982, Hospital treatment of alcoholism: A profile of middle income Americans, *Alcoholism: Clin. Exp. Res.*, 6:377–383.

Miller, S., Helmrick, E., Berg, L., Nutting, P., and Schorr, G., 1975, Alcoholism: A statewide program evaluation, *Am. J. Psychiat.*, 131:274–281.

Mishara, B. L., and Kastenbaum, R., 1980, *Alcohol and Old Age*, Grune & Stratton, Inc., New York.

Mogar, R. E., Wilson, W. M., and Helm, S. T., 1970, Personality subtypes of male and female alcoholic patients, *Int. J. Addict.*, 5:99–114.

Moore, M. H., and Gerstein, D. R. (eds.), 1981, *Alcohol and Public Policy: Beyond the Shadow of Prohibition,* National Academy Press, Washington, D.C.

Moore, R. A., 1971, The prevalence of alcoholism in a community general hospital, *Am. J. Psychiat.,* 128:638–639.

Moore, M. A., Merson, M. H., Charache, P., and Shepard, R. H., 1977, Characteristics and mortality of outpatient-acquired pneumonia, *Johns Hopkins Med. J.,* 140:9–14.

Moos, R. H., 1969, Typology of menstrual cycle symptoms, *Am. J. Obstet. Gynecol.,* 103:390–401.

Morales, A., 1972, Police deployment theories and the Mexican American community, in *Voices from el Grito* (O. Romano, ed.), Quinto Sol, Berkeley, Calif.

Morey, L. C., and Blashfield, R. K., 1981, Empirical classifications of alcoholics: A review, *J. Stud. Alc.,* 42:925–937.

Morgan, M. Y., and Sherlock, S., 1977, Sex-related differences among 100 patients with alcoholic liver disease, *Br. Med. J.,* 1:939–941.

Morrissey, E. R., and Schuckit, M. A., 1978, Stressful life events among women seen at a detoxication center, *J. Stud. Alc.,* 39:1559–1576.

Mulford, H. A., 1977, Women and men problem drinkers, *J. Stud. Alc.,* 38:1624–1639.

Mulvihill, J. J., Klimas, J. T., Stoker, D. C., and Risenberg, H. M., 1976, Fetal alcohol syndrome, *Am. J. Obstet. Gynecol.,* 125:937–941.

Mulvihill, J. J., and Yeager, A. M., 1976, Fetal alcohol syndrome, *Teratology,* 13:68–72.

National Safety Council, 1979, *Accident Facts,* National Safety Council, Chicago.

Nelson, L., 1977, Alcoholism in Zuni, New Mexico, *Prev. Med.,* 6:152–166.

Neville, J. N., Eagles, J. A., Samson, G., and Olson, R. E., 1968, Nutritional status of alcoholics, *Am. J. Clin. Nutrition,* 21:1329–1340.

Neugarten, B. L., 1975, The future and the young-old, *Gerontology,* 15:4–9 (part 2).

NIAAA, 1978, *Spanish Clients Treated in NIAAA Funded Programs: Calendar Year 1977,* National Institute on Alcohol Abuse and Alcoholism, Rockville, Md.

———, 1981a, *Black Clients Treated in NIAAA Funded Categorical Programs: Calendar Year 1979,* National Institute on Alcohol Abuse and Alcoholism, Rockville, Md.

———, 1981b, *Indian Clients Treated in NIAAA Funded Programs: Calendar Year 1980,* National Institute on Alcohol Abuse and Alcoholism, Rockville, Md.

Noonan, J. A., 1976, Congenital heart disease in the fetal alcohol syndrome, *Am. J. Cardiol.,* 37:160.

Oetting, E. R., and Beauvais, F., 1982, *Drug Use among Native American Youth: Summary of Findings (1975–1981),* Western Behavioral Studies, Ft. Collins, Colo.

Ouellette, E. M., and Rosett, H. L., 1976, A pilot prospective study of the fetal alcohol syndrome at the Boston City Hospital, Part II: The infants, *Ann. N.Y. Acad. Sci.,* 273:123–129.

Padilla, E. R., Padilla, A. M., Morales, A., and Omedo, E. L., 1979, Inhalant, marijuana, and alcohol abuse among barrio children and adolescents, *Int. J. Addict.*, 14:945–964.

Paine, H. J., 1977, Attitudes and patterns of alcohol use among Mexican Americans: Implications for service delivery, *J. Stud. Alc.*, 38:544–553.

Palmer, H. P., Ouellette, E. M., Warner, L., and Leichtman, S. R., 1975, Congenital malformations in offspring of a chronic alcoholic mother, *Pediatr.*, 53:490–494.

Parker, F. B., 1972, Sex-role adjustment in women alcoholics, *Q. J. Stud. Alc.*, 33:647–657.

Parsons, O. A., and Farr, S. P., 1981, The neuropsychology of alcohol and drug abuse, in *Handbook of Clinical Neuropsychology* (S. B. Filskov and T. J. Boll, eds.), pp. 320–365, John Wiley & Sons, New York.

Pascarelli, E. F., and Fisher, W., 1974, Drug dependence in the elderly, *Int. J. Aging. Hum. Dev.*, 5:347–356.

Pequignot, G., Chabert, C., Eydoux, H., and Courcoul, M. A., 1974, Increased risk of liver cirrhosis with intake of alcohol, *Rev. Alcohol,* 20:191.

Perlow, W. E., Bacarona, E., and Lieber, C. S., 1977, Symptomatic intestinal disaccharidase deficiency in alcoholics, *Gastroenterology,* 72:680–684.

Pfeiffer, E., 1977, Psychopathology and social pathology, in *Handbook of the Psychology of Aging* (J. E. Birren and K. W. Schaie, eds.), Van Nostrand, New York.

Pitts, F. N., Jr., and Winokur, G., 1966, Affective disorder. VII: Alcoholism and affective disorder, *J. Psychiatr. Res.,* 4:37–50.

Podolsky, E., 1963, The woman alcoholic and premenstrual tension, *J. Am. Med. Wom. Assoc.,* 18:816–818.

Polich, J. M., 1979, Alcohol problems among civilian and military youth, in *Youth, Alcohol, and Social Policy* (H. T. Blane and M. E. Chafetz, eds.), pp. 59–86, Plenum Press, New York.

Polich, J. M., Armor, D. J., and Braiker, H. B., 1980, *The Course of Alcoholism: Four Years after Treatment,* The Rand Corporation, Santa Monica, Calif.

Randall, C. L., Taylor, J., and Walker, D. W., 1977, Ethanol-induced malformations in mice, *Alcoholism: Clin. Exp. Res.,* 1:219–224.

Rachal, J. V., Hubbard, R. L., Williams, J. R., and Tuchfield, B. S., 1976, Drinking levels and problem drinking among junior and senior high school students, *J. Stud. Alc.,* 37:1751–1761.

Rachal, J. V., Maisto, S. A., Guess, L. L., and Hubbard, R. L., 1982, Alcohol use among youth, in *Alcohol Consumption and Related Problems,* Alcohol and Health Monograph No. 1, pp. 55–95, National Institute on Alcohol Abuse and Alcoholism, Rockville, Md.

Rachal, J. V., Williams, J. R., Brehm, M. L., Cavanaugh, B., Moore, R. P., and Echerman, W. C., 1975, *A National Study of Adolescent Drinking Behavior, Attitudes, and Correlates,* National Institute on Alcohol Abuse and Alcoholism, Rockville, Md.

Rainwater, L., 1970, *Behind Ghetto Walls: Family Life in a Federal Slum,* Aldine Press, Chicago.

Rankin, J. G., Smith, W., Popham, R. E., and de Lint, J., 1975, Epidemiology of alcoholic liver disease—Insights and problems, in *Alcoholic Liver Pathology* (J. M. Khanna, Y. Israel, and H. Kalant, eds.), Addiction Research Foundation, Toronto.

Rathbone-McCuan, E., 1980, Elderly victims of family violence and neglect, *Soc. Casework*, 61:296–304.

Rathbone-McCuan, E., Lohn, H., Levenson, J., and Hsu, J., 1976, *Community Survey of Aged Alcoholics and Problem Drinkers*, National Institute on Alcohol Abuse and Alcoholism, Rockville, Md.

Rathod, N. H., and Thompson, I. G., 1971, Women alcoholics: Clinical study, *Q. J. Stud. Alc.*, 32:42–45.

Reed, T. E., Kalant, H., Gibbons, R. J., Kapur, B. M., and Rankin, J. G., 1976, Alcohol acetaldehyde metabolism in Caucasian, Chinese, and Amerinds, *Can. Med. Assoc. J.*, 115:851–855.

Reinhold, L., Hütteroth, H., and Schulte-Wisserman, H., 1975, Das fetale Alkohol-Syndrom: Falbericht über 2 Geschwister [The fetal alcohol syndrome: Case of two siblings], *Müch. Med. Wochenschr.*, 117:1731–1734.

Rimmer, J., Pitts, F. N., Reich, T., and Winokur, G., 1971, Alcoholism: II. Sex, socioeconomic status, and race in two hospitalized samples, *Q. J. Stud. Alc.*, 32:942–952.

Rimmer, J., Reich, T., and Winokur, G., 1972, Alcoholism: V. Diagnosis and clinical variation among alcoholics, *Q. J. Stud. Alc.*, 33:658–666.

Robertson, L. S., and Zader, P. L., 1977, *Driver Education and Fatal Crash Involvement* of Teen-aged Drivers, Insurance Institute for Highway Safety, Washington, D.C.

Robins, L. N., 1980, Epidemiology of adolescent drug use and abuse, in *Psychopathology of Children and Youth: A Cross-Cultural Perspective* (E. F. Purcell, ed.), pp. 223–242, Josiah Macy, Jr., Foundation, New York.

Robins, L. N., and Guze, S. B., 1971, Drinking practices and problems in urban ghetto populations, in *Recent Advances in Studies of Alcoholism* (N. K. Mello and J. H. Mendelson, eds.), pp. 825–842, National Institute on Alcohol Abuse and Alcoholism, Rockville, Md.

Roebuck, J. B., and Kessler, R. G., 1972, *The Etiology of Alcoholism: Constitutional, Psychological, and Sociological Approaches*, Charles C Thomas, Springfield, Ill.

Roizen, J., 1982, Estimating alcohol involvement in serious events, in *Alcohol Consumption and Related Problems*, Alcohol and Health Monograph No. 1, pp. 111–134, National Institute on Alcohol Abuse and Alcoholism, Rockville, Md.

Room, R., 1972, Drinking patterns in large U.S. cities: A comparison of San Francisco and national samples, *Q. J. Stud. Alc.*, Suppl. 6:28–57.

Root, A. W., Reiter, E. O., Andriola, M., and Duckett, G., 1975, Hypothalamic-pituitary function in the fetal alcohol syndrome, *J. Pediatr.*, 87:585–587.

Rosenberg, L., Slone, D., Shapiro, S., Kaufman, D. W., Miettienen, O. S., and Stolley, P. D., 1981, Alcoholic beverages and myocardial infarction in young women, *Am. J. Pub. Health*, 71:82–85.

Rosenblatt, S. M., Grass, M. M., Bromer, M., Lewis, E., and Malenowski, B., 1971, Patients admitted for treatment of alcohol dependence syndrome: An epidemiological study, *Q. J. Stud. Alc.*, 32:104–115.

Rosett, H. L., 1980, The effects of alcohol on the fetus and offspring, in *Alcohol and Drug Problems in Women*, vol. 5, *Research Advances in Alcohol and Drug Problems* (O. J. Kalant, ed.), pp. 595–652, Plenum Press, New York.

Rosett, H. L., Ouellette, E. M., and Weiner, L., 1976, A pilot prospective study of the fetal alcohol syndrome at the Boston City Hospital, Part I: Maternal drinking, *Ann. N.Y. Acad. Sci.,* 273:118–122.

Rosin, A., and Glatt, M. M., 1971, Alcohol excess in the elderly, *Q. J. Stud. Alc.,* 32:52–59.

Ruebner, B. H., Edin, M. D., Miyai, K., and Keio, M. D., 1961, The low incidence of myocardial infarction in hepatic cirrhosis, *Lancet,* 2:1435–1436.

Rushing, W. A., 1969, Suicide and the interaction of alcoholism (liver cirrhosis) with the social situation, *Q. J. Stud. Alc.,* 30:93–103.

Russell, M., 1977, Intrauterine growth in infants born to women with alcohol-related diagnoses, *Alcoholism: Clin. Exp. Res.,* 1:225–231.

Saghir, M. T., and Robins, E., 1973, *Male and Female Homosexuality: A Comprehensive Investigation,* Williams & Wilkins Company, Baltimore.

Sanchez-Dirks, M., 1978, Drinking practices among Hispanic youth, *Alc. Health Res. World,* 3:21–27.

Sander, L. W., Snyder, P. A., Rosett, H. L., Lee, A., Gould, J. B., and Ouellette, E., 1977, Effects of alcohol intake during pregnancy on newborn state regulation: A progress report, *Alcoholism: Clin. Exp. Res.,* 1:233–241.

Sandmaier, M., 1980a, *The Invisible Alcoholics,* McGraw-Hill Book Company, New York.

————, 1980b, Women helping women: Opening the door to treatment, in *Alcoholism in Women* (C. C. Eddy and J. L. Ford, eds.), Kendall/Hunt Publishing Co., Dubuque, Iowa.

Saule, H., 1974, Fetales Alkohol-Syndrome: Ein Falbericht [Fetal alcohol syndrome: One case], *Klin. Pediatr.,* 186:452–455.

Saunders, B., 1980, Psychological aspects of women and alcohol, in *Women and Alcohol* (Camberwell Council on Alcohol, ed.), pp. 67–100, Tavistock Publications, London.

Schaefer, J. M., 1982, Ethnic and racial variations in alcohol use and abuse, in *Special Population Issues,* Alcohol and Health Monograph No. 4, pp. 293–311, National Institute on Alcohol Abuse and Alcoholism, Rockville, Md.

Schmidt, W., and de Lint, J., 1972, Causes of death of alcoholics, *Q. J. Stud. Alc.,* 33:171.

Schmidt, W., and Popham, R. E., 1980, Sex differences in mortality: A comparison of male and female alcoholics, in *Research Advances in Alcohol and Drug Problems,* vol. 4, *Alcohol and Drug Problems in Women* (O. J. Kalant, ed.), pp. 365–384, Plenum Press, New York.

Schottenfeld, D., Gantt, R. C., and Wynder, E. L., 1974, The role of alcohol and tobacco in multiple primary cancers of the upper digestive system: A prospective study, *Prev. Med.,* 3:277–293.

Schuckit, M. A., 1972, Sexual disturbance in the woman alcoholic, *Human Sexuality,* 6:44–65.

————, 1973, Depression and alcoholism in women, in *Proceedings of the First Annual Alcoholism Conference of the National Institute on Alcohol Abuse and Alcoholism,* pp. 355–363, Washington, D.C.

————, 1978, Alcoholism in women, *Advances in Alcoholism,* 1:1–3.

————, 1979, Inpatient and residential approaches to the treatment of alcoholism, in *The Diagnosis and Treatment of Alcoholism* (J. H. Mendelson and N. K. Mello, eds.), pp. 257–282, McGraw-Hill Book Company, New York.

————, 1980, Phenomenology and treatment of alcoholism in the elderly, in *Phe-*

nomenology and Treatment of Alcoholism (W. E. Fann, I. Karacen, A. D. Pokorny, and R. L. Williams, eds.), Spectrum Publications, Jamaica, N.Y.

Schuckit, M., Pitts, F. M., Jr., Reich, T., King, L. J., and Winokur, G., 1969, Alcoholism. I: Two types of alcoholism in women, *Arch. Gen. Psychiat.,* 20:301–306.

Schuckit, M. A., Goodwin, D. A., and Winokur, G., 1972, A study of alcoholism in half-siblings, *Am. J. Psychiat.,* 128:1182–1136.

Schuckit, M. A., and Miller, P. L., 1976, Alcoholism in elderly men: A survey of a general medical ward, *Ann. N.Y. Acad. Sci.,* 273:558–571.

Schuckit, M. A., and Morrissey, E. R., 1976, Alcoholism in women: Some clinical and social perspectives with an emphasis on possible subtypes, in *Alcoholism Problems in Women and Children* (M. Greenblatt and M. A. Schuckit, eds.), pp. 5–35, Grune & Stratton, Inc., New York.

————, 1979, Drug use among alcoholic women, *Am. J. Psychiat.,* 136:607–611.

Schuckit, M. A., Morrissey, E. R., and O'Leary, M. R., 1977, Alcohol problems in elderly men and women, *Addict. Dis.,* 3:405–416.

Schuckit, M. A., and Pastor, P. A., 1978, The elderly as a unique population, *Alcoholism: Clin. Exp. Res.,* 2:60–67.

————, 1979, Alcohol-related psychopathology in the aged, in *Psychopathology in the Aging* (O. J. Kaplan, ed.), pp. 211–227, Academic Press, New York.

Scida, J., and Vannicelli, M., 1979, Sex-role conflict and women's drinking, *J. Stud. Alc.,* 40:28–44.

Sclare, A. B., 1970, The female alcoholic, *Br. J. Addict.,* 65:99–107.

Seixas, F. A., 1978, Racial differences in alcohol metabolism: Facts and their interpretation—a seminar, *Alcoholism: Clin. Exp. Res.,* 2:59–92.

————, 1979, Drug/alcohol interactions: Overt potential dangers, *Geriatrics,* 17:89–102.

Sherfey, J. M., 1955, Psychopathology and character structure in chronic alcoholism, in *Etiology of Chronic Alcoholism* (O. Diethelm, ed.), pp. 16–42, Charles C Thomas, Springfield, Ill.

Shinar, D., McDonald, S. T., and Treat, J. R., 1978, Interaction between driver mental and physical conditions and errors causing traffic accidents: An analytic approach, *J. Safety Res.,* 10:16–23.

Shore, J. H., Kinzie, J. D., Hampson, J. L., and Pattison, E. M., 1973, Psychiatric epidemiology of an Indian village, *Psychiatry,* 36:70–81.

Siassi, I. G., Crocetti, H., and Spiro, R., 1973, Drinking patterns and alcoholism in a blue collar population, *Q. J. Stud. Alc.,* 34:917–926.

Sieber, M. F., 1979, Social background, attitudes, and personality in a three-year follow-up of alcohol consumers, *Drug Alc. Depend.,* 4:407–417.

Siegal, H. A., Peterson, D. M., and Chambers, C. D., 1975, The emerging skid row: Ethnographic and social notes on a changing scene, *J. Drug Issues,* 5:160–166.

Simpson, L. V., and Simpson, M. L., 1976, The Spanish-speaking social service worker: Attitudes towards the alcoholic and alcoholism, *Drug Forum,* 7:7–9.

Slater, A. D., and Albrecht, S. L., 1972, The extent and costs of excessive drinking among the Uintah-Ouray Indians, in *Native Americans Today: Sociological Perspectives* (H. M. Bahr, B. A. Chadwick, and R. C. Day, eds.), pp. 358–367, Harper & Row, New York.

Smart, R. G., 1979a, Priorities in minimizing alcohol problems among young people, in *Youth, Alcohol, and Social Policy* (H. T. Blane and M. E. Chafetz, eds.), pp. 229–261, Plenum Press, New York.

————, 1979b, Young alcoholics in treatment: Their characteristics and recovery rates at follow-up, *Alcoholism: Clin. Exp. Res.*, 3:19–23.

Smart, R. G., and Finley, J., 1976, Increases in youthful admissions to alcohol treatment in Ontario, *Drug. Alc. Depend.*, 1:83–87.

Smith, J. W., 1977, Alcohol disorders of the heart and skeletal muscles, in *Alcoholism: Development, Consequences, and Interventions*, pp. 136–143, C. V. Mosby Company, St. Louis.

Smith, S. L., 1975, Mood and the menstrual cycle, in *Topics in Psychoneuroendocrinology* (E. J. Sacher, ed.), pp. 19–58, Grune & Stratton, Inc., New York.

Snyder, P. K., and Way, A., 1979, Alcoholism and the elderly, *Aging*, 291:8–11.

Sokol, R. J., Miller, S. I., and Reed, G., 1980, Alcohol abuse during pregnancy: An epidemiologic model, *Alcoholism: Clin. Exp. Res.*, 4:135–145.

Spain, D. W., 1945, Portal cirrhosis of the liver: A review of 250 necropsies with reference to sex differences, *Am. J. Clin. Path.*, 15:215.

Spitzer, R. L., Endicott, J., and Robins, E., 1978, *Research Diagnostic Criteria (RDC) for a Selected Group of Functional Disorders*, New York State Psychiatric Institute, New York.

Stack, C. B., 1974, *All Our Kin*, Harper & Row, New York.

Statistical Abstract of the United States, 1981, U.S. Department of Commerce, Bureau of the Census, U.S. Government Printing Office, Washington, D.C.

Steiner, M., and Carroll, B. J., 1977, The psychobiology of premenstrual dysphoria: Review of theories and treatments, *Psychoneuroendocrin.*, 2:321–335.

Sterne, M. W., 1967, Drinking patterns and alcoholism among American Negroes, in *Alcoholism* (D. J. Pittman, ed.), pp. 66–99, Harper & Row, Publishers, New York.

Stewart, O. C., 1964, Questions regarding American Indian criminality, *Human Organization*, 23:61–66.

Stratton, R., Zeiner, A., and Paredes, A., 1978, Tribal affiliation and prevalence of alcohol problems, *J. Stud. Alc.*, 39:1166–1177.

Streissguth, A. P., 1976a, Maternal alcoholism and the outcome of pregnancy: A review of the fetal alcohol syndrome, in *Alcohol Problems in Women and Children* (M. Greenblatt and M. A. Schuckit, eds.), pp. 251–272, Grune & Stratton, Inc., New York.

————, 1976b, Psychological handicaps in children with fetal alcohol syndrome, *Ann. N.Y. Acad. Sci.*, 273:140–145.

————, 1978, Fetal alcohol syndrome: An epidemiologic perspective, *Amer. J. Epidemiol.*, 107:462–478.

Summerskill, W. H. J., Davidson, C. S., Dible, J. H., Mallory, G. K., Sherlock, S., Turner, M. D., and Wolfe, S. H., 1960, Cirrhosis of the liver: A study of alcoholic and nonalcoholic patients in Boston and London, *New Engl. J. Med.*, 262:1.

Tamerin, J. S., Tolor, A., and Harrington, B., 1976, Sex differences in alcoholics: A comparison of male and female alcoholics, self and spouse perceptions, *Am. J. Drug Alc. Abuse.*, 3:457–472.

Technical Systems Institute, 1977, Final report: Drinking practices and alcohol-related problems of Spanish-speaking persons in three California locales, Alhambra, Calif.

————, 1980, An executive summary of the Final Report on Drinking Practices and Alcohol-Related Problems of Spanish-speaking Persons in Three California Locales, Alhambra, Calif.

Tenbrinck, M. S., and Buchin, S. Y., 1975, Fetal alcohol syndrome: Report of a case, *JAMA,* 232:114–1147.

Thomas, R. K., 1981, The history of North American Indian alcohol use as a community-based phenomenon, *J. Stud. Alc.,* Suppl. 9:29–39.

Tokuhata, G. K., Digon, E., and Ramaswamy, K., 1971, Alcohol sales and socio-economic factors related to cirrhosis of the liver mortality in Pennsylvania, *HMSMHA Health Reports,* 86:253–264.

Tracey, D. A., and Nathan, P. E., 1976, Behavioral analysis of chronic alcoholism in four women, *J. Consult. Clin. Psychol.,* 44:832–842.

Trevino, M. E., 1975, Machismo alcoholism: Mexican-American machismo drinking, in *Research, Treatment, Prevention* (M. E. Chafetz, ed.), pp. 295–302, U.S. Government Printing Office, Washington, D.C.

Trotter, R. T., and Chavira, J. A., 1978, Discovering new models for alcohol counseling in minority groups, in *Modern Medicine and Medical Anthropology in the United States-Mexico Border Populations* (B. Velirovic, ed.), pp. 164–171, Pan-American Health Organization Scientific Publication No. 359, Washington, D.C.

United States Bureau of the Census, 1979, Population characteristics: Persons of Spanish origin in the United States, Current Population Reports, Series P-20, No. 339, U.S. Government Printing Office, Washington, D.C.

Vaillant, G. E., 1980, Natural history of male psychological health: VIII. Antecedents of alcoholism and "orality," *Am. J. Psychiat.,* 137:181–186.

————, 1982, Natural history of male alcoholism, IV. Paths to recovery, *Arch. Gen. Psychiat.,* 39:127–133.

Vanecek, R., 1976, Atherosclerosis and cirrhosis of the liver, *Bull. WHO,* 53(516):567–570.

Vestal, R. E., McGuire, E. A., Tobin, J. D., Andres, R., Norris, A. H., and Mezy, E., 1977, Aging and ethanol metabolism, *Clin. Pharmacol. Therap.,* 21:343–354.

Victor, M., Adams, R. D., and Collins, H. G., 1971, *The Wernicke-Korsakoff Syndrome,* Blackwell Scientific Publications, Oxford.

Vitols, M. M., 1968, Culture patterns of drinking in Negro and white alcoholics, *Dis. Nerv. Sys.,* 29:391–394.

Wall, J. H., 1937, A study of alcoholism in women, *Am. J. Psychiat.,* 93:943–952.

Waller, P. F., 1970, The youthful driver, some characteristics and comparisons, *Beh. Res. Highway Safety,* 1:3.

Waller, S., and Lorch, B., 1978, Social and psychological characteristics of alcoholics: A male-female comparison, *Int. J. Addict.,* 13:201–212.

Wanberg, K. W., and Horn, J. L., 1970, Alcoholism symptom patterns of men and women: A comparative study, *Q. J. Stud. Alc.,* 31:40–61.

Wanberg, K. W., and Knapp, J., 1970, Differences in drinking symptoms and behavior of men and women alcoholics, *Br. J. Addict.,* 64:347–355.

Wanberg, K. W., Lewis, R., and Foster, F. M., 1978, Alcoholism and ethnicity: A comparative study of alcohol use patterns across ethnic groups, *Int. J. Addict.,* 13:1245–1262.

Warner, R. H., and Rosett, H. L., 1975, The effect of drinking on offspring: An historical survey of the American and British literature, *J. Stud. Alc.*, 36:1395-1420.

Wechsler, H., 1979, Patterns of alcohol consumption among the young: High school, college, and general population studies, in *Youth, Alcohol, and Public Policy* (H. T. Blane and M. E. Chafetz, eds.), pp. 39-58, Plenum Press, New York.

Wechsler, H., and McFadden, M., 1976, Sex differences in adolescent alcohol and drug use: A disappearing phenomenon, *J. Stud. Alc.*, 36:1208-1223.

Weibel, J. C., 1982, American Indians, urbanization, and alcohol: A developing urban Indian ethos, in *Special Population Issues,* Alcohol and Health Monograph No. 4, pp. 331-358, National Institute on Alcohol Abuse and Alcoholism, Rockville, Md.

Weibel-Orlando, J. C., Long, J., and Weisner, T. S., 1982, *A Comparison of Urban and Rural Indian Drinking Patterns in California,* Alcohol Research Center, UCLA Neuropsychiatric Institute, Los Angeles, Calif.

Weiss, N. S., 1976, Recent trends in violent deaths among young adults in the United States, *Am. J. Epidemiol.*, 103:416-422.

Weissman, M. M., and Klerman, G. L., Sex differences and the epidemiology of depression, *Arch. Gen. Psychiat.* 34:98-111.

Weissman, M., and Myers, J., 1980, Clinical depression in alcoholism, *Am. J. Psychiat.*, 137:372-373.

Westermeyer, J., 1972a, Chippewa and majority alcoholism in the Twin Cities: A comparison, *J. Nerv. Men. Dis.*, 155:322-327.

⸺, 1972b, Options regarding alcohol use among the Chippewa, *Am. J. Orthopsychiat.*, 42:398-403.

⸺, 1974, "The drunken Indian": Myths and realities, *Psychiat. Ann.*, 4:29-36.

⸺, 1976, Use of a social indicator system to assess alcoholism among Indian people in Minnesota, *Am. J. Drug. Alc. Abuse*, 3:447-456.

⸺, 1981, Research on treatment of drinking problems: Importance of cultural factors, *J. Stud. Alc.*, Suppl. 9:44-59.

Westermeyer, J., and Peake, E., 1983, A ten-year follow-up of alcoholic Native Americans in Minnesota, *Am. J. Psychiat.*, 140:189-194.

Westie, K. S., and McBride, D. C., 1979, The effects of ethnicity, age, and sex upon processing through an emergency alcohol health care delivery system, *Br. J. Addict.*, 74:21-29.

White, R., 1948, *The Abnormal Personality,* Ronald Press, New York.

Whitehead, P. C., and Ferrence, R. G., 1976, Women and children last: Implications of trends in consumption for women and young people, in *Alcoholism Problems in Women and Children* (M. Greenblatt and M. A. Schuckit, eds.), pp. 163-192, Grune & Stratton, New York.

Wilkinson, P., 1980, Sex differences in morbidity of alcoholics, in *Research Advances in Alcohol and Drug Problems,* vol. 4, *Alcohol and Drug Problems in Women* (O. J. Kalant, ed.), pp. 331-384, Plenum Press, New York.

Wilkinson, P., Santamaria, J. N., and Rankin, R. G., 1969a, Epidemiology of alcoholic cirrhosis, *Aust. Ann. Med.*, 18:222-226.

⸺, 1969b, Epidemiology of alcoholism: Social data and drinking patterns of a sample of Australian alcoholics, *Med. J. Aust.*, 1:1020.

Wilkinson, P., Kornaczewski, A., Rankin, R. G., and Santamaria, N. J., 1971, Physical disease in alcoholism: Initial survey of 1,000 patients, *Med. J. Aust.*, 1:1217-1223.

Williams, R. R., 1976, Breast and thyroid cancer and malignant melanoma promoted by alcohol-induced pituitary secretion of prolactin, TSH, and MSH, *Lancet,* 1:966–999.

Wilsnack, S., 1973, Sex-role identity in female alcoholics, *J. Abnorm. Psychol.,* 82:253:261.

————, 1976, The impact of sex-roles on women's alcohol use and abuse, in *Alcohol Problems in Women and Children* (M. Greenblatt and M. A. Schuckit, eds.), pp. 37–63, Grune & Stratton, Inc., New York.

Wilsnack, S. C., and Wilsnack, R. W., 1979, Sex roles and adolescent drinking, in *Alcohol, Youth, and Public Policy* (H. T. Blane and M. E. Chafetz, eds.), pp. 183–224, Plenum Press, New York.

Wilson, G. T., 1981, The effects of alcohol on human sexual behavior, in *Advances in Substance Abuse: Behavioral and Biological Research* (N. K. Mello, ed.), pp. 1–40, JAI Press, Greenwich, Conn.

Wilson, G. T., and Lawson, D. M., 1976, Effect of alcohol on sexual arousal in women, *J. Abnorm. Psychol.,* 5:489–497.

Winokur, G., and Clayton, P. J., 1968, Family history studies, IV: Comparison of male and female alcoholics, *Q. J. Stud. Alc.,* 29:885–891.

Winokur, G., Reich, T., Rimmer, J., et al., 1970, Alcoholism, III: Diagnosis and familial psychiatric illness in 259 alcoholic probands, *Arch. Gen. Psychiat.,* 23:104–111.

Wolff, P. H., 1972, Ethnic differences in alcohol sensitivity, *Science* 175:449–450.

————, 1973, Vasomotor sensitivity to ethanol in diverse Mongoloid populations, *Am. J. Hum. Genet.,* 25:193–206.

Wolin, S., Bennett, L., Noonan, D., and Teitelbaum, M., 1980, Disrupted family rituals: A factor in the intergenerational transmission of alcoholism, *J. Stud. Alc.,* 41:199–214.

Wood, H. P., and Duffy, E. L., 1966, Psychological factors in alcoholic women, *Am. J. Psychiat.,* 123:341–345.

Woodruff, R. A., Guze, S. B., and Clayton, P. J., 1973, Alcoholics who see a psychiatrist compared with those who do not, *Q. J. Stud. Alc.,* 34:1162–1171.

Wu, C. F., Sudhakar, G., Jaferi, G., Ahmed, S. S., and Regan, T. J., 1976, Preclinical cardiomyopathy in chronic alcoholism: A sex difference, *Am. Heart J.,* 91:281–286.

Zax, M., Gardner, E. A., and Hart, W. T., 1964, Public intoxication in Rochester: A survey of individuals charged during 1961, *Q. J. Stud. Alc.,* 25:669–678.

Zeiner, A. R., Paredes, A., and Cowden, L., 1976, Physiological responses to ethanol among the Tarahumara Indians, *Ann. N.Y. Acad. Sci.,* 273:151–158.

Zeiner, A. R., Paredes, A., and Christiansen, H. D., 1979, The role of acetaldehyde in mediating reactivity to an acute dose of ethanol among different racial groups, *Alcoholism: Clin. Exp. Res.,* 2:11–18.

Zimberg, S., 1978, Treatment of the elderly alcoholic in the community and in an institutionalized setting, *Addict. Dis.,* 3:417–427.

Zucker, R. A., 1976, Parental influences upon drinking practices of their children, in *Alcohol Problems in Women and Children* (M. Greenblatt and M. A. Schuckit, eds.), pp. 211–238, Grune & Stratton, Inc., New York.

————, 1979, Developmental aspects of drinking through the young adult years, in *Alcohol, Youth, and Public Policy* (H. T. Blane and M. E. Chafetz, eds.), pp. 91–146, Plenum Press, New York.

CHAPTER 5

The Selection of Treatment Modalities for the Alcoholic Patient

E. Mansell Pattison, M.D.
Professor and Chairman, Department of Psychiatry and Health Behavior,
Medical College of Georgia
Augusta, Georgia

The purpose of this chapter is to describe the differential selection of the most appropriate treatment for a person's specific alcohol problems. Differential diagnosis and differential treatment have a long tradition in the health sciences. Although there are generic and global aspects to any health intervention, the health practitioner seeks to refine diagnostic and treatment procedures, eliminate ineffective or inappropriate treatments, reduce the cost, effort, inefficiency, and undesirable side effects of nonspecific treatments, and attain the most efficient, potent, and effective specific treatment interventions possible. In the case of the alcoholism syndrome we have begun the task of definition and refinement. However a caveat is in order: The scientific study of the alcoholism syndrome has received significant attention for only the past 20 years. Even 10 years ago treatment interventions were global and nonspecific. Consequently we are in the early stages of formulating specific treatment methodologies. So although we are aware of the task before us, it is not possible to present rigorous and precise differential treatment strategies, and this chapter can give only rough first approximations. Details of the clinical approach of this chapter are presented in Pattison and Kaufman (1982).

I. TOWARD A MULTIVARIANT MODEL OF THE ALCOHOLISM SYNDROME

Prior to World War II, few alcoholism treatment programs existed, and the problem of alcoholism was generally hidden in dim recesses away from public view. There were alcoholism conditioning sanitaria, state hospital wards, and a few clinics, but few scientific guidelines and little clinical experience to guide the pioneers in this field. A review of alcoholism treatment in 1942 by Voegtlin and Lemere (1942) was both skeptical and pessimistic, citing a rehabilitation rate of perhaps no more than 30%. In contrast, a national survey by Armor et al. (1976) reports a 70% rehabilitation rate. The survey also reports, however, a bewildering array of treatment methods, with seemingly scant rationale and no general scientific approach. One might conclude that many treatments are *offered,* but few are *selected.*

It is not surprising that many methods were tried, many types of facilities were organized, many philosophies developed. No one had answers, so the best approach was to "give it a try." As a result, the treatment of alcoholism became a highly idiosyncratic enterprise, with each clinician or program isolated clinically, programmatically, and ideologically from other treatment approaches. What is surprising is the persistence of this fragmented approach and the consideration of treatment as a "personal monopoly."

This monopolistic approach gave rise to a "competitive monolithic" array of treatment entrepreneurs. Babow (1975) comments: "Particular treatment modalities or treatment programs . . . are praised as 'the only effective way' by their enthusiasts and denigrated by advocates of competing models." The result is a lack of professional and public accountability, an antiscientific bias against the accumulation of evidence, and the failure to develop cooperation among treatment resources. Babow concludes: "A vicious circle thus operates in which a program policy of rigid ideology tries to shut off anyone or anything that does not fit."

A study of alcoholism treatment personnel by Einstein et al. (1970) illustrates this problem. The authors report that treatment personnel focus on only one aspect of the alcoholism syndrome and then pursue one personal line of rehabilitation. They conclude: "Is it reasonable to expect that effective treatment and/or prevention of a condition as complex as alcoholism can be achieved by such a simplistic approach?"

Similarly, Hadley and Hadley (1972) studied the social climate of 10 different alcoholism treatment programs. Not only were attitudes and social behaviors different in each program, within each program the staff members held individual philosophies and treatment approaches at variance with one another and with their common program. In a factor analytic study of dimensions of change in alcoholic rehabilitation, Pemper (1976) isolated six sociopsychological variables, but found that treatment personnel focused on only one variable—personal maladjustment.

An alternative approach to treatment which became popular is the eclectic, laissez-faire multiple-treatment philosophy of "a little bit of everything for everybody." Such an indiscriminate barrage of interventions can be confusing, congesting, contaminating, and contentious. More seriously, in a methodological review of treatment programs, Costello (1975) found that multiple indiscriminate programs such as these had the lowest rehabilitation rates, the highest dropout rates, and the largest number of overt treatment failures.

Basic to all these programs is the lack of a coherent scientific formulation of the alcoholism syndrome. The first major attempt in this direction was made by E. M. Jellinek (1960) in *The Disease Concept of Alcoholism.* Although Jellinek was circumspect in his formulations, his ideas were rapidly assimilated into the field and became part of a revised corpus of "conventional wisdom" that supported the concept of the "unitary" syndrome of alcoholism. Roughly, the unitary concept proposes that there is a unitary phenomenon called alcoholism, in which all persons so afflicted are substantially the same; they experience a similar progressive deterioration, and they will respond to a singular treatment, resulting in one specific outcome—abstinence. This unitary concept has been implemented by numerous isolated treatment personnel, each preferring the singular treatment to achieve one simple outcome (Kalb and Propper, 1976).

Although major scientific advances have been made in both our understanding of the alcoholism syndrome and our treatment methodologies, we have been reluctant to abandon the unitary approach to alcoholism in clinical practice (Verden and Shatterly, 1971). In constructing an alternative "multivariant" model of alcoholism (cf. Pattison, 1966, 1968, 1974, 1976), we must ask: What alcoholism syndromes at which stage of their development and in what kinds of patients respond under what conditions in what short- and long-range ways to what measures administered by whom? In his examination of alcoholism models, Kissin (1977) firmly endorses the multivariant model as the most adequate conceptual approach to alcoholism treatment. And, in fact, most recent alcoholism researchers now conceptualize alcoholism in terms of this model (Davis and Schmidt, 1977; Larkin, 1975; Pomerleau et al., 1976; Ruggels, 1975; Willems et al., 1973).

The following multivariant model of alcoholism has been set forth by Pattison, Sobell, and Sobell (1977) in a series of formal propositions, which, although they require further experimental clarification and validation, do present a framework for a multivariant approach to treatment.

A. Formal Model Propositions

Proposition 1: Alcohol dependence subsumes a variety of syndromes defined by drinking patterns and the adverse consequences of such drinking.

> *Corollary A:* These syndromes are defined as any combination of deleterious physical, psychological, or social consequencs that follow the use of alcohol by an individual.

> *Corollary B:* These syndromes can vary along a continuum from minimal consequences to severe and even fatal consequences.

> *Corollary C:* These syndromes, jointly denoted as alcohol dependence, are best considered as serious health problems.

> *Corollary D:* In specific circumstances it may be desirable for sociocultural, legal, political, and therapeutic goals to label alcohol dependence as a "disease," perhaps especially at the time of acute physical symptomatology. At the same time the alcohol dependent person may appropriately be labeled as "sick." Such circumstances should be carefully delineated and limited in application to specific situations.

Proposition 2: An individual's use of alcohol can be considered as a point on a continuum from nonuse, to nonproblem drinking, to various degrees of deleterious drinking.

> *Corollary A:* There may be preexisting differences between individual reactions to alcohol or vulnerability to adverse consequences of alcohol use, as a function of genetic, biological, psychological, and sociocultural factors. Such factors may increase or decrease the possibility that one may encounter problems in the use of alcohol.

> *Corollary B:* Differing susceptibility to alcohol does not in and of itself produce alcohol dependence. Any person who uses alcohol can develop a syndrome of alcohol dependence.

> *Corollary C:* There is no natural dichotomy between alcoholic and nonalcoholic but rather a continuous spectrum of drinking patterns that may result in different combinations of deleterious consequences.

Proposition 3: The development of alcohol problems follows variable patterns over time.

Corollary A: Alcohol problems may develop gradually over time, leading to increasingly severe consequences, or such problems may develop rapidly.

Corollary B: Alcohol problems do not necessarily proceed inexorably to severe fatal stages but may remain static at any level of severity.

Corollary C: Alcohol problems may be partially or completely reversed through either a natural process or a treatment program.

Proposition 4: Abstinence bears no necessary relation to rehabilitation.

Corollary A: A person may be totally abstinent without improvement in other areas of life function which were related to deleterious use of alcohol.

Corollary B: A person may demonstrate little change in his patterns of alcohol use yet make major improvements in other areas of life function, which were related to his use of alcohol.

Corollary C: A person may change his patterns of alcohol use so that his drinking no longer constitutes a problem in and of itself.

Proposition 5: Psychological dependence and physical dependence on alcohol are separate and not necessarily related phenomena.

Corollary A: Psychological dependence on alcohol is a syndrome of learned patterns of alcohol use.

Corollary B: Genetic, biological, psychological, and sociocultural factors may increase or decrease a person's vulnerability to develop a pattern of psychological dependence. None of these factors in isolation is necessarily sufficient to cause psychological dependence.

Corollary C: The consumption of a small amount of alcohol by a person once labeled "alcoholic" does not necessarily initiate a physical need that in turn causes further drinking.

Corollary D: An individual may experience a strongly felt need to drink in certain situations and not in others, which may be exacerbated by the consumption of small amounts of alcohol.

Proposition 6: Continued drinking of large doses of alcohol over an extended period of time is likely to initiate a process of physical dependence.

Corollary A: The state of physical dependence is marked by increased tolerance to alcohol, and may be manifest by the symptoms of an alcohol withdrawal syndrome of varying severity.

Corollary B: Any person who consumes a sufficient amount of alcohol over time will eventually develop some degree of physical dependence. This varies over a wide continuum: The increased tolerance of the nonproblem light drinker, to the hangover of the occasional intoxicated drinker, to severe withdrawal symptoms of the chronic heavy drinker.

Corollary C: The development of physical dependence is related primarily to amount and frequency of alcohol intake, not to a unique metabolic processing of alcohol.

Corollary D: A state of physical dependence may exist without any other adverse consequences of drinking, except the physiological sequelae.

Corollary E: There may be individual differences in biological sensitivity to the effects of alcohol, but such differences are neither necessary nor sufficient to establish physical dependence.

Corollary F: The state of physical dependence does not appear to be a permanent state but may vary with subsequent patterns of drinking after physical dependence is established. The degree of physical dependence appears to be reversible.

Proposition 7: The population of individuals with alcohol problems is multivariant.

Corollary A: While the range of types of problems and severity of problems may be arbitrarily defined into categories for research or clinical utility, such typologies must be recognized as relatively arbitrary heuristic classifications.

Corollary B: Treatment intervention must be multivariant. Individual treatment plans need to address: (1) the severity of the person's alcohol use; (2) the particular problems and consequences associated with the individual drinking pattern; and (3) the person's ability to achieve specific treatment goals.

Corollary C: Comprehensive rehabilitation requires a variety of services that range from information and education to intensive long-term care. Available services, methods, and goals should be flexible enough to meet individual needs and abilities to participate.

Proposition 8: Alcohol problems are typically interrelated with other life problems, especially when alcohol dependence is long established.

Corollary A: Rehabilitation should aim at specific changes in drinking behavior suitable to each individual.

Corollary B: Rehabilitation should aim at specific changes in problem areas of life function, in addition to efforts aimed at drinking behavior per se.

Corollary C: Rehabilitation must take into account individual preferences, goals, choice of treatment, degree of disability, and ability to attain goals.

Proposition 9: Because of the documented strong relationship between drinking behavior and environmental influences, emphasis should be placed on treatment procedures that relate to the drinking environment of the person.

Corollary A: The alcohol dependent individual may require temporary removal from his environment (i.e., hospital, supportive residential facility, etc.), with a planned return to his natural environment.

Corollary B: To avoid further problems and achieve some stable level of existence, some alcohol dependent individuals may require a quasipermanent, sheltered living environment.

Corollary C: Rehabilitation is likely to require direct involvement in the environment. This should begin with an analysis of the alcohol dependent person's interactions with his environment and proceed to planned environmental interventions with family, relatives, friends, and others in the social network.

Proposition 10: Treatment and rehabilitation services should be designed to provide for continuity of care over an extended period of time. This continuum of services should begin with effective identification, triage, and referral mechanisms, extend through acute and chronic phases of treatment, and provide follow-up aftercare.

Proposition 11: Evaluative studies of treatment of alcohol dependence must take into account the initial degree of disability, the potential for change, and an inventory of individual dysfunction in diverse life areas, in addition to drinking behavior. Assessment of improvement should include both drinking behavior and behavior in other areas of life function, consistent with presenting problems. Degrees of improvement must also be recognized. Change in all areas of life function should be assessed on an individual basis. This necessitates using pretreatment and posttreatment comparison measures of treatment outcome.

B. Clinical Implications of the Multivariant Model

The multivariant model states that a number of series of factors are involved in alcoholism treatment. Our goal is to *match* a particular patient with the appropriate treatment facility, in which he or she will be matched with the appropriate personnel, who in turn will match treatment interventions to the needs of the person (Gottheil, et al., 1981).

This is a large order, and in fact most reviewers of treatment methods report that no large-scale, clear indicators for selective treatment-matching can be determined from the data (Armor et al., 1976; Baekeland, 1977; Baekeland et al., 1975; Costello, 1975; Emrick, 1974, 1975). However, in view of the widespread indiscriminate utilization of treatment methods, such a conclusion from global reviews is not surprising (Crawford and Chalopsky, 1977; Swint and Nelson, 1977).

On the other hand, small-scale, discrete research projects have demonstrated the utility of developing a match of patient-facility-therapist-method. For example, Pattison et al. (1969, 1973) have shown that different types of alcoholics present themselves at different facilities, receive distinctly different treatments, and achieve different treatment outcomes. This data suggests that some covert "matching" already occurs. Similar findings in other research projects have demonstrated some predictors for matching (Kissin, et al., 1970; Trice et al., 1969). Perhaps the clearest illustration of the potential value of the "matching" concept is provided by McLachlan (1974), who reported:

> When the patient was matched to both therapy and aftercare environments 77% were recovered; when matched to either the aftercare or therapy environment alone 61% and 65% were recovered; when mismatched to both therapy and aftercare only 38% were recovered.

One simple way of looking at these factors is in terms of "life health," or the total adaptation of the person. We can divide this into five parts: Drinking Health, Emotional Health, Interpersonal Health, Vocational Health, and Physical Health. So in a given alcoholism syndrome the person may have disability of varying severity in each area of life health. The successful outcome of treatment would be assessed in terms of relative improvement in each area of life health where disability exists.

It must be emphasized that the relationship between Drinking Health and the other areas of life health is not a simple cause and effect. For changes in Drinking Health do not necessarily relate to areas of improvement in other life health areas. Conversely, there may be improvement in the other four life health areas not closely related to improvement in the Drinking Health area. This is illustrated by Bowman et al. (1975) who found that changes in drinking accounted for only 50% of the variance in treatment outcome.

This means that the clinician must construct treatment goals and implement treatment methods relevant to each area of impairment. And the success of treatment must be assessed in terms of multiple outcome variables. For example, Lowe and Thomas (1976) evaluated successful outcome in three areas. In their alcoholic population at follow-up, 70% had achieved vocational rehabilitation, 62% psychosocial behavioral rehabilitation, and 34% abstinence. Thus we can see that successful rehabilitation is not a unitary phenomenon. It is probably rare that there is either total failure or total success. A more accurate appraisal might yield different degrees of rehabilitation in different life health areas for different alcoholism syndromes.

II. VARIABILITY IN THE ALCOHOLISM SYNDROME

When Jellinek (1960) proposed that the disease concept of alcoholism be used, he meant the term "concept" quite deliberately to indicate a wide panoply of patterns of alcohol abuse and misuse. In fact he reserved the use of the term "disease" for only one type of alcohol addiction, which merited definition as a disease. The other four types of alcohol abuse were considered to be alcohol problems. Unfortunately, the "conventional wisdom" of the field soon wrenched the Jellinek formulation out of context to produce the unitary concept of alcoholism described before (Robinson, 1972).

Yet even giving due credit to the circumspection of Jellinek, he did assume some relative uniformity and consistency among his five types of alcoholism. And he clearly formulated a relatively consistent and uniform pattern for the gamma alcoholic—the alcohol addict.

The question of whether alcoholism is to be considered a disease is *not at debate*. Rather, the issue is whether alcoholism is a unitary phenomenon or a multivariant syndrome. A syndrome can be defined as "a group or set of concurrent symptoms which together can be considered a disease." To consider alcoholism a disease does not necessarily require a unitary set of symptoms, nor does it necessarily require a uniform clinical course. A syndrome is a concatenation of symptoms that can be usefully aggregated to describe a clinical problem. Thus to formulate alcoholism as a syndrome does not do violence to the clinical utility of defining alcoholism as a disease (Robinson, 1976).

A major classification advance has been made in the American Psychiatric Association *Diagnostic and Statistical Manual* (DSM-III) which clearly identifies alcoholism as a distinct syndrome apart both from other psychiatric disorders and from personality disorders. As Solomon (1982) observes: "Alcoholism can exist apart from, concurrent with, or as a complication of other psychiatric disorders."

Let us return to the Jellinek proposition that there are five distinct subtypes of alcoholism, one of which—the addictive gamma alcoholic— is distinctly different from the others. Since 1960 extensive research on a wide variety of alcoholic populations had rather conclusively demonstrated that there are no distinct categories of alcoholics. Certainly the five subtypes proposed by Jellinek have not been validated. Rather, there are pattern clusters—that is, certain sets of symptoms, behaviors, and disabilities tend to cluster out on factor-analytic studies. Thus one can generate subtypes of alcoholics. But these subtypes are composed of complex personality, social, and drinking variables, not simply categories such as Jellinek proposed. Further, this research has not validated the Jellinek concept of the gamma addictive alcoholic. Rather, degrees of severity of alcohol use are complexly intertwined with other psychosocial variables. The existence of the "true" gamma addictive alcoholic has thus proved nonexistent (Horn and Wanberg, 1969, 1970; Horn et al., 1974; Hurwitz and Lelos, 1968; Mogar et al., 1970). Consequently we conclude that the syndrome of alcoholism has one constant feature: *a significant life problem associated with the use of alcohol.* Beyond that, we find multiple preexistent and consequent variables associated with a given person's alcohol problem.

Second, let us consider the extent to which the clinical course of the alcoholism syndrome can be considered unitary. Jellinek proposed that there were distinct clinical phases leading to alcohol addiction. He postulated a sequence of 43 specific symptoms of alcoholism, with three symptoms—blackouts, loss of control, and prolonged intoxication (binges)— serving as markers to identify the onset of each major phase—the prodromal phase, the crucial phase, and the chronic phase, respectively. Jellinek, however, cautioned: "Not all symptoms . . . occur necessarily in the same sequence."

The Jellinek model suffers from many methodological problems. His notion of a unitary phase sequence was derived from his interpretation of an open-ended questionnaire distributed only to AA members via their in-house newsletter, "The Grapevine." Of those questionnaires returned, only 98 (6.13%) were adequate for analysis. Thus the sample consisted of a small group of persons willing to respond to an open-ended questionnaire who were self-identified as recovered alcoholics from one organization. Among the inadequacies of this method is the fact that the sampling methodology is highly biased and the returns are not representative of the sample. Second, as Seiden (1960) has pointed out, members of AA are nonrepresentative of the alcoholic population in general. The technique used retrospective reconstruction and self-report. It is likely that the ideology of AA greatly influenced the nature of the reconstructed symptom development. Third, the questions were open-ended and the data were coded by Jellinek in a post hoc manner. Thus preexisting assumptions or biases may have influenced the analysis of the data. Finally, several more refined research studies have failed to confirm Jellinek's analysis. A reanalysis of the Jellinek data by Park (1973) using new statistical techniques revealed that the original Jellinek data did not support a phase sequence of symptoms. Orford (1974) assessed a large sample of alcoholics in England and found a large variation in ordering of symptoms, unrelated to Jellinek's postulates. Similarly, in his own data from Finland, Park (1973) found:

> If there be three phases in the development of alcohol addiction . . . a sizeable proportion of experiences do not occur in the phases to which they are assigned. . . . The presumed manifestations of alcoholism do not necessarily develop in the order given by Jellinek.

Finally, although a specific set of sequential symptoms cannot be substantiated, can we concur with the unitary concept that in the alcoholism syndrome there is a relatively common progressive course of illness such that we consider characteristic early, middle, and late stages of alcoholism common to all?

A majority of observations on this issue have come from clinicians working within circumscribed clinical populations and without comparative or longitudinal data. Thus this clinical data is subject to the distortions of a severely disabled population, retrospective analysis, and lack of generalizability to larger populations of alcohol users.

In contrast, in large-scale national and regional epidemiological surveys of drinking practices, which have followed individuals with varying degrees of drinking problems over time, it has been shown that: (1) people move in and out of symptomatic drinking; (2) severity of drinking problems may remain constant and nonprogressive; and (3) remissions and progressions significantly vary with time, place, and circumstance (Cahalan, 1970; Cahalan and Room, 1974; Cahalan et al., 1969; Mulford and Miller, 1960; Polich et al., 1980).

In a study of problem drinking over only a four-year span, Clark and Cahalan (1976) found that there was a substantial turnover in the number of persons who moved into or out of the problem drinking population. Thus entry into the category of problem drinker does not necessarily imply an inexorable progression toward middle and late stages of the alcoholism syndrome. The abuse of alcohol does not necessarily in itself move from one stage to another. As Chandler et al. (1971) conclude: "It may be useful to call alcoholism a disease, but the notion is simplistic in the extreme if it ignores the probably vital influence of social circumstances and personality in patterning the consequences of abnormal drinking."

In still another fashion, the development or cessation of drinking problems may be related to stages of life and life circumstances rather than to the use of alcohol per se. For example, Fillmore (1974) followed up a group of college students who then had drinking problems. After 20 years she found that 68% of the males and 67% of the females had become nonproblem drinkers, while 10% of those who had been abstainers in college now were problem drinkers. Similarly, Goodwin et al. (1975) followed a group of 451 army men in Vietnam subsequent to their return to civilian life. They found that most of those with drinking problems in Vietnam discontinued their abusive use of alcohol and had no subsequent problems associated with alcohol. Hyman (1976) conducted a 15-year follow-up and found the majority of young severe drinkers had become moderate drinkers or abstainers.

A different pattern is described by Blum and Levine (1975) for "reactive" alcoholics. In contrast to the "progressive" pattern in which the person moves from early to middle late stages of alcoholism in mid-life, they have found that "reactive" alcoholics develop a significant alcohol syndrome only in mid-life, a syndrome associated with acute life stress and inability to cope effectively at this point in the life cycle.

And then there is the pattern of alcoholism problems emerging only toward the end of the life cycle among the aged. In this case there may have been a life history of nonproblem drinking. However the stresses of retirement and aging may precipitate significant alcoholism problems among the aged (Gaitz and Baer, 1971; Schuckit, 1977; Simon et al., 1968).

Not all of this data indicates that there is no progression of severity in the alcoholism syndrome. Orford and Hawker (1974) found that a small number of clusters of events can be seen as a clinical sequence: First, the onset of psychological dependence; second, tremor, morning drinking, and amnesia; and third, aspects of alcoholic psychosis. Orford and Hawker conclude:

> There is a characteristic ordering of new events or symptoms in the development of alcoholism, but we would argue strongly that the extensions of this notion to include a wide range of events encompassing psychophysiological,

social, and treatment events is not feasible and has served only to obscure a number of more basic and relatively circumscribed processes.

So if we observe the alcoholism syndrome throughout a continuing clinical course, we can indeed separate that clinical course into early, middle, and late stages (Mulford, 1977). The point is that the alcoholism syndrome is not necessarily an invidious progressive "disease." Rather, significant symptoms associated with alcohol use will vary with each person in accord with his or her own life history. Garitano and Ronall (1974) suggest that we can view the alcoholism syndrome as the particular expression of the use of alcohol embedded in the "life-style" of a given person.

A more complex, but perhaps clinically useful approach to the alcoholism syndrome is to organize areas of dysfunction into factors. Thus, a given alcoholic person can be described clinically in terms of a "pattern of factors." Different alcoholics might be high or low on certain factors, thus profiling distinct clinical patterns of alcoholism. Let us consider the following 10-factor profile.

Factor 1: Alcohol consumption   This refers to consumption patterns per se in terms of quantity, frequency, and volume (QFV) over time. Streissguth, et al. (1977) have shown eight different subtypes of alcoholismic behavior based on different QFV patterns, while Armor and Polich (1982) report a high correlation of QFV measures with other signs and symptoms of different patterns of alcohol abuse.

Factor 2: Drinking behavior   This involves the actual social behavior of drinking. Several subitems are present:

a. The salience or preoccupation with obtaining alcohol
b. The sense of need, desire, or craving for drinking
c. The attempt to constrict, control, or avoid drinking
d. The experience of inability to control drinking behavior
e. The pursuit of drinking in the face of high costs of physical, interpersonal, social, vocational, psychological losses in life.

Factor 3: Psychic dependence   This refers to the dependence on alcohol to achieve desired psychic change. Psychic dependence is a "particular state of mind." Clinically, I have found it useful to ask two diagnostic questions here:

a. Does your personality change or do you experience yourself change when you are drinking?
b. Do you operate or behave as a person in a different fashion when you drink?

The person with psychic dependence recognizes and affirms a change in psychic operation when drinking and will answer yes to both questions. It is this change in a "particular state of mind" that the alcoholic desires and which the use of alcohol helps him or her to achieve.

Factor 4: Physical dependence   This refers to the pharmacologic phenomenon of the development of tolerance and the possible occurrence of withdrawal symptoms.

Factor 5: Physical consequences   This involves both the acute consequences of drinking (intoxication syndrome) and chronic organ system damage due to direct and indirect effects of alcohol.

The direct effects of alcohol may produce organic mental disorders (acute and chronic), while organ system disorders represent the indirect effects of alcohol on body metabolism, the secondary complications of an alcoholic life style in severe, chronic, heavy drinkers.

Factor 6: Emotional consequences   Here we see the effect of drinking behavior on psychic operation: the emergence of paranoid ideation, homosexual fantasy, shame, guilt, regressive ego defenses, altered reality testing, anxiety states, panic attacks, alternating grandiose narcissism and reactive self-deprecation and depression. These may appear while drinking, after drinking, or as a chronic state.

Factor 7: Interpersonal consequences   This would include problems in maintaining intimate relationships with spouse, children, friends, and relatives. Differential changes in relationships from nondrinking associations to drinking associations would be included.

Factor 8: Vocational consequences   These involve work performance, maintenance of vocational skills and abilities, and continuity of work functions.

Factor 9: Informal social consequences   These include problems of social behavior that disrupt the person's social sphere, including embarrassing social behavior, offensive social behavior, violation of proprieties, failure to meet social obligations, and loss of friendships.

Factor 10: Legal consequences   Here we find antisocial behavior—criminality, violent behavior, drunken driving, and accidents—that leads to formal social-legal responses: arrests, legal suits, court actions.

Some alcoholics would score high on almost all 10 factors. Others may score high on factors 1–5, yet have few adverse consequences. These are so-called "high-competency" alcoholics. Others, high in factors 8–10, may misuse alcohol, in turn experience adverse consequences, but show little if any dependency characteristics of factors 1–5. These latter persons might well not be diagnosed as alcoholic and may not require treatment, but they do require social interventions to modify their misuse of alcohol. The drunk driver is a good example of this type.

In summary, we have proceeded a significant way toward specification of different factors that may be combined in a particular alcoholism syndrome. Patient assessment must distinguish not only the presence of each factor, but the degrees to which each factor contributes to the alcoholism syndrome of a specific patient. In turn, this may lead to more precise treatment selection.

III. VARIABILITY OF ALCOHOLIC POPULATIONS

Early attempts to clarify and define the "alcoholic personality" have failed. Blane (1968) considers the concept of a personality structure *unique* to alcoholics and *only to* alcoholics a straw man. Or as Keller (1972) put it: "Alcoholics are different in so many ways that it makes no difference."

It is important to differentiate between the attempt to define a uniformity among all alcoholics—which has failed—and the attempt to define a number of personality factors which might predict individual vulnerability to alcoholism or individual response to treatment. Recent research has repeatedly demonstrated such great diversity in personality structure that one cannot find specific personality attributes, traits, or mechanisms that would predict alcoholism (Horn et al., 1974; Rohan, 1976). Likewise, personality variables alone are not reliable predictors for treatment (Donovan et al., 1975; Gellens et al., 1976; Hague et al., 1976; O'Leary et al., 1975). Thus the use of psychological tests to predict or select treatment has not been successful (Jacobson, 1976; Neuringer and Clopton, 1976).

Nevertheless, we may consider the relationship of personality structure as it may interrelate to different alcoholism syndromes. Vaillant (1982) has reported on the often insignificant effect of prior personality on the development of alcoholism, yet development levels of personality organization may affect how a person uses and responds to alcohol (Thornton et al., 1981; Zucker, 1979). Let us review five levels of personality organization in relation to the primary psychic function of alcohol use and estimate how many alcoholics may fall in each level (Pattison, 1983).

Level 1: The inadequate, immature personality   These are persons who often inhabit skid row. They are passive-dependent, with immature and primitive interpersonal relations. They use alcohol as a symbolic representation of maternal presence and love. The psychic equation that bottle equals breast is probably accurate. They are usually not dependent on alcohol, do not engage in serious adverse behavior, and drink only when alcohol is readily available. I estimate this to be 5% of the alcoholic population.

Level 2: The borderline personality   These people are fixated at the 18- to 24-month level of personality organization. Alcohol is a transitional object—symbolizing the absent and longed-for mother. They use alcohol for self-soothing purposes, and they may develop dependence. They are typically conflicted about their alcohol use, highly ambivalent, both hating and desiring alcohol. They make up about 10–15% of the alcoholic population.

Level 3: The sociopathic and narcissistic personalities   They represent the 2- to 3-year development level. They use alcohol as a primary pleasure, and may or may not become alcohol dependent. They are about 15% of the alcoholic population.

Level 4: The neurotic character   At the 3- to 5-year level, they experience conflict in establishing nonconflictural and stable interpersonal object relations. Variations in personality structure include paranoid, histrionic, obsessional, and schizoid. They use alcohol as an "internal" coping device, to resolve neurotic conflicts within themselves. They comprise 15–20% of the alcoholic population.

Level 5: Relatively mature personality structure   This is probably the bulk of alcoholics—50%. They use alcohol as an "external" coping device when faced with acute life crisis, or when faced with life losses such as those in old age, or as part of a culturally sanctioned pattern of alcohol abuse. They often demonstrate *personality regression* after a period of drinking. With attainment of sobriety and rehabilitation, they often return to mature levels of personality operation.

In the above analysis, then, we conclude that alcoholics exist at several levels of personality organization and development and that the distribution of alcoholics across personality level is definable. The consumption of alcohol serves very different psychic functions at each level. During the acute phases of alcoholism, it may not be possible to determine personality structure because of the direct effects of alcohol and the severity of personality regression that has occurred. Thus, although there is no alcoholic personality, there is a significant relationship between type of personality and type of alcoholism syndrome.

Another population variable is social class. Again the evidence suggests that social class and other social variables alone do not predict alcoholism or response to treatment (Robinson, 1976). However, social class variables are loosely related to different alcoholism syndromes, to response to treatment, and to selection of treatment by professional personnel (Kalb, 1975; Schmidt et al., 1968; Wanberg and Horn, 1973). It is possible to examine certain types of populations who have some common characteristics which may assist in the development of appropriate treatment interventions, however.

Women are a distinct population who appear to vary on both psychological and social dimensions from men in terms of alcoholism syndromes (Beckman, 1975; Greenblatt and Schuckit, 1976). Similarly, we must consider alcoholism syndromes in children and adolescents in terms of their own life-stage settings (Bacon and Jones, 1968; Freedman and Wilson, 1964; Mandell and Ginzburg, 1976).

Ethnic populations constitute an important variable with regard to patterns of alcohol use, attitudes toward alcohol, and response to treatment programs (Westermeyer, 1972, 1976). Although our information is still minimal, there is recent data on alcoholism syndromes among blacks (Vitol, 1968; Zimber et al., 1971), Mexican-Americans (Paine, 1977), Alaskan natives (Miller et al., 1975), and American Indians (Brod, 1975; Shore and Fummetti, 1972).

Another way of looking at alcoholic populations is in terms of the populations who constitute the clientele of specific treatment facilities. In 1969, Pattison et al. reported on clientele at three different alcoholism treatment facilities. They found that the successful cases at each facility were substantially different from one another, constituting unique subpopulations. Each facility subpopulation improved, but improved in different patterns. Subsequently, Pattison et al. (1973) studied the populations presenting *before* treatment at four different treatment facilities. They found that the subpopulations were not just the result of treatment but were distinct preexistent subpopulations upon entering each facility. Other researchers have published confirming studies (Edward et al., 1974; English and Curtin, 1975; Orford et al., 1974, 1975; Tomsovic, 1968).

Finally, within a given treatment facility and its subpopulation there is variation in terms of the needs of that population. Therefore, we must further divide the subpopulation of a facility into smaller population categories. Here we begin to approach individual differences in perceived needs (Hart, 1977), as well as motivations for treatment and attitudes toward different treatment methods and personnel (Kammeier et al., 1973; Pisani, 1969; Price and Curlee-Salisbury, 1975).

In conclusion, there is no unitary population of alcoholics. We must consider the important dimensions of age, sex, and ethnicity that influence alcoholism syndromes. Further, when we examine different treatment facilities, we can observe certain population subtypes that tend to be represented in a specific facility. This type of subpopulation combines psychological, social, and cultural variables, which together describe a relatively distinct clinical subgroup. But within the subpopulation we must also include individual need assessment and individual orientation toward treatment options if we are to make the best selection of treatment (Zimberg, 1982).

IV. VARIABILITY OF TREATMENT SYSTEMS

As we have already seen, different subpopulations of alcoholics tend to appear at different treatment facilities. Research studies have focused primarily on the alcoholic population, while there has been relatively little systematic study of the treatment facilities themselves. Bromet et al. (1976) have pioneered in evaluating the "social climate" of different treatment facilities. Although only exploratory, their studies demonstrate that different treatment facilities have the same overall goal of alcoholism rehabilitation but that ideology, operation, and climate vary.

Are there certain characteristics in common among treatment facilities that relate to effective function? The best indicators come from a comprehensive review by Costello (1975a, 1975b) of comparative treatment methods. He found that the most effective treatment programs had the following characteristics: (1) a well-organized treatment philosophy that was implemented in consistent and logical fashion; (2) inpatient resources for medical care and for nonmedical rehabilitation; (3) an aggressive postdischarge follow-up; (4) collateral counseling and participation, i.e., involvement with and assistance for the significant people in the life of the alcoholic; (5) aggressive outreach with community agencies, both to bring alcoholics into the program through community contacts and to effect transition back into community resources; (6) adjunctive use of Antabuse; and (7) behaviorally oriented interventions, in addition to purely verbal therapies.

In short, effective treatment facilities are *systems of treatment* that have coherent organization and aggressive intake and follow-up procedures and that provide a wide spectrum of carefully constructed treatment options. With this perspective, we can briefly examine some of the systems of alcoholism treatment.

A. The Alcoholism Information and Referral Center

So-called AIR has been promoted for three decades as a major resource in the rehabilitation of alcoholics. There has been concerted effort to establish AIR centers in all communities of at least 50,000 population. The underlying motive is admirable: AIR would provide information to the community about alcoholism, help the community to identify alcoholics, and provide a central resource for effective referral.

Few studies have been conducted on AIR activity (Corrigan, 1974; Edwards et al., 1967). These suggest that AIR does provide significant services. Alcoholics and their kin may seek help, referral, direct counseling, and other assistance. Corrigan has shown that AIR may be a pivotal agency in terms of referral and catalysis of rehabilitation efforts.

However, AIR has not been an unqualified success. First, many AIRs are staffed by recovered alcoholics who may not be aware of different community resources and who push all alcoholics to follow their own pattern of rehabilitation. Such AIR staff may polarize and alienate their relationship with available community resources. More often, the AIR staff member may be a health educator whose skills lie in administration and community organization. Such personnel are not skilled in diagnosis and therapy. Yet the people who come to AIR are seeking help and therapy. Thus AIR is often a "liaison treatment program," staffed by personnel who have no preparation or skills in providing treatment. Then there is the problem of inadequate community resources. AIR staff often come to a town, establish good working relationships in the community, make their AIR viable, and then find that they have no primary care resources. The community rises up in arms: They have alcoholics, they have identified alcoholics, but now there are no treatment resources available. As a result AIR might be discredited, disenfranchised, and the staff deposed.

Another problem AIR faces is the appropriate utilization of resources. In our study of AIR, we found that less than 20% of the referrals for treatment were successful, whereas more than 60% of the alcoholics eventually sought treatment at an identified facility. In other words, AIR was not making a successful referral. This represents a major slippage in the effective operation of the social system of alcoholism treatment.

An effective AIR turns out to be both a referral agency and a first-line treatment center. Thus personnel must have some clinical skills, the AIR must relate to all aspects of community resources, and effective function will be reflected in appropriate referrals.

B. The Physician and the General Hospital

The alcoholic in the medical care system usually does not present a primary complaint of alcoholism. The alcoholic may seek medical care for major *complications* of alcohol abuse, such as hepatic, cardiac, dermatologic, or peripheral neurological complaints. Such persons often do not consciously link their medical illness with their alcohol abuse. A second group present in medical setting with severe *consequences* of alcoholism such as fractures and head trauma due to falls, burns, or peripheral palsies accrued while intoxicated, or a variety of acute or chronic brain syndromes. Such patients may recognize that their medical problems are directly tied to their drinking but are not likely to complain of their alcoholism. A third group recognize their alcoholism problems, may seek medical help for their alcoholism, but *disguise* their situation in somatic complaints such as insomnia, nervousness, tremors, anxiety, anorexia, dyspepsia, etc.

Respectable "community alcoholics" appear regularly in the everyday caseload of the physician. In a survey of 3376 internists, Jones and Helrich (1972) found that only 3% of internists saw no alcoholics, whereas 16% of internists saw over 20 alcoholics during a one-month period. Significantly, *half were women*. Dunn and Clay (1971) report that 10% of general physician and internist case loads were alcoholic. The *Medical Times* (1975) states that 70% of physicians in private practice saw at least 10 alcoholics per month, although 76% of these alcoholics initially denied that they had alcoholism problems.

How effective is the physician outpatient management of alcoholism? There is little empirical data to answer this question. Dunn and Clay (1971) studied the visiting staff utilization of a general hospital alcoholism program. Only 40% of the staff referred patients for treatment. Of those that referred, 65% were general physicians and 21% internists. Of the nonusers 61% were surgeons.

The incidence of alcoholics in hospital populations is even higher than in private outpatient settings. The incidence of hospitalized patients who can be identified as having moderate to severe alcoholism problems ranges from 27% to 60% (Barchha et al., 1968; Gomberg, 1975; Kearney, 1968). Hagnell and Tunvig (1972) found that the highest incidence of alcoholism is associated with respiratory, cardiac, endocrine, and urogenital illness. In another study, McCusker et al. (1971) found alcoholism among 100% of patients with seizures, 67% with respiratory disease, 53% with liver disease, and 25% with cardiovascular disease. It is obvious that alcoholic patients are widely distributed across most clinical services of a hospital.

At particular high risk are tuberculous patients. Lennon et al. (1970) reported 80% of tuberculars as alcoholic. The tubercular-alcoholic is also a poor risk patient. Rhodes et al. (1969) found that 86 of 90 such patients were major medical and behavioral problems.

The problem of effective identification of the hospitalized alcoholic is highlighted by the study of McCusker et al. (1971). They found that only 55% of alcoholics were so diagnosed on admission, and that at discharge only 45% were still diagnosed as alcoholic!

The major problem of medical management in the hospital is "overmanagement." Finer (1972) has detailed the excessive use of medications, diagnostic procedures, and unduly prolonged hospitalization for uncomplicated medical problems associated with alcoholism. Finer points out that this process often fosters undue dependency on medical strategems by the alcoholic, may reinforce a focus on somatic complaints, and may foster continued denial of the major underlying problem of alcoholism. The physician must be wary lest good medical treatment of the complications of alcoholism obscure the treatment of the alcoholism. Treating the physical complications of alcoholism without dealing with the underlying condition itself is simply not good medical care.

The problem of the alcoholic patient in surgery needs to be emphasized. The debilitated alcoholic may be vulnerable to complications of anesthesia and may also respond poorly to postoperative recovery procedures. An excellent clinical text by Lowenfels (1971) details these problems clearly.

Management of the alcoholic in the emergency room is still a neglected area of good patient care. A study by Dorsch et al. (1969) found that of identified alcoholics at an emergency service, 16% were referred to alcoholism treatment resources, 20% were hospitalized, and *61% received no treatment and no referral*. This is a major gap in the medical care system where diagnosis, initial treatment, and referral should be instituted (Anderson and Weisman, 1970).

1. Types of Hospital Alcohol Programs

In 1956 the American Medical Association and the American Hospital Association officially declared alcoholism an admissible diagnosis for admission and treatment in general hospitals. Since then there has been widespread acknowledgment of the successful admission and management of alcoholics on a nonsegregated basis on general medical and surgical wards. Contrary to popular staff expectation, alcohol patients have proven not to be disruptive nor untoward management problems. Such a minimal program should have psychiatric and internist consultation support and preferably a solid social work staff to provide triage after medical treatment into an alcoholism rehabilitation program (Galanter et al., 1976).

Alcoholism wards for acute detoxification are usually revolving doors with high recidivism and low staff morale if they are not directly linked to and part of a comprehensive alcoholism rehabilitation program. The isolated detoxification ward is probably an inept and obsolescent approach to detoxification as outlined previously. However, general hospitals should provide medical detoxification management capability to back up outpatient detoxification and social detoxification programs (Catanzaro, 1971).

Finally, a number of hospitals have launched alcoholism rehabilitation programs. Many such programs have been developed and are operating successfully. These are not strict medical units but are actually hospital-related rehabilitation programs (Champ, 1974; Hansen, 1972; Mann,

1965). Such programs usually do not offer definitive rehabilitative programs but can serve as an initial treatment and triage center linked to community rehabilitation programs.

2. Outpatient Methods of Management by the Physician

The physician is usually not in a position to provide definitive rehabilitation programs for alcoholics. However there are several specific services the physician can offer in his office practice (Pattison, 1977).

1. The physician can provide a regular contact program of disulfiram maintenance with motivated patients who need to maintain abstinence but do not desire or require other avenues of rehabilitation.

2. The physician can maintain regular contact with patients who are not yet willing to accept treatment. Over time, the physician, by virtue of his positive doctor-patient relationship, may be able to guide the patient into a rehabilitation program.

3. The physician can safely manage acute intoxication and mild withdrawal syndromes and use this contact to guide the patient into rehabilitation.

4. The physician can be an effective diagnostic and triage agent.

5. The physician is in an excellent position to *involve the spouse and family members* in the process of rehabilitation. The alcoholic behavior patterns have direct impact on spouse and family. Conversely, the spouse and family are likely either to exacerbate and play into the perpetuation of the alcoholism behavior or contribute signally to changes and effective rehabilitation. Therefore, effective management of the alcoholic and effective treatment are likely to be directly related to the degree of effective family involvement.

6. All of these services do require that the physicians become acquainted with their local community resources. They should learn what types of AA groups are available so that they can refer the willing patient to a group suited to his/her needs. They should be able to effectively hospitalize and manage alcoholic patients who require inpatient care. They should have personal information about the facilities, admission requirements, fees, and suitability of different community rehabilitation programs so that they can counsel the alcoholic in terms of the program best suited for him or her.

7. The physician can effectively promote increased awareness and acceptance of the importance of careful evaluation of alcohol use among his/her patients.

C. The Mental Hospital

Over the past 20 years many state and private psychiatric hospitals have developed special alcoholism wards, units, and programs. In a nationwide survey, Moore and Buchanan (1966) found wide variation in methods, philosophy, populations, and results. Their survey revealed rather meager success rates in most programs. Cahn (1970) found most hospital programs were underfunded, were accorded low status, and tended to be staffed by second-class personnel. In a careful methodological study of a state hospital alcoholism program, Ludwig et al. (1970) came to the conclusion that such programs were probably ineffective and inappropriate.

Although there are the exceptional programs, there are major problems with the social system of mental hospitals that militate against alcoholism programs therein. First, the population that is triaged into the state hospital system are typically lower-middle class who have major social and vocational disabilities. They are not candidates for intensive psychotherapy, nor are they in need of confinement. They need relocation within the social context of community life. But the mental hospital is rarely equipped to provide social and vocational rehabilitation. Second, the mental hospital is dominated by a medical model of professional hierarchies—to a greater or lesser degree they are controlling institutions. This role model of sickness plays into the central psychodynamic conflicts of the alcoholic. The aura of the institution conveys the message that in the patient role, the alcoholic should obey orders, remain dependent on others, not assume responsibilities for daily life management, etc. In fact, the very process of seeking admission involves a role shift from a competent community life to an incompetent inmate life. Third, the alcoholic may learn to adapt and adjust within the milieu of the hospital. That is not his or her problem. At issue is the capacity to adapt in the community. The problem and the result is similar to our national experience with hospitals for drug addiction. The addict can live in the "hospital world," but he or she cannot translate that life-style into the "real world."

Therefore, in view of the overall poor results as well as the psychosocial characteristics of the mental hospital, there is serious question as to the advisability of alcoholism programs in mental hospitals, except in unusual circumstances.

D. The Alcoholism Rehabilitation Hospital

In the past 20 years a new type of alcoholism inpatient program has appeared. These are inpatient hospital programs, typically free-standing nonprofit organizations. One prototype is the Hazelton Foundation in

Minnesota. The alcoholic is admitted to the hospital for a 3–6 week period. Detoxification and other medical treatment is provided if necessary. But these medical regimes are seen as adjunctive services. The orientation is nonmedical, with ex-alcoholics trained as counselors making up the bulk of the staff. A type of therapeutic milieu is maintained. Basic lectures on alcoholism are provided, followed by group counseling. But such counseling is based on understanding and dealing with the alcoholism problem per se rather than on a psychodynamic insight type of psychotherapy. AA meetings are usually part of the community life. Family sessions are often part of the total program. And the alcoholic usually assumes responsibilities for some planning of programs, activities, and on-going maintenance.

Although there are almost no published empirical data on these facilities, I have observed a number of such programs. They serve a middle-class working clientele. Often these are alcoholics who cannot stop their drinking. The period of hospitalization interrupts their cycle of drinking and gives them some distance from which to observe their ongoing life situation. The facility, via contact with the family, assists in a renegotiation of the total life situation of the alcoholic.

These programs avoid the sick-role model of alcoholism. They focus on the alcoholismic behavior. They recruit staff who are dedicated to the field of alcoholism rehabilitation; thus there is a sense of "elan," commitment, and surety of purpose. Often these programs maintain alumni programs so that after discharge the alcoholic and his or her family continue in regular contact with the therapeutic program. The programs emphasize personal responsibility and individual involvement, with reliance on education and strong group identification. Hospitalization is seen as a therapeutic interruption, not as a retreat or asylum.

These inpatient programs are probably quite appropriate for the population that has viable social competence. Many of these programs have established working relations with business and industry programs so that nominated alcoholics on the job can be deployed from work for this brief hospitalization and then returned to work. However, such programs would be less effective for populations requiring major social and vocational rehabilitation. And such programs would not be effective at all for alcoholics with high degrees of denial and defensiveness, nor for those requiring a major realigning of psychological coping styles.

E. The Aversion-Conditioning Hospital

The method of aversion conditioning has been employed in the treatment of alcoholism longer than any other method. Based on the Pavlovian concepts of aversive stimuli conditioning of behavior, the procedure has been incorporated into a relatively uniform and institutionalized treatment pattern. Thimann (1966) has reviewed the program at the Washington Hospital in Massachusetts, one of the oldest and most successful programs. There are little empirical data on these private institutions, compared to most evaluative research on public-facility alcoholism programs.

In general, these hospitals are private institutions run for profit. Their programs are usually costly, running as high as several thousand dollars. The clientele tend to be upper class and socially competent with a strong medical orientation, often negatively oriented toward psychological parameters of alcoholism. These facilities are typically well appointed, with a medical hospital pattern of service. The alcoholic is a client-patient who is there to be treated. The length of stay may run 10–14 days. For the first several days the patient is provided alcohol ad libitum while a medical evaluation is made. Then a series of aversion-conditioning treatments is conducted, after which the patient is discharged. Some hospitals provide varying degrees of counseling. In his program, Thimann describes careful attention to family counseling and continuing rehabilitation plans. However, the Washington Hospital program is probably atypical. In most hospitals with this type of program, alcoholism is viewed as a physical/medical problem, requiring physical treatment, not as a personal problem requiring psychological treatment. Some of the hospitals provide follow-up and continuing programs, but many clients apparently simply come in for treatment and then leave again.

As with all treatment programs, these hospitals claim a high degree of success. However there are no well-controlled follow-up studies.

Although the rationale for this type of treatment facility is based on the assumption that the alcoholic is "successfully conditioned," there are no controlled studies to indicate that the conditioning routine is indeed "conditioning." Alcoholics do improve and remain abstinent after hospitalization. However, there are many variables involved in placing oneself in the role definition of alcoholic, of entering a treatment facility, and of participation in the socialization into a "treated alcoholic" role as well as the various informal and formal counseling and discussion experiences that may be conducted along with the conditioning. Even if the aversion conditioning is a placebo procedure, the total gestalt of the treatment facility does provide a powerful intervention for some types of alcoholics. As illustrated later, for socially and psychologically competent alcoholics with high field dependence and high denial and strong ego defenses, this procedure may be an ego-syntonic treatment method, congruent with their life-style and ego-coping style. However, this type of facility serves a unique subpopulation of alcoholics, and is quite expensive. It therefore has limited usefulness in an overall community system of care.

F. The Halfway House

The need for transitional care facilities in the community became evident 20 years ago in the wake of attempts to move patients from the total hospital milieu into community life. Gradually the concept of partial institutional support came into the field of alcoholism. The movement has spread to the point where a national organization of alcoholism halfway house personnel has been formed. In general, the halfway house clientele are alcoholics who have lost both social and psychological competence. They are isolated, homeless, and jobless, with loss of self-esteem and inability to cope with life. They have "hit bottom." However, they are to be distinguished from the skid row habitué who has typically never participated in society. The halfway house may be seen as a transitional agency that provides a means whereby the decompensated alcoholic can regain social and psychological functioning and return to society. The halfway house typically provides shelter, food, clothing, and a well-structured living milieu where everyone assumes a responsible share in the conduct of everyday living. The director and staff are typically exalcoholics, usually with no specialized training except on-the-job experience. Usually there are strong links with Alcoholics Anonymous. Although these programs are sometimes given bureaucratic sponsorship, they are typically nonprofit community programs supported by people in the alcoholism movement. Some of the larger programs have a graded series of programs, a one-fourth house, a one-half house, and a three-fourths house. These programs provide varied degrees of external support to the alcoholic during the process of resocialization.

The programs are nonmedical and nonprofessional in nature. They may use professional personnel for adjunctive medical treatment and some supportive counseling. But the major focus is on the "therapeutic milieu" of life in the house.

The halfway house movement has provided a very important addition to the overall social system of alcoholism care, meeting the needs of a class of alcoholics that either revolved through legal agencies, welfare agencies, and mental hospitals, or finally landed on skid row (Rubington, 1977).

The services of different halfway houses reflect a certain commonality of concern. However, the effectiveness of halfway houses appears to vary widely. In a recent study, Baker et al. (1976) have been able to classify two major types of programs. The "shelter" programs do provide a medium for resocialization, whereas the "shackle" programs tend to reinforce the deviant role of the alcoholic and perhaps even use him.

The "shelter" programs have the following characteristics: They (1) are nonprofit organizations, (2) utilize community hospital facilities, (3) maintain advisory and control boards, (4) use professional counselors in therapy whenever possible, (5) maintain open business books and welcome inspections, and (6) engage in few illicit activities.

The "shackle" programs are characterized by (1) profit making, (2) the attempt to supply medical care, at cost, to the alcoholic, (3) a totally autonomous director, (4) lack of ties with professionals or professional organizations, (5) secrecy in financial concerns, (6) discouragement of governmental aid contingent upon inspections, and (7) illicit activities.

The major problem in placing the halfway house program in perspective in the social system of care is financial stability. Most programs have been shoestring operations. Yet public subsidy is seen as a threat to the movement. The halfway house movement has been a nonprofessional and nonbureaucratic enterprise. The problem with subsidy is the issue of professional control and bureaucratic institutionalization. Many fear that this will destroy the personal commitment and involvement that has created the movement and the programs.

This raises a basic issue regarding many community-based programs, namely, the assets and liabilities of a professional versus lay program. The staff of a halfway house are alcoholics themselves. They are living demonstrations of the success of the program. The program is often their life. They create a program in which they offer a model to the incoming alcoholic. In one sense, this has been described as a reconstituted family. It is doubtful that a professionally oriented program could recreate this living reality. Thus the problem becomes one of providing professional support without bringing along the professional ideology (Otto and Orford, 1978).

G. Vocational Rehabilitation Clinics

As experience with community rehabilitation programs has increased, it has become evident that emotional or social rehabilitation is often ineffective without major attention to vocational rehabilitation. It cannot be assumed that an alcoholic can return to employment and self-sustenance just because he or she once held a job or had a trade. For those alcoholics who have endured a lengthy period of vocational deterioration, previous vocational skills may no longer be appropriate. Typical employment agencies and vocational rehabilitation agencies are often negatively oriented toward the alcoholic and unwilling to devote the necessary effort to collaborate with alcoholism treatment facilities. As a result, many states have developed specialized positions for alcoholism vocational rehabilitation, placing such counselors on the staff of various treatment facilities. Other states have used vocational rehabilitation monies to directly support alcoholism treatment clinics under the rubric of vocational rehabilitation.

Free-standing vocational rehabilitation programs are more vulnerable to difficulty than liaison programs. The vocational rehabilitation counselor is usually not equipped to provide intensive counseling or to work with family relationships. Further, in most states vocational rehabilitation is limited by statutes to the period leading to employment. Once the alcoholic is employed, the services of the counselor are terminated or limited. This model of service is appropriate to physical illness and disability but is hardly adequate for the chronic and relapsing difficulties of the alcoholic. For the alcoholic on the road to rehabilitation, successful employment placement is merely the first step, with continuing support and guidance a requisite. Another problem is that various subpopulations of alcoholics have very different vocational rehabilitation needs. Therefore, a free-standing vocational rehabilitation program is beset with divergent needs within one facility. Therefore, the more optimum public-policy strategy would be to augment the services of various alcoholism facilities with vocational rehabilitation services geared specifically to the needs of alcoholics (Plant, 1979; Roman and Trice, 1976).

H. The Alcoholism Outpatient Clinic

Beginning in the 1940s, community-based outpatient clinics for alcoholics were begun under various governmental agencies. These "Yale-plan clinics" became the prototype for many community alcoholism programs. An extensive comparative study of these clinics was conducted by Gerard and Saenger (1966). They found extremely wide variation in staffing, treatment philosophy, and treatment goals. They concluded that more attention must be given to specifying treatment methods and goals to meet the needs of the different populations that each clinic served.

Outpatient clinic programs vary most widely in methodology among all facilities, ranging from ambulatory detoxification, to drug clinics, to discussion groups and AA meetings, to all varieties of psychotherapy techniques. Some outpatient programs are run in conjunction with inpatient services and day/night partial hospitalization programs.

Thus one can hardly discuss outpatient programs in terms of methodology. However, one can make observations about the populations they serve. An outpatient program by its very structure assumes a degree of ongoing life function. An alcoholic must be able typically to work and live somewhere in order to avail himself of ambulatory services.

Thus we would expect a higher degree of ego competence in those seeking outpatient care in contrast to those entering a halfway house. A major problem in many communities, however, is that an outpatient clinic may be the only available facility. Hence the outpatient facility is pushed to treat alcoholics who need more social and vocational rehabilitation than an outpatient program can appropriately provide. An outpatient program also has less leverage on the alcoholic in terms of ongoing drinking behavior, and hence less opportunity to interrupt drinking than the specialized shortstay alcoholism facility. Thus the alcoholic who needs at least some brief high external support and control will not find it in an outpatient program, even though many programs are perhaps forced to attempt such supportive control. Alcoholics in this situation are an inappropriate load on an outpatient program and undercut its effectiveness.

I. Community Human Service Agencies and Agents

Alcoholics are found everywhere in the community subsystems of human services. Often they are not identified as alcoholic, or if so identified they are not dealt with as alcoholics. Unfortunately the alcoholism may exacerbate the problems for which the alcoholic seeks services, or the alcoholism may underlie the need for services. For example, alcoholics comprise a major part of the case load of welfare workers, of probation officers, and of public health nurses. Were all these personnel to refer their alcoholic clientele to community alcoholism facilities the load would be overwhelming! Indeed the same general principle is involved in the community mental health approach to community care. Care-givers in the social systems of the community are involved with more clientele than specialized care facilities can ever hope to provide services for. The major alternative developed thus far is to provide specialized consultation to care-giving agencies and care-giving personnel so that they can appropriately identify and manage alcoholics within the conceptual framework of their own services.

It is of some note that more effective care may be provided within an agency framework than by referral to an alcoholism facility. For example, in a project with public health nurses, Pattison (1965) found that alcoholic families dropped out of an alcoholism clinic, but the public health nurses maintained contact and were able to effect substantial rehabilitation. Although the concept of mental health consultation has received relatively widespread acceptance in community mental health programs, it has not been generally implemented in regard to community alcoholism programming. It is a program concept that merits further elaboration.

Careful attention also should be given to other care-giving agents in the community who are not part of the agency structure of care. A major example is the community clergy, who provide counseling, guidance, and assistance to many alcoholics and their families. Professional antagonism toward the so-called nonprofessional skills of clergy often overlooks the fact that there is a sizable manpower resource that provides a major input into the total community response to alcoholism (Clinebell, 1968).

J. The Police-Court System

Among community services, the protective legal services play a major role in response to human problems. Putting aside the problem of the skid row habitué, the police are agents of both identification and response. The drinking driver is a good example of police identification-response. In addition, to the local court come many complaints involving alcoholism, including family abuse, child neglect, separation and divorce proceedings, bad debt complaints, etc.

Various alcoholism programs have been established in liaison with the police and court systems. Such programs have not always carefully distinguished between clientele with alcoholism problems who are part of the ongoing social system and the skid row habitué who also ends up in the police-court system and is outside the social system. For those within the social system, the police-court system may be a locus for identification and action (Glaser and O'Leary, 1966). The notion of enforced treatment or rehabilitation has a negative connotation within the mental health arena. Yet enforced participation in alcoholism rehabilitation programs is not only possible but may be more effective than voluntary treatment for comparable populations. More effective collaboration between the police-court system and community treatment agencies merits exploration and evaluation (Dittman et al., 1967).

K. The Skid Row System of Agencies

One of the common stereotypes of the alcoholic is the skid row bum. However, the skid row habitué is not primarily an alcoholic, although he may use and even abuse alcohol. The skid row man is typically socially inept, with minimal ego-coping skills and has always operated on the edge of society. The various facilities of skid row appear to differ radically. For example, we have the Salvation Army Center, the flop-house hotel, the jail, the police work-farm for trustees and alcoholics, the evangelical missions, and the jailhouse medical and psychiatric programs.

The alcoholics who habitate skid row differ in their social, vocational, and psychological makeup from alcoholics who are participant in the society at large. They absorb a great deal of time, space, and energy in the police-court system (Bahr, 1973). Yet the police-court system—the "revolving door"—is but part of a circuit that involves all of the other agencies (Spradley, 1970). The skid row person is unable to care for himself effectively, and thus he wanders or is pulled or pushed from one agency, one program, and one subsystem of skid row to the next. He does not seek anything different from the Salvation Army, the flop-house, the jail, or the hospital; he looks for shelter, warmth, and a bit of quiet and repose. The title of Wiseman's (1970) book on skid row life is an apt summary: *Stations of the Lost*. The work of both Spradley and Wiseman illustrates that although the skid row agencies are superficially variable, they all fulfill the same covert sociological function—to provide a sheltered living place for men on the margin of society.

The term *rehabilitation* in this context is a misnomer. These men have never achieved primary socialization. In contrast to halfway house clientele who have experienced loss of socialization and require resocialization, the skid row man requires primary psychological and social orientation. Programs for this visible minority group of alcoholics might best be considered in terms of extended sheltered domiciliary care, which would provide enough external structure that such men might achieve some partial entry into society (Bibby and Maus, 1974; Fry and Miller, 1975; Wright, 1975).

It is one of the ironies of comprehensive alcoholism program development that the visible skid row man is usually perceived in the community as the primary target for alcoholism programs. This is the alcoholic subpopulation that will require the most expensive, long-term total care, the population with the lowest probability of success, and the population most atypical of the total alcoholic population. Thus to link a nascent alcoholism program in a community to the skid row problem is to hitch the wagon to a political dead horse. Given the skepticism and negative attitude toward alcoholism problems, the new alcoholism program that hopes to demonstrate its effectiveness must not only address the alcoholic subpopulations more amenable to rehabilitation, but it must also educate the community in regard to the true nature of the skid row problem, which is primarily a social problem, not simply an alcoholism problem (Cook, 1975).

L. The Business and Industry System

It has been estimated that in any work force of more than 100, 10–15% of the employees will have symptomatic alcoholism. This is often expressed in high accident rates, higher rates of sick leave, and lowered rate of productivity. The so-called half-time employee represents a considerable cost to the company. Thus many companies have embarked on in-house alcoholism programs. These range from an alcoholism coordinator for the company or plant to comprehensive rehabilitation programs conducted within a plant on company time. In general, these programs have been highly effective in comparison to general community programs. Those programs are most effective when they employ very specific sanctions. That is, the worker is confronted with effects of alcoholism on his work performance and he is faced with participation in rehabilitation or termination of employment. Many companies have included alcoholism in their health insurance programs, thus affording the worker an opportunity to obtain outside treatment (Heyman, 1976; Schramm and De Fillippi, 1975; Williams and Moffet, 1975).

Although the details of such programs vary, here we can note that the resources of business and industry are considerable. In an overall schema of development of comprehensive community resources, one should consider the opportunity to assist business and industry in the development of their own personnel resources, to develop adequate insurance funding for alcoholism rehabilitation, and to develop working liaison between community facilities and the major labor markets of the community. The principle of early identification and early intervention within the social system of the identified alcoholic seems most appropriate to this major subpopulation of alcoholics. Similar relations to community resources have been established in military alcoholism programs (Conroy et al., 1971; Rock and Donley, 1975).

M. Alcoholics Anonymous as a Treatment System

Strictly speaking, Alcoholics Anonymous is not a treatment facility, but it can be considered as a treatment institution without walls. In the past there has been considerable rhetoric about AA, in which opinions have been polarized. On the one hand AA has been touted as the paradigm for the rehabilitation of the alcoholic and perhaps our major treatment resource. On the other hand, AA has been disparaged and deprecated as a nonprofessional and rigid ideological sect.

More careful empirical studies reveal that AA is neither a panacea for alcoholism, nor is it a miscreant resource. People who affiliate successfully with AA are likely to be neither upper class nor of the lowest social class. They are likely to be part of the large middle class of America and not otherwise socially deviant in class, race, or social identity save for their alcoholism. Successful affiliators are likely to be field dependent, affiliative in nature, with loss of social status while retaining psychological competency. In a word, AA provides a means of regaining lost social esteem and social status, while providing a framework for resocialization and the development of a new ideology of life (Allen and Dootjes, 1968; Bebbington, 1976; Edwards et al., 1967: Jones, 1970; Trice and Roman, 1970).

It is clear that AA appeals to, recruits from, and is likely to be a successful resource for a specific subpopulation of alcoholics. Baekeland et al. (1975) estimate that the success rate in AA approximates 34%, which is not nearly as high as popular statements. Thus AA is one of several community systems which has value to the subpopulation it serves best. However, because of its basic ideology, AA operates best in cooperation with other treatment facilities, rather than as an intrinsic part of treatment programs (Kurtz, 1979).

V. VARIABILITY OF TREATMENT METHODS

As we have already noted, it has been difficult to determine which specific treatment methods are more effective than others. However, we have noted that different populations tend to seek treatment facilities that would offer them treatment options compatible with their own desires and needs. Recently, Bromet et al. (1977) and Cronkite and Moos (1977) have published large-scale studies which indicate that treatment method selection is more important to successful outcome than previously realized. Thus there is evidence to support more careful differentiation among treatment methods. We shall briefly review available evidence that might guide us toward rational use of the treatment methods available. But first some general principles.

First, the concept of "motivation" is quite misleading. It is tempting to accept only persons into treatment who verbalize some appropriate cliché about wanting help or wanting to stop drinking. However, as Rossi and Filstead (1976) point out, this is only a means of stating how professionals demand that patients present themselves, or as they call it, the "professional's secular morality." For if the alcoholic person mouths motivational statements, it is assumed that this is a "good" patient who will do well in treatment. Whereas a person who does not profess the correct motivation is a "bad" patient who is not likely to do well. In fact, recent data suggest that initial statements of motivation are highly misleading, not highly correlated with successful treatment or long-term outcome (Rossi and Filstead, 1976; Baekeland, 1977). As Pattison et al. (1973) reported in their study of four different treatment facilities, different persons present with different motivations for different kinds of change. Thus it is misleading to ask if a person with alcohol problems is motivated. Rather, we need to ask each person what types of change they desire. We can then capitalize on the existent motivation that does actually bring a person to treatment.

Second is the issue of "coercion." Again, it has long been assumed that only if a person voluntarily seeks treatment himself can effective treatment occur. However, this overlooks the fact that there are many elements of coercion in life: from spouse, children, other relatives, friends, employers, as well as self. And there can be legal coercions as well. Thus, like motivation, this tends to be a spurious issue. It is clinically more useful to determine what coercive forces are impacting on a person so that he comes to a treatment setting. Where legal or economic coercion has been employed to "force" people into treatment, it is remarkable that such alcoholic persons do as well or better than those who allegedly seek treatment voluntarily (Mills and Hetrick, 1963; Rosenberg and Liftik, 1976; Smart, 1974).

Third is the issue of selecting treatment according to the *specific phase of treatment*. Thus we need to consider emergency treatments, initial intake treatment methods, selection of ongoing treatments, and termination and follow-up methods of treatment. Thus rather than ask What is *the* treatment of alcoholism? we might better ask Which treatments are most appropriate to what phase of a longitudinal rehabilitation process?

Fourth is the *target* of treatment. As indicated earlier, we may consider treatments that will impact on five areas of health of the alcoholic person: drinking behavior per se, emotional/psychological function, interpersonal relations, vocational function, and physical health. Each of these five areas may be appropriately addressed. But each area is likely to require different target interventions. Just providing vocational rehabilitation is no more sensible than just providing medical care, etc. So we can see that we do *not* treat "alcoholism," but rather specific areas of dysfunction.

Finally, there is the problem of "over-treatment." By this I mean a shotgun approach of a little bit of everything. It is *not* true that if a little bit of treatment is good, a lot of treatment is better. Nor is it true that all therapies help, so mixing lots of therapies together can do no harm. Such a shotgun approach may merely confuse the patient. More important, neither patients nor the therapists may develop solid commitments to a treatment approach. Or no one person may assume responsibility to monitor carefully and guide a patient toward a successful therapeutic experience but rather let the patient drift among many therapists and programs. As we have noted, such unsystematic treatment programs have poor results.

In conclusion, multiple treatment methods do have a place, and indeed the need for multiple treatments is stressed here. However, we need to define "multiple treatments" as: the appropriate selection of treatment methods in accord with the phase of rehabilitation; the selection of target areas where disability exists and treatment intervention is likely to be useful; and the matching of treatment methods with the patient's own personal proclivity. It does *not* mean exposing the patient to everything in the hope that something will "take."

A. Psychotherapy Methods

Although there are numerous personalized accounts of the psychotherapy of alcoholics, it is remarkable that there is little systematized study of psychotherapy methods for alcoholism. In fact, the general tenor of the field has seemed to play down the use of psychotherapy as an effective treatment method (Blum and Blum, 1967; Hill and Blane, 1967). A few books have addressed psychotherapy in terms of particular schools of psychotherapy, such as transactional analysis (Steiner, 1971), psychoanalysis (Hayman, 1966), and eclecticism (Forrest, 1975). Yet these efforts ignore the fact that psychotherapy is a generic approach to intrapsychic function that can range from brief crisis intervention, to short-term supportive therapies, to long-term insight-oriented psychoanalytic approaches. In a real sense, the psychotherapy of alcoholic persons has been approached from a generic perspective rather than a specific person-situation perspective in which the specific psychotherapeutic modality is selected to meet the need of the person. Despite this lack of "specified psychotherapies," Emrick (1975) found that nonspecific psychotherapy was effective in 30–60% of selected populations, and Baekeland et al. (1975) found a 41.6% success rate for psychotherapy with groups of patients with relatively poor prognoses.

With certain selected groups of patients who have stable home and work situations, who are psychologically minded, and who are personally oriented toward psychotherapy, individual outpatient psychotherapy can be successfully implemented. Gerard and Saenger (1966) have demonstrated that one can successfully identify such "psychotherapy alone" candidates, although they are probably a minority of outpatients.

The major caveat about outpatient psychotherapy is its frequent failure. Where outpatient psychotherapy is a modality offered in a comprehensive alcoholism program, it has better likelihood for success. However, for the general private psychotherapist there are several major pitfalls. As Glasscote et al. (1967) have clearly pointed out, the private psychotherapist usually is inexperienced in conducting psychotherapy with alcoholics, is likely to have a preexistent negative attitude toward alcoholics, and does not know how to use other resources. But perhaps most important, the psychotherapist is likely to *ignore the drinking*. The drinking behavior is treated solely as a symptom that will disappear in the course of successful psychotherapy. This orientation often leads to failure. It is important to emphasize that even with good candidates for psychotherapy, the therapist must deal with *both* the drinking behavior and the psychological and emotional functions of the patient (Zimberg et al., 1978).

The more common problem is the outpatient alcoholic who has multiple problems in many areas of life, who is not oriented toward individual in-depth psychotherapy, or who requires an institutional program. In this case, as Blane (1977) points out: "Psychotherapy does not occur in isolation but includes the participation of family members and other significant persons and is often conducted, in various combinations, with other forms of treatment." To the above, I would add that we need to develop much more precise and specific psychotherapeutic techniques directed toward specific targets of psychic change in specific alcoholics. This might range from crisis intervention techniques that assist in anxiety reduction, reduce initial shame and guilt, and orient the alcoholic at intake to a promising new reality, to educational psychotherapies that do not directly challenge defenses yet avoid rationalizations and denial, and thence onward into more personal psychotherapeutic encounters.

In sum, psychotherapy has acquired an unwarranted negative reputation in the treatment of alcoholics. With a certain minority of outpatients, it may be the sole treatment of choice; but in the majority of instances specific psychotherapeutic interventions must be interwoven with other forms of treatment.

B. Group Psychotherapies

Our discussion of individual psychotherapy can be generally applied to group psychotherapy. Cahn (1970) found in a national survey that group therapy was a widely preferred method in alcoholism programs. Yet there has been little empirical research to support the popularity of group therapy as a method of choice. Several reviews indicate the scant literature, which is primarily clinical description (Doroff, 1977; Mullan and Sanguiliano, 1966). What is lacking is a clear differentiation of types of group methods which can be selectively used for specific therapeutic goals with different types of patients (Pattison, 1965, 1970). This is not to say that group therapies are not useful but rather that we need to construct specific guidelines for this therapy.

C. Family Therapies

Although the family has long been recognized as an important aspect of the alcoholism syndrome, it is striking that alcoholism treatment programs have lagged behind most mental health programs in using family therapy approaches to treatment (Janzen, 1977). The family can be seen as both cause and consequence. That is, conflicts within the family can exacerbate personal conflict and perpetuate drinking behavior (Burton and Kaplan, 1968). On the other hand, problems with spouse and family are often the consequence of drinking behavior, rather than a cause (Orford et al., 1975).

Since the family environment has been shown to be a major determinant of successful treatment outcome (Moos et al., 1977), the family context is more often than not an important *target* for interpersonal interventions (Orford, 1975). Optimally this should begin at the time of intake, with involvement of the spouse. For as Pattison et al. (1965) have shown, it is easier to involve the spouse early in the rehabilitation process than later. Then one can proceed to involvement of other members of the family in a variety of family-oriented therapeutic activities, including marital couples groups, whole family therapy, and multiple family therapies (Berman, 1968; Scott, 1970; Shipp, 1963; Steinglass, 1976, 1977).

An important extension of the family therapy model has been to include both the formal kin and informal friend, neighbor, and co-worker relationships that compromise the psychosocial kinship network or "social network" of the identified alcoholic. These therapeutic techniques identify the significant people in the life of the alcoholic and bring them together for cohesive and collaborative support of the identified alcoholic person. This methodology is generally termed "social network therapy" (Catanzaro et al., 1977; Finlay, 1966; Pattison et al., 1975; Sands and Hansen, 1971; Ward and Faillace, 1970).

Again, as with all psychotherapies, there is little empirical data on the effectiveness of such methods. However, there is abundant clinical evidence to support further careful clinical development (Kaufman and Pattison, 1981).

D. Drug Therapies

A variety of pharmacotherapeutic agents have been used to treat alcoholism over time. As Mottin (1973) has clearly demonstrated in his review of drug treatments, a specific drug has often been introduced with the hope that it would be the "magic bullet" to cure alcoholism. Yet it is apparent that no drug can "treat" all five areas of life health. Drugs can indeed be useful to treat specific "target symptoms," but it is fallacious to assume that a drug can "cure" alcoholism (Kissin, 1975).

Nevertheless, there is a certain subgroup of alcoholics who have been identified as positive responders to drug treatment. In particular Kissin and his coworkers have found that certain alcoholics who have social stability, including stable family and work relations, and who are not psychologically minded, yet form dependent relationships with authority figures, can develop a therapeutically useful relationship with a drug-dispensing doctor or nurse (Kissin and Platz, 1968; Kissin et al., 1968, 1970). Here the actual pharmacologic action of the drug is probably not of critical importance—in their studies a minor tranquilizer in modest doses was dispensed. The drug is more properly seen as a symbolic vehicle for the clinician-patient interaction (Ornstein and Whitman, 1965). This is not merely a placebo response but is actually a "treatment gestalt" of giving and receiving. It works well with patients who feel comfortable with a medical model of alcoholism, who can effectively respond to an emotionally low-level intensity of interaction with authority figures, and for whom the drug-treatment setting provides an ego-syntonic style of interaction. Rosenberg (1974) has described similar results, although he found decreasing effectiveness after 4–5 months if no further personal elements of therapy were introduced. It is a misnomer to call this "drug therapy" in the narrow sense; it might be better termed "drug-mediated" psychotherapeutic intervention.

The more general picture of drug treatment of alcoholism is one of misuse and faddish claims devoid of empirical validity. This is highlighted by a review of 89 drug treatment studies by Viamontes (1972). He found that 94.5% of uncontrolled studies showed positive results, but only 5.8% of controlled drug studies showed positive results. Many sensationalistic drug fads have recently passed through the alcoholism treatment scene, which upon careful study have not proven of significant value. These have included LSD (Ludwig et al., 1970), the antitrichomonad Flagyl (Goodwin and Reinhard, 1972), multivitamins and multiple other miscellaneous drugs (Charnoff, 1970; Kaplan et al., 1972).

One of the serious issues in the use of drugs in the treatment of alcoholics is that it conveys the message to the alcoholic that the drug he has been using—alcohol—can appropriately be replaced by another drug. This may interfere with an effective treatment program and play into an alcoholic's denial and other defenses. Bissell (1975) comments:

> Arguments are still advanced at times that, if one does not prescribe sedatives for a highly manipulative patient, he will simply get his drugs from another doctor and fall into hands less expert than ours. This same reasoning

could be applied whenever one is asked to give penicillin for a viral pharyngitis, but that does not justify our doing so. It is also agreed that giving drugs makes the patient more likely to keep coming back to us. Many a street-corner pusher would agree. I do think we need to give our patients a substitute for alcohol, but I don't think that substitute can be another sedative. I think it has to be our concern, our time, our caring, and ourselves.

The problem of drug substitution by the alcoholic is a major treatment problem. And indeed it is well documented that alcoholics can develop mixed drug dependencies or switch drug dependencies from one to another (Freed, 1973). This includes dependencies on amphetamines (Kipperman and Fine, 1974), barbiturates (Devenyi and Wilson, 1971), and narcotics (Chessick et al., 1961), as well as the minor tranquilizers, which have become the major offender.

In addition to the perpetuation of drug dependency, the problem of mixed and switched drug dependencies can pose critical medical problems. Such drug combinations can exacerbate physical illnesses, create perplexing drug side effects, and produce drug withdrawal syndromes which are both difficult to diagnose and to manage medically. A large technical literature exists on these alcohol-drug combinations and attendant complications (Polacsek et al., 1972).

One clinical population of timely concern here are narcotic addicts who are being treated on methadone-maintenance programs. A significant number of these patients also develop alcohol problems. Not only is the drug combination problematic, but combined treatment is often difficult. Here the use of disulfiram (Antabuse) has been reported to be salutary in maintaining control over the use of alcohol and safe in combination with methadone (Charuvastra et al., 1976; Liebson et al., 1973; Pugliese et al., 1975; Schut et al., 1973).

Turning now to specific classes of drugs, the selection of specific types of drugs can be considered in terms of target symptoms.

1. Antipsychotic Drugs

The so-called major tranquilizers or antipsychotic drugs have been widely prescribed for alcoholics to modify agitation and anxiety. On a short-term basis, following withdrawal from alcohol, there appears to be only minimal justification for the use of this class of drugs to treat severe agitation. The major objections are that these drugs have a high incidence of side effects, produce behavioral retardation, increase depression, and may even precipitate psychotic symptoms as a side effect (Baekeland, 1977).

The one clear indication for these drugs is in persons who have *both* a psychotic disorder and an alcoholism problem. In such cases the alcohol may have acted as an antipsychotic agent and the cessation of drinking may result in florid psychotic symptoms. Here the major tranquilizers have a place in treating the psychosis.

2. Antidepressant Drugs

The rationale for the use of antidepressant drugs for alcoholics is that depression is a major psychopathological symptom among alcoholics. During acute withdrawal the alcoholic person is typically depressed, while the chronic alcoholic person has rather uniform elements of depression. However, there are major problems associated with the use of antidepressants.

First, the depression of acute withdrawal is severe and limited in time (to the first several days of withdrawal), whereas antidepressant drugs take at least a week and usually two to three weeks before they have any demonstrable effect.

Second, the depression of the chronic alcoholic is more a characterological coping style than a neurotic reaction. Antidepressant drugs are not effective for characterological types of depression, while the evidence is highly equivocal that antidepressants significantly affect neurotic depression.

Third, in the face of the fact that antidepressants are not demonstrably effective for the types of depression typically experienced by alcoholics and that antidepressants have significant side effects, as well as the issues of expense and the symbolic meaning of more drug-taking, it does not appear that antidepressants should be routinely used.

Fourth, there is a small group of alcoholic persons who have *preexistent* severe mental disorders, including unipolar and bipolar types of manic-depressive syndromes. In these highly selected instances, as in the case of the antipsychotics, the use of antidepressant drugs may be useful in treating the manic-depressive disorder.

Recent studies on affective disorders has demonstrated that a small group of alcoholics have a life history of either unipolar or bipolar affective disorder. They may concurrently develop an alcoholism syndrome. Alcohol may also be used as self-medication. In a depressive state the person may drink to relieve depression, while in a manic state alcohol may be indiscriminately consumed or alternatively used as a sedative. Differential diagnosis is critical here because almost all acute alcoholics demonstrate some depression. This does not justify the diagnosis of an affective disorder, however. The drug lithium is an effective prophylactic against the recurrence of manic and bipolar affective episodes so it may be a vital part of treatment for such patients. However, the use of lithium for the treatment of alcoholism or for depression per se is *not* indicated (Goodwin and Erickson, 1979).

3. *Antianxiety and Sedative Drugs*

In this class the target symptoms are anxiety and restlessness. The drug classes include: the minor tranquilizers such as meprobamate, the tranquilizer-muscle relaxants such as the benzodiazepenes, and the sedatives such as the barbiturates and chloral hydrate. As noted earlier, the major problem with this group of drugs is that they can readily be used to produce mixed alcohol-drug dependencies, or the alcoholic can switch from alcohol to one of these drugs.

During the initial first few days of acute withdrawal, the use of these drugs can be beneficial in controlling anxiety, agitation, and restlessness. Under these conditions of careful daily supervision, these drugs can be safely employed without undue pharmacologic or psychodynamic problems. However, the continued use of this class of drugs after perhaps the first week of withdrawal treatment has no justification except for those carefully selected patients described earlier who are placed in a "drug-mediated" therapeutic program. Finally, the routine use of such drugs as an initial treatment procedure appears strongly contraindicated, because of the factors discussed (Solomon, 1982).

4. *Alcohol-Aversive Drugs*

A major class of drugs that has found clinical utility are the drugs which in combination with alcohol produce an uncomfortable physiological reaction. Chief among these is disulfiram (Antabuse). When first introduced to the United States in the 1950s, Antabuse was used in similar fashion to apomorphine—to induce an adverse reaction to the simultaneous intake of alcohol. Thus Antabuse was used as an aversive-conditioning agent. However, it was soon found that Antabuse did not produce as dramatic a reaction as the older method of using apomorphine. Further, it was found that success rates with Antabuse were not related to an initial conditioning experience. Therefore, for the most part, the use of an initial series of conditioning sessions has been abandoned as a method of Antabuse treatment. Most clinicians now describe the adverse reaction that occurs when one takes Antabuse regularly and then consumes alcohol. The alcoholic is then given a supply of Antabuse with the instruction to take his daily pill. Thus the alcoholic knows that if he drinks he will experience an adversive physiological reaction. It is proposed that the alcoholic is thereby "protected from drinking."

However, this is only part of the picture. There is an interesting and widespread mythology that Antabuse somehow "prevents" the alcoholic from drinking, or that while taking Antabuse this medication produces a distaste for alcohol. Although there is no evidence for this interpretation, I have found this belief widespread among both alcoholics and practitioners.

But Antabuse has no effect as a pharmacological agent, save for the adverse reaction after consumption of alcohol. One might presume that this negative reaction might serve as a deterrent to drinking. However, a frequent clinical observation is that an alcoholic who has enough impetus to drink will do so, regardless of the reaction. In fact, in hostile, negatively oriented treatment situations where the alcoholic is forced to take Antabuse, he may deliberately drink to provoke the reaction, as if to prove that the therapist cannot control him.

It is clear that the forced administration of Antabuse is a therapeutic fallacy. The alcoholic for whom Antabuse is effective is the one who is motivated to stop drinking, who forms a positive relationship with the therapist, and for whom Antabuse is seen not as a control but as an aid to his own self-motivation. In an interesting paper, Usdin et al. (1952) collected fantasies of alcoholics taking Antabuse. Those with a negative view of the drug as a control had dreams and fantasies of stomachaches and vomiting, whereas those with a positive view reported images of mild drinking and small therapists sitting inside their stomachs. Billet (1964) has described Antabuse as a method of "ego reinforcement" to the alcoholic who already wants not to drink. The daily ingestion of Antabuse is probably one of its major psychodynamic advantages. There is a saying that goes, "You only have to make one decision a day about drinking—whether to take the pill or not." This is very similar to an AA aphorism which states that the alcoholic makes only one decision—not to drink today.

It is clear that Antabuse is not a panacea, and the widespread indiscriminate use of routine Antabuse administration to all alcoholic patients has no clinical justification. However, reviews of alcoholism programs have shown that programs which have Antabuse available as a treatment *option* are likely to have higher success rates. That is, the judicious use of Antabuse can be a useful adjunct while other aspects of a treatment program are concurrently underway. The current evidence suggests that the person who will positively respond to Antabuse administration is one who (1) has a positive stated desire to abstain from alcohol, (2) tends to be obsessive-compulsive and not prone to severe depression, (3) is socially stable and socially competent, (4) is usually not highly introspective, (5) has a propensity to form dependent relationships with trusted figures, and (6) tends to drink sporadically rather than continually and compulsively (Baekeland et al., 1971; Gerrein et al., 1973; Lubetkin et al., 1971).

E. Behavioral Therapies

The most important development in treatment methods of the past 10 years has been the rapid expansion of behavioral methodologies. Classic aversive conditioning of alcoholics has been used worldwide for at least 50 years or more. Typically this took the form of the administration of a drug like apomorphine which was injected into the patient just at the time he or she took a drink at the experimental bar rail. The adverse reaction, typically vomiting, sweating, temperature, some confusion, etc., was thought to "condition" the alcoholic to associate drinking with the conditioned experience of sickness. Hence the alcoholic would avoid drinking. There are many conceptual and experimental flaws in this simplistic view. Nevertheless, the conditioning approach did prove useful to a specific subpopulation of alcoholics and remains a viable treatment alternative.

During the 1960s a variety of new techniques for producing conditioned aversion to alcohol were developed (Franks, 1966). Since that time, however, it has been shown that simple aversion-conditioning techniques are less powerful than more personalized behavioral techniques (Caddy and Lovibond, 1976; Elkins, 1975). These latter "broad spectrum" behavioral approaches are predicated on the careful analysis of the total life behavior of the alcoholic person, the definition of target behaviors to be changed, and the development of multiple behavioral interventions in which the alcoholic patient himself consciously participates (Cheek, 1972; Hamburg, 1971; Hedberg and Campbell, 1974; Hunt and Azrin, 1973). In addition, these latter approaches emphasize the need to construct individualized behavioral programs based on the specific target behaviors of each alcoholic (Sobell and Sobell, 1973). Because most of this work has been conducted on an experimental basis, there are no clear clinical guidelines that indicate what specific types of alcoholic populations might differentially respond to a behavioral approach (Litman, 1976; Nathan and Briddel, 1977). However, just as in the case of the psychotherapies, we might rather ask where behavior methods might be appropriately used as part of a treatment program for what areas of Life Health intervention, rather than as an ideological approach to treatment.

Recent work in behavioral therapies has focused on the analysis of the real-life cues to which the alcoholic responds to drinking, on strategies for teaching and practicing life skills, and on cognitive reorganization of the alcoholic's patterns of thought. In short, the behavioral therapies have moved from a mechanistic approach to a psychological approach. Currently, a wide range of behavioral strategies are being implemented and evaluated (Nathan et al., 1978; Nathan and Hay, 1982).

VI. VARIABILITY IN TREATMENT PERSONNEL

The issue of effective treatment for alcoholism has focused primarily on the selection of alcoholic clients, facilities, or treatment methods. Yet treatment may be significantly affected by the selection of the treatment personnel. This is an area devoid of systematic attention, much less of empirical data. As noted earlier, some data suggest that there are widely disparate and contradictory ideologies and attitudes among alcoholism personnel, even within the same programs. Only recently has concerted attention been focused on the specific manpower problems in the field of alcoholism (Blacker, 1977; Blume, 1977).

First, the field of alcoholism services has been ignored by health professionals in general, and by mental health professionals in particular. Repeated surveys of professional agencies and professional attitudes indicate that there is a general negativism towards alcoholics, that generic service agencies ignore or screen out alcoholics, much less make measured efforts to help them, and that professionals avoid choosing services to alcoholics as a professional option.

The result has been a curious and perhaps tragic vacuum. For the bulk of alcoholism services manpower has come from the ranks of volunteers and paraprofessional personnel. Until at least 1950, most alcoholism programs and services were nonprofessional in nature. As Cahn (1970) has documented, what alcoholism services were developed tended to be staffed by second-class professional staff, with second-class funding, resulting in second-class programs operating in the back-waters of professional developments.

Second, the training of mental health professionals has rarely included much preparation in the field of alcoholism (Einstein and Wolfson, 1970). Hence, professional recruitment has been difficult. Perhaps the bulk of professional recruits have been those who have been alcoholics themselves, achieved sobriety, and then sought professional training to return to the field of their personal experience. The influence of this type of professional has not been critically evaluated.

One response to this professional vacuum has been the development of specialized professional-training programs for alcoholism counselors. These range from new careers training of recovered alcoholics to B.A. and M.A. level academic curricula. Although such programs are personally successful, we must question their overall national value if they continue apart from a more general manpower development program. Such specialized alcoholism personnel would have little lateral mobility into other human service jobs, they would have little vertical mobility except on an idiosyncratic basis within a specific program; and they have ambiguous professional status and sanction at this time. On the other hand, if such professional training programs do interdigitate with more general manpower training and manpower personnel series, they could offer a highly potent specialized manpower development track for personnel directed toward alcoholism services (Staub and Kent, 1973).

Third, a major problem in the development of manpower, from a professional point of view, is the fragmented professional orientation toward alcoholism. Some medical professionals view alcoholism solely as a biological problem; some psychiatric professionals view alcoholism solely as a neurotic emotional problem; some psychological professionals view alcoholism solely as a conditioned behavioral problem, etc. In sum, there is no widely accepted frame of reference within which professional training can be developed. Hence we have partisan professionalism rather than scientific professionals. Until a more adequate conceptual base for manpower preparation is developed, we may expect difficulties in the recruitment and training of adequate manpower.

A further complication in the manpower field is the split between the lay and professional approaches to alcoholism treatment. Kalb and Propper (1976) describe the differences in terms of the cognitive style and commitments of the two manpower groups. According to them, the professionals use an analytical-objective-inductive cognitive style, whereas the lay personnel use an intuitive-subjective-deductive style. And they point out that lay personnel often have a strong personal commitment to a personalized treatment style, whereas the professional is likely to lack intense personal commitment and look at treatment methods as a scientific problem. The result, say Kalb and Propper, is a conflict of power and ideology between two manpower pools in the field.

Other aspects of manpower issues are reflected in the rather unique types of personnel who are often recruited into the alcoholism field.

A. Alcoholics Anonymous

One of the most misunderstood groups of personnel are the members of AA who have been lonely pioneers. At times the AA movement has been seen as the only manpower resource in the field of alcoholism. Yet AA has also been disparaged as nonprofessional or even antiprofessional.

These views overlook the social psychology of all self-help groups. Hans Toch (1965) in his extensive study of nonprofessional self-help movements has found that there are certain universal characteristics. One, self-help movements arise when professional helpers do not provide effective services. Two, therefore the deviant distressed people turn to each other for help. Three, they discover that they can help themselves. Four, because they can help themselves they conclude that professionals cannot help them. Five, because they have developed an effective self-help method they conclude that their method can help anyone similarly afflicted. Six, they conclude that their method is effective, and if a person fails in their system, it is the failure of the person, not the system. Seven, they conclude that their self-developed conceptual interpretation of the deviant problem is correct, as proved by the efficacy of their self-help method.

Now it is important to note that all self-help groups have an intrinsic antiprofessional bias, have a nonscience-based conceptual frame of reference, and a self-fulfilling prophecy justification of their method. All of these ingredients are necessary for a self-help group. These attitudes are the social glue that coalesce such groups and promote the group solidarity and commitment that make them successful.

It is important not to attempt to scientificize or professionalize a self-help movement. The mode of collaboration with mutual respect for differing methods and differing concepts allows both the self-help movement efforts and professional efforts to exist side by side and complement each other. In line with our discussion thus far, Alcoholics Anonymous provides an entree for certain types of alcoholics, whereas professional programs provide entree for other types. Both are part of an overall community system. But it would be a mistake to demand agreement on methods and concepts.

B. The Ex-alcoholic as an Alcoholism Worker

In our initial discussion it was pointed out that one facet of manpower development was the recruitment of indigenous community workers, who both knew their community and were to be afforded a career providing escape from the poverty ghetto. The same motif is found in the recruitment of the indigenous recovered alcoholic. Certainly, it has been advantageous in providing workers who are familiar and comfortable in working in alcoholism territory. Wiseman (1970) pointed out in her book on skid row, *Stations of the Lost,* that recruitment into alcoholism programs as an alcoholism worker is indeed a career method of escape from the alcoholism ghetto.

The disadvantages are that rarely are new careers afforded ex-alcoholics. They have jobs and careers so long as they can trade on their expertise as ex-alcoholics (Trice and Roman 1970). That expertise also limits them in terms of providing expertise in other areas of human service. There are exceptions, of course. The other major disadvantage is that ex-alcoholics tend to operate within a limited frame of reference, an alcoholic's view of the world. They may therefore continue to function with many biases, prejudices, and distortions of the complex world of human services that may limit their effectiveness or constrain the purview of their programs.

C. The Ex-alcoholic as a Professional

As noted, a number of ex-alcoholics have been recruited into professional ranks. Often they are dedicated and conscientious workers. They have often assumed positions of major leadership in the field of alcoholism. I have had the opportunity to train, supervise, and collaborate with many such professionals. On the basis of my personal observation, I conclude that they have made major contributions to the field of alcoholism.

On the other hand, the ex-alcoholic as a professional may sometimes work at a personal disadvantage. For example, the ex-alcoholic usually enters into professional training with relatively set views about alcoholism. He/she is not seeking professional training so much to learn about alcoholism as to acquire professional credentials. Such a person may be disinterested in those aspects of professional training and knowledge that he or she does not see as pertinent to the field of alcoholism. Because of this personal investment in recovery, the ex-alcoholic may be emotionally resistant to professional knowledge that challenges a personal view of recovery and rehabilitation. And, finally, the most personal and poignant dimension may be that the ex-alcoholic is torn inside between a commitment to a view of alcoholism that undergirds his or her continuing personal stability and a commitment to intellectual and scientific knowledge and its concurrent professional integrity. As one professional told me: "When I work, I view alcoholism scientifically, but when I live, I view alcoholism the way I know I have to live."

The ex-alcoholic professional may bring certain insights, understandings, and compassion to the professional field, while at the same time having less personal freedom to look at alcoholism problems dispassionately and perhaps innovate new approaches.

D. The Culturally Indigenous Alcoholism Worker

In the past 20 years, the mental health field has become painfully aware of the culture biases of our community mental health programs. Most mental health services have operated from white middle-class biases. This problem, from my observations, is even more accentuated in alcoholism services.

For example, alcoholism is the number-one health problem on American Indian reservations. Yet most of the typical urban alcoholism services are inappropriate and ineffective when applied to Indian reservation programs. The successful Indian programs have relied upon indigenous Indian personnel from the local community on the reservation or in the urban Indian ghetto. The same holds true for alcoholism services located in black or Chicano urban ghettos and barrios.

In recognition of this fact, recent urban programs have been developed that are based in ethnic communities, staffed by indigenous community personnel, with program structure geared to life-styles and values systems of the community. One of the major manpower issues that faces the alcoholism field is the recruitment, training, and effective utilization of minority personnel in appropriately designed service programs (Rosenberg et al., 1976).

E. Implications

These descriptions suggest the importance of matching personnel to programs, so that the skills, values, and ideologies of the staff match the values, ideology, and programmatic goals of the facility program. Where this does not occur, staff are likely to provide services not congruent with program goals (Mogar et al., 1969). Or staff attitudes may be shaped by external factors that bias treatment services. For example, Smart et al. (1969) studied a large alcoholism program in which careful treatment recommendations, based upon individual need assessment, were made at diagnostic intake. Yet they found that the actual treatment received was based on social class biases of the staff, which ignored the needs of the individual alcoholics.

Within a comprehensive treatment program, then, we recommend that careful attention be given to matching treatment personnel, in terms of their specific skills and values, with individual alcoholic clients who need those specific treatment skills and share similar values (Baekeland and Lundwall, 1975; Larkin, 1974). Then collaborative and mutually committed therapeutic relationships are likely to develop. Several studies suggest that effective therapist performance is directly linked to therapist involvement, commitment, and active pursuit of treatment goals (Howard et al., 1970; McNair et al., 1962). To achieve this, the therapist must be matched as appropriately as possible to clients with whom he or she can engage in a therapeutic process. As Goldstein (1962) has pointed out, matching of therapist-client values and goals is the most powerful predictor of successful outcome.

VII. CLIENT-FACILITY-METHOD-PERSONNEL MATCHES: AN EXAMPLE

As an illustration of how matching can occur among all four dimensions in the development of alcoholism rehabilitation programs, the following short vignettes summarize data from a study by Pattison et al. (1973). Table 1 shows how each population gave a different definition of alcoholism, had different self-defined treatment goals, and was provided different treatment by different personnel.

A. The Aversion-Conditioning Hospital

This population has the highest education (college), has achieved the highest socioeconomic status, has maintained intact marriages, and has the healthiest interpersonal and vocational health scores. These are all indicators of capacity for successful social competence. MMPI data indicate a constellation of personality traits requisite for social skills, because they are oriented toward social acceptance, externalization of problems, and somatization of anxiety. In other words, these people are able to keep life conflict outside themselves, or at least generally out of conscious awareness. They seek a treatment program that will restore flagging social acceptance, are sensitive to social sanctions, and turn to appropriate social resources.

This population of alcoholics is relatively "less sick," and hence has less need for, or room for, improvement in total life rehabilitation. Alcoholism for them is still seen as an external problem. Alcoholism has not severely disrupted their social and vocational life. If these people feel that they have reached their most desperate point, that level is not nearly as low as for alcoholics at the other facilities. These are "high bottom" alcoholics. Further, being socially sensitive they may seek treatment earlier in their career of alcoholism before disintegration has occurred, with more social and vocational pressures present to push them into treatment. Although they have been drinking as long as the alcoholics at other facilities, they appear to have more capacity to defend against overt alcoholism.

For this population alcoholism is a disease, a medical problem akin to heart trouble or a broken leg, not a reflection of personal conflict. The medical view of alcoholism is a psychodynamic and sociodynamic stance that allows them to maintain their characteristic life-style.

The facility in turn reflects the needs and perceptions of this population. The population is "high-class," and the treatment is "high-priced." The medical orientation of the hospital conveys the message that medical personnel will "do something" to the person to rid him of the unpleasant affliction—alcoholism. The aversion treatment philosophy allows the subjects to maintain their image of adequate, successful individuals. Further, this facility does little in the way of social and vocational rehabilitation, since little is needed in this area; nor does it provide much psychological treatment. Overtly this facility does not define alcoholism as a

Table 1
Matching Variables in Four Alcoholism Programs

Facility	Aversion Hospital	Outpatient Clinic	Halfway House	Police Farm
Definition of alcoholism	Medical allergy	Neurotic symptom	Life problem	Secondary nuisance
Treatment goals	Abstinence	Emotional restructure	New life-style	Stay dry and sober
Treatment methods	Aversion-conditioning	Psychotherapy	Group socialization milieu	Sheltered, structured living
Staffing:	1. Medical professional 2. Technical aides	1. Mental health professional 2. Technical aides 3. Community counselors	1. Paraprofessional 2. Volunteers	1. Paraprofessional

psychological problem. Yet the facility would probably be less successful if it did attempt psychological treatment because this would challenge the major defense systems of this population.

B. The Alcoholism Outpatient Clinic

This population provides evidence of less social competence. They have a high-school education, have more middle-class jobs, have married but experienced more divorces, and have intermediate interpersonal and vocational health scores. The MMPI data indicate a capacity for moderate defenses against anxiety but not sufficient to prevent breakthrough of anger, depression, and feelings of inadequacy and passivity. This population experiences conflict while still maintaining a reasonable degree of social competence. They are still socially sensitive and look to socially respectable resources; however, they are more negativistic and pessimistic.

They see alcoholism as a personal problem, yet fear that it will overwhelm their lives more than it has. The definition of alcoholism as an expression of neurotic conflict is an apt summation of their personal experience of being alcoholic. In this population there is less need to maintain status by using a medical rationalization as the aversion hospital alcoholics do. Yet alcoholism is disrupting their lives and hence undercuts their capacity to deny that alcoholism is a personal problem.

The outpatient clinic is the most eclectic of the facilities. It has a physician and nurse to manage withdrawal symptoms. Disulfiram and psychotropic drugs are prescribed, and patients are informed of and encouraged to attend Alcoholics Anonymous. Yet the main modality is psychotherapy. Treatment is addressed to the personal conflicts that cause the patient to abuse alcohol and to dealing with the consequences of drinking in order to provide insight and strengthen ego adaptive skills. These alcoholics do not seek dramatic life rehabilitation, but they cannot afford to "close over" and deny the personal nature of their alcoholism. This facility does not provide shelter and life maintenance, because this population still can maintain social competence. Nor does this facility focus on abstinence as its treatment goal, since the supposition is that symptomatic alcoholism will disappear with the resolution of life conflict. This is a feasible treatment approach for this population. In contrast, abstinence must be a treatment goal for the aversion-hospital alcoholics since life conflict is maintained outside awareness. Abstinence is also required for halfway house and police farm alcoholics, because they lack sufficient social competence to go ahead with the business of living life while simultaneously coping with their drinking style—abstinence for them is a precursor to rehabilitation.

C. The Alcoholism Halfway House

This population demonstrates the effects of diminished social competence. They have only partial high school education, have held laboring and technical jobs, have often suffered marital disintegration, and have less healthy interpersonal and vocational health scores. Their MMPI data show characterological traits of inability to cope adequately with conflict and stress. They seek succor and repress anger in order to get others to help them. Manipulation of others to provide for them becomes a major coping style in their lives. They experience a breakdown of coping mechanisms and turn to others, the clergy or institutions, to rehabilitate them.

These are the "low bottom" alcoholics. They possessed enough social competence to achieve a degree of successful social adaptation before alcoholism caught up with them. But they have suffered huge steps downward from their previous jobs and family relationships. Although not on skid row, they are close to it. Alcoholism for this population is not an isolated affliction but a major disruption of their entire life. The use of the medical model of alcoholism is not a defense this population can use. Even if they stopped drinking immediately they would still face immense problems of social and vocational rehabilitation. Neither can they employ the model of alcoholism as a neurosis, because alcoholism is a total life problem, not just a neurotic affliction. Further, the psychological "set" of this population would not fit them for the usual methods of middle-class psychotherapy, because they are faced with the real-life exigencies of just existing. Alcoholism is a problem of life, a need to start over, a spiritual renewal, and a destruction of the self which means that a new style of life adaptation must be carved out.

The halfway house facility reflects the definitions and needs of this population. There is heavy reliance on Alcoholics Anonymous philosophy, including the need to surrender one's previous life-style, to start over, to begin to live one day at a time, and the quasireligious conversion to becoming a new man. The AA philosophy emphasizes the need to change one's whole orientation toward life and toward oneself, and this matches very well the fact that alcoholism has destroyed their lives and that major construction of a new pattern of living is needed. Similarly, the program does not emphasize denial or strengthening of ego skills to dispatch neurosis. Rather it starts by providing nurturance and gratification of daily needs and desires; it sets limits and defines behavior—very necessary for persons with limited ego strength. The facility provides a setting for resocialization and only secondarily is psychological enquiry made. This is social rehabilitation, followed by vocational rehabilitation.

D. The Police Farm Work Center

This population lies at the lowest end of the social competence scale. These people are the socially inept. They have completed only grade school, have held transient laboring jobs, and have usually never married. Their interpeı sonal and vocational health scores are the unhealthiest of all the groups. Their MMPI data reveal a lack of capacity to cope with stress. They show little capacity to deal with internal conflict save via direct action. Hence, they show psychopathic qualities, nonconformity, overt hostility, and yet despair and depression. There is little strength in themselves which they can call upon; hence they can only look to external agencies and personnel to cope with life. Alcoholism is for them just another piece of problematic behavior with which they cannot cope. They see little difference between treatment methods or facilities. They have no hope that life can be different. Their only goal is to achieve some respite in life by living in an institution that will provide them with support and nurturance that they cannot give themselves. They will pass from one institution to the next. Within an institution that provides necessary supports they can function; outside a supportive institution, they cannot.

The facility provides a program that in actuality meets the immediate needs of this population, although the treatment goals of the facility may be more ambitious than appropriate. The subjects live in the work farm for 60 days isolated from society and from liquor. The subjects are provided with guided and supervised living experiences, and some realistic work experience is provided. It is the type of facility, were it a long-term domiciliary, that could provide a sheltered living base where this population might function at a modest level of self-care. The facility makes no major effort at gradual social reentry; it does not provide significant psychological counseling. These additions would doubtless be of little value to the recipients. In contrast to the halfway house alcoholics where the problem is "resocialization," the problem here is primary "socialization," which would also require significant augmentation of basic psychological coping skills, basic vocational training, and entry into society. The facility provides a short-term "drying out" and a brief surcease from the buffeting rounds of skid row life, which may be the appropriate level of intervention for this population.

VIII. SELECTION OF TREATMENT AS A COMMUNITY PROCESS

Thus far we have examined selection of treatment from the point at which the alcoholic person appears at a treatment facility. However, our discussion has pointed up the fact that *no one* facility represents the total community involvement in response to alcoholism. Some facilities are indirectly and covertly involved with alcoholism, whereas other facilities offer explicit alcoholism services. Thus it is important to consider both the formal and informal network of community services involved in alcoholism problems.

A. Community Epidemiology

The selection of treatment is based upon the needs of different alcoholism subpopulations that exist in a community and the existent resources. Where the resources do not match the needs we will find services that are not appropriately utilized and alcoholics for whom appropriate services do not exist. Thus it is important to first approach the treatment of alcoholism from the perspective of the total community (Catanzaro, 1968; Cross, 1968; Goldfarb and Hartman, 1975; Holder and Stratas, 1972).

Edwards (1973) has described in detail the principles of an epidemiological approach, which describes the incidence, prevalence, location, and needs of the various alcoholism subpopulations of the community. Community surveys are needed to determine social indicators of alcohol problems in the community (Westermeyer and Bearman, 1973). Then the identification of subpopulations and potential resources must be made in order to construct rational plans for overall community priorities for specific types of services (Biegel et al., 1974).

A community epidemiology approach addresses the following issues. What are the different subpopulations of alcoholics in the community? How many persons are in each subpopulation? Where is each subpopulation located? What facilities and resources exist to meet the rehabilitation needs of each subpopulation? To what extent do existing community resources fail to provide appropriate treatment resources for which subpopulations? What treatment resources need to be developed to meet the needs of which subpopulations? And finally, in what order of priority should treatment resources be developed in the community over time?

B. Facility Epidemiology

With the above perspective then, each individual facility must then determine where it fits most appropriately in the community collage of treatment resources. Each facility must identify the subpopulations it can best serve in relation to total community resources (Costello et al., 1976) and then determine base line data on its capacity to provide services, so that it can set realistic goals (Costello et al., 1973).

As with the community, Selig (1975) proposes that the agency establish its own epidemiological framework for program development. He suggests an eight-step process:

1. Value orientation (establishment of explicit assumptions basic to the program)
2. Problem identification (the extent of the problem, its history, its function in the system, attitudes about it)
3. Goal setting (explicit goals identified as immediate, intermediate, and long range with estimates of time needed to accomplish each level)
4. Goal-measuring criteria
5. Program planning
6. Program implementation
7. Assessment
8. Feedback (information learned from evaluation put back through the process and the program adapted accordingly)

C. Referral Processes and Problems

Studies of the career of alcoholics in various community agencies reveal that they are the "unwanted clients." Thus, although the alcoholic appears in the case load of many community agencies and caregivers, he or she is provided perfunctory treatment and shunted aside with "referral" to another agency (Cohen and Krause, 1971; Hunter, 1963). The result is that alcoholics often receive "nontreatment" when they do enter the network of commnity services (Pittman and Gordon, 1958). Their contacts with community agencies result in a dead-end blockade to further steps toward rehabilitation (Sterne and Pittman, 1965). Or they trudge from one frustrating blockade experience to the next as they follow the referral. Pittman and Sterne (1963) describe this referral wandering as "the Carousel." Obviously this is wasteful of the time and effort of the facilities and is certainly not therapeutic for the alcoholic.

Another aspect of referral involves the referral process itself, which is a psychodynamic interaction. The mere statement of the existence of a treatment resource cannot be considered a referral. Instead we must consider the referral process as part of the treatment process. This includes forming an initial relationship with the alcoholic so that he or she experiences this initial contact as useful and hopeful. Then an initial assessment must be made of the situation of the alcoholic, assisting him or her to identify the alcohol problem and to make a differential assessment, a diagnosis, of the type of alcoholism problems and associated life health problems which will require rehabilitation procedures. Once this assessment has been made, then appropriate referral to a treatment resource can take place. This would involve contact with the referral agency, discussion with the alcoholic client, and establishment of appropriate procedures so that the alcoholic can actually arrive at the referral agency. The referral process is complex, and the establishment of an effective referral network in the community requires a program of agency education, agency consultation, and ongoing working communication among the various agencies involved.

It is inappropriate to consider that one central agency will be "the" referral agency for a community, for this overlooks the fact that many alcoholics enter the community system for care through the portals of other agencies.

Another aspect of the referral process involves making an accurate assessment of where the alcoholic will accept referral that will "take." In an unpublished research project, Pattison and his co-workers studied the careers of more than 600 alcoholics in one community over a five-year period. They found that only 20% of the alcoholics followed through on referral and sought treatment at the primary referral facility. However, more than 60% of the alcoholics in the sample eventually sought treatment at one or more of the 22 facilities studied. One might argue that the alcoholic was not "motivated" at the time of referral. However, the weight of other studies described herein suggests that the referral process is very imprecise and ineffective. We may suggest that if referral were a more effective process, the alcoholic might be brought to a facility that was a good match, resulting in a successful entry into the rehabilitation system.

Another example of imprecision came out of the above study. In not one instance was a treatment facility found that referred the alcoholic to another treatment facility as a more appropriate match. It appears as if all alcoholism treatment facilities accept all alcoholics. The result is that the treatment facilities have a high level of "noise" in their system. Alcoholics are being run through a treatment program which is inappropriate and which has a high level of nonsuccess treatment cases, while the alcoholic experiences another episode of treatment failure. Changes in this interfacility relationship are requisite if we are to improve the overall effectiveness of a community system of rehabilitation.

D. Relations between Agencies and Programs

Comprehensive alcoholism rehabilitation has been considered in terms of either multiple competitive agencies or a single agency offering multiple treatments to all. The alternative model for a comprehensive community program is a *multiple-complementary* model. By this time it should be clear that this does not imply unitary views on the causes, treatment, or models of alcoholism. In fact, the failure to discriminate appropriately among the different prevailing viewpoints has been dysfunctional in terms of selective referral, selective treatment, and selective evaluation (Jongsma, 1970).

The relationship between alcoholism agencies, then, is a subset of the necessary relations between all community agencies. Many communities have developed interagency alcoholism councils, with varying degrees of bureaucratic function. Although their structure will vary from one community to another, there is one major issue that will affect treatment programs. That is, the degree to which an alcoholism coordinating agency reflects one ideological view or the degree to which it promotes recognition, respect, and need for involvement with divergent philosophies. I have observed community councils dominated by psychiatric, medical, or AA ideology, for example, to the exclusion of other views. The result is often functionally to exclude those segments of the community that are not ideologically congruent. This produces a dominant system of alcoholism services and a deviant system of alcoholism services. This sets the stage for antagonism rather than collaboration. And the relationship between agencies is then acted out with the alcoholic client as the pawn. In this situation, although there may be excellent resources and facilities, the destructive interaction of the social system may undercut the utilization of rehabilitation resources.

E. Relations between Programs and the Community

The health and welfare of alcoholism rehabilitation is intimately related to social and cultural attitudes (Linsky, 1970, 1972). An alcoholism treatment program that does not have community acceptance and support will atrophy. A program that does not have community sanction for innovative approaches or fails to meet felt community needs will experience negative community sanctions.

Finally, a comprehensive treatment program must involve itself in preventive programs. At first glance one might assume that a clinical treatment program is not directly related to preventive programs. To some extent this will vary among rehabilitation facilities. However, many treatment programs, whose mission is clinical rehabilitation, are directly involved with prevention issues. For example, the identified alcoholic represents a person who is influencing his or her family, spouse, and children. These "significant others" represent a high-risk group, both for the development of alcoholism and for other psychosocial disabilities (Wilkinson, 1970).

The referral network provides an opportunity for clinical personnel to establish working relations with community groups that shape attitudes toward drinking patterns; this might include churches, schools, and health agencies. Likewise, clinical working relationships may provide contact with business and industry groups that affect policies in regard to employee drinking patterns, food servicing patterns, advertisement policy, and the variety of legal processes and procedures related to alcohol use in the community.

IX. PHASE SEQUENCES OF TREATMENT: A MODEL

The frame of reference we have established now makes it feasible to consider selection of treatment not as one single event, but a *series of decision points* throughout the entire *community system* of alcoholism treatment. Thus we view selection of treatment from a *longitudinal* point of view as well as at a cross-sectional point in time.

Table 2 represents the rehabilitation process as a flowchart, in which alcoholic clients enter the alcoholism treatment system through multiple ports of entry. From this point onward we can identify seven phases of treatment, each of which involves selective treatment decisions. Ultimately the alcoholic client will exit from the treatment system back into multiple ongoing involvements in community relationships.

As illustrated, Phase A (identification) and Phase B (triage) involve Type I treatment decisions, which are *definitional*. That is, the decisions involve defining persons with alcohol problems, defining the nature of the problems, defining the appropriate resources for referral. These decision points are located in multiple agencies throughout the community, and may include churches, hospitals, social welfare agencies, business and industry, legal agencies, mental health services, etc. These decisions are the most generalized.

The next three phases, Phase C (entry), Phase D (initial treatment), and Phase E (goals and method selection) involve Type II treatment decisions, which are *procedural*. That is, the decisions revolve around methods to involve the alcoholic initially in the treatment process and

Table 2
Phase Sequences of Treatment

Phase A: Identification	Phase B: Triage	Phase C: Entry	Phase D: Initial Treatment	Phase E: Goals and Method Selection	Phase F: Treatment Maintenance/ Monitoring	Phase G: Termination and Follow-up
Agency 1		Facility 1				
Agency 2		Facility 2	R_x 1		Method 1	Community involvement 1
Agency 3	Decision process		R_x 2	Decision process	Method 2	Community involvement 2
Agency 4		Facility 3	R_x 3		Method 3	Community involvement 3
Agency n		Facility n				

Community →

Type I decisions (Definitional)	Type II decisions (Procedural)	Type III decisions (Evaluative)
Decision points located within multiple community agencies	Decision points located within alcoholism treatment facility	Decision points located within individual person with alcoholism syndrome

then conduct appropriate individual assessment as to which particular treatment goals and methods should be provided from among the options available within the treatment program. These decision points are located within each treatment facility; and the decisions are intermediate in specificity.

The final two phases, Phase F (treatment maintenance/monitoring) and Phase G (termination and follow-up), involve Type III treatment decisions, which are *evaluative*. That is, these decisions involve regular review of the client's progress toward stated treatment goals, appropriate utilization of specific treatment methods, assessment of individual progress toward termination, and specific individual plans for reinvolvement in community life. These decision points are therefore located within each individual, while the decisions are the most specific of all.

Thus we see that the rehabilitation process as a system involves multiple levels of decision making which range from the community to the individual. Different types of decisions are involved in each phase of the rehabilitation process, while the decisions become increasingly specific throughout the process. It is obvious that highly specific decisions in the early phases are just as inappropriate as highly global and generalized decisions are inappropriate in the later stages of rehabilitation. Optimally, decisions about treatment should be made within the overall framework of rehabilitation. In this manner, we can clearly define *what types of treatment decisions need to be made in each phase*.

Now we shall consider each phase in turn.

X. PHASE A: IDENTIFICATION

The person with alcohol problems is likely to appear in many service settings where identification can be made. The major problem is a stereotyped public image of alcoholism which equates the alcoholism syndrome solely with the skid row image of the alcoholic. However, this is a misleading stereotype, for it is estimated that only 5% of alcoholics are on skid row, and only 5% of the persons on skid row are alcoholic (Plaut, 1967). Thus the skid row alcoholic is *atypical*. The more typical alcoholic is likely to be employed, married, a church, lodge, or club member, and a respectable member of the community. Since the alcoholic person does not look or act like the stereotyped public image, the diagnosis is likely to be overlooked.

A second problem is a restricted focus on the most severe or end stages of alcohol syndromes. Thus, the person with mild to moderate alcohol problems is often not identified unless specific attention is given to careful diagnosis.

A third problem is that traditional diagnostic criteria emphasize frequency or quantity of drinking. Both are misleading. Increased frequency and quantity lead to high-risk drinking and are associated with a higher probability of alcoholismic dysfunction. Yet people with mild and moderate alcohol problems do not necessarily drink with abnormal frequency or in abnormal quantity.

The National Council on Alcoholism (1972) has published a set of diagnostic criteria guidelines. There are two sets of criteria: physical-clinical and behavioral-attitudinal-psychological. Unfortunately these guidelines only pinpoint late stages of severe alcoholism.

A diffuse but simple diagnostic criterion is this: *Alcoholism is any degree (mild, moderate, severe) of alcohol use which results in physical, emotional, interpersonal, or vocational dysfunction, or where alcohol is used to any degree in order to maintain or improve function*. In order to use this criterion, one must take a careful alcohol-use history. The history should detail the frequency, quantity, and circumstances of the patient's alcohol use. More importantly, this history should detail three specific items. (1) Does the person feel differently or experience himself or herself differently when drinking? (2) Does the person behave differently when drinking? (3) Does the person demonstrate any adverse consequences of drinking in terms of physical, emotional, interpersonal, or vocational function? The normal person who drinks in a moderate low-risk fashion will answer negatively to these three items. Where there is some degree of positive response we must *at least* assume that the person is engaging in high-risk drinking, and then we must explore detailed evidence for mild, moderate, or severe dysfunction in relation to alcohol use (Zimberg, 1982).

A word must be said about the accuracy of an alcohol-use history. It is popular to assert that alcoholics deny their alcoholism. This is true. But the denial is superficial. The alcoholic is fearful of judgment, rejection, or dismissal. Sobell and Sobell (1975) found that the accuracy of alcoholics' self-reports is directly related to the consequences of that report. The alcoholic gives an inaccurate history if the consequences will be negative; whereas where there may be positive consequences, the alcoholic does give highly accurate self-reports. Thus the challenge is to let the alcoholic know the positive benefits of providing an accurate history of his or her alcohol use.

The identification phase of treatment is often overlooked. Yet if adequate identification does not occur, several adverse consequences may follow: (1) The alcoholic may be reinforced in his or her rationalization, denial, or avoidance of facing his or her alcohol-related problems. (2) The alcoholic person may receive inappropriate or adverse treatment, as for example, the prescription of other addictive drugs. (3) There may be selective inattention to symptoms that further delay diagnosis of the alcoholism. (4) The alcoholic person may experience frustrating and demoralizing failure to gain appropriate attention and investigation of his or her alcohol problems. For example, Chafetz (1967) reports one emergency room study in which the alcoholic was seen diagnostically by 8–16 different persons before a diagnosis of alcoholism was made.

A variety of diagnostic tests for alcoholism have been developed, many of which have screening utility (Jacobson, 1976). However, the major problem is not screening adequacy, but rather the lack of knowledge about alcoholism syndromes and adequate use of diagnostic acumen among the initial contact agents in community agencies (Baekeland and Lundwall, 1977). Negativistic and nihilistic attitudes of these community contact agents is another major barrier to effective identification (Chafetz et al., 1962; Wolf et al., 1965).

Nevertheless, identification services can be effective. Corrigan (1974) found that in one Alcoholism Information and Referral center, 68% of those who called about their own alcohol problems and 57% of those others called about actually did enter the treatment system.

XI. PHASE B: TRIAGE REFERRAL

Once identification has been made, the next step involves referral to the appropriate treatment facility. However referral involves more than just the provision of information. Referral is an active process. The fact that identification alone is not sufficient is highlighted by Baekeland and Lundwall (1977), who recount that a family agency only referred 1 of 40 identified alcoholic clients, a welfare agency referred only 1 of 102, a police desk only 1 of 55, a social service department none. They go on to point out that 55% of community agencies had no systematic referral procedure, and that a hospital emergency room had only 5% successful referrals.

It is not that the alcoholic may not eventually show up somewhere at an alcoholism treatment facility, for Chameides and Yamamoto (1973) have shown that people eventually do find their way to community resources. But rather, the issue is whether the initial referral agencies are moving alcoholics to the facility that may most appropriately meet their needs.

To assure success, initial contact agents must develop a collaborative relationship with the alcoholic person, so that the alcoholic is receptive to referral. Second, there must be a mutual exploration with the alcoholic client of his or her perceptions, needs, and desires about the type of facility and treatment which are acceptable to the alcoholic. Third, the alcoholic must be given necessary assistance to make contact with the referral agency. This might even include making transportation available to get the alcoholic to the facility. Fourth, the more specific the time, place, and person who will meet the alcoholic at the referral facility the better. Fifth, it is important that the initial contact agent know the different programs and contact persons at those programs, so that personal arrangements can be made with the referral agency.

Admittedly some alcoholic clients will be difficult referral problems. However, they often experience high degrees of social alienation, and extra motivational effort on the part of the initial contact referral agents may likely pay off in a positive response (Calicchia and Barresi, 1975; Muller and Brunner-Orne, 1967). In addition to the above steps, it is important to eliminate waiting lists, for the longer an alcoholic waits before entry into the treatment system, the less likely he or she is to enter the system at all or succeed in treatment (Wanberg and Jones, 1977). Some programs have found that telephone and letter contact is an important additional means of moving the alcoholic into initial treatment (Cantazaro and Green, 1970; Koumans et al., 1965, 1967).

XII. PHASE C: PROGRAM ENTRY

Obviously, different alcohol treatment facilities vary in their requirements for admission to a program. In such specific programs the entry problem involves determination of whether the person meets the requirements. If he or she does not, that facility becomes an initial contact agency with responsibility to arrange effective triage referral to an appropriate alternative resource, so that the alcoholic does not get caught in agency revolving doors (Gallant et al., 1973).

On the other hand, let us consider the types of treatment decisions that are involved in alcoholism programs that receive several types of alcoholism syndromes on an open, public-access basis. Here we are faced with a relatively nonselected population.

The important first issue is to immediately receive the alcoholic into a personally oriented milieu. This is the principle of "immediate involvement." If extensive legal, fiscal, historical, and evaluative procedures are the first reception for the alcoholic, he or she is not likely to return. Rather the entry must be viewed as a *clinical emergency,* in which the first order of business is to respond to the immediate needs of the alcoholic person. Thus the point of entry is of critical importance (Mayer et al., 1965).

Several issues must be addressed at entry:
1. The personal anxiety, isolation, and alienation of the client should be reduced through the personal relationships of the entry personnel.
2. Denial and rationalization should be firmly resisted, but in such a manner as to affirm self-esteem and self-respect. Interactions that evoke shame or guilt should be avoided.
3. An initial attitude of hope and positive expectation should be offered.
4. Immediate needs for acute medical or psychiatric care should be assessed.
5. Immediate needs for amelioration of withdrawal symptoms should be provided.
6. Where clients need food, clothes, or housing, such resources should be available in collaboration with community resources.

Overall then, the entry phase involves general decisions relative to the immediate needs of the alcoholic. The goals at this point are to respond to emergency needs and to involve the alcoholic in a receptive emotional climate.

A. Decisions about Hospitalization

Specific criteria for hospitalization should be employed. An alcoholic should be admitted to an acute psychiatric hospital or a general hospital psychiatric unit when:

1. the patient is psychotic;
2. or the patient is severely depressed;
3. or the patient displays extreme behavior disorder.

In other words, psychiatric hospitalization should be provided when the patient has a psychiatric problem other than *his or her alcoholism,* and when the psychiatric problem is acute (Freed, 1969). It must be noted that almost all acutely ill alcoholics will demonstrate some degree of depression, thought disorganization, and behavior disorder. But these transient disturbances must be differentiated from an essentially psychotic rather than drunk demeanor. One exception is the so-called "24-hour schizophrenia syndrome" in which the patient appears to have classic psychotic schizophrenic symptoms while intoxicated. After a 24-hour sobering-up period the psychotic manifestations vanish. It is virtually impossible to make this differential diagnosis except after the fact.

An acute general hospital admission is indicated when the patient:

1. is unconscious or has evidence of a head injury;
2. is seriously hemorrhaging;
3. is in serious withdrawal with impending delirium tremens (not just drunk);
4. has a disulfiram-alcohol reaction;
5. has a fever;
6. is jaundiced or shows other signs of liver disease;
7. is convulsing;
8. is dehydrated or shows significant malnutrition and vitamin deficiency;
9. has any significant medical pathology judged serious enough for general hospital care.

Put simply, acute general hospital admission is necessary for any medical disorder, other than alcoholism, serious enough to require admission (Anderson and Weisman, 1970; Twerski, 1969).

Acute alcoholism syndromes are a confusing diagnostic melange. We can separate these syndromes into three groups: simple intoxication, acute withdrawal, and psychotic withdrawal.

The psychotic syndrome group includes alcoholic paranoia, alcoholic hallucinosis, alcoholic schizophreniform psychosis, and delirium tremens. In this group the paranoid and schizophreniform symptoms usually appear during the period of actual intoxication and disappear with sober-

Table 3
Differences between Intoxication and Major Withdrawal in the Alcoholic Patient

	Intoxication	*Major Withdrawal*
Frequency	Common	Less common
Onset	Immediately after drinking	24–72 hr after cessation
Duration	Hours	of drinking
Symptoms and	Slurred speech, staggering	Days
signs	gait, stupor	Tremor, hallucinations,
Blood alcohol level	Elevated	delirium, seizures
Response to alcohol	Aggravates the symptoms	Not elevated
Mortality	Rare	Decreases the symptoms
		10% with severe DT

ing up; whereas the clouding of sensorium, hallucinations, and motoric-seizure symptoms usually appear after sobering up. Yet this division of symptoms is not neat and clean, for Gross et al. (1972) find an overlap of about 50% of symptoms in these clinical categories.

There is a similar overlap in the symptomatology of intoxication and withdrawal states. Acute simple intoxication does indeed produce psychic and somatic distress, as anyone with a "hangover" can attest to. Mild withdrawal includes the symptoms of insomnia, irritability, and tremor, whereas major withdrawal in addition includes anxiety, agitation, diaphoresis, and disorientation. Acute intoxication can trigger seizures in epileptogenic vulnerable persons. Seizures are rare in mild withdrawal states. Major withdrawal states have a high probability, if untreated, of progressing to delirium tremens with the familiar seizures and hallucinations. The major differences are shown in Table 3.

One must also consider the other causes for delirium and psychotic symptomatology that may be the major etiology despite the fact that the patient has been drinking, or even is intoxicated, as shown in Table 4.

The intensity and severity of intoxication and withdrawal symptoms vary with the preceding alcohol exposure. Mild reactions to withdrawal appear during the sobering up period and usually dissipate within 48 hours. In severe withdrawal reactions, the symptoms begins to exacerbate as the blood alcohol level is falling and become most manifest in 48–60 hours. Delirium tremens occurs in less than 5% of hospitalized patients in major withdrawal. The mortality rate from delirium tremens has been at about 15% in the past, although the rate is dropping due to improved supportive treatment.

Most acutely intoxicated alcoholics are *not* withdrawal risks (Alsen, 1975). In the past expensive inpatient detoxication hospital units were built to provide for the management of withdrawal. Such units are rela-

Table 4
Common Nonalcoholic Causes for Delirium

Medical	Surgical	Metabolic	Drug	
			Intoxication	*Withdrawal*
Infection (particularly pneumonia)	Head trauma	Hypoxia	Bromides	Barbiturates
Thyrotoxicosis	Postanesthesia confusional states	Uremia	Steroids	"Tranquilizers"
Hypoparathyroidism	Brain tumor	Hypoglycemia	Stimulants	Opiates
Congestive heart failure	Fat embolus	Hepatic encephalopathy	Atropine	
	Pancreatitis	Water intoxication	Psychedelics	

tively unnecessary, however, because only a very small group of alcoholics require hospitalization for acute symptomatology and/or withdrawal management (Hague et al., 1976; Kissin, 1977; Knott and Fink, 1976).

In many parts of the country the need for detoxification triage and a simultaneous entry into a rehabilitation program have given rise to "social detoxification" centers. The management is similar to the outpatient regime described above, and they provide a 24-hour care capacity to interrupt the drinking and initiate intensive therapeutic encounter where patients are not likely to enter and remain in an outpatient program (O'Briant et al., 1973; Siegal, 1975).

B. Immediate Entry Decisions

As an example of the process of intake, Feldman et al. (1975) give the following description.

When a patient is accepted at clinic intake, a routine initial blood alcohol concentration breath test (BAC) is taken. If the client has no history of immediate drinking, has a BAC of zero, and shows no signs of withdrawal, medical evaluation is bypassed and the client enters the rehabilitation program. However, if the BAC is elevated or there is any complaint of withdrawal symptoms, the patient is referred for medical evaluation before entering into the rehabilitation program.

Medical evaluation is based on assessment of both the clinical state and the BAC. Because of the known high tolerance to alcohol in alcoholics, we do not depend solely on clinical symptoms. Thus a patient with a BAC of over 0.10 is routinely observed on site and monitored with sequential BACs until the BAC drops below 0.10.

The criteria for clinical management are outlined in Table 5. A patient with minimal clinical withdrawal symptoms and a BAC of 0 to 0.10 is not considered in medical danger. After medical evaluation, this type of patient is returned to intake for entry into the rehabilitation program the same day.

A patient with minimal withdrawal symptoms and a BAC of 0.10 to 0.30 is retained in the medical unit for observation and sequential BACs until it drops below 0.10. Outpatient detoxification procedures are initiated if this is clinically indicated. The patient is then returned to intake for triage into the rehabilitation program the same day.

Simple intoxication is clearly separated from clinical withdrawal symptoms. If there are clinical signs of simple intoxication without withdrawal symptoms, regardless of blood level, or if the BAC is over 0.30, regardless of degree of intoxication, the patient is remanded to his or her home or to a recovery station in the community to sober up. The family at

Table 5
Criteria for Medical Triage

Description of Clinical Withdrawal Symptoms	Blood Alcohol Concentration (BAC)	Initial Treatment Decision
Minimal	0	Return to rehabilitation intake
Minimal or none	Less than 0.10	Return to rehabilitation intake
Minimal	0.10–0.30	Medical observations; BAC monitor until BAC is less than 0.10; detoxification regimen; return to rehabilitation intake
None None (whether clinically intoxicated or not)	0.10–0.30 More than 0.30	Remand to home or recovery station to sober up; alert caretakers; set intake appointment for when sober
Moderate: psychomotor agitation, modest elevation in blood pressure, somatic complaints	Any level	Medical observation; BAC monitor until BAC is less than 0.10; detoxification regimen; return to rehabilitation intake
Severe: hallucinations, severe psychomotor agitation, convulsions, disorientation, marked elevation in blood pressure	Any level	Hospitalization

home or the staff at the recovery station are alerted to the patient's condition and advised to return the patient if withdrawal symptoms appear. The patient is given a return appointment for medical and intake evaluation the next day, when he or she is sober.

Patients with moderate clinical withdrawal symptoms, regardless of BAC level, are retained in the medical unit for observation and sequential BAC monitor. The patient is retained until clinical withdrawal symptoms moderate and the BAC has dropped below 0.10. Whenever possible this type of patient is then moved immediately into the rehabilitation program. Outpatient detoxification procedures are initiated and the patient is followed regularly in the medical unit while concomitantly involved in the rehabilitation program.

Referral to a private contracting alcoholism hospital is recommended if any of the following symptoms or combination of symptoms are considered clinically incompatible with outpatient detoxification: hallucinations, disorientation, impending delirium tremens, severely elevated blood pressure, acute emotional crisis posing a risk to life functions, or severe concomitant medical illness.

The acute detoxification services are provided by a staff of registered nurses with a physician consultant always available. A nursing assessment evaluates current physical withdrawal symptoms, current emotional stability, and associated medical complications. This assessment typically takes 30 to 40 minutes. A clinical treatment decision is then reached, with physician consultation if required. The medical unit retains and monitors the patient if necessary and returns the patient to initial rehabilitation program intake if possible. If the decision is for outpatient detoxification management, the alcoholic is provided with day-to-day medication management. Medication includes minor tranquilizers and anticonvulsants as indicated.

After careful observation and BAC monitor indicate that the patient may be released, he or she is given a return appointment for the next day to see one of the nurses on duty. The next visit also involves an evaluation by a nurse and appropriate medication and observation. Visits may be daily or spaced according to clinical indication until the patient is no longer symptomatic.

Every effort is made to integrate the detoxification program into the rehabilitation program from the moment the acute alcoholic presents himself or herself. The alcoholic is immediately met by an intake alcoholism counselor. This counselor obtains an assessment of the alcoholic's clinical state. An alcoholism history as well as personal, family, social, medical, and vocational histories are also obtained. If medical evaluation is required, the alcoholic is taken to the medical unit. After release from the medical unit, the alcoholic returns to the intake counselor, who then collects any intake data not obtained previously.

The intake counselor introduces the new alcoholic patient to one of the daily "new patient groups." This group provides an orientation to the clinic and a brief discussion about the nature of alcoholism and the goals of rehabilitation. The new alcoholic returns daily to the new patient group for more didactic information, socialization with other new patients, and involvement with the problem of alcoholism that is kept at a low level of emotional intensity. At the same time the new alcoholic is introduced in the Social Learning Center (SLC). The SLC provides an opportunity to meet alcoholics involved in rehabilitation, reading, recreation, and informal learning activities that focus on interaction with others in appropriate everyday activities. Emphasis is given to the experience of normal daily interaction.

Within the first week the intake counselor reviews the initial status of the new alcoholic at a staff conference, presenting a preliminary report of family resources, requirements for food, clothing, and housing, and needs for psychological, social, medical, and vocational services.

By the end of the second week the new alcoholic has usually passed through the subacute phases of withdrawal and has experienced intensive participation in the new patient group and in SLC activities. A second case review is made at this time and a definitive treatment plan is negotiated with the alcoholic client. Subsequent rehabilitation based upon individual needs for psychological, medical, social, and vocational services is then initiated.

Thus, upon first presentation of himself or herself for treatment, the acute alcoholic enters a total treatment program that simultaneously involves necessary acute detoxification services, subacute management, and immediate triage into a sequential rehabilitation program (Stinnett, 1982).

XIII. PHASE D: INITIAL TREATMENT PROCESSES

Although the entry phase is in itself part of the treatment process, the focus of the entry phase is upon the immediate life situation of the alcoholic. As we move into the initial process of treatment, the problem shifts to the transition of the alcoholic person from that of an outsider to becoming a member of the treatment environment. If the alcoholic person does not find a "place" for himself or herself in this new therapeutic arena, there is a high likelihood that he or she will drop out of treatment after initial contacts. The magnitude of the dropout problem is exemplified in a review by Baekeland and Lundwall (1977). They found that in inpatient settings the dropouts ranged from 13–40%, while in outpatient settings dropouts ranged from 52–75%. They report that the alcoholic most likely to drop out of an inpatient program is in a more advanced stage of alcoholism, has more passive-aggressive and psychopathic features, is more apt to deny his hostility, suspicion, and interpersonal problems, and depends on alcohol for relief of feelings of resentment, anxiety, or depression. In contrast the outpatient dropout is typically field dependent, counterdependent, highly symptomatic, a socially isolated lower-class person of poor social stability, who is highly ambivalent about treatment and has psychopathic features.

A. Remedies against Early Dropout

Although alcoholics may present themselves initially for treatment because of acute problems, the acute motivation will shortly wear off. Thus the initial treatment phase must support and enhance more durable motivations to continue in treatment. For example, Gerard and Saenger (1966) found that only 20% of "motivated" outpatient alcoholics returned after four visits. In fact, *initial* expressed motivation is *not* an accurate predictor of either continuance in treatment or successful outcome. Rather, Gerard and Saenger (1966) found that three variables predicted retention: (1) The patient received medications; (2) the patient was immediately involved in peer group activities; and (3) the family and significant others were quickly involved in the rehabilitation process.

Along similar lines, Baekeland and Lundwall (1977) offer seven commandments to involve the alcoholic person: (1) Eliminate waiting lists and offer immediate entry. (2) Satisfy the patient's dependency needs by offering as wide a range of ancillary services as possible. (3) Offer a variety of treatment modalities to the patient and apply that which is best suited to him or her rather than that which is easiest or simply happens to be available. (4) Explain clearly to the patient the aims, scope, probable results, side effects, and duration of the kind of treatment to which he or she is assigned and make sure the patient understands his or her role in it. (5) Find out whether the patient has previously dropped out of treatment. If he or she has, explore the reasons for it thoroughly and right away. Do not allow the patient to store up unverbalized resentments, and let the person know he or she can express negative feelings toward the program, methods, or personnel without fear of retribution. (6) Maintain contact with significant others and enlist their help. (7) In more symptomatic patients, put a major emphasis on rapid symptom relief, and do not withhold medication during initial treatment where it may help.

B. General Treatment Processes

Now it is important to emphasize the *general* aspects of treatment during this initial phase. If the alcoholic person experiences any significant withdrawal symptoms, there may be important cognitive and affective impairment for several weeks. Just because the alcoholic is sober does not mean that there are not important mental impairments that will interfere with perception, feelings, thought, and judgment. And even if there is no organic impairment, there still may be considerable anxiety, confusion, depression, fear, anger, apathy, withdrawal, suspicion, resentment, frustration, and alienation. This long list merely highlights the very real turmoil the alcoholic person is likely to experience during the initial treatment phase. Thus the initial phase is *not* the time to introduce complex and long-term treatment planning. Rather, we should emphasize general treatment experiences that are: (1) supportive, (2) symptom-relieving, (3) reality-oriented, (4) nonthreatening, and (5) option-oriented.

In other words, the initial treatment phase is a *preparatory* treatment experience. As Hoehn-Saric et al. (1964) have shown, patients are more apt to engage successfully in therapy if they participate in preliminary educational and socialization experiences that prepare them to consider more definitive treatment experiences. Orne and Wender (1968) term this "anticipatory socialization."

There are several means by which general treatment experiences can be offered to the alcoholic person. First, initial intake group experiences can provide a nonthreatening opportunity to learn about alcoholism problems, share experiences with others, and become acquainted with other patients (Gallant et al., 1966; Pattison et al., 1965). Second, educational lectures and informational orientation sessions can provide objective information and reality orientation without personally challenging the unstable emotional equilibrium of the new patient (Pattison et al., 1971; Suchotliff and Meyer, 1975). Third, recreational, occupational, and socialization activities with groups of patients can provide a natural vehicle for promoting interpersonal relationships among fellow patients and with staff (Androes and Whitehead, 1966; Cantor, 1969; Slaughter and Torno, 1968). This process of relationship building is aptly termed "familization" by Catanzaro et al. (1973). Fourth, spouses, family, relatives, and friends can be brought into the treatment milieu to participate in both formal and informal groups, discussions, and socialization experiences (Berman, 1968; Corder et al., 1972; Pattison et al., 1965; Sands and Hanson, 1971; Wedal, 1965).

In sum, the initial treatment phase does not focus on the individual alcoholic, but rather seeks to involve the alcoholic person with the program, the program staff, with other patients, and with significant others. In this manner, a new social environment is created which can support and engender a *shared motivation* toward continuation in treatment.

XIV. PHASE E: SELECTION OF GOALS AND METHODS OF TREATMENT

To follow a typical pattern of treatment sequences, once the alcoholic person has had several weeks to attain physical, cognitive, and emotional stability, it is time to develop a more specific and definitive long-term rehabilitation treatment plan.

During the initial treatment phase many programs have found it useful to introduce the alcoholic person to the various types of treatment methods and treatment goals that may be considered; Ewing (1977) calls this the "cafeteria experience." The important emphasis here is on *collaborative* treatment planning, in which the alcoholic actively participates in assessing his or her treatment needs, realistic and appropriate treatment goals, and acceptable and desirable treatment methods.

A. Principles of Differential Assessment

Again it is important to reiterate that long-term treatment planning must focus on multiple areas of life function. A focus on change in drinking behavior alone is not likely to affect other areas of life function. And conversely, treatment plans which ignore the drinking per se are likely to fail. For our purposes, I shall continue to use the five life health areas of Drinking Health, Emotional Health, Interpersonal Health, Vocational Health, and Physical Health. However, I should note that there are numerous ways to define treatment-specific target areas. The important point is to focus on particular areas of the individual alcoholic's life that will become targets for change (Belasco, 1971; Costello, 1975; Selig, 1975).

The first step is a functional analysis of the behavior of the individual alcoholic (Sobell et al., 1976). This involves a careful inventory in specific terms of where, when, how, and why the person drinks. In addition, this should include an assessment of how drinking changes the person's behavior, how others respond, and how the alcoholic reacts to his or her own drinking. Thus one develops a picture of the *functional use of alcohol* in this person (Bowman et al., 1975; Little et al., 1977; Shelton et al., 1969).

The second step is to assess where this person is in life. That is, we must assess the person's life, functional ability, coping capacity, and resources aside from the drinking behavior per se. Drinking behavior may be part of an early, middle, or late drinking career (Clark, 1976; Fillmore, 1975; Hymen, 1976; Mulford, 1977).

The third step is to assess the alcoholic's personally expressed needs (Hart, 1977). This can then be used to determine what changes are both *possible* and personally *desirable*. One can then construct a *relative change index* (Stallings and Oncken, 1977). This means a definition of three items for each area of life health:

1. The degree of *disability* in each area of life health;
2. The degree to which change is *feasible* in each area of life health;
3. The degree to which this individual wishes to *commit* himself or herself and *personally work* toward attainment of those goals.

This then produces a systematic frame of reference within which specific treatment interventions can be planned for *each* area of life health, taking into account both the *degree of impairment* and the *potential for change*.

This process can be illustrated by reference to the four treatment facilities previously described. In Table 6 I list a differential assessment of disability for each area of Life Health for each of the four populations. As can be seen, at the time of admission all were quite different in terms of their profiles of differential disability. In the same table I list the degree of expected change. Note that again we have different profiles of expected change. The ACH population are "high bottom" alcoholics. They have little disability in most areas, and hence have little need for improvement in most areas and will show modest evidence of changes in their life as a result of treatment. The major change to be expected is in their drinking. The OPC population has more disability and will show more improvement and change in their total Life Health. The HWH population has severe disability in almost every area, but they also have a high potential for rehabilitation. These are the classic alcoholics whose lives have been disintegrated by alcoholism. They will show the most dramatic improvement and change. The PWF population are the skid row, "low bottom" alcoholics. They too have great dysfunction in all areas of Life Health. But unlike the HWH population, they have little potential for rehabilitation. Hence we can predict little improvement or change. This chart illustrates the necessity to describe carefully the precise disabilities for each subpopulation of alcoholics, and also the need to describe the degree of potential improvement that can be expected.

Finally, it is important to note that not all alcoholics are impaired, or impaired to the same extent, in each area of Life Health. Neither does impairment in one area necessarily bear a high correlation with impairment in other areas of Life Health. But if we do consider selection of treatment methods and goals in terms of specific target areas, it is then possible to construct *individual specific treatment profiles*.

B. Definition of Drinking Goals

Over the past 15 years one of the major changes in alcoholism treatment has been a reexamination of treatment goals in terms of drinking behavior. Although controversial, this is an important area of treatment selection to examine in detail (Pattison, 1976a, 1976b).

The importance of initial abstinence has been repeatedly demonstrated to correlate highly with continuing in treatment and eventual successful outcome of treatment (Armor et al., 1977; Baekeland, 1977). However, as we move from the initial phase of treatment into definitive

Table 6
Differential Treatment Goal Profiles for Four Alcoholic Groups

Target Health Area	Aversion Hospital		Outpatient Clinic		Halfway House		Police Farms	
	Disability on Admission	Predicted Degree Improvement	Disability on Admission	Predicted Degree Improvement	Disability on Admission	Predicted Degree Improvement	Disability on Admission	Predicted Degree Improvement
Drinking	4	4	4	4	4	4	4	2
Interpersonal	1	1	2	2	4	4	4	1
Emotional	1	1	3	3	4	4	4	1
Vocational	0	0	1	1	4	4	4	1
Physical	1	1	0	0	2	2	4	3

Disability ratings are on a scale of 0–4, with 0 = no disability, and 4 = highest disability.
Degree of improvement ratings are on a scale of 0–4, with 0 = no improvement, 4 = greatest degree of improvement.

individual treatment plans, it then becomes appropriate to consider individual potential, interest, and commitment to different types of drinking goals. A drinking goal which is neither possible nor desirable for a given alcoholic may be pursued by the staff, but not by the patient. Therefore, it is important to emphasize that collaborative agreement on drinking goals in treatment is just as important as collaborative agreement in other target areas of planned intervention (Orford, 1973; Popham and Schmidt, 1976).

The criterion goal of total abstinence implies that if the alcoholic achieves abstinence he will also demonstrate improvement in the other four areas of Life Health. However, empirical data do not support this assumption. Pattison et al. (1966, 1968) presented empirical and clinical data to illustrate that abstinent alcoholics often did not exhibit improvement in these other areas of Life Health, and in fact some abstinent alcoholics showed *deterioration* in these other four areas. The most significant study has been that by Gerard et al. (1962). In their evaluation of a group of totally abstinent "successes" they found 43% independent successes. Thus abstinence does *not* necessarily indicate *rehabilitation*.

Case Example: This 56-year-old white salesman had been a compulsive drinker since age 18. He had asthma and stuttered. He was plagued with guilt feelings and inability to express himself in social situations. He was in treatment for 5 years. He had been abstinent for 2 years, yet he continually feared a relapse. He felt psychotherapy helped him understand his conflicts, but he ascribed his sobriety to intensive participation in AA. Although he enjoyed his sobriety, he had multiple neurotic complaints that interfered with social function; so he stayed at home most of the time, where his wife sheltered him. He could not work effectively because of his inhibitions, and he was so dependent on his wife that he could not assume any assertive role with her. Any anxiety or frustration would precipitate psychosomatic symptoms.

In this case, we see a man who is abstinent, but who has major dysfunctions in the emotional area, vocational area, interpersonal area, and physical area.

On the other side of the abstinence coin, it had been assumed that alcoholics who did drink were not successfully treated. This assumption was not examined in most of the earlier evaluation studies which did not examine other Life Health areas. It was merely assumed that if an alcoholic was not abstinent, he or she was not rehabilitated. A series of reports, beginning with Davies in 1962, have shown that alcoholics do develop the capacity to change their drinking patterns and attain a successful life adjustment (Pattison, Sobell, and Sobell, 1977; Heather and Robertson, 1981).

In summary, the use of total abstinence as the outcome criterion of alcoholism treatment is misleading. It may be associated with improvement, no change, or deterioration in other critical areas of total Life Health.

The focus on abstinence tends to obscure attention that should be given to treatment methods aimed at rehabilitation in other areas of Life Health. And abstinence may be neither a necessary nor a desirable goal in terms of a drinking outcome.

Therefore, we shall turn to consideration of several subsets of drinking goals that can be considered.

1. The Abstinence Subset

Although we have challenged the use of abstinence as the sole or primary criterion for evaluation of treatment outcome, abstinence may be a feasible outcome goal. However, two caveats must be made. First, abstinence should only be considered as a subset goal for the drinking variable and not be used as an inferential indication of change in any of the other areas of Life Health. Second, abstinence is only one of several possible subsets in the Drinking Health variable outcome. There is no logical justification for assuming that abstinence is a more desirable or superior drinking outcome than any other drinking outcome, per se. Rather, it may be more appropriate to determine the circumstances under which abstinence is the necessary or desirable drinking outcome and the circumstances where it may be a less desirable outcome or where it may be desirable but not achievable. In the latter case, one would accept a different drinking outcome as successful.

2. The Social Drinking Subset

"Social drinking" is a vague and ambiguous term, for it merely states that one drinks among other people. It does not specify the meaning, function, amount, or result of drinking. Hayman (1967) calls this "The Myth of Social Drinking," for the rubric of social drinking may only obscure, justify, and rationalize many dysfunctional, dyssocial, and psychopathological forms of alcoholismic drinking in social settings. This does not seem to be an appropriate or useful concept. Therefore, I suggest we discard the term "social drinking."

3. The Attenuated Drinking Subset

Recognition that continued drinking might not indicate a poor rehabilitation has occasioned research that differentiates between the drinking variable and other Life Health variables.

One of the best studies, from a methodological point of view, was conducted by Ludwig et al. (1970). They found that although 80–90% of patients returned to their previous patterns of pathological drinking, there was sustained improvement in all other areas of Life Health. They conclude: "Return to drink need not be automatically equated with return to all the maladaptive behaviors which lead to mental hospitalization in the first place. . . . Most patients are able to carry on most of their other social tasks, at least at a higher level than that noted on hospital admission."

Other recent studies support the concept that following treatment the alcoholic may show no change in his drinking pattern, or only modest improvement, and yet profit from treatment as evidenced by better adjustment in the other four areas of Life Health. For example, Mayer and Myerson (1971) report on alcoholics who achieved stability and drank less even though still experiencing episodes of insobriety. Gillis and Keet (1969) report that 58% of their sample showed significant improvement in life adjustment although still drinking. At the same time the *extent* of pathological drinking was reduced from 70% of drinking episodes to 20% of drinking episodes. In this same sample some 47% had improved drinking habits without deterioration, while 23% improved in drinking but showed some deterioration of overall function. Fitzgerald et al. (1971) found that of their alcoholic sample, 22% with good adjustment were abstinent, 19% with good adjustment were drinking, while 18% with poor adjustment were drinking. Kish and Hermann (1971) report 22% of improved alcoholics were abstinent, while 26% of improved alcoholics were occasionally or regularly engaged in alcoholismic drinking.

This is suggestive evidence that some moderation in the amount of alcohol intake, the frequency of drinking, the degree of intoxication (all measures of increased control) do have a correlation with improvement in other areas of Life Health. We do not know which particular measures of modification of pathological drinking may be more significant for overall adaptation. But the evidence is beginning to accumulate that continued pathological drinking may not be a dire indicator of treatment failure. Further, the goal of modification or attenuation of the degree of pathological drinking may be an acceptable goal in conjunction with improvement in other areas of Life Health. It may not be an ideal goal, but it may suffice to return an alcoholic to a degree of successful life function. On the other hand, if we ignore these facts, we may fail to help an alcoholic achieve at least some degree of improvement, or fail to help him or her see and utilize the real gains he or she may have made in several areas. And finally, it may avert our attention from the fact that successful treatment does not have to be all or nothing. Degrees of improvement are realistic goals.

Thus it is possible to set as a treatment goal the modification of the severity of the drinking pattern, such that the alcoholic continues to drink in an alcoholic fashion, but in an attenuated fashion. The result may be a shift from an incapacitating alcoholic state to a pattern of successful adaptation despite ongoing alcoholismic drinking.

In summary, the subset of attenuated drinking defines a drinking goal in which *pathological drinking is not eliminated, but is attenuated.*

> *Case example:* This 46-year-old single male lives with his widowed mother. For five years his drinking increased until he had no control over his drinking intensity. He drank daily, usually to intoxication, often until he passed out. His job as a warehouseman was in jeopardy. He was "fed up" with his drinking, while his mother urged that he seek treatment. He had several interviews at an Alcoholism Information Center, but he refused any further treatment. His drinking subsequently subsided. He stated that the few interviews were enough for him to see his problems and alter his behavior. Now 4 years later he drinks only on specific occasions, usually alone. He will usually drink to intoxication on those occasions, but he does not pass out anymore. He is no longer absent from work and has no problems in job performance.

4. The Controlled Drinking Subset

The development of behavior modification programs for alcoholics has stimulated attention in regard to a drinking goal that is defined not by attenuation, but by the establishment of control over the drinking situation, the frequency of drinking, or the amount of alcohol drunk. This does not mean that the meaning or functional use of alcohol has necessarily been changed, but rather that the alcoholic is able to control his or her drinking within limits that are not dysfunctional.

Many behavior modification programs build learning procedures for change in both drinking and other areas of Life Health. All make an attempt to analyze the pattern of drinking with the alcoholic, specify the changes to be made, and program a reinforcement schedule to achieve the desired behavior goals. Usually there is no attempt to change the internal motivation, meaning, or function of drinking alcohol.

Perhaps an illustration by analogy will help here. Suppose that we have a voyeur who peeps into the neighbors' windows every night. Eventually he is caught and enters a treatment program. The voyeur might be taught to control his "peeping-tom" impulses so that he no longer prowls the neighborhood. His basic sexual problems are not changed, but he has increased his control over his impulse to peep. Still further, he might be taught to satisfy his voyeuristic impulses by going to strip-tease shows rather than peering into windows. Again his sexual problem remains unchanged, but he learns a more socially adaptive means of gratifying his sexual impulses.

In similar fashion, behavior modification may not change the basic psychological problems that lead to impulsive alcoholismic drinking.

However, the behavior modification program may increase the control over the impulses, or provide alternative means of gratifying the impulses. (The defense mechanism of displacement can be seen elsewhere. For example, many abstinent alcoholics have displaced their addiction to alcohol with an addiction to food, candy, coffee, and cigarettes.)

Since alcoholismic drinking results in manifold disruptions in a person's capacity to function, it may be only necessary to control the alcoholismic behavior in some instances in order to affect substantial rehabilitation. Also, in this case, even if the basic conflicts and impulses remain unchallenged and untouched, the achievement of controlled drinking may be possible. The notion that the alcoholic has a "craving" for drink that will lead to alcoholismic drinking if he or she starts with one drink, is unsubstantiated by much recent research. The alcoholic can and does control his or her drinking, and can be taught to increase that control. However, it should be noted that control of drinking per se, just like abstinence or moderation of drinking per se, does not necessarily imply that there will be improvement in other areas of Life Health.

Case example: A 36-year-old machinist had drunk heavily since adolescence. Drinking became a compulsive daily routine that threatened to disrupt his job and marriage. He was in therapy for two years during which he noticed a change in his pattern of drinking. He now drinks about once a week and does not experience a compulsion to drink more. However, when he feels depressed he feels the urge to go and get drunk. He avoids drinking at bars because he would drink more with buddies than he would at home.

Case example: A 45-year-old musician had drunk compulsively for twenty years. He had been in psychoanalysis for five years which improved his emotional adaptation, but his drinking worsened to the point that he could not perform in public. During the course of two years of therapy focused on drinking behavior change, he learned to limit himself to one drink before a performance and to avoid drinking at parties. He occasionally would drink to intoxication at home when severely depressed.

In both of these cases the alcoholic changed his overt pattern of drinking. To the casual observer neither now drank in an alcoholic fashion. However, in both cases, they were aware of their continued impulse to use alcohol in order to cope with life, and both had to maintain specific conscious limits on where and how much they drank. The meaning of drinking was not changed, but the actual drinking was changed.

5. The Normal Drinking Subset

Many reports have now been published that indicate that a certain proportion of alcoholics, perhaps 10–15%, develop normal drinking either after treatment, or with changes in life circumstances. However, many of these reports do not provide enough clinical data to determine whether the change in drinking pattern was "attenuated," controlled, or normal drinking.

In both the "attenuated" drinking outcome and the "controlled" drinking outcome the alcoholic continues to use alcohol as a functional drug, although he or she is able to increase control over its use. In other words, the alcoholic has not changed his or her symbolic perception of the meaning of drinking. The same is true for the typical abstinent alcoholic, who differs from the above two categories only in that he or she maintains total control over drinking. Although the abstinent alcoholic may not have taken a drink for 10 or 20 years, he or she is still vulnerable to abuse of alcohol should he or she even drink small amounts. So for example, many abstinent alcoholics may say: "What? Stop with one drink? Who would want to do that? That would spoil drinking. If I could only take one drink, I wouldn't want to learn that. It's all or nothing. So it's better to be abstinent." The one drink breaks the defensive control barrier and there are no stopping places beyond; thus the common observation that the abstinent alcoholic cannot take a drink without risking loss of control and starting alcoholismic drinking again.

In contrast, achieving a normal drinking pattern involves a change in the symbolic meaning of drinking. It is worth noting that many alcoholics have never been normal drinkers. They drank in alcoholic fashion from the time of their first drink, even though they exercised control over their alcoholic behavior. Thus they did not perceive themselves, nor did others perceive them as drinking in this fashion because they considered their drinking pattern to be "appropriate social drinking."

We commonly observe that alcoholics will report 20 years of "social drinking" after which they "suddenly" became alcoholic. Careful analysis of their social drinking behavior reveals that actually they engaged in controlled alcoholismic drinking for 20 years, conducted in social settings where the drinking was not defined as aberrant. So in actuality we have a 20-year history of prodromal alcoholism with gradual development of secondary effects that reaches such a manifest level that the person is suddenly labeled an overt alcoholic.

The import for treatment is that the alcoholic does not return to normal drinking, for he or she has never been a normal drinker. Rather the alcoholic must learn normal drinking for the first time in his or her life and must change the symbolic meaning of alcohol and change his or her use of alcohol. Most treatment programs have not made such goals explicit. Thus the number of alcoholics who develop attenuated, controlled, or normal drinking may not reflect what can be achieved in treatment. There are some indications, however, Gerard and Saenger (1966) report, that the normal drinking outcome appears to vary with treatment philosophy and whether normal drinking is made a specific goal. DeMorsier and Feldmann (1952) followed 500 cases in which 15% achieved a social cure as a deliberate goal. A social cure was defined as avoiding the psychological bad effects of drinking, changing their attitude toward drinking, and drinking only in a family and social context.

> *Case example:* This 30-year-old mechanic had drunk heavily for ten years. For six years he had been unable to work steadily because of his drinking. His marriage had been stormy and his wife had left him at the time he entered treatment. At that point he was depressed and suicidal. Individual and conjoint marital therapy resulted in resolution of marital conflict. He stopped drinking and obtained a steady job. He resumed drinking only at family gatherings with his wife's full acceptance. He experienced no compulsion to drink. He had no desire to get drunk, and he felt no need to drink as a way of coping with his life.

In summary, differential drinking-goal profiles are just beginning to be introduced into rational treatment selection and planning. The clinical and experimental data are too sparse to justify very specific guidelines. However, an example of how we may approach such differential selection is illustrated in Table 7, which again uses our four treatment facilities as a model for analysis.

XV. PHASE F: TREATMENT MAINTENANCE/MONITORING

Once a definitive long-term treatment plan has been agreed upon and developed, then a process of treatment maintenance must be developed. It cannot be assumed that once an alcoholic person has agreed upon and commenced treatment that no further treatment decisions need be made.

Blane (1977) has pointed out that the early, middle, and late stages of treatment each contain pitfalls and problems. This is particularly true for the alcoholic, where major disappointments, frustration, relapses, and continuing real life problems may be very much part of the rehabilitation process. In particular, Wellman (1955) has pointed out the sense of "fatigue" that an alcoholic may experience after six months or so, when the realistically difficult road toward rehabilitation may seem endless.

During this time then, it is important to regularly *monitor* the progress of the alcoholic in terms of achievement in *each* target area of intervention. In this manner, both the alcoholic patient and the treatment personnel can determine where actual progress has been made, which can serve to realistically maintain treatment morale. Where progress is *not*

Table 7
Possible Differential Drinking Goals for Four Alcoholic Groups

Drinking Goals	Aversion Hospital	Outpatient Clinics	Halfway House	Police Farm
Abstinent	Primary X	X	Primary X	Problematic X
Social*	–	–	–	–
Attenuated	Problematic X	Problematic X	Problematic X	Primary X
Controlled	X?	X?	X?	
Normal		Primary X		

X Primary: Goal most likely to be achieved in terms of treatment offered.
X Problematic: Goal that may be achieved but is unlikely or difficult to attain because of the psychosocial problems of that alcoholic group.
X? Goal that may be achievable, but sufficient data not yet available.
* Social drinking subset is listed here only to indicate that it is a vacuous goal that has no operational meaning.

being made, this offers an opportunity to reexamine both goals and intervention methods for that target area. *Renegotiation* of treatment experience suggests modification. Larkin (1974) has described the use of the Problem Oriented Record as one useful clinical device to carefully and regularly monitor patient progress in each area of targeted intervention.

Thus clinical assessment at regular intervals provides a series of treatment decision points. This can alert treatment staff to undue drug prescriptions (Rosenberg, 1974), undue psychological dependence (Rosenberg and Amodeo, 1974), failure to participate (Baekeland and Lundwall, 1975), or failure to move toward stated goals (Matijevic and Parenovic, 1973).

When patients fail to keep appointments it is imperative that treatment staff initiate immediate contact. For if allowed silently to drop out, the alcoholic is likely to relapse. On the other hand, aggressive efforts to retain patients are likely to be successful. For example, Panepinto and Higgins (1969) found that immediate phone calls reduced dropouts from 79% to 28%.

In summary, this phase of treatment involves:
1. Regular assessment of progress in each target area of intervention;
2. Renegotiation of treatment goals and methods when necessary and appropriate;
3. Aggressive follow-up on patients who do not involve themselves, fail to attend scheduled treatment, or are otherwise nonparticipatory.

XVI. PHASE G: TERMINATION AND FOLLOWUP

In many ways the alcoholism syndrome can be viewed as a "life-style." Thus as the person's life becomes more involved and revolves around the use of alcohol, that person begins to live the "world of alcoholism." Just because the person stops abusing alcohol does not automatically lead to an effective new life. In fact, one major aspect of alcoholism rehabilitation involves reentry and reinvolvement in the "world of nonalcoholics." Thus rehabilitation of the alcoholic is more than just the application of effective treatments. It also involves assisting the alcoholic to effectively move back into normalized interpersonal and community life. Roman and Trice (1968) term this "delabelling."

This requires that the alcoholic patient be carefully prepared for a new life-style. This is where Alcoholics Anonymous has perhaps made its most outstanding contribution, in teaching its members how to live in society. Most professional treatment programs have neglected this aspect of rehabilitation. Thus it is not unusual to see "treatment" of the alcoholic described as something that is "done" for a "period of time."

An alternative concept is to view professional treatment programs as one phase of rehabilitation. Thus, when therapeutic relationships are terminated, the alcoholic person is established in ongoing relationships with others in his or her ongoing life who continue to provide emotional, psychological, and social support, feedback, correction, sustenance, guidance, and nurturance. This is the "natural psychosocial support system," which everyone needs (Pattison, 1976).

From this point of view, the final phase of rehabilitation involves selection of appropriate means and methods to provide these ongoing psychosocial support systems for the alcoholic after formal treatment termination.

One method for provision of ongoing support and guidance is through affiliation with Alcoholics Anonymous. For those persons who accept AA, this can be a very feasible follow-up procedure.

A second method is the provision of follow-up group therapy or group alumni meetings (Pokorny et al., 1973; Gillis and Keet, 1969; Hansen and Teilmann, 1954; Moore and Ramseur, 1960; Ritson, 1971). Follow-up letters and phone calls are also used to keep in contact with patients after formal termination (Tarleton and Tarnower, 1960).

A third method is to explore deliberately the psychosocial relationships of the alcoholic patients, and then proceed to develop and enrich those community relationships, so that by the time of termination an effective network has been established to receive the alcoholic person. In this case, then, it is possible to effect a gradual transition from the social environment of the treatment facility to the social environment of the community (Dalton et al., 1972; Dubourg, 1969; Finlay, 1966; Hunt and Azrin, 1973; Ward and Faillace, 1970). The importance of this final phase of rehabilitation is shown by Simpson and Webber (1971) who term this the "field program" of rehabilitation, that is, planning the means to move the alcoholic patient out into the field of the community.

XVII. GUIDELINES FOR TREATMENT SELECTION

Our current state of knowledge about treatment is still too global and imprecise to formulate exact treatment guidelines. Our measurement and evaluation methods are too crude to assess our methods accurately. Nevertheless, the accumulation of research to date does strongly suggest the value of *matching* subpopulations of alcoholics with the most appropriate *facilities, methods,* and treatment *personnel* (Pattison, 1982).

Further, our analysis of *phases* of rehabilitation point up the value of selective treatment decisions appropriate to each phase of treatment.

Finally, our data on treatment planning emphasize the importance of long-term *individual* treatment plans. Treatment should involve the alcoholic person in a collaborative planning process that defines specific target areas of disability, degrees of impairment, potential for change, individual preferential choice of goals and methods for intervention in each target area, and regular sequential assessment of treatment progress in each target area.

I should like to conclude this chapter with some *clinical* principles which are based on the research data reviewed herein. These are summary guidelines that the *working clinician* might reasonably employ in making treatment decisions.

A. Facility Principles

One, each clinical facility should examine their own population clientele to determine what type of alcoholic subpopulation they predominantly serve.

Two, each facility should determine which treatment methods they can best offer that are relevant to the population they serve.

Three, the facility should discard treatment methods that are irrelevant to their population and discard treatment methods that they cannot effectively deliver.

Four, clientele should be *prescreened* so that only those alcoholics are accepted into a program to whom realistically relevant services can be given.

Five, a facility should provide effective *referral* and *transfer* mechanisms for the inappropriate clientele, so that those alcoholics are successfully placed in a program suited for them elsewhere.

Six, a facility should provide a *group* of alternative treatment approaches so that the alcoholic client may select the treatment approach most suited to his or her personal preference.

Seven, the alcoholic client should be actively engaged in the process of *mutual selection* of treatment methods and selection of treatment goals.

Eight, a treatment program should provide continuity of care through each phase of rehabilitation or, if necessary, provide careful transfer of the alcoholic from phase to phase to different facilities. Programs that deal with only one phase of alcoholism rehabilitation without specific linkages are likely to be ineffective.

Nine, a facility should provide ancillary services, directly or in careful collaboration with other community agencies. These include provision of shelter, food, clothes, welfare support, legal aid, and vocational rehabilitation.

Ten, inpatient alcoholism programs are likely to be ineffective if they do not provide for continuing outpatient care after discharge.

Eleven, short-term inpatient programs of less than 3–4 weeks are likely not to engage alcoholics in a rehabilitative process; whereas lengthy programs of over six weeks are likely to foster withdrawal from self-sufficiency and create dependency upon the institution.

Twelve, programs that offer indiscriminate treatment, without specific individualized treatment plans, or offer only a general domicile milieu, are likely to be ineffective, whereas carefully organized, logical treatment programs with specific individual plans are likely to be more effective.

B. Population Principles

One, simple psychological and social data are likely to provide better indicators for treatment selection than any available complex tests and measurements.

Two, a history of prior attainment of successful social and psychological adaptation is positively correlated with treatment success, regardless of the treatment.

Three, clients who are currently functioning well in psychological, social, vocational, and physical areas of life but who are nevertheless drinking in an abusive pattern may likely not accept psychological treatment, but may be good candidates for aversive-conditioning hospital programs, or alcoholism hospital programs that stress the medical and disease aspects of alcoholism.

Four, clients who are functioning reasonably well in psychological, social, vocational, and physical areas of life but in addition experience some self-defined emotional distress are likely to accept various forms of psychotherapy and are probably good candidates for broad-spectrum behavioral approaches.

Five, clients who have a past history of reasonable life function, but are seriously impaired at present in their ability to be self-sustaining, may likely need vocational assistance, short- to medium-term living facilities, and careful attention to the restoration of family and community relationships.

Six, clients who have always been seriously impaired in life, such as the prototype skid row alcoholic, will need supportive types of care over a long period of time. Intensive psychotherapy, aversive-conditioning, disulfiram, tranquilizers and antidepressants, and behavior modification approaches, all are probably inappropriate here.

C. Treatment Method Principles

One, Alcoholics Anonymous appears to be a limited resource that should not be used indiscriminately. Alcoholics who are guilt-prone, desire group affiliations in life, have a prior history of positive social relations, and who tend to develop dependent relations are likely to affiliate with AA.

Two, the use of disulfiram (Antabuse) seems best suited for those who have a stable social and vocational history, are personally motivated to refrain from drinking after some years of problem drinking, and are able to establish and maintain a positive relationship with the treatment staff who dispense the drug. Major elements of depression seem a contraindication, as well as evidence of impulsiveness. The more careful, controlled, obsessive-compulsive person is a better treatment risk.

Three, broad-spectrum behavioral treatment methods, and marital/family psychotherapeutic methods appear to offer the best potential for long-term, intensive treatment methods. These methods seem best suited for persons who are relatively functional despite their alcohol abuse, or who have prior good function, with a potential to reestablish their prior level of life adaptation. Methods that link the patient with his or her community life appear most promising.

Four, drug maintenance may be feasible where the patient is socially stable but is psychologically more dependent and positively oriented toward authority figures.

Five, where there has been severe impairment of ability to function, and a major loss of social, family, job, and community ties, the treatment of choice seems to be reality-based retraining for life. Reeducation, vocational training, structured living settings, specified social responsibilities, supervised use of time, energy, and money, etc. all appear paramount.

Six, the management of acute detoxification problems remains a major issue that challenges us. Available data indicate that many detoxification problems can be handled on an outpatient basis. On the other hand, many of the people seen for detoxification are not medical problems, but present the problem of social vagrancy and public intoxication.

D. Treatment Goal Principles

One, the first task is to engage the individual alcoholic in personal contact and establish a working agreement to participate in a rehabilitation program.

Two, only *after* engagement should a careful preliminary evaluation be made, which should include the suitability of the client for the program.

Three, evaluation should include an assessment of the degree of impairment in terms of major areas of life function—which I have for convenience termed Drinking Health, Psychological Health, Social Health, Vocational Health, and Physical Health.

Four, evaluation would determine degree of impairment, the stage in the person's life and alcoholism career, and what the *potential* is for change.

Five, evaluation should then lead to a client-worker mutual decision and treatment plan for each area of impairment where change is *desired* and *possible.*

Six, the treatment plan should include both specific *goals* and specific *methods* and means to achieve those goals for each area of life where change is planned.

Seven, the client and worker should develop specific times for *review* of treatment progress, so that there is ongoing feedback to both the alcoholic client and the treatment staff as to areas of progress and areas where plans need revision or more specific attention. The result then is a plan that can be monitored and revised in the light of actual clinical progress by the alcoholic client as well as by the treatment staff.

There is no panacea nor one ideal method that will produce successful treatment of the alcoholic person. Yet the pessimism of prior years about alcoholism treatment is no longer justified. The alcoholism syndrome is varied and complex. And so too must treatment selection be varied and individualized. I find the experimental and clinical data persuasive that significant and effective treatment can be accomplished. But diffuse, global, or heterogeneous treatment is not the answer. Rather, successful treatment requires the careful application of rational, organized, and selective treatment programs.

REFERENCES

Allen, L. R., and Dootjes, I., 1968, Some personality characteristics of an alcoholic population, *Percept. Mot. Skills,* 27:707–712.

Alsen, M., 1975, Outpatient treatment of acute withdrawal states, *Br. J. Addict.,* 70 (suppl. 1):56–63.

Anderson, R. H., and Weisman, M. N., 1970, *The Alcoholic in the Emergency Room,* National Council on Alcoholism, New York.

Androes, L., and Whitehead, W. A., 1966, The "buddy system" in the hospital treatment of alcoholism, *Q. J. Stud. Alc.,* 27:524–529.

Armor, D. J., and Polich, J. M., 1982, Measurement of alcohol consumption, in

Encyclopedic Handbook of Alcoholism (E. M. Pattison and E. Kaufman, eds.), Gardner Press, New York.

Armor, D. J., Johnson, P., Polich, S., and Stanbul, H., 1977, *Trends in U.S. Adult Drinking Practices,* The Rand Corporation, Santa Monica, Calif.

Babow, I., 1975, The treatment monopoly in alcoholism and drug dependence: A social critique, *J. Drug Issues,* 5:120–128.

Bacon, M., and Jones, M. B., 1968, *Teen-Age Drinking,* T. Y. Crowell, New York.

Baekeland, F., 1977, Evaluation of treatment methods in chronic alcoholism, in *The Biology of Alcoholism.,* vol. 5, *Treatment and Rehabilitation of the Chronic Alcoholic* (B. Kissin and H. Begleiter, eds.), ch. 10, pp. 385–440, Plenum Press, New York.

Baekeland, F., and Lundwall, L. K., 1975, Dropping out of treatment: A critical review, *Psychol. Bull.,* 82:738–783.

———, 1977, Engaging the alcoholic in treatment and keeping him there, in *The Biology of Alcoholism,* vol. 5, *Treatment and Rehabilitation of the Chronic Alcoholic* (B. Kissin and H. Begleiter, eds.), ch. 4, pp. 161–196, Plenum Press, New York.

Baekeland, F., Lundwall, L. K., and Kissin, B., 1975, Methods for the treatment of chronic alcoholism: A critical appraisal, in *Research Advances in Alcohol and Drug Problems,* vol. 2 (Y. Israel, ed.), ch. 7, pp. 247–328, John Wiley & Sons, New York.

Baekeland, F., Lundwall, L. K., Kissin, B., and Shanahan, T., 1971, Correlates of outcome in disulfiram treatment of alcoholism, *J. Nerv. Ment. Dis.,* 153:1–9.

Baekeland, F., Lundwall, L. K., and Shanahan, T. J., 1973, Correlates of patient attrition in the outpatient treatment of alcoholism, *J. Nerv. Ment. Dis.,* S157:99–107.

Bahr, H. M., 1973, *Skid Row: An Introduction to Disaffiliation,* Oxford University Press, New York.

Baker, T. B., Sobell, M. B., Sobell, L. C., and Cannon, D. S., 1976, Halfway houses for alcoholics: A review, analysis and comparison with other half-way house facilities, *Inter. J. Soc. Psychiat.,* 22:130–139.

Barchha, R., Stewart, M. A., and Guze, S. B., 1968, The prevalence of alcoholism among general hospital ward patients, *Am. J. Psychiat.,* 125:681–684.

Bebbington, P. E., 1976, The efficacy of alcoholics anonymous: the elusiveness of hard data, *Br. J. Psychiat.* 128:572–580.

Beckman, L. J., 1975, Women alcoholics: A review of social and psychological studies, *J. Stud. Alc.,* 36:797–824.

Belasco, J. A., 1971, The criterion question revisited, *Br. J. Addict.,* 66:39–44.

Berman, K K., 1968, Multiple conjoint family groups in the treatment of alcoholism, *J. Med. Soc. New Jersey,* 65:6–8.

Bibby, R. W., and Mauss, A. L., 1974, Skidders and their servants: Variable goals and functions of the skid road rescue missions, *J. Sci. Stud. Relig.,* 13:421–436.

Biegel, A., 1974, Planning for the development of comprehensive community alcoholism services: Organizational approaches, *J. Drug Issues,* 4:142–148.

Biegel, A., Hunter, E. J., Tamerin, J. S., Chapin, E. II., and Lowery, M. J., 1974, Planning for the development of comprehensive alcoholism services, I, The prevalence survey, *Am. J. Psychiat.,* 131:1112–1116.

Biegel, A., McCabe, T. R., Tamerin, J. S., Lowery, M. J., Chapin, E. H., and Hunter, E. J., 1974, Planning for the development of comprehensive community alcoholism services, II, Assessing community awareness and attitudes, *Am. J. Psychiat.*, 131:1116–1121.

Billet, S. L., 1964, The use of antabuse: An approach that minimizes fear, *Med. Ann. D.C.*, 33:612–615.

Bissell, L., 1975, The treatment of alcoholism: What do we do about long-term sedatives, *Ann. N.Y. Acad. Sci.*, 252:396–399.

Blane, H. T., 1968, *The Personality of the Alcoholic: Guises of Dependency*, Harper & Row, New York.

———, 1977, Psychotherapeutic approach, in *The Biology of Alcoholism*, vol. 5, *Treatment and Rehabilitation of the Chronic Alcoholic* (B. Kissin and H. Begleiter, eds.), ch. 3, pp. 105–160, Plenum Press, New York.

Blacker, E., 1977, Training for professionals and nonprofessionals in alcoholism, in *The Biology of Alcoholism*, vol. 5, *Treatment and Rehabilitation of the Chronic Alcoholic* (B. Kissin and H. Begleiter, eds.), ch. 13, pp. 567–592, Plenum Press, New York.

Blum, E. M., and Blum, R. H., 1967, *Alcoholism: Modern Psychological Approaches to Treatment*, Jossey-Bass, San Francisco.

Blum, J., and Levine, J., 1975, Maturity, depression, and life events in middle-aged alcoholics, *Addict. Behav.*, 1:37–45.

Blume, S., 1977, Role of the recovered alcoholic in the treatment of alcoholism. In *The Biology of Alcoholism*, vol. 5, *Treatment and Rehabilitation of the Chronic Alcoholic* (B. Kissin and H. Begleiter, eds.), ch. 12, pp. 545–563, Plenum Press, New York.

Bowman, R. S., Stein, L. I., and Newton, J. R., 1975, Measurement and interpretation of drinking behavior, *J. Stud. Alc.*, 36:1154–1172.

Brod, T. M., 1975, Alcoholism as a mental health problem of native Americans, *Arch. Gen. Psychiat*, 32:1385–1393.

Bromet, E., and Moos, R. H., 1977, Environmental resources and the post-treatment functioning of alcoholic patients, *J. Hlth. Soc. Behav.*, 18:326–338.

Bromet, E., Moos, R. H., and Bliss, F., 1976, The social climate of alcoholism treatment programs, *Arch. Gen. Psychiat.*, 33:910–916.

Bromet, E., Moos, R. H., Bliss, F. and Wuthman, C., 1977, The post-treatment functioning of alcoholic patients: Its relation to program participation, *J. Consult. Clin. Psychol.*, in press.

Burton, G., and Kaplan, H. M., 1968, Marriage counseling with alcoholics and their spouses, II, The correlation of excessive drinking with family pathology and social deterioration, *Br. J. Addict.*, 63:161–170.

Caddy, G. R., and Lovibond, S. H., 1976, Self-regulation and discriminated aversive-conditioning in the modification of alcoholics drinking behavior, *Behav. Ther.*, 7:223–230.

Cahalan, D., 1970, *Problem Drinkers: A National Survey*, Jossey-Bass, San Francisco.

Cahalan, D., and Room, R., 1974, *Problem Drinking Among American Men*, Rutgers Center for Alcohol Studies, New Brunswick, N.J.

Cahalan, D., Cisin, I. H., and Crossley, H. M., 1969, *American Drinking Practices: A National Survey of Behavior and Attitudes*, monog. 6., Rutgers Center for Alcohol Studies, New Brunswick, N.J.

Cahn, S., 1970, *The Treatment of Alcoholics: An Evaluative Study*, Oxford University Press, New York.

Callichia, J. P. and Barresi, R. M., 1975, Alcoholism and alienation, *J. Clin. Psychol.*, 31:770–775.

Canter, F., 1969, A self-help project with hospitalized alcoholics, *Inter. J. Grp. Psychother.*, 19:16–27.

Catanzaro, R. J., 1971, Establishing alcoholism treatment programs in a general hospital, *J. Drug Issues*, 1:47–51.

Catanzaro, R. J. (ed.), 1968, *Alcoholism: The Total Treatment Approach*, C. C Thomas, Springfield, Ill.

Catanzaro, R. J., and Green, W. G., 1970, WATS telephone therapy: A new follow-up technique for alcoholics, *Am. J. Psychiat.*, 126:1024–1027.

Catanzaro, R. J., Pisani, V. C., Fox, R., and Kennedy, E. R., 1973, Familization therapy, *Dis. Nerv. Syst.*, 34:212–218.

Chafetz, M. E., 1967, Motivation for recovery in alcoholism, in *Alcoholism, Behavioral, Research, Therapeutic Approaches* (R. Fox, ed.), Springer, New York.

Chafetz, M. E., Blane, H. T., Abram. H. S., Golner, J., Lacy, E., McCourt, W. F., Clark, E., and Meyers, W., 1962, Establishing treatment relations with alcoholics, *J. Nerv. Ment. Dis.*, 134:395–409.

Chameides, W. A., and Yamamoto, J., 1973, Referral failures: A nine-year followup, *Am. J. Psychiat.*, 130:1157–1158.

Champ, R. L., 1974, Establishing an alcoholism treatment program in a community hospital, *Hosp. Prog.*, 55:76–77.

Chandler, J., Hensman, C., and Edwards, G., 1971, Determinants of what happens to alcoholics, *Q. J. Stud. Alc.*, 32:349–363.

Charnoff, S. M., 1970, Long-term treatment of alcoholism with amitryptaline and emylcamate, *Q. J. Stud. Alc.*, 31:289–294.

Charuvastra, C. V., Panell, J., Hopper, M., Ehrmann, M., Blakis, M., and Ling, W., 1976, The medical safety of the combined usage of disulfiram and methadone; pharmacological treatment for heroin addicts, *Arch. Gen. Psychiat.*, 33:391–393.

Cheek, F. E., 1972, Broad spectrum behavioral training in self-control for drug addicts and alcoholics, *Behav. Res. Ther.*, 3:515–520.

Chessick, R. D., Loof, D. H., and Price, H. G., 1961, The alcoholic-narcotic addict, *Q. J. Stud. Alc.*, 22:261–268.

Clark, W. B., and Cahalan, D., 1976, Changes in problem drinking over a four-year span, *Addict. Behav.*, 1:251–259.

Clinebell, H. J., Jr., 1968, *Understanding and Counseling the Alcoholic Through Religion and Psychology*, rev. ed., Abingdon Press, Nashville, Tenn.

Cohen, P. C., and Krause, M. K., 1971, *Casework with Wives of Alcoholics*, Family Services Association of America, New York.

Conroy, R. W., Friedberg, B. and Krizaj, P., 1971, A community plan for military alcoholics, *Am. J. Psychiat.*, 128:774–777.

Cook, T., 1975, *Vagrant Alcoholics*, Routledge & Kegan Paul, Boston.

Corder, B. F., Corder, R. F., and Laidlaw, N. D., 1972, An intensive treatment program for alcoholics and their wives, *Q. J. Stud. Alc.*, 33:1144–1146.

Corrigan, E. M., 1974, *Problem Drinkers Seeking Treatment*, Monog. 8., Rutgers Center for Alcohol Studies, New Brunswick, N.J.

Costello, R. M., 1975a, Alcoholism treatment and evaluation, I, In Search of methods, *Inter. J. Addict.*, 10:251–275.
————, 1975b, Alcoholism treatment and evaluation, II, Collation of two year followup studies, *Inter. J. Addict.*, 10:857–868.
Costello, R. M., Bechtel, J. E., and Giffen, M. B., 1973, A community's efforts to attack the problem of alcoholism, II, Base rate data for future program evaluation, *Inter. J. Addict.*, 8:875–888.
Costello, R. M., Giffen, M. B., Schneider, S. L., Edgington, P. W., and Manders, K. R., 1976, Comprehensive alcohol treatment planning, implementation and evaluation, *Inter. J. Addict.*, 11:553–570.
Crawford, J.J., and Chalopsky, A. B., 1977, The reported evaluation of alcoholism treatment 1968–1971: A methodological review, *Addict. Behav.*, 2:63–74.
Cronkite, R., and Moos, R. H., 1977, Evaluating alcoholism treatment programs: An integrated approach, submitted for publication.
Cross, J. N., 1968, *Guide to the Community Control of Alcoholism*, American Public Health Association, New York.
Dalton, M. S., Chegwidden, M. J., and Duncan, D., 1972, Wisteria House: Results of transition of alcoholics from treatment unit to community house, *Inter. J. Soc. Psychiat.*, 18:213–216.
Davies, D. L., 1962, Normal drinking in recovered alcohol addicts, *Q. J. Stud. Alc.*, 23:94–104.
Davis, C. S., and Schmidt, M. R. (eds.), 1977, *Differential Treatment of Drug and Alcohol Abuses*, ETC Publ., Palm Springs, Fla.
De Morsier, G., and Feldman, H., 1952, Le traitment de l'alcoolisme par l'apormorphine: Etude de 500 cas., *Schweiz. Arch. Neurol./Psychiat.*, 70:434–440.
Devenyi, P., and Wilson, M., 1971, Abuse of barbituates in an alcoholic population, *Can. Med. Assoc. J.*, 104:219–221.
Dittman, K. S., Crawford, G. G., Forgy, E. W., Moskowitz, H., and MacAndrew, C. D., 1967, A controlled experiment in the use of court probation for drunk arrests, *Am. J. Psychiat.*, 124:160–163.
Donovan, D. M., Hague, W. H., and O'Leary, M. R., 1975, Perceptual differentiation and defense mechanisms in alcoholics, *J. Clin. Psychol.*, 31:356–359.
Dorsch, G., Talley, R., and Bynder, H., 1969, Response to alcoholics by the helping professions and community agencies in Denver, *Q. J. Stud. Alc.*, 30:905–919.
Dubourg, G. O., 1969, Aftercare for alcoholics: A followup study, *Br. J. Addict.*, 64:155–163.
Dunn, J. H., and Clay, M. L., 1971, Physicians look at a general hospital alcoholic service, *Q. J. Stud. Alc.*, 32:162–167.
Edwards, G., 1973, Epidemiology applied to alcoholism, *Q. J. Stud. Alc.*, 34:28–56.
Edwards, G., Fisher, M. Y., Hawker, A., and Hensman, C., 1967, Clients of alcoholism information centers, *Br. Med. J.*, 4:346–349.
Edwards, G., Hensman, C., Hawker, A., and Williamson, V., 1967, Alcoholics Anonymous: The anatomy of a self-help group, *Soc. Psychiat.*, 1:195–204.
Edwards, G., Kyle, E., and Nicholls, P., 1974, Alcoholics admitted to four hospitals in England, *Q. J. Stud. Alc.*, 35:499–522.
Einstein, S., and Wolfson, E., 1970, Alcoholism curricula: How professionals are trained, *Inter. J. Addict.*, 5:295–307.

Einstein, S., Wolfson, E., Gecht, P., 1970, What matters in treatment: Relevant variables in alcoholism, *Inter. J. Addict.*, 5:54–67.

Elkins, R. L., 1975, Aversion therapy for alcoholism: Chemical, electrical, or verbal imagery, *Inter. J. Addict.*, 10:157–209.

Emrick, C. D., 1974, A review of psychologically oriented treatment for alcoholism, I, The use and interrelationships of outcome criteria and drinking behavior following treatment, *Q. J. Stud. Alc.*, 35:534–549.

————, 1975, A review of psychologically oriented treatment of alcoholism, II, The relative effectiveness of different treatment approaches and the effectiveness of treatment versus no-treatment, *J. Stud. Alc.*, 36:88–108.

English, G. E., and Curtin, M. E., 1975, Personality differences in patients at three alcoholism treatment agencies, *J. Stud. Alc.*, 36:52–61.

Ewing, J. A., 1977, Matching therapy and patients—The cafeteria plan. *Br. J. Addict.*, in press.

Feldman, D. J., Pattison, E. M., Sobell, L. C., Graham, T., and Sobell, M. B., 1975, Outpatient alcohol detoxification: Initial findings on 564 patients, *Am. J. Psychiat.*, 132:407–412.

Fillmore, K. M., 1975, Relationships between specific drinking problems in early adulthood and middle age: An exploratory 20-year follow-up study, *J. Stud. Alc.*, 36:887–907.

Finer, J. J., 1972, Overmanagement of the alcoholic patient, *J. Am. Med. Assoc.*, 219:622.

Finlay, D. G., 1966, Effect of role network pressure on an alcoholics approach to treatment, *Social Work*, 11:71–77.

Fitzgerald, B. J., Pasework, R. A., and Clark, R., 1971, Four-year followup of alcoholics treated in a rural state hospital, *Q. J. Stud. Alc.*, 32:636–642.

Forrest, G. G., 1975, *The Diagnosis and Treatment of Alcoholism*, Charles C Thomas, Springfield, Ill.

Franks, C. M., 1966, Conditioning and conditioned aversion therapies in the treatment of alcoholism, *Inter. J. Addict.*, 1:61–98.

Freed, E. X., 1969, The dilemma of the alcoholic patient in a psychiatric hospital, *J. Psychiat. Nurs.*, 7:113–116.

————, 1973, Drug abuse by alcoholics: A review, *Inter. J. Addict.*, 8:451–473.

Freedman, A. M., and Wilson, E A., 1964, Childhood and adolescent addictive disorders, *Pediatrics*, 34:283–292.

Fry, L. J., and Miller, J., 1975, Responding to skid row alcoholics: Self-defeating arrangements in an innovative treatment program, *Social Problems*, 22:675–688.

Gaitz, C. M., and Baer, P. E., 1971, Characteristics of elderly patients with alcoholism, *Arch. Gen. Psychiat.*, 24:372–378.

Galanter, M., Karasu, T. B., and Wilder, J. F., 1976, Alcohol and drug abuse consultation in the general hospital: A systems approach, *Am. J. Psychiat.*, 138:930–934.

Gallant, D. M., Bishop, M. P., Stoy, B., Faulkner, M. A., and Paternostro, L., 1966, The value of a "first contact" group intake session in an alcoholism clinic: Statistical confirmation, *Psychosomatics*, 7:349–352.

Gallant, D. M., Bishop, M. P., Mouledoux, A., Faulkner, M. A., Brisolara, A., and Swanson, W. A., 1973, The revolving-door alcoholic: An impasse in the treatment of the chronic alcoholic, *Arch. Gen. Psychiat.*, 28:633–635.

Garitano, W. A., and Ronall, R. E., 1974, Concepts of life-style in the treatment of alcoholism, *Inter. J. Addict.,* 9:585–592.

Gellens, H. K., Gottheil, E., and Alterman, A. I., 1976, Drinking outcomes of specific alcoholic subgroups, *J. Stud. Alc.,* 37:986–989.

Gerard, D. L., and Saenger, G., 1966, *Outpatient Treatment of Alcoholism,* University of Toronto Press, Toronto.

Gerard, D. L., Saenger, G., and Wile, R., 1962, The abstinent alcoholic, *Arch. Gen. Psychiat.,* 6:83–95.

Gerrein, J. R., Rosenberg, C. M., and Manohar, V., 1973, Disulfiram maintenance in outpatient treatment of alcoholism, *Arch. Gen. Psychiat.,* 28:798–802.

Gillis, L. S., and Keet, M., 1969, Prognostic factors and treatment results in hospitalized alcoholics, *Q. J. Stud. Alc.,* 30:426–437.

Glaser, D., and O'Leary, V., 1966, *The Alcoholic Offender,* U.S. Department of Health, Education, and Welfare, Washington, D.C.

Glasscote, R. M. (ed.), 1967, *The Treatment of Alcoholism: A Study of Programs and Problems,* Joint Information Service, Washington, D.C.

Goldfarb, C., and Hartman, B., 1975, A total community approach to the treatment of alcoholism, *Dis. Nerv. Syst.,* 36:409–414.

Goldstein, A. P., 1962, *Therapist Patient Expectancies in Psychotherapy,* Pergamon Press, New York.

Gomberg, E., 1975, Prevalence of alcoholism among ward patients in a Veterans Administration hospital, *J. Stud. Alc.,* 36:1456–1467.

Goodwin, D. W., and Erickson, C. K. (eds.), 1979, *Alcoholism and Affective Disorders,* Spectrum Books, New York.

Goodwin, D. W., and Reinhard, J., 1972, Disulfiram-like effects of trichomonad drugs: A review and double-blind study, *Q. J. Stud. Alc.,* 33:734–470.

Goodwin, D. W., David, D. H., and Robins, L. N., 1975, Drinking amid abundant illicit drugs: The Vietnam case, *Arch. Gen. Psychiat.,* 32:230–233.

Gottheil, E., McLellan, A. T., and Druley, K. A. (eds.), 1981, *Matching Patient Needs and Treatment Methods in Alcoholism and Drug Abuse,* Charles C Thomas, Springfield, Ill.

Greenblatt, M., and Schuckit, M. A. (eds.), 1976, *Alcoholism Problems in Women and Children,* Grune & Stratton, New York.

Gross, M. M., Rosenblatt, S. M., Malenowksi, B., Broman, M., and Lewis, E., 1972, Classification of alcohol withdrawal syndromes, *Q. J. Stud. Alc.,* 33:400–407.

Hadley, P. A., and Hadley, R. G., 1972, Treatment practices and philosophies in rehabilitation facilities for alcoholics, *Proc. Am. Psychol. Ass.,* 80:729–730.

Hagnell, O., and Tunvig, K., 1972, Mental and physical complaints among alcoholics, *Q. J. Stud. Alc.,* 33:77–84.

Hague, W. H., Donovan, D.M., and O'Leary, M. R., 1976, Personality characteristics related to treatment decisions among inpatient alcoholics: A nonrelationship, *J. Clin. Psychol.,* 32:476–479.

Hague, W. H., Wilson, L. G., Dudley, D. L., and Cannon, D. S., 1976, Postdetoxification drug treatment of anxiety and depression in alcohol addicts, *Dis. Nerv. Syst.,* 37:354–359.

Hamburg, S., 1971, Behavior therapy in alcoholism: A critical review of broadspectrum approaches, *J. Stud. Alc.,* 36:69–97.

Hansen, H. A., and Teilmann, K., 1954, A treatment of criminal alcoholics in Denmark, *Q. J. Stud. Alc.*, 15:245–287.

Hansen, P. L., 1972, The development of an alcoholism unit in a private general hospital, *Minn. Med.*, 55:577–579.

Hart, L., 1977, Rehabilitation need patterns of men alcoholics, *J. Stud. Alc.*, 38:494–511.

Hayman, M., 1966, *Alcoholism: Mechanism and Management*, Charles C Thomas, Springfield, Ill.

———, 1967, The myth of social drinking, *Amer. J. Psychiat.*, 124:585–592.

Heather, N., and Robertson, I., 1981, *Controlled Drinking*, Methuen, London.

Hedberg, A. G., and Campbell, L., 1974, A comparison of four behavioral treatments of alcoholism, *J. Behav. Ther. Exp. Psychiat.*, 5:251–256.

Heyman, M. M., 1976, Referral to alcoholism programs in industry: Coercion, confrontation and choice, *J. Stud. Alc.*, 37:900–907.

Hill, M. J., and Blane, H. T., 1967, Evaluation of psychotherapy with alcoholics: A critical review, *Q. J. Stud. Alc.*, 28:76–104.

Hoehn-Saric, R., Frank, J. D., Imber, S. D., Nash, E. H. Jr., Stone, A. R. and Battle, C. C., 1964, Systematic preparation of patients for psychotherapy, I, Effects of therapy behavior and outcome, *J. Psychiat. Res.*, 2:267–281.

Horn, J. L., and Wanberg, K. W., 1969, Symptom patterns related to excessive use of alcohol, *Q. J. Stud. Alc.*, 30:35–58.

———, 1970, Dimensions of perception of background and current situation of alcoholic patients, *Q. J. Stud. Alc.*, 31:633–658.

Horn, J. L., Wanberg, K. W., and Adams, G., 1974, Diagnosis of alcoholism: Factors of drinking, background, and current conditions in alcoholics, *Q. J. Stud. Alc.*, 35:147–175.

Howard, K., Rickels, K., Mack, J. E., Lipman, R. S., Covi, L., and Baum, N. C., 1970, Therapeutic style and attrition from psychiatric drug treatment, *J. Nerv. Ment. Dis.*, 150:102–110.

Hunt, G. M., and Azrin, N. H., 1973, A community reinforcement approach to alcoholism, *Behav. Res. Ther.*, 11:91–104.

Hunter, G., 1963, Alcoholism and the family agency with special reference to early phase and hidden types, *Q. J. Stud. Alc.*, 24:61–79.

Hurwitz, J. I., and Lelos, D., 1968, A multilevel interpersonal profile of employed alcoholics, *Q. J. Stud. Alc.*, 29:64–76.

Hyman, M. M., 1976, Alcoholics fifteen years later, *Ann. N.Y. Acad. Med.*, 273:613–623.

Jacobson, G. R., 1976, *The Alcoholisms: Detection, Diagnosis, and Assessment*, Human Sciences Press, New York.

Janzen, C., 1977, Families in the treatment of alcoholism, *J. Stud. Alc.*, 38:114–130.

Jellinek, E. M., 1952, Phases of alcohol addiction, *Q. J. Stud. Alc.*, 13:673–684.

———, 1960, *The Disease Concept of Alcoholism*, Hillhouse Press, Highland Park, N.J.

Jones, R. K., 1970, Sectarian characteristics of alcoholics anonymous, *Sociology*, 4:181–195.

Jones, R. K., and Helrich, A. R., 1972, Treatment of alcoholism by physicians in private practice: A national survey, *Q. J. Stud. Alc.*, 33:117–131.

Jongsma, K., 1970, An experiment in cooperation between agencies and clinics in the treatment of persistent chronic alcoholism, *Br. J. Addict.*, 65:297–304.

Kalb, M., 1975, Social class, length of treatment contacts, and the outpatient treatment of alcoholism, *Br. J. Addict.*, 70:253–262.

Kalb, M., and Propper, M. S., 1976, The future of alcohology: Craft or science? *Am. J. Psychiat.*, 133:641–645.

Kammeier, M. L., Lucero, R. J., and Anderson, D. J., 1973, Events of crucial importance during alcoholism treatment as reported by patients: A preliminary study, *Q. J. Stud. Alc.*, 34:1172–1189.

Kanas, T. E., Cleveland, S. E., Pokorny, A. D., and Miller, B. A., 1976, Two contrasting alcoholism treatment programs: A comparison of outcomes, *Inter. J. Addict.*, 11:1045–1062.

Kaplan, R., Blume, S., Rosenberg, S., Pitrelli, J. and Turner, W. J., 1972, Phenytoin, Metronidazole, and multivitamins in the treatment of alcoholism, *Quart. J. Stud. Alc.*, 33:97–104.

Kaufman, E., and Pattison, E. M., 1981, Differential methods of family therapy in the treatment of alcoholism, *J. Stud. Alc.*, 42:951–971.

Kearnes, T. R., 1968, Alcohol and general hospital patients, *Am. J. Psychiat.*, 125:681–684.

Keller, M., 1972, The oddities of alcoholics, *Q. J. Stud. Alc.*, 33:1147–1148.

Kipperman, A., and Fine, E. W., 1974, The combined abuse of alcohol and amphetamines, *Am. J. Psychiat.*, 131:1273–1280.

Kish, G. B., and Hermann, H. T., 1971, The Fort Meade alcohol treatment program: A followup study, *Q. J. Stud. Alc.*, 32:628–325.

Kissin, B., 1975, The use of psychoactive drugs in the long-term treatment of chronic alcoholism, *Ann. N.Y. Acad. Sci.*, 252:385–395.

——, 1977, Theory and practice in the treatment of alcoholism, in *The Biology of Alcoholism*, vol. 5, *Treatment and Rehabilitation of the Chronic Alcoholic* (B. Kissin and H. Begleiter, eds.), ch. 1, pp. 1–51, Plenum Press, New York.

Kissin, B., and Platz, A, 1968, The use of drugs in the long-term rehabilitation of chronic alcoholics, in *Psychopharmacology: A Review of Progress 1957–1967* (D. H. Efron, ed.), U.S. Public Health Service Publication 1836, Washington, D.C.

Kissin, B., Charnoff, S. M., and Rosenblatt, S. M., 1960, Drug and placebo responses in chronic alcoholics, *Psychiat. Res. Repts.*, 24:44–60.

Kissin, B., Platz, A., and Su, W. H., 1970, Social and psychological factors in the treatment of chronic alcoholics, *J. Psychiat. Res.*, 8:13–27.

Knott, D. H., and Fink, R. D., 1975, Problems surrounding emergency-care services for acute alcoholics, *Hosp. & Comm. Psychiat.*, 26:42–43.

Koumans, A. J. R., Muller, J. J., and Miller, C. F., 1965, Use of letters to increase motivation for treatment in alcoholics, *Psychol. Repts.* 16:1152.

——, 1967, Use of telephone calls to increase motivation for treatment in alcoholics, *Psychol. Repts.*, 21:327–328.

Kurtz, E., 1979, *Not God—A History of Alcoholics Anonymous,* Hazelden Foundation, Center City, Minn.

Larkin, E. J., 1974, *The Treatment of Alcoholism: Theory, Practice, and Evaluation,* Addiction Research Foundation, Toronto.

Lennon, B. E., Rekosh, J. H., Patch, V. C., and Howe, L. P., 1970, Self-reports of drunkenness arrest: Assessing drinking problems among men hospitalized for tuberculosis, *Q. J. Stud. Alc.*, 31:90–96.

Liebson, I., Bigelow, G., and Flamer, R., 1973, Alcoholism among methadone patients: A specific treatment method, *Amer. J. Psychiat.*, 130:483–485.

Linsky, A., 1970, The changing public views of alcoholism, *Q. J. Stud. Alc.*, 31:692–704.

————, 1972, Theories of behavior and the social control of alcoholism, *Soc. Psychiat.*, 7:47–52.

Litman, G. K., 1976, Behavior modification techniques in the treatment of alcoholism: A review and critique, in *Research Advance in Alcohol and Drug Problems*, vol. 3 (Y. Israel, ed.), ch. 8, pp. 359–400, John Wiley & Sons, New York.

Little, R. E., Schultz, F. A. and Mandell, W., 1977, Describing alcohol consumption: A comparison of three methods and a new approach, *J. Stud. Alc.*, 38:544–562.

Lowe, W. C., and Thomas, S. D., 1976, Assessing alcoholism treatment effectiveness: A comparison of three evaluative measures, *Q. J. Stud. Alc.*, 37:883–889.

Lowenfels, A. B., 1971, *The Alcoholic Patient in Surgery*, The William & Wilkins Company, Baltimore.

Lubetkin, B. S., Rivers, P. C. and Rosenberg, C. M., 1971, Difficulties of disulfiram therapy with alcoholics, *Q. J. Stud. Alc.*, 32:168–171.

Ludwig, A. M., Levine, J., and Stark, L. H., 1970, *LSD and Alcoholism: A Clinical Study of Treatment Efficacy*, Charles C Thomas, Springfield, Ill.

McCusker, J., Cherubin, C. E., and Zimberg, S., 1971, Prevalence of alcoholism in a general municipal hospital population, *N.Y. St. Med. J.*, 71:751–756.

McLachlan, J. F. C., 1974, Therapy strategies, personality orientation, and recovery from alcoholism, *Can. Psychiat. Ass. J.*, 19:25–30.

McNair, D. M., Callahan, D. M., and Lorr, M., 1962, Therapist-type and patient response to psychotherapy, *J. Consult. Psychol.*, 26:425–429.

Mandell, W., and Ginzburg, H. M., 1976, Youthful alcohol use, abuse and alcoholism, in *The Biology of Alcoholism*, vol. 5, *Treatment and Rehabilitation of the Chronic Alcoholic* (B. Kissin and H. Begleiter, eds.), ch. 5, pp. 167–204, Plenum Press, New York.

Mann, G. A., 1965, An alcoholic treatment center in a community general hospital, *Hosp. Prog.*, 50:125–128.

Matijevic, I., and Paunovic, N., 1973, Rehabilitation of alcoholics in a club of treated alcoholics, *Alcoholism (Zagreb)* 9:50–54.

Mayer, J., and Myerson, D. J., 1971, Outpatient treatment of alcoholics: Effects of status stability and nature of treatment, *Q. J. Stud. Alc.*, 32:620–627.

Mayer, J., Needham, M. A., and Myerson, D. J., 1965, Contact and initial attendance at an alcoholism clinic, *Q. J. Stud. Alc.*, 26:480–485.

Medical Times, 1975, *An Alcohol Abuse Manual for Family Physicians*, Special Issue No. 103(6).

Miller, P. M., 1973, Behavioral assessment in alcoholism research and treatment: Current techniques, *Inter. J. Addict.*, 8:831–837.

Miller, S. I., Helmick, E., Berg, L., Nutting, P., and Shorr, G., 1975, An evaluation of alcoholism treatment services for Alaskan natives, *Hosp. & Comm. Psychiat.*, 26:829–831.

Mills, R. B., and Hetrick, E. S., 1963, Treating the unmotivated alcoholic: A coordinated program in a municipal court, *Crime & Delinq.*, 9:36–59.

Mogar, R. E., Helm, S. T., Snedeker, M. R., Snedeker, M. H., and Wilson, W. M., 1969, Staff attitudes toward the alcoholic, *Arch. Gen. Psychiat.*, 21:449–454.

Mogar, R. E., Wilson, W. M., and Helm, S. T., 1970, Personality subtypes of male and female alcoholic patients, *Inter. J. Addict.*, 5:99–113.

Moore, R. A., and Buchanan, T. K., 1966, State hospitals and alcoholism: Nationwide survey of treatment techniques and results, *Q. J. Stud. Alc.*, 27:459–468.

Moore, R. A., and Ramseur, F., 1960, Effects of psychotherapy on open-ward hospital inpatients with alcoholism, *Q. J. Stud. Alc.*, 21:233–252.

Moos, R. H., Bromet, E., Tsu, V., and Moos, B., 1977, Family characteristics and the outcome of treatment for alcoholics, *Q. J. Stud. Alc.*, 40:78–88 (1979).

Mottin, J. L., 1973, Drug-induced attenuation of alcohol consumption: A review and evaluation of claimed, potential or current therapies, *Q. J. Stud. Alc.*, 34:444–472.

Mulford, H. A., 1977, Stages in the alcoholic process: Toward a cumulative, nonsequential index, *J. Stud. Alc.*, 38:563–583.

Mulford, H. A., and Miller, D. E., 1960, Drinking in Iowa, IV, Preoccupation with alcohol, and definitions of alcoholism, heavy drinking, and trouble due to drinking, *Q. J. Stud. Alc.*, 21:279–291.

Mullan, H., and Sanguiliano, I., 1966, *Alcoholism: Group Psychotherapy and Rehabilitation*, Charles C Thomas, Springfield, Ill.

Muller, J., and Brunner-Orne, M., 1967, Social alienation as a factor in the acceptance of outpatient psychiatric treatment by the alcoholic, *J. Clin. Psychol.*, 23:513–518.

Nathan, P. E., and Briddell, D. W., 1977, Behavioral assessment and treatment of alcoholism, in *The Biology of Alcoholism*, vol. 5, *Treatment and Rehabilitation of the Chronic Alcoholic* (B. Kissin and H. Begleiter, eds.), pp. 301–349, Plenum Press, New York.

Nathan, P. E., and Hay, W. M., 1982, *Clinical Case Studies in the Behavioral Treatment of Alcoholism*, Plenum Press, New York.

Nathan, P. E., Marlatt, G. A., and Lorberg, T. (eds.), 1978, *Alcoholism: New Directions in Behavorial Research and Treatment*, Plenum Press, New York.

National Council on Alcoholism, 1972, Criteria for the diagnosis of alcoholism, *Ann. Intern. Med.*, 77:249–258.

Neuringer, C., and Goldstein, B., 1976, The use of psychological tests for the study of the identification, prediction, and treatment of alcoholism, in *Empirical Studies of Alcoholism* (G. Goldstein and C. Neuringer, eds.), pp. 7–30, Ballinger, Cambridge, Mass.

Novick, L. F., Hudson, H., and German, E., 1974, In-hospital detoxification and rehabilitation of alcoholics in an inner city area, *Am. J. Publ. Hlth.*, 64:1089–1094.

O'Briant, R. B., Lennor, H. L., Allen, S. D., and Ransom, D. C., 1973, *Recovery from Alcoholism: A Social Treatment Method*, Charles C Thomas, Springfield, Ill.

O'Leary, M. R., Donovan, D. M., and Hague, W. H., 1975, Relationship between locus of control and defensive style among alcoholics, *J. Clin. Psychol.*, 31:360–363.

Orford, J. A., 1973, A comparison of alcoholics whose drinking is totally uncontrolled and those whose drinking is mainly controlled, *Behav. Res. Ther.*, 11:565–576.

——, 1974, Notes on ordering of onset of symptoms in alcohol dependence, *Psychol. Med.*, 4:281–288.

——, 1975, Alcoholism and marriage: The argument against specialism, *J. Stud. Alc.*, 36:1537–1563.

Orford, J. A., and Hawker, A., 1974, Investigation of an alcoholism rehabilitative halfway house, II, Complex questions of client motivation, *Br. J. Addict.*, 69:315–323.

Orford, J. A., Guthrie, S., and Nicholls, P., 1975, Self-reported coping behavior of wives of alcoholics and its association with drinking outcomes, *J. Stud. Alc.*, 36:1154–1163.

Orford, J. A., Hawker, A., and Nicholls, P., 1974, An investigation of an alcoholism rehabilitative halfway house, I, Types of clients and modes of discharge, *Br. J. Addict.*, 69:213–224.

——, 1975, An investigation of an alcoholism rehabilitative halfway house, IV, Attractions of the halfway house for residents, *Br. J. Addict.*, 70:179–186.

Orford, J. A., Oppenheimer, E. D., Egert, S., Hensman, C., and Guthrie, S., 1976, The cohesiveness of alcoholism-complicated marriages and its influence on treatment outcome, *Br. J. Psychiat.*, 128:318–339.

Orne, M. T., and Wender, P. H., 1968, Anticipatory socialization for psychotherapy methods and rationale, *Am. J. Psychiat.*, 124:1202–1212.

Ornstein, P., and Whitman, R. M., 1965, On the metapharmacology of psychotropic drugs, *Comp. Psychiat.*, 6:166–175.

Otto, S., and Orford, J., 1978, *Not Quite Like Home: Small Hostels for Alcoholics and Others*, John Wiley & Sons, New York.

Paine, H. J., 1977, Attitudes and patterns of alcohol use among Mexican-Americans: Implications for service delivery, *J. Stud. Alc.*, 38:544–553.

Panepinto, W. C., and Higgins, M. J., 1969, Keeping alcoholics in treatment: Effective follow-through procedures, *Q. J. Stud. Alc.*, 30:414–419.

Park, P., 1973, Developmental ordering of experiences in alcoholics, *Q. J. Stud. Alc.*, 34:473–488.

Pattison, E. M., 1965a, Treatment of alcoholic families with nurse home visits, *Family Process*, 4:75–94.

——, 1965b, Evaluation of group psychotherapy, *Inter. J. Grp. Psychother.*, 15:382–397.

——, 1966, A critique of alcoholism treatment concepts; with special reference to abstinence, *Q. J. Stud. Alc.*, 27:49–71.

——, 1968, A critique of abstinence criteria in the treatment of alcoholism, *Inter. J. Soc. Psychiat.*, 14:260–267.

——, 1969, The relationship of adjunctive and therapeutic recreation services to community mental health programs, *Therap. Rec. J.*, 3:16–25.

——, 1970, Group psychotherapy and group methods in community mental health programs, *Inter. J. Grp. Psychother.*, 20:516–539.

——, 1974, Rehabilitation of the Chronic Alcoholic, in *The Biology of Alcoholism*, vol. 3, *Clinical Pathology* (B. Kissin and H. Begleiter, eds.), pp. 587–658, Plenum Press, New York.

————, 1976a, Non-abstinent drinking goals in the treatment of alcoholism: A clinical typology, *Arch. Gen. Psychiat.*, 33:923–930.

————, 1976b, A conceptual approach to alcoholism treatment goals, *Addict. Behav.*, 1:177–192.

————, 1976c, Non-abstinent drinking goals in the treatment of alcoholism, in *Research Advances in Alcohol and Drug Problems,* vol. 3 (Y. Israel, ed.), pp. 401–455, John Wiley & Sons, New York.

————, 1976d, Psychosocial systems therapy, in *The Changing Mental Health Scene* (R. G. Hirschowitz and B. Levy, eds.), pp. 127–152, Spectrum Publications, New York.

————, 1977. Management of alcoholism in medical practice, *Med. Clin. No. Amer.*, 61:797–809.

Pattison, E. M. (ed.), 1982, *Selection of Treatment for Alcoholics,* Rutgers Press, New Brunswick, N.J.

Pattison, E. M., and Kaufman, E., 1982, *Encyclopedic Handbook of Alcoholism,* Gardner Press, New York.

Pattison, E. M., 1983, Types of alcoholism reflective of character disorders, in *Character Pathology* (M. Zales et al., eds.), Bruner/Mazel, New York.

Pattison, E. M., Courlas, P. G., Patti, R., Mann, B., and Mullen, D., 1965, Diagnostic-therapeutic intake groups for wives of alcoholics, *Q. J. Stud. Alc.*, 26:605–616.

Pattison, E. M., Headley, E. B., Gleser, G. C., and Gottschalk, L. A., 1968, Abstinence and normal drinking: An assessment of changes in drinking patterns in alcoholics after treatment, *Q. J. Stud. Alc.*, 29:610–633.

Pattison, E. M., Bishop, L. A., and Linsky, A. S., 1968, Changes in public attitudes on narcotic addiction, *Am. J. Psychiat.*, 125:160–167.

Pattison, E. M., Coe, R., and Rhodes, R. A., 1969, Evaluation of alcoholism treatment: Comparison of three facilities, *Arch. Gen. Psychiat.*, 20:478–488.

Pattison, E. M., Rhodes, R. S., and Dudley, D. L., 1971, Response to group treatment in patients with severe chronic lung disease, *Inter. J. Grp. Psychother.*, 21:214–225.

Pattison, E. M., Coe, R., and Doerr, H. O., 1973, Population variation among alcoholism treatment facilities, *Inter. J. Addict.*, 8:199–229.

Pattison, E. M., DeFrancisco, D., Frazier, H., Wood, P. E., and Crowder, J., 1975. A psychosocial kinship model for family therapy, *Am. J. Psychiat.*, 132:1246–1251.

Pattison, E. M., Sobell, M. B., and Sobell, L. C., 1977, *Emerging Concepts of Alcohol Dependence,* Springer, New York.

Pemper, K., 1976, Dimensions of change in the improving alcoholic, *Inter. J. Addict.*, 11:641–649.

Pisani, V. D., 1969, Assessing inpatient attitudes toward an alcoholism treatment center, *Q. J. Stud. Alc.*, 30:640–644.

Pittman, D. J., and Gordon, C. W., 1958, *Revolving Door,* The Free Press, Glencoe, Ill.

Pittman, D. J., and Sterne, M. W., 1963, *Alcoholism: Community Agency Attitudes and the Impact on Treatment Services,* U.S. Public Health Service publication 1273, Washington, D.C.

Plant, M. A., 1979, *Drinking Careers: Occupations, Drinking Habits, and Drinking Problems,* Tavistock, London.

Plaut, T. F., 1967, *Alcohol Problems: A Report to the Nation*, Oxford University Press, New York.

Pokorny, A. D., Miller, B. A., Kanas, T., and Valle, J., 1973, Effectiveness of extended aftercare in the treatment of alcoholism, *Q. J. Stud. Alc.*, 34:435–443.

Polacsek, E., Barnes, T., Turner, N., Hall, R., and Weise, C., 1972, *Interaction of Alcohol and Other Drugs*, Second Revised Edition, Addiction Research Foundation, Toronto.

Polich, J. M., Armor, D. J., and Braiker, H. B., 1980, *The Course of Alcoholism Four Years After Treatment*, John Wiley & Sons, New York.

Pomerleau, O., Pertschuk, M., and Stinnet, J., 1976, A critical examination of some current assumptions in the treatment of alcoholism, *J. Stud. Alc.*, 37:849–867.

Popham, R. E., and Schmidt, W., 1976, Some factors affecting the likelihood of moderate drinking by treated alcoholics, *J. Stud. Alc.*, 37:868–882.

Price, R. H., and Curlee-Salisbury, J., 1975, Patient-treatment interactions among alcoholics, *J. Stud. Alc.*, 36:659–669.

Pugliese, A., Martinez, M., Maselli, A., Zalick, D. H., 1975, Treatment of alcoholic methadone-maintenance patients with disulfiram, *J. Stud. Alc.*, 36:1584–1588.

Rhodes, R. J., Hames, G. H., and Campbell, M. D., 1969, The problems of alcoholism among hospitalized tuberculous patients: Report of a national questionnaire survey, *Am. Rev. Resp. Dis.*, 99:440–442.

Ritson, B., 1971, Personality and prognosis in alcoholism, *Br. J. Psychiat.*, 118:79–82.

Robinson, D., 1972a, The alcohologist's addiction—Some implications of having lost control over the disease concept of alcoholism, *Q. J. Stud. Alc.*, 33:1028–1042.

———, 1972b, *From Drinking to Alcoholism: A Sociological Commentary*, John Wiley & Sons, New York.

Rock, N. L., and Donley, P. J., 1975, Treatment program for military personnel with alcohol problems, II, The program, *Inter. J. Addict.*, 10:467–480.

Rohan, W. P., 1976, Quantitative dimensions of alcohol use for hospitalized problem drinkers, *Dis. Nerv. Syst.*, 37:154–159.

Roman, P. M., and Trice, H. M., 1968, The sick role, labelling theory, and the deviant drinker, *Inter. J. Soc. Psychiat.*, 14:245–251.

———, 1976, Alcohol abuse and work organizations, in *The Biology of Alcoholism*, vol. 4, *Social Aspects of Alcoholism* (B. Kissin and H. Begleiter, eds.), pp. 445–513, Plenum Press, New York.

Rosenberg, C. M., 1974, Drug maintenance in the outpatient treatment of chronic alcoholism, *Am. J. Psychiat.*, 30:373–377.

Rosenberg, C. M., and Amodeo, M., 1974, Long-term patients seen in an alcoholism clinic, *Q. J. Stud. Alc.*, 35:660–666.

Rosenberg, C. M., and Liftik, J., 1976, Use of coercion in the outpatient treatment of alcoholism, *J. Stud. Alc.*, 37:58–65.

Rosenberg, C. M., Gerrein, J. R., Manohar, V., and Liftik, J., 1976, Evaluation of training of alcoholism counselors, *J. Stud. Alc.*, 37:1236–1246.

Rossi, J. J., and Filstead, W. J., 1976, Treating the treatment issues: Some general observations about the treatment of alcoholics, in *Alcohol and Alcohol Prob-*

lems: New Thinking and New Directions (W. J. Filstead, J. J. Rossi, and M. Keller, eds.), pp. 193–228, Ballinger, Cambridge, Mass.

Ruggels, W. L., Armor, D. J., and Polich, J. M., 1975, *A follow-up study of clients at selected alcoholism treatment centers funded by NIAAA*, Stanford Research Institute, Menlo Park, Calif.

Sands, P. M., and Hanson, P. G., 1971, Psychotherapeutic groups for alcoholics and relatives in an outpatient setting, *Inter. J. Grp. Psychother.*, 21:23–33.

Schmidt, W., Smart, R. G., and Moss, M. K., 1968, *Social class and the treatment of alcoholism*, University of Toronto Press, Toronto.

Schramm, C. J., and DeFillippi, R. J., 1975, Characteristics of successful alcoholism treatment programs for American workers, *Br. J. Addict.*, 70:271–275.

Schuckit, M. A., 1977, Geriatric alcoholism and drug abuse, *Gerontologist*, 17:168–174.

Schut, J., File, K., and Wohlmuth, T., 1973, Alcohol use by narcotic addicts in methadone maintenance treatment, *Q. J. Stud. Alc.*, 34:1356–1359.

Scott, E. M., 1970, *Struggles in an Alcoholic Family*, Charles C Thomas, Springfield, Ill.

Seiden, R. H., 1960, The use of alcoholics anonymous members in research on alcoholism, *Q. J. Stud. Alc.*, 21:506–509.

Selig, A. L., 1975, Program planning, evaluation, and the problem of the alcoholic, *Am. J. Publ. Hlth.*, 65:72–75.

Shelton, J., Hollister, L. E., and Gocka, E. F., 1969, The drinking behavior interview: An attempt to quantify alcoholic impairment, *Dis. Nerv. Syst.*, 30:464–467.

Shipp, T. J., 1963, *Helping the Alcoholic and His Family*, Prentice-Hall, Englewood Cliffs, N.J.

Shore, J. H., and Fumetti, B. V., 1972, Three alcohol programs for American Indians, *Am. J. Psychiat.*, 128:1450–1454.

Siegel, H. H., 1973, *Alcohol Detoxification Programs*, Charles C Thomas, Springfield, Ill.

Simon, A., Epstein, L. J., and Reynolds, L., 1968, Alcoholism in the geriatrically mentally ill, *Geriatrics*, 23:125–131.

Simpson, W. S., and Webber, P. W., 1971, A field program in the treatment of alcoholism, *Hosp. & Comm. Psychiat.*, 22:170–173.

Slaughter, L. D., and Torno, K., 1968, Hospitalized alcoholic patients, IV, The role of patient-counselors, *Hosp. & Comm. Psychiat.*, 19:209–210.

Smart, R. G., 1974, Employed alcoholics treated voluntarily and under constructive coercion: A follow-up study, *Q. J. Stud. Alc.*, 35:196–209.

Smart, R. G., Schmidt, W., and Moss, M. K., 1969, Social class as a determinant of the type and duration of therapy received by alcoholics, *Inter. J. Addict.*, 4:543–556.

Sobell, M. D., and Sobell, L. C., 1973, Individualized behavior therapy for alcoholics, *Behav. Ther.*, 4:49–72.

Sobell, L. C., and Sobell, M. B., 1975, Outpatient alcoholics give valid self-reports, *J. Nerv. Ment. Dis.*, 161:32–42.

Sobell, M. B., Sobell, L. C., and Sheahan, D. B., 1976, Functional analysis of drinking problems as an aid in developing individual treatment strategies, *Addict. Behav.*, 1:127–132.

Solomon, J., 1982, *Alcoholism and Clinical Psychiatry*, Plenum Press, New York.

Spradley, J. P., 1970, *You Owe Yourself a Drunk: An Ethnography of Urban Nomads,* Little, Brown and Company, Boston.

Stallings, D. L., and Oncken, G. R., 1977, A relative change index in evaluating alcoholism treatment outcome, *J. Stud. Alc.,* 38:457–464.

Staub, G. E., and Kent, L. M. (eds.), 1973, *The Para-Professional in the Treatment of Alcoholism,* Charles C Thomas, Springfield, Ill.

Steiner, C., 1971, *Games Alcoholics Play,* Grove Press, New York.

Steinglass, P., 1976, Experimenting with family treatment approaches to alcoholism, 1950–1975: A review, *Family Process,* 15:97–123.

Steinglass, P., 1977, Family therapy in alcoholism, in *The Biology of Alcoholism,* vol. 5, *Treatment and Rehabilitation of the Chronic Alcoholic* (B. Kissin and H. Begleiter, eds.), pp. 259–300, Plenum Press, New York.

Sterne, M. W., and Pittman, D. J., 1965, The concept of motivation: A source of institutional and professional blockage in the treatment of alcoholics, *Q. J. Stud. Alc.,* 26:41–57.

Stinnett, J. L., 1982, Outpatient detoxification of the alcoholic, *Inter. J. Addict.,* 17:1031–1046.

Streissguth, A. P., Martin, D. C., and Buffington, V. E., 1977, Identifying heavy drinkers: A comparison of eight alcohol scores obtained on the same sample, in *Currents in Alcoholism,* vol. 2 (F. A. Seixas, ed.), Grune & Stratton, New York.

Suchotliff, L., and Meyer, S., 1975, The educational process as a treatment modality in a drug rehabilitation program, *Am. J. Psychiat.,* 132:195–197.

Swint, J. M., and Nelson, W. B., 1977, Prospective evaluation of alcoholism rehabilitative efforts, *J. Stud. Alc.,* 38:1386–1404.

Tarleton, G. H., and Tarnower, S. M., 1960, The use of letters as part of a psychotherapeutic relationship: Experiences in a clinic for alcoholics, *Q. J. Stud. Alc.,* 21:82–89.

Thimann, J., 1966, *The Addictive Drinker,* Philosophical Library, New York.

Thornton, C. C., Gottheil, E., Gellens, H. K., and Alterman, A. I., 1981, Developmental level and treatment response in male alcoholics, in *Matching Patient Needs and Treatment Methods in Alcoholism and Drug Abuse* (E. Gottheil, et al., eds.), Charles C Thomas, Springfield, Ill.

Toch, H., 1965, *The Social Psychology of Social Movements,* Bobbs-Merrill, Indianapolis, Ind.

Tomsovic, M., 1968, Hospitalized alcoholic patients: A two-year study of medical, social and psychological characteristics, *Hosp. & Comm. Psychiat.,* 19:197–204.

Trice, H. M., and Roman, P. M., 1970, Delabelling, relabelling, and alcoholics anonymous, *Social Problems,* 17:538–542.

———, 1970, Sociopsychological predictors of affiliation with alcoholics anonymous: A longitudinal study of treatment success, *Social Psychiatry,* 5:51–59.

Trice, H. M., Roman, P. M., and Belasco, J. A., 1969, Selection for treatment: A predictive evaluation of an alcoholic treatment regimen, *Inter. J. Addict.,* 4:303–317.

Twerski, A. J., 1969, When to hospitalize the alcoholic, *Hosp. Prog.,* 4:47–55.

Uecker, A. E., and Boutilier, L. R., 1976, Alcohol education for alcoholics: Relation to attitude changes and post-treatment abstinence, *J. Stud. Alc.,* 37:965–975.

Usdin, G. L., Rond, P. C., Hinchcliffe, J. A., and Ross, W. D., 1952, The meaning of disulfiram to alcoholics in group psychotherapy, *Q. J. Stud. Alc.*, 13:590–599.

Vaillant, G. E., 1983, *The Natural Course of Alcoholism*, Harvard University Press, Cambridge, Mass.

Verden, P., and Shatterley, D., 1971, Alcoholism research and resistance in understanding the compulsive drinker, *Ment. Hyg.*, 55:331–336.

Viamontes, J. A., 1972, Review of drug effectiveness in the treatment of alcoholism, *Am. J. Psychiat.*, 128:1570–1571.

Vitols, M. M., 1968, Culture patterns of drinking in Negro and white alcoholics, *Dis. Nerv. Syst.*, 29:391–394.

Voegtlin, W. L., and Lemere, F., 1942, The treatment of alcohol addiction: A review of the literature, *Q. J. Stud. Alc.*, 2:717–803.

Wanberg, K. W., and Horn, J. L., 1973, Alcoholism syndromes related to sociological classification, *Inter. J. Addict.*, 8:99–120.

Wanberg, K. W., and Jones, E., 1973, Initial contact and admission of persons requesting treatment for alcohol patients, *Br. J. Addict.*, 68:281–285.

Wanberg, K. W., Horn, J. L., and Foster, F. M., 1977, A differential assessment model for alcoholism: The scales of the alcohol use inventory, *J. Stud. Alc.*, 38:512–543.

Ward, R. F., and Faillace, L. A., 1970, The alcoholic and his helpers: A systems view, *Q. J. Stud. Alc.*, 31:684–691.

Wedel, H. L., 1965, Involving alcoholics in treatment, *Q. J. Stud. Alc.*, 26:468–479.

Wellman, M., 1955, Fatigue during the second six months of abstinence, *Can. Med. Assoc. J.*, 72:338–342.

Westermeyer, J., 1972, Chippewa and majority alcoholism in the Twin Cities: A comparison, *J. Nerv. Ment. Dis.*, 155:322–327.

Westermeyer, J., 1976, Clinical guidelines for the cross-cultural treatment of chemical dependency, *Am. J. Drug Alc. Abuse*, 3:315–322.

Westermeyer, J., and Bearman, J., 1973, A proposed social indicator system for alcohol-related problems, *Prevent. Med.*, 2:438–444.

Westermeyer, J., and Lang, G., 1975, Ethnic differences in use of alcoholism facilities, *Inter. J. Addict.*, 10:513–520.

Wilkinson, R., 1970, *The Prevention of Drinking Problems: Alcoholic Control and Cultural Influences*, Oxford University Press, New York.

Willems, P. J. A., Letemendia, F. J. J., and Arroyave, F., 1973, A categorization of the assessment of programs and outcomes in the treatment of alcoholism, *Br. J. Psychiat.* 122:649–654.

Williams, R. L., and Moffat, G. H. (eds.), 1975, *Occupational Alcoholism Programs*, Charles C Thomas, Springfield, Ill.

Wiseman, J. P., 1970, *Stations of the Lost: The Treatment of Skid Row Alcoholics*, Prentice-Hall, Englewood Cliffs, N.J.

Wolf, I., Chafetz, M. E., Blane, H. T., and Hill, M. J., 1965, Social factors in the diagnosis of alcoholism in social and non-social situations, I, Attitudes of physicians. *Q. J. Stud. Alc.*, 26:72–79.

Wright, D. E., 1975, Alternative housing for the recovery of the skid row alcoholic, *Am. Arch. Rehab. Ther.*, 23:59–66.

Zimberg, S., 1982, *The Clinical Management of Alcoholism*, Brunner/Mazel, New York.

Zimberg, S., Lipscomb, H., and Davis, E. B., 1971, Sociopsychiatric treatment of alcoholics in an urban ghetto, *Am. J. Psychiat.*, 127:1670–1674.

Zimberg, S., Wallace, J., and Blume, S. B. (eds.), 1978, *Practical Approaches to Alcoholism Psychotherapy*, Plenum Press, New York.

Zucker, R. A., 1979, Developmental aspects of drinking through the young adult years, in *Youth, Alcohol, and Social Policy* (H. T. Blane and M. L. Chafetz, eds.), Plenum Press, New York.

CHAPTER 6

Treatment of Alcoholism in Office and Outpatient Settings

Marc A. Schuckit, M.D.
Professor of Psychiatry
University of California, San Diego, School of Medicine
Director of the Alcohol Treatment Program
Veterans Administration Medical Center
San Diego, California

I. INTRODUCTION

There are no magic cures for alcoholism. However, with consistent and careful help, almost all alcoholics will improve, and 60% to 70% of the most stable group will still be abstinent a year after treatment (Schuckit, 1984).

Thus, the average clinician's fear that "nothing will work with the alcoholic" is erroneous. This bias probably comes from observing the small cadre of the most obvious alcoholics seen in central city hospitals— individuals who appear with cirrhosis or pancreatitis and come for treatment in an intoxicated state. These "skid row" alcoholics have a poor prognosis (perhaps 10% will be "dry" a year later), and this leads to subsequent unwarranted pessimism.

NOTE: Supported by the Veterans Administration Medical Research Service, NIAAA grant #PHSAA04353, and Joan and Ray Kroc.

The clinician plays a *central* role in the alcoholic's recovery. You are a "gatekeeper" who helps the alcoholic by confrontation, maximizing proper medical functioning, and introducing him or her to rehabilitation. Rehabilitation is straightforward and consists of maneuvers to maximize motivation toward abstinence (e.g., education of the patient and his or her family) and to help the patient establish a new life pattern without alcohol (e.g., by counseling).

In choosing patients for treatment it is important to distinguish clearly between information on drinking patterns, data regarding alcohol problems (which may be temporary and disappear on their own), and information on alcoholism. Ninety percent or more of the population of most Western countries drink at some time during their lives, and a subsequent minority (perhaps up to 40% of men) experience a single drunk-driving arrest, arguments with friends because of drinking, or skipping work or school because of a hangover or desire to drink—problems which tend to disappear with time alone (Cahalan, 1970; Fillmore, 1975). However, the comments offered in Chapters 6 and 7 deal with alcoholism, i.e., serious, persistent and pervasive alcohol-related problems which predict the persistence of such serious difficulties.

Outpatient treatment involves a series of steps of recognition, confrontation, and then offering care (see Figure 1). Therapeutic options include outpatient or (preferably) inpatient detoxification if needed and possible referral to an inpatient facility or to structured outpatient rehabilitation. Treatment involves enhancing the patient's motivation and helping him or her through recovery by individual or (preferably) group psychotherapy which probably places an emphasis on simple "day-to-day" life adjustment and education on alcohol. Patients will also benefit through family counseling and referral to Alcoholics Anonymous (AA).

To understand alcoholic rehabilitation, it is important that you read both Chapter 6 and Chapter 7. This overview begins with a general discussion which serves as a basis for both outpatient and residential efforts. For convenience, the alcoholic is noted as "he," but the term refers equally to men and women.

A. The Clinical Importance of Alcoholism

Alcoholism and related problems are major forces in our lives. Somewhere between 5% and 10% of the adult male population and between 2% and 5% of adult women meet the criteria for alcoholism, with an additional 30% to 40% of young men demonstrating isolated alcohol problems of limited severity (Cahalan and Cisin, 1968; Cahalan et al., 1972). Thus, whether you are engaged in industrial counseling, police work, or health

Is the problem alcohol-related?

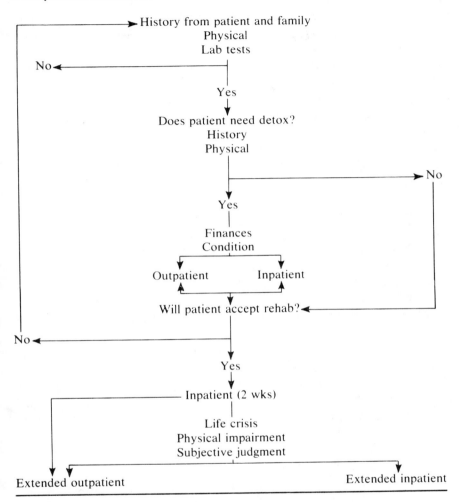

Figure 1
Decisions in Alcoholism Treatment

clinic work, or are a physician in private practice, alcoholism is an important factor to watch for in the patients you see. Because alcohol so adversely affects most body systems, the rate of alcoholism and alcohol-related problems is even higher in medical and surgical patients than in the general population, with between 20% and 35% of medical and surgical inpatients meeting fairly rigid criteria for alcoholism (Barchha et al., 1968; Moore, 1971). Therefore, at least one out of every five men and women walking into your office experience serious alcohol-related pathology which may significantly shorten his life.

This patient is likely to look like everyone else, for the average alcoholic is a middle-class individual—only about 3% to 5% of alcoholics reside on skid row (Haglund and Schuckit, 1982). Furthermore, the alcoholic patient is likely to present a variety of medical and psychological problems, only admitting to alcohol-related pathology if directly questioned (as discussed in greater depth later in this chapter).

Therefore you should know about alcoholism. It has an impact on both our private lives and our professional experiences, and without recognizing the disorder, you are likely to miss much medical and psychological pathology and may have great difficulty in putting a patient's entire clinical picture together in an adequate manner.

B. How Best to Define Alcoholism

While specific biases are briefly presented here, a more thorough discussion of the definition of alcoholism appears in Chapter 1. There is probably no one best definition. The different diagnostic schemes outline slightly different populations, but there is a great deal of overlap. Each approach has inherent assets and liabilities, and the final choice depends upon the goals and biases of the investigator or clinician. The *quantity-frequency-variability* scheme (Cahalan, 1969) defines heavy drinkers by a high correlation between those in the highest drinking categories and those demonstrating life problems related to alcohol. However, it may be difficult to establish accurate drinking practices, especially for the heaviest drinkers, who may be experiencing alcohol blackouts (Goodwin et al., 1970). A second definition involves *psychological dependence,* meaning evidence of a life-style centering around alcohol (including such things as taking drinks before going to a party, etc.), but this is very subjective and thus of limited usefulness. A third definition centers around *physical addiction,* usually defined as the occurrence of an abstinence syndrome when the alcohol intake is decreased. (Sellers and Kalant, 1976). In its full-blown form, the physical withdrawal syndrome probably occurs in only 5% to 15% of individuals going through some sort of withdrawal (Victor, 1966), and the sole use of this definition results in isolation of only a severely ill group.

The definition of greatest use to the clinician evaluates the occurrence of a significant alcohol-related life problem, including a marital separation or divorce related to alcohol, *or* multiple arrests related to alcohol, *or* physical evidence that alcohol has harmed health, *or* loss of a job related to drinking (Schuckit et al., 1969). It is this type of definition, as shown in Figure 2, which has been most frequently applied to follow-up studies of alcoholics, and it allows one to outline the probable future course and make some generalizations about treatment. An individual fitting this definition is probably drinking heavily and showing psychological dependence and might have physical dependence.

If the purpose in diagnosis is prediction of future course and selection of treatment (Goodwin & Guze, 1979; Guze, 1970), then it makes sense that an individual demonstrating only alcoholism (as defined above) will run a different course from someone showing alcoholism in the midst of another disorder. Therefore, *primary* (or uncomplicated) alcoholism means serious alcohol problems occurring in an individual demonstrating no preexisting major psychiatric disorder, while *secondary* alcoholism (or complicated alcoholism) is an alcoholic picture beginning after another major psychiatric disorder has developed (Schuckit, 1973). A series of investigations demonstrate that between 60% and 70% of inpatients meet the rigorous criteria for primary alcoholism (Schuckit et al., 1969; Schuckit, 1973). Of those who demonstrate preexisting psychiatric disorders (i.e., secondary alcoholism), the most frequently appearing diagnoses are the antisocial personality and primary affective disorder.

The *antisocial personality* as used here is defined as serious antisocial problems in all four major life areas (family, peers, police, and school) beginning prior to age 16 and before the first alcoholic major life problem (Robins, 1966; Schuckit, 1973). Approximately 20% of the group of male alcoholics entering either a private or public alcoholic treatment facility and 5% of women alcoholics entering similar facilities meet the criteria for primary antisocial personality and secondary alcoholism (Schuckit, 1984). *Primary affective disorder* is outlined by Goodwin and Guze (1979) to mean a persistent depression lasting for weeks on end, accompanied by serious changes in body functioning (e.g., constipation, insomnia, lethargy, etc.) and mind functioning (e.g., inability to concentrate, the future looking hopeless, unable to feel joy, etc.). If the picture develops prior to the onset of serious alcohol-related life problems or during an extended period of abstinence (arbitrarily, three months or more), the person is labeled as primary affective disorder and secondary alcoholism (Schuckit et al., 1969). Twenty percent to 25% of a group of women alcoholics and 5% of a group of male alcoholics demonstrate this picture of primary affective disorder and secondary alcoholism (Schuckit et al., 1969). *Process* (or *nuclear*) *schizophrenia* as defined by Goodwin and Guze (1979) is only seen in 3% to 5% of alcoholic inpatients, and other major diagnoses make up less than 1% or 2% each (Winokur et al., 1970).

There is evidence that the individual with a primary antisocial personality and secondary alcoholism runs the course of the antisocial per-

1. Ask all patients about alcohol-related life problems:
   Marital separation or divorce *or*
   Job loss or layoff *or*
   Multiple arrests *or*
   Physical evidence of alcohol-harmed health

   Diagnosis of alcoholism

2. Then screen for preexisting psychiatric disorders, especially affective disorder and the antisocial personality

Has antisocial problems in all four life areas beginning before age 16	Has extended periods of depression (or mania) before onset of first alcoholic life problem (or during an extended abstinence)	No major preexisting psychiatric problems
Primary antisocial personality	Primary affective disorder	Primary alcoholism
Secondary alcoholism	Secondary alcoholism	

Figure 2
The Diagnosis of Alcoholism

sonality with many more serious problems than the primary alcoholic, while those with primary affective disorder and secondary alcoholism have a more benign course for their alcohol problems (although they run a much higher risk for suicide) (Schuckit and Winokur, 1972). More information on the treatment of secondary alcoholics is given in this and the subsequent chapters.

C. Alcoholism as a "Disease"—The Natural History

Health care deliverers' patients come to you asking for help with symptoms or constellations of problems. Because they look to you as the "expert" and are likely to follow some of your recommendations, it is important that you carefully choose the best mode of intervention (if any intervention is appropriate). One way to do this is to evaluate the clinical picture objectively and compare it to information in the literature in order to best predict the future course and most rationally select treatment (Guze, 1970). If a disorder can be objectively defined in a manner that allows establishment of prognosis and selection of treatment, for all *practical* purposes it becomes a "disease." Thus, this section "sidesteps" the question of whether alcoholism is a syndrome, a phenomenon, or a true disease by stating that it is a problem involved in the differential diagnosis of many medical and psychiatric disorders. The actual label used is up to each individual clinician.

If the definition of primary alcoholism based on major life problems is used and those patients who demonstrate alcohol problems in the midst of other obvious psychiatric disorders (secondary alcoholism) are excluded, there does appear to be a predictable natural course for primary alcoholism as shown in Table 1. The average alcoholic demonstrates his first major life problem related to drinking in his late twenties to early or middle thirties (Haglund and Schuckit, 1982), and this event can arbitrarily be considered the age of onset of alcoholism. Controlling for socioeconomic stratum (SES) and the occurrence of other major preexisting psychiatric disorders, the age estimates appear to be similar for men and women (Schuckit and Morrissey, 1976). Most alcoholics present for treatment in their early forties with alcohol problems which have been going on for almost a decade (Schuckit, 1977b).

One important aspect of the course of alcoholism is its fluctuating nature. As demonstrated by Ludwig (1972), at any given month after treatment, approximately one-half of alcoholics report abstinence with a mean of four months of being "dry" in the year-and-a-half following release from therapy. Thus, the usual alcoholic doesn't begin his drinking in his late teens and demonstrate the first problem by the early thirties

Table 1
The Natural History of Primary Alcoholism

1. Age of first drink	12–14
2. Age first intoxicated*	14–18
3. Age first minor alcohol problem*	18–25
4. Usual age of first major problem	28–30
5. Usual age entering treatment	40
6. Usual age of death	55–60
Leading causes: heart disease	
cancer	
accidents	
suicide	
7. In any year, abstinence alternates with active drinking	
8. "Spontaneous remission" rate *or*	10–30%
Response to nonspecific intervention	

*These ages are about the same in the general population.

only to stay drunk until he dies. Rather, spontaneous periods of abstinence and marked decreases in drinking can be expected to alternate with times of drinking problems.

A number of longitudinal investigations (Schmidt and deLint, 1972; Sundby, 1967) have shown that the alcoholic dies 10 to 15 years earlier than the general population, even when one controls for such factors as SES. The leading causes of death in approximate decreasing order are heart disease, cancer, accidents, and suicide, as discussed in other areas of this chapter and the overview of medical disorders in Chapter 2.

Finally, as part of the natural history of alcoholism, one can expect that as high as 10% to 30% of individuals who meet the criteria for alcoholism will learn to abstain or seriously limit their alcohol intake even without exposure to formal treatment (Lemere, 1953; Vaillant and Milofsky, 1982; Kendell and Staton, 1966; Drew, 1968). A variety of approaches have documented this phenomenon, including follow-ups of individuals in treatment who didn't initially seem to respond, comparisons of those who entered versus those who were denied treatment, and information on general population alcoholics who have never received therapy.

Thus, once someone has been diagnosed as a primary alcoholic, you know something about the problems you can expect during the subsequent course of their illness and, as discussed later in this and subsequent chapters, you can make some rational decisions about treatment. This information, along with the data tending to indicate that alcohol is a genetically influenced disorder, as discussed in Chapter 3, allows the health care deliverer to feel comfortable looking at alcoholism as a disease. This is a practical decision, not one based on meticulous semantic arguments which are of theoretical (but somewhat limited clinical) value.

D. A General Treatment Philosophy

This chapter has emphasized that it is important for the clinician to choose a definition of alcoholism and stick with it, understanding the biases involved in choosing that particular approach. Before interfering in the lives of individuals with alcohol problems, it is important for us to understand the expected course of their disorder and to have some manner of choosing among the various treatment approaches available. In addition, there are a number of elements in the "art" of treating alcoholism which have no scientific basis but which help you in carrying out your therapeutic efforts.

While we must try to motivate people, it may be impossible to force them to do things they don't want to do. In that light, it helps to recognize that the major responsibility for improvement rests with the patient and not the health care deliverer. As a clinician, you can identify the most important parts of the problem, share what you see as the course and potential treatment with the patient, and strongly urge him or her to take advantage of the care that is available. If you try to take responsibility for the patient's life (something you can never successfully do anyway), you run the risk of playing a game most patients have already used with friends and relatives for years (Berne, 1965). Therefore, confront and suggest and continue to see the patient no matter what his decision is. Do not assume the role of the omnipotent healer.

II. OUTPATIENT TREATMENT WITH THE ALCOHOLIC

With these issues clearly in mind, you can use some general rules in formulating your own treatment approaches, although you may have to modify them for each patient. Treatment follows common-sense guidelines based on the issues of diagnosis and natural history discussed above. This section briefly reviews some general rules which will help the clinician identify the alcoholic, carry out adequate detoxification, confront and attempt to motivate the unwilling patient, and carry out proper referral as well as outpatient rehabilitation.

A. Presentation of the Alcoholic in a General Outpatient Practice

The average alcoholic is likely to appear in clinical settings in a sober state, looking well groomed and having no smell of alcohol about him. He or she will complain of a variety of medical and emotional problems which must be properly diagnosed if the clinician hopes to avoid unexpected calls in the middle of the night and nonresponse to ill-advised treatments which should never have been given to an alcoholic in the first place (e.g., sleeping pills). Thus, it is in the clinician's best interest to identify the alcoholic in order to save himself or herself time and inconvenience and to be certain that he or she is offering the maximal amount of care at the minimal risk.

Since it can be very difficult to identify the alcoholic, it is best for the clinician to consider the possibility of alcoholism in *every* patient. Each individual should be asked about his pattern of life problems (e.g., recent accidents, driving arrests, difficulty getting along with spouse or friends, problems on the job, etc.). This is then followed by a brief attempt to establish whether the life problems are related to alcohol or other substance intake—i.e., information on the quantity and frequency of drinking may be best established after the pattern of life problems. If the patient meets or comes close to the criteria for alcoholism, the next step is to establish whether the problem is primary or represents a secondary manifestation of depressions unrelated to drinking or antisocial behaviors occurring in all life areas and beginning prior to the age of 16. These secondary alcoholics have different prognoses and additional treatment needs as discussed elsewhere in this text.

The interested clinician might also consider using a brief paper-and-pencil screening test, such as the 25-item Michigan Alcohol Screening Test (MAST), which might correctly identify up to 95% of alcoholics (Selzer, 1971; Lancet, 1980a). An even shorter 10-question form of the MAST has also been shown to identify over 90% of the alcoholics appearing in general psychiatric hospitals (Bernadt et al., 1982). Of course, gathering additional information from the spouse or other relevant resource person can be very helpful.

The usual blue-collar or white-collar working alcoholic or housewife also presents with a variety of medical problems and aberrant laboratory tests. While these are not diagnostic of alcoholism, they help to raise your suspicion that the patient is at even higher risk for alcoholism than the average person you see.

1. Medical Problems

The easiest series of screening tests involve simple blood markers. Many alcoholics will have mild elevation in uric acid, free fatty acid, mean corpuscular volume, and/or gamma glutamyl transferase (White-head, et al., 1978; 1981a). Another approach is to evaluate the pattern of 25 fairly commonly used blood tests which, according to one report using a mathematical formula, may be used to correctly identify over 85% of alcoholics versus controls (Ryback et al., 1980). While many clinicians will be unwilling to use such sophisticated formulas, the simple combination of the brief MAST and observation of the blood tests specifically noted above can be very useful. The remainder of this section on medical problems gives a rapid overview of some of the more dramatic aspects of the physiological toxicity of ethanol with the hope that you have read Chapter 2, and that those interested will go on to read some of the excellent review books such as those by Becker et al. (1974) and Kissin and Begleiter (1971a, 1971b).

Most readers are familiar with the alcohol-related *digestive system* problems of cirrhosis (only seen in about 15% of identified alcoholics) and pancreatitis (seen in an even lower percentage). Additional problems are that alcoholics and heavy drinkers show high rates of cancers of all areas of the digestive tract, especially the esophagus and stomach (Hakulinen et al., 1974), high rates of ulcer disease (Iber, 1971), and elevated rates of gastritis (Lieber, 1975). Of course, any evidence of serious pathology in the digestive tract should raise the possibility of alcoholism.

The *neurologic system* is another frequent problem area in alcoholics (Freund, 1976). Deterioration of the nerves of muscle and sensation in the hands and feet (peripheral neuropathy) is seen in about 10% of alcoholics, and should raise the clinician's suspicion about alcoholism, even in the elderly (Schuckit, 1977d). Levels of confusion, especially of recent onset, can be related to simple intoxication, especially for individuals with preexisting brain disease such as might occur after repeated trauma or in the elderly—making alcohol intake part of the differential diagnosis of all recent onset states of confusion and disorientation, especially in the elderly (Schuckit, 1983). Confusion associated with autonomic nervous system dysfunctioning (e.g., increased pulse, respirations, body tempera-ture, and tremors) can be seen in alcoholics as part of the withdrawal syndrome—with 5% to 10% of hospitalized alcoholics showing significant confusion (Sellers and Kalant, 1976), a problem which tends to be tran-sient and disappear within four to five days. An additional confused state is associated with vitamin deficiencies, especially those of thiamine (the Wernicke-Korsakov's syndrome) and possibly niacin—problems which should improve with vitamin supplementation but which might not totally reverse (Victor et al., 1971; Lishman, 1981). The rapid development of problems with coordination may herald alcoholic cerebellar degeneration (Victor et al., 1959) and there are additional exceedingly rare but dramatic (alcohol-related) neurologic disorders which may result in rapid death—including central pontine myolinoysis and Marchiava-Bigiami syndrome (Dreyfus, 1974).

The association between alcoholism and more permanent decreased *intellectual functioning* is not very clear. The majority of alcoholics presenting for detoxification show some signs of intellectual impairment and 40–70% may show increased brain ventricular size (probably indicating decreased brain tissue) (Lancet, 1981; Lishman, 1981; Wilkinson, 1982). While some investigators feel that there is a correlation between increased brain ventricular size and decreased functioning on neuropsychological testing, not all agree, and it is probable that most alcoholics will recover in both parameters after several months of abstinence (Zelazowski, et al., 1981; Wilkinson, 1982). The etiology of these neuropsychological changes is unknown, but it probably represents a combination of trauma, vitamin deficiencies, and a direct neurotoxic effect of alcohol (Walker et al., 1980; Lishman, 1981). While most intellectual deficits disappear with time, there may be a decrease in abstract reasoning when alcoholics are compared to age-matched controls. This has led some authors to advance a theory of more rapid "brain aging" in alcoholics, although the evidence regarding this hypothesis is contradictory (Ryan, 1982).

Another area of medical difficulties, probably noted in more than one-quarter of alcoholics, involves the *cardiovascular system* (Wu et al., 1976). While it has been recognized that low doses of alcohol (less than two drinks a day or less than one ounce of absolute alcohol daily) may increase blood high-density lipoproteins (HDLs) which may decrease the risk for heart disease, enhanced risk comes with higher levels of alcohol intake (Lancet, 1980). Alcohol can adversely affect the heart functioning of individuals with cardiac disease, even at relatively low doses (Gould et al., 1971; Parker, 1974), but the ready reversibility of this pathology usually allows people who don't drink heavily to escape serious consequences. Ethanol raises the blood pressure (Klatsky et al., 1977), increases the blood fats (including cholesterol) (Cameron et al., 1975), and is a direct toxin to heart muscle (Wu et al., 1976). The result is more atherosclerosis, hypertensive heart disease, and cardiomyopathy in the alcoholic than in the general population (Horowitz, 1975; Pader, 1973). Individuals presenting with blood pressure problems which are difficult to regulate, elevated blood fats that don't come under control, or unusual signs of heart disease, including cardiomyopathy, should be considered at high risk for also having alcoholism.

The elevated risk for *cancers* of the digestive tract extends to cancers of the head and neck where, in one series, over 50% of individuals presenting with cancers above the epiglottis met the criteria for alcoholism (Lowry, 1975). Similarly, and perhaps related to high rates of smoking, alcoholics demonstrate an elevated incidence of cancer of the lung (Lundby, 1967). The reasons for this might rest with the irritant effects of alcohol, potential carcinogens present in alcohol or its congeners, or the alcohol-induced decreased functioning of white blood cells hypothesized to be important in controlling tumors (Lundby et al., 1975). However, patients entering your care for cancer of the head and neck, lung, or digestive tract are at high risk for alcoholism, and it may save a great deal of postoperative problems (including unanticipated withdrawal) if patients and their families are routinely queried about alcohol-related life difficulties.

High levels of alcohol also cause deterioration of skeletal *muscle* with a resulting muscle inflammation or wasting seen mainly in the shoulders and hips (Becker et al., 1975, pp. 56–58). In addition to those mentioned earlier, other blood tests noted to occur with even low doses of alcohol include impairment in *clotting* due to low levels of platelets and clotting proteins (Lieber, 1973), a decreased production of red blood cells with a resulting *macrocytic anemia* (Eichner and Hillman, 1971), and a lowered level of production and impairment in the functioning of *white blood cells* (Liu, 1973), which might be responsible for the high rate of infection among alcoholics. Thus, unexplained muscle pains or weaknesses, elevated uric acid levels, abnormal blood indices, or recurrent infections should increase your already high level of suspicion that a patient is at risk for alcoholism.

This review of medical problems could go on to fill an entire text. The important things are that alcohol and alcoholism affect many of the body systems and that the clinician should be aware of the possible role of alcoholism in explaining unusual clinical pictures and unusual responses to treatment. In addition, a host of medical signs and symptoms, including cancers of the upper digestive tract, macrocytic anemia, sporadically elevated uric acid levels, etc., should raise the index suspicion of alcoholism. These are important clues that help us recognize the 95% of the alcoholics who do not belong to skid row and who make up as much as one-third of the patient load of the usual physician and surgeon.

2. Psychiatric and Emotional Problems

A general life crisis or specific emotional problem might precipitate the alcoholic into seeking help. These encompass a variety of areas, including sexual difficulties such as menstrual irregularities, frigidity (Schuckit, 1972), or impotence, and disturbances in sleep or appetite. Interpersonal problems with the spouse, employer, or friends might also

Table 2
Differential Diagnosis of Sadness or Psychosis in an Alcoholic

A. Alcohol and sadness
   R/O primary affective disorder with secondary alcohol misuse
   R/O pharmacologic effect of alcohol producing sadness in the primary alcoholic
   R/O sadness in response to a real life crisis

B. Alcohol and psychosis
   R/O primary schizophrenia with secondary alcohol misuse (<5% of patients)
   R/O alcoholic paranoia—rapid onset of paranoid delusions in a clear sensorium
   R/O alcoholic hallucinosis—rapid onset of auditory hallucination in a clear sensorium
   R/O drug-induced psychosis—e.g., hypnotics or stimulants

be perceived by the alcoholic as a crisis for which to seek help. It is important to consider the possibility that alcohol is a major or ancillary factor in all patients presenting with life problems.

Alcohol can cause problems that mimic almost any psychiatric disorder (Schuckit, 1983). Even after screening out the secondary alcoholics, a level of confusion remains regarding depressive symptoms (Schuckit, 1977b), as noted in Table 2. Alcohol in high doses causes a picture of sadness in almost anyone (Warren and Raynes, 1972; Tamerin and Mendelson, 1970), with a level of depression that can result in spur-of-the-moment suicides (deLint and Levinson, 1975). However, unlike primary affective disorder, alcohol-induced sadness will disappear within days to weeks of cessation of drinking (Gibson and Becker, 1973a). Not only do alcoholics get sad, the diagnostic confusion is further complicated by the increased level of drinking which is seen in the majority of manic patients and at least one-third of patients in depressive episodes (Schuckit, 1977b; Morrison, 1974). It is probably not possible to diagnose primary affective disorder in the presence of heavy drinking unless a careful history of prior affective episodes unrelated to alcoholism is obtained (Schuckit et al., 1969). Sadness, which disappears with abstinence, should be recognized as a frequent presenting symptom for alcoholics.

Alcohol in high doses can also cause a picture of paranoia and/or auditory hallucinosis in the presence of a clear sensorium (Victor and Hope, 1955). As shown in Table 2, this picture can be clinically identical to paranoid schizophrenia, amphetamine psychosis, or the psychosis associated with barbiturate abuse (Ellinwood, 1971). Alcoholism must be part of the differential diagnosis for an individual presenting with a rapid onset of a psychotic picture. Alcoholic paranoia or hallucinosis usually clears within days to weeks of abstinence, even without antipsychotic medications.

A high level of anxiety is part of the withdrawal syndrome from alcohol and can also be seen in the midst of active drinking. In addition, there is evidence of a protracted abstinence syndrome going on for six months after primary withdrawal—a picture which is also characterized by high levels of anxiety (Johnson et al., 1970). Thus, alcoholism must be considered as part of a differential diagnosis of any individual who presents with what appears to be global anxiety, anxiety neurosis, obsessive-compulsive neurosis, or phobic neurosis (Goodwin and Guze, 1979).

The specific level of association between alcoholism and psychiatric disorders is dependent upon the diagnostic scheme used and the reasons for labeling. When a model using objective criteria for psychiatric syndromes to outline disorders with a known natural course is used, it can be seen that alcoholism must be considered as part of the differential diagnosis of almost all psychiatric pictures. Recognition of this can aid in accurate diagnosis and proper selection of treatment. It is important to take a careful history of alcohol (and drug) use from all patients and their families—regardless of their presenting complaint.

B. Confrontation

As the therapist or physician involved, the best way to head off future problems is to share your concerns with the patient. One approach is to use the patient's presenting complaint as your entrée to the alcohol area, sharing your thoughts, educating him or her about the future problems that can be expected unless drinking is modified, and telling the person that it appears as if he or she has reached a point in life where alcohol is causing significant problems. (*Note:* you might choose not to use the term "alcoholism" directly at this stage.) For instance, to a man coming in for a checkup because he isn't "feeling well" you might say that you are very concerned about how he feels, share with him the laboratory tests and physical findings that are abnormal, and tell him that alcohol has probably caused much of the damage. You might then share your knowledge of the course of alcohol problems and explore possible avenues for attacking the problem.

A related problem is what to do with the patient who refuses to recognize the problem and stop drinking. One goal in this situation is to keep "the door open" by encouraging the patient and his family to maintain contact, while at the same time being careful that the patient recognizes he is responsible for his own actions. In effect, what you are saying to the patient and the family is: "I care what happens to you. While I have told you the risks involved, the decision about drinking is yours, and I can't make you do what you don't want to do. I am available for you if you decide you need me." At the same time, the family may benefit from counseling and perhaps referral to a self-help group such as Alanon for the wife and Alateen for the teenage children.

An additional approach has been suggested by some clinicians, but it has some inherent dangers (Twerski, 1983). It is possible to take the education of family and friends a step further and advise them of their option of gathering all "significant others" together at one time and carrying out a confrontation with the patient. In effect, each individual would say to the patient, "I love you, but I must tell you what I think alcohol is doing to you. It is very important that you stop." While this might result in the patient entering care, there is also the possibility that the patient will ignore the help, take offense at the confrontation, and become isolated from his support system. Therefore, the family should be prepared for the possibility that this intense confrontation will backfire. Perhaps the more intensive intervention is best reserved for those individuals who are at an extremely important crisis point in their lives regarding their drinking (e.g., those whose medical problems are likely to result in a risk of death in the near future and/or those who are about to lose major support systems).

A more conservative approach is to invite the "denying" patient back to "review some other tests" in several weeks. This gives him the opportunity of thinking things over and perhaps decreasing his own denial. Should he continue to deny, you might work with family and significant others while treating the patient for the problems alcohol is causing in the hopes that he will come to you when the next crisis occurs.

Finally, those patients who refuse to stop but admit that they might "cut down" should be reminded that the average alcoholic successfully cuts down scores of times, but sooner or later escalates his drinking and subsequent problems. The patient who absolutely refuses to stop might be offered guidelines telling him that he cannot drink more than two drinks (e.g., 4 oz of wine, 12 oz of beer, or 1.5 oz of 80 proof beverage equals one drink) in any 24-hour period—working with both patient and significant others so that they are likely to come back to you when the next crisis occurs as the drinking escalates.

C. Detoxification

Once the alcoholic has been identified and confronted, the next relevant clinical decision is whether detoxification is required. Because alcoholics have such serious medical problems and because the alcohol withdrawal syndrome (as is true with all depressant drugs) is potentially serious (Sellers and Kalant, 1976), it is best to hospitalize the patient for withdrawal from alcohol. While outpatient detoxification holds promise for the future because of its low cost, this regimen requires further evaluation before it can be used routinely.

Outpatient withdrawal programs can be used when the patient refuses to be hospitalized or does not have available funds. If you choose to do detoxification outside the hospital, it is first important that all patients be screened for serious medical problems that might require hospitalization (Feldman et al., 1975; Tennant, 1977). Then, some level of "guess work" will be needed to establish the degree of withdrawal symptomatology one can expect. This can be obtained by correlating the degree of withdrawal symptomatology with the blood alcohol level, taking into consideration whether the blood ethanol is increasing or decreasing. Thus, an individual showing severe shakes and autonomic nervous system dysfunction (see Chapters 6 and 8 for more thorough discussions of these) and a blood alcohol level of 125 mg/dl which is decreasing rapidly can probably be expected to soon enter more serious withdrawal. Other patients showing slight or moderate symptoms with a zero blood alcohol level and reporting of a last drink 12 hours ago might be less likely to enter serious withdrawal.

A complete outpatient detoxification program regimen has been outlined by Feldman et al. (1975), where, through careful screening, only half of the patients required active detoxification with only 20% of these needing inpatient treatment. Under their program, the majority of patients successfully completed outpatient detoxification and half entered rehabilitation programs. Clinical management includes a thorough medical evaluation upon entering care, careful monitoring of blood alcohol levels before the patient is released on the first day, and the judicious use of antianxiety drugs (as discussed in Chapters 6 and 8). It is advisable that medications, if used at all, be stopped after three to five days in a manner similar to that explained in Chapter 7. This is to avoid possible dangerous drug interaction or abuse of the depressant drugs.

A clinical example may be helpful at this point. This "typical" middle-class alcoholic is a 43-year-old man who has a pattern of many years of drinking "too many" martinis in the evening and drinking great quantities on weekends. He probably comes to see you for some relatively nonspecific complaint, but you are able to establish a history of serious alcohol-related problems and a recent crisis (possibly a second drunk-driving arrest or a serious argument with a spouse regarding his drinking). The physical examination is basically normal except for a mild hypertension, a slightly enlarged liver, and perhaps a mild elevation in the GGT and/or mean corpuscular volume. Despite having had his last drink 12 hours before, the only evidence of withdrawal is a mild tremor and a slight increase in the pulse rate—all other vital signs are basically normal. The patient refuses to enter the hospital, and you decide (after your careful physical examination) to carry out outpatient detoxification by giving the patient multiple vitamins, 100 mg of thiamine per day, and a CNS depressant. You might choose a benzodiazepine—for example, 25-mg chlordizepoxide tablets to be taken three or four times a day as given by his spouse. It is best to give a one- or at most a two-day supply and see the patient for perhaps 15 minutes each day over the next four to five days, warning both the patient and the spouse that they should go to an emergency room immediately if there is any great intensification of the signs of withdrawal (spelling out what they might expect). Each subsequent day over the next four to five days, the patient will be given approximately 20% less of the CNS depressant until day 5 when the medication can be stopped.

D. When to Use Inpatient Treatment

After a patient has been diagnosed, confronted, and, if necessary, undergone detoxification, you are faced with a decision about the best setting for rehabilitation. There is no magic cure for alcoholism and no specific formula for selecting a particular type of therapy, although some guidelines are presented in Chapter 5 by Dr. Pattison.

The bias of Chapters 6 and 7 is that there is no convincing evidence that inpatient rehabilitation is any more effective for the average alcoholic than outpatient care (assuming the confrontation and detoxification have been carried out). In an outpatient setting, the patient has the opportunity of learning real-life lessons in a real-life setting and does not face the problems of "reentry adjustment" seen after release from an inpatient facility. While the inpatient treatment offers the advantage of forced abstinence, it has additional dangers, not the least of which is the higher expense. Therefore, until better data is available, it is probably wise to attempt to use outpatient rehabilitation whenever possible.

Selection of an inpatient or outpatient mode will be based on a series of patient preferences and characteristics. These range from your *opinion* of what is "the best" approach for this patient to the preferences of the individual and his family, financial considerations, and your prior experiences with this individual.

In short, valid reasons for considering referral of the patient for *inpatient* treatment include the following:

1. Serious Medical Problems

If your patient is suffering from liver or heart disease or other chronic medical problems, you might choose to use a general hospital to begin rehabilitation. Similarly, an individual with a state of confusion which doesn't clear after detoxification may be best handled in a sheltered environment such as an alcohol treatment center or psychiatric hospital where he can take advantage of the program as his confusion lifts.

2. Emotional Problems in the Primary Alcoholic

As mentioned briefly above, alcohol can cause evanescent syndromes of severe depression, psychosis, organicity, and even mania (Schuckit, 1977a). These pictures, while expected to clear within days to weeks, can make it difficult (if not impossible) for the patient to function adequately outside the hospital. In this instance, you might ideally choose an alcohol treatment program which is either part of a psychiatric hospital or in a medical hospital where a psychiatrist is available. For this type of patient, nonpsychiatrists will probably choose to order a psychiatric evaluation.

3. Inpatient Treatment of Secondary Alcoholism

To use the diagnosis of primary affective disorder to predict future course, one should note only depressive episodes occurring before the onset of alcohol problems or during a protracted abstinence (arbitrarily three months or more). Sadness occurring during active drinking is likely to lift without antidepressant treatment.

The treatment of choice for patients with primary affective disorder and secondary alcoholism is *probably* (there is little data here) tricyclic-like antidepressants (like trazadone or nortriptyline) which are usually best given by a psychiatrist (Hollister, 1973, pp. 72–110). If the patient is suicidal or incapacitated by his symptoms, treatment is best done in an inpatient setting. Patients demonstrating a history of mania (Winokur et al., 1969) are *probably* best treated with Lithium (Hollister, 1973, pp. 56–71; Merry et al., 1976). Antidepressants and lithium, however, have not been proven to be of clinical use in primary alcoholics without persistent depression (Viamontes, 1972).

The other usual case of secondary alcoholism is the primary antisocial personality. The importance of recognizing the diagnosis is more to predict course than to choose a treatment. The usual mode of therapy takes place in an outpatient setting, as discussed below. The rare primary schizophrenic (Winokur et al., 1970) with alcohol problems is often treated as an outpatient. This is also discussed in a later section.

In all of these cases, the patient will be given detoxification, if needed, and may undergo inpatient or outpatient alcoholic rehabilitation. However, the prognosis is probably that of the primary disorder, and additional care for their first-appearing psychiatric problem will be needed.

4. Severe Life Crisis Problems

Patients often enter treatment because of a precipitating event. For an alcoholic this is frequently a life crisis such as an accident, increased difficulties with a spouse, job or legal problems, etc. (Gibson and Becker, 1973b). If the life crisis has been too great, the individual may be unable to cope in a nonstructured atmosphere. Under these circumstances, one can choose to use an inpatient alcohol program based on the common-sense assumption that there are not enough supports otherwise available. Here, the inpatient mode is perhaps justified, not because it has been proven to be more effective, but because it is a common-sense solution to a life crisis situation.

5. Either Patient or Therapist Preference

While there are no hard rules about selecting the type of patient most likely to benefit from inpatient care, an individual might have a strong preference for such treatment. The therapist might also choose to use an inpatient setting through a totally subjective evaluation or because prior attempts at outpatient treatment have been unsuccessful. One would hope that this subjective approach would be used most carefully, as inpatient treatment is not without its dangers and should be used only when justified.

6. Other Patient Characteristics

The list of reasons given here is not exhaustive. There may be other patient or familial patterns which justify inpatient care.

E. Setting Up an Outpatient Treatment Regimen

1. A General Approach

In alcoholism rehabilitation, there is no evidence that any one specific style of rehabilitation is essential. What seems to be more important is consistent care following common-sense rules in helping the patient to establish a life-style free of alcohol. This care is given at a decreasing frequency over a 6- to 12-month period (e.g., meetings once a week for three months, then once every other week for three months, then once a month for six months). What follows in this subsection are some brief thoughts on outpatient rehabilitation. These notes are complemented by the information given in Chapter 7 inasmuch as outpatient and inpatient rehabilitation approaches overlap.

A number of these guidelines follow the bias of trying to keep costs in money and pain as low as possible. First establish a "contract" with the patient, sharing with him the fact that he is responsible for his own drinking behavior but that you strongly suggest abstinence. For those alcoholics who will accept abstinence, it is the safest goal in attempting to avoid future alcohol problems. On the other hand, we shouldn't neglect the fact that other areas of life difficulties may exist, even if drinking ceases.

Then set up a series of meetings, usually beginning with a frequency of once a week, even if only for 15 minutes. At these, the patient's problems will be the primary concern, but consider also working with family members. To be "cost effective," establish an outpatient alcoholic group, meeting with the patients approximately once a week for at least three months, followed by decreasing frequency of sessions over the subsequent year.

You can utilize whatever mode of therapy you are most comfortable with. However, if you have little formal training in psychotherapy, the counseling sessions should center on the "here and now."

A number of important topics should be stressed during the counseling sessions:

1. There is a need to structure and "fill in" the free time which is generated by the lack of drinking. Most alcoholics have little idea of what they will do with the evening and weekend hours they used to spend intoxicated.
2. Interactions with significant others should be emphasized. The spouse, children, and friends are likely to be angry and frustrated by the patient's past actions while drunk. Therefore, family counseling sessions carried on both with and without the patient can be an important focus of treatment.
3. The circle of peers is an area of concern inasmuch as the patient may find it difficult to stop drinking if drunkenness is the accepted behavior among his friends. Such "friends" may find abstinence in the patient threatening to their own self-images and may do whatever they can to undercut treatment.
4. Some patients will need active vocational rehabilitation to either establish a vocation or develop working skills. The emphasis should be on learning jobs which do not carry a high level of risk for drinking; certain sales positions, for example, or bartending should be avoided.

2. Alcoholics Anonymous

You should encourage patients to take part in Alcoholics Anonymous (AA), and you might help establish an AA group in your area if none is yet available (although they seem to be almost everywhere). This group, composed of individuals who are themselves recovering from alcoholism (the term can still be applied after many years of abstinence), establishes a milieu where an alcoholic has help available 24 hours a day, seven days a week, by just picking up the phone (O., 1976). Especially during early phases of recovery, patients should be encouraged to attend as many AA meetings as possible, even daily if needed. At such gatherings, members have a chance to share their own experiences of recovery which demonstrates to the patient that he is not alone and that a better life-style is possible. AA also offers help in the form of group discussions for the children of alcoholics (Alateen) and for the spouses (Alanon).

Members of AA range from the unskilled and unemployed to bank presidents and professionals. Each AA group has its own personality, and the patient might experiment with different groups before deciding on the one in which he is most comfortable.

Some professionals may have had bad experiences with overzealous members of AA who feel that the only people qualified to treat alcoholics are recovering alcoholics. The possibility of running into this type of rigidity can be discussed with patients before referral, but the potential disadvantages of patients receiving advice of this sort is outweighed by the potential benefits of their association with this group. AA can be looked at as an adjunct to your own efforts at confrontation and rehabilitation. Most established alcohol rehabilitation programs use AA in parallel with their active treatment.

3. Medications

Many alcoholics improve or totally stop drinking with time alone (Schuckit, 1977a; Schuckit, 1977b). As a result, the administration of any treatment to a group of alcoholics is associated with some level of success. The crucial step is to show that the therapeutic regimen caused the outcome and that it was not the result of a "spontaneous cure" or a nonspecific response to intervention. Therefore, new treatments must be evaluated as part of studies where nonspecific factors are controlled by random assignment of subjects to the new regimen versus a standard treatment. Without controlled trials, treatments that pose the threat of potential dangers, like those involving metronidazole (Flagyl) (Goodwin and Reinhard, 1972) and LSD (Ludwig, et al., 1970), are erroneously touted as new cures.

In dealing with the alcoholic, what is *not* done is sometimes as important as what *is* done. As is discussed in Chapters 7 and 8, there are few medications that are justified in treating the outpatient alcoholic. Sleeping pills and antianxiety drugs, even though the patient may demand them, have no place in the treatment of alcoholism after withdrawal is completed. These drugs carry with them the dangers of addiction and of adverse interactions with other depressant drugs such as alcohol, and, at least for most hypnotics, potential dangers in overdosage (Shuckit, 1975).

Disulfiram (Antabuse) is a promising drug in the treatment of alcoholism (Kitson, 1977; Baekeland et al., 1971), but it, too, has some attendant dangers (Kitson, 1977; Keeffe and Smith, 1974; Rainey, 1977; Price and Silberfarb, 1976), and the drug cannot be given to patients with serious medical disorders. The restrictions are based on the common-sense assumption that because the alcohol-antabuse reaction involves vomiting and a drop in blood pressure it should not be given to individuals with serious heart disease, a history of strokes, diabetes, etc. In addition to the alcohol-Antabuse reaction, the drug alone has other side effects, including fatigue (perhaps seen in 50% of patients), a metallic taste in the mouth, and a skin rash, with more serious and life-threatening problems (such as seizures, psychoses, confusion, neuritis, etc.) seen in only a very small percentage of patients (Schuckit, 1981b).

Antabuse and related drugs do not decrease the drive to drink but, because the effects of the medication last up to 72 hours or more after the drug is taken, help to enhance the abstinence rate by decreasing the chance that the patient will go back to drinking on the spur of the moment (Sellers et al., 1981; Gerrein, 1973; Wilson, 1976). The drug is usually given orally in the daily dose of 250 mg and is maintained for three months to a year, depending upon clinical need. While controlled studies comparing Antabuse with no additional treatment make this drug look promising, comparisons of the effect of usual doses with placebo doses (e.g., 500 mg versus 1 mg of disulfiram) show few differences, raising the possibility that the psychological deterrent is more important than the actual effects of the drug (Fuller and Williford, 1980). A number of evaluations have looked at a long-lasting subcutaneous implant, and while patients treated this way appear to do better than those without any procedures, there may be a high level of placebo effect as blood levels are low or nonexistent after a period of weeks (Wilson, 1975; Wilson et al., 1980; Bergstrom et al., 1982).

When an alcoholic drinks while taking disulfiram, there is great individual variability in the intensity of the reaction. Most of the symptoms occur because of an accumulation of acetaldehyde and appear to be the result of dilation of blood vessels and a decrease in the blood pressure along with gastrointestinal upset and anxiety. The time course of the reaction probably relates to the length of the time acetaldehyde circulates, but most individuals report beginning to feel ill within a matter of minutes after drinking and stay symptomatic for the next 30 to 60 minutes.

No perfect treatment for the alcohol-Antabuse interaction has been developed. Most clinicians recommend symptomatic therapy in which dangerous hypotension is treated conservatively with the Trandelenberg position and oxygen, while others have advocated the use of antihistamines to block histamine release and ascorbic acid to speed up acetaldehyde metabolism (Schuckit, 1981b). An additional treatment specific toward the reaction itself but still considered experimental is the administration of 4-methylpyrazole in a dose of 7 mg/kgm intravenously as this drug results in an 80% inhibition of the conversion of ethanol to acetaldehyde. Methylpyrazole can also be given orally, and one dose may be sufficient to control the reaction (Lindros et al., 1981).

Sleep problems can be approached by informing the patient that you understand his difficulty, but that medications are likely to cause more problems than they cure. Therefore, the patient is "prescribed" a regimen of going to sleep at the same time every night (watching television or reading if he can't fall asleep) and getting up at exactly the same time every morning—even if he's only slept for 15 minutes. He must avoid caffeine after 5:00 P.M. and must not take naps. Soon the patient finds that his body begins to readjust to a new sleep cycle.

The treatment of *anxiety* is not magical either. It involves helping the patient to recognize when symptoms of anxiety are developing because often these are ignored until the patient is ready to "explode." The next step in treating the anxiety (which reflects a secondary abstinence syndrome as well as situational difficulties) is to "experiment" with each individual until the behavior which best decreases anxiety is discovered. For some people this will be reading, and for others meditation, biofeedback, exercise, religion, and so on.

F. Referral to Established Outpatient Resources

With a moderate amount of training, most clinicians are well qualified to do outpatient alcoholic rehabilitation. A step-by-step approach to recognition, confrontation, detoxification, and rehabilitation is given in this and the subsequent chapter. However, because some clinicians may prefer to refer the patient elsewhere for rehabilitation, some brief guidelines are offered here.

Most county governments maintain a series of outpatient counseling facilities, and a number of private facilities are usually available. Before choosing among them, it is best to visit those which have the best reputation. The competence of a program may be difficult to judge, but you should utilize the same basic rules outlined in the next chapter on evaluation of inpatient treatment programs. Look for a program run by individuals who appear to be well-educated regarding alcoholism, who are actively interested in their clients' welfare, who attempt to work with the patient and the family, utilizing all available resources to help the individual, but who stay clear of the more fancy, expensive, and potentially dangerous drugs or psychotherapies. Solid programs usually use a psychotherapeutic approach of group counseling, with an emphasis on the patient's current life problems.

III. SUMMARY

The clinician's job is to learn how to recognize alcoholism, to establish the most successful way of confronting the alcoholic (with the mode of confrontation depending on the personality of the particular physician and patient as well as the circumstances), and then to carry out maneuvers to increase motivation, maximize health, and increase ease of readjustment without alcohol. There are no magic cures, but there appear to be a number of nonspecific helping mechanisms which may be invoked. In this approach, the patient is responsible for his own actions, but the clinician is responsible for doing all that he or she can to help accomplish the realistic goals discussed in this and the subsequent chapter. This is done by increasing your level of knowledge about alcoholism, recognizing the high prevalence of the problem, destroying inaccurate stereotypes of the alcoholic, and gaining a modest level of expertise on handling the patient with alcohol problems.

Even before you begin treatment, it is important that you outline your definition of alcoholism (and the biases inherent in that definition) and the problems that you can expect to encounter in the course of treatment of the individual patient (i.e., the natural history of the disorder). You should also identify those alcoholics with serious pre-existing psychiatric disorders (i.e., secondary alcoholics) and either give them proper treatment yourself or refer them to a psychiatrist if appropriate.

The alcoholic is likely to present to the general practitioner with a variety of medical or psychological problems. The diagnosis is made by having a high index of suspicion (remembering that up to one-third of your patients will have alcohol-related medical problems), especially for those with complex or changing clinical pictures. Specific problems indicating a high risk for alcoholism include a high MCV or GGT, peripheral neuropathy, impotence, insomnia, depression, life crises, repeated accidents, etc.

Once your suspicion is aroused, it is best to take a few minutes to ask about the history of life problems related to alcohol in order to determine whether the individual fits the definition of alcoholism. It is also a good idea to gather a history from both the patient and another resource person, such as the spouse, to be certain that the information obtained is as accurate as possible.

Confrontation involves taking advantage of the area of the patient's concerns (e.g., life problems, accidents, general health problems, etc.). A first confrontation is likely to involve letting the patient know that he is responsible for his own actions and that he seems to have reached a point in life where alcohol is causing significant problems. If he wishes to maximize the chances of living a normal life, it is important that he stop drinking. If the patient refuses to stop, it is probably important to "keep the door open" in the hopes that the "denial" will decrease with time and that the patient will look to you for help when the next crisis appears. It is also important to educate the family and other significant resource persons and to give them the kind of general support they may need in learning to cope with the patient's alcoholism and to help maximize the chances of recovery.

Once the patient has agreed to treatment, detoxification is the next step, and this can sometimes be carried out as an outpatient, especially for individuals in relatively good health who do not show obvious signs of serious withdrawal. Rehabilitation then involves a series of general helping maneuvers which maximize motivation towards abstinence and help the patient establish a pattern of day-to-day life interactions in the absence of alcohol. Such nonspecific mechanisms can easily be carried out by the average clinician and probably had best be attempted on an outpatient basis, at least at first. Patients who have failed in outpatient care in the past and/or who have special needs may be referred for inpatient care.

Much of the information presented here represents common-sense conclusions about offering treatment to the huge number of alcoholics we all see in our clinical practices. It is hoped that you can use the general guidelines offered here and modify them for the particular needs of your own individual setting. You are encouraged to go on and read the next chapter for an overview of the types of treatments which can be offered alcoholics in inpatient settings.

REFERENCES

Baekeland, F., Lundwall, L., Kissin, B., and Shanahan, T., 1971, Correlates of outcome in disulfiram treatment of alcoholism, *Nerv. Men. Dis.*, 153:1–9.

Barchha, R., Stewart, M. A., and Guze, S. B., 1968, The prevalence of alcoholism among general hospital ward patients, *Am. J. Psychiat.*, 125:133–136.

Becker, C. E., Roe, R. L., and Scott, R. A., 1974, *Alcohol as a Drug*, The Williams & Wilkins Company, Baltimore.

Bergstrom, B., Ohlin, H., Lindblom, P. E., and Wadstein, J., 1982, Is disulfiram implantation effective? *Lancet*, 1:49–50.

Bernadt, M. W., Mumford, J., Taylor, C., Smith B., and Murray, R. M., 1982, Comparison of questionnaire and laboratory tests in the detection of excessive drinking and alcoholism, *Lancet,* 1:325.

Berne, E., 1964, *Games People Play: The Psychology of Human Relationships,* Grove Press, Inc., New York.

Cahalan, D., 1969, A multivariate analysis of correlates of drinking, *Soc. Prob.,* 17:234–247.

Cahalan, D., 1970. *Problem drinkers.* Jossey-Boss, Inc., San Francisco.

Cahalan, D., and Cisin, I. H., 1968, American drinking practices, *Q. J. Stud. Alc.,* 29:130–151.

Cahalan, D., Cisin, I. H., Gardner, G. L., and Smith, G. C., 1972, A study to measure the extent and patterns of alcohol use and abuse in the U.S. Army, *U.S. Army Report,* 73:6.

Cameron, J. L., Zuidema, G. D., Margolis, S., 1975, A pathogenesis for alcoholic pancreatitis, *Surgery,* 77:754–763.

deLint, J., and Levinson, T., 1975, Mortality among patients treated for alcoholism: A 5-year follow-up, *Can. Med. Assn. J.,* 113:385–387.

Drew, L. R. H., 1968, Alcoholism as a self-limiting disease, *Q. J. Stud. Alc.,* 29:956–167.

Dreyfus, P. M., 1974, Diseases of the nervous system in chronic alcoholics, in *The Biology of Alcoholism,* vol. 3 (B. Kissin and H. Begleiter, eds.), pp. 265–290, Plenum Press, New York.

Eichner, E. R., and Hillman, R. S., 1971, The evolution of anemia in alcoholic patients, *Am. J. Med.,* 50:218–232.

Ellinwood, E. H., Jr., 1971, Assault and homicide associated with amphetamine abuse, *Am. J. Psychiat.,* 127:90–95.

Feldman, D. J., Pattison, E. M., Sobell, L. C., Graham, T., and Sobell, M. B., 1975, Outpatient alcohol detoxification: Initial findings on 564 patients, *Am. J. Psychiat.,* 132:407–412.

Fillmore, K. M., 1975, Relationships between specific drinking problems in early adulthood and middle age, *J. Stud. Alc.,* 36:882–907.

Freund, G., 1976, Diseases of the nervous system associated with alcoholism, in *Alcoholism, Interdisciplinary Approaches to an Enduring Problem* (R. E. Tarter and A. A. Sugerman, eds.), Addison-Wesley Publishing Co., Reading, Mass.

Fuller, R. K., and Williford, W. O., 1980, Life-table analysis of abstinence in a study evaluating the efficacy of disulfiram, *Alcoholism: Clin. Exp. Res.,* 4:298–301.

Gerrein, J. R., Rosenberg, C. M., and Manohar, V., 1973, Disulfiram maintenance in outpatient treatment of alcoholism, *Arch. Gen. Psychiat.,* 28:798–802.

Gibson, S., and Becker, J., 1973a, Changes in alcoholics' self-reported depression, *Q. J. Stud. Alc.,* 34:389–836.

———, 1973b, Alcoholism and depression, *Quart. J. Stud. Alc.,* 34:400–408.

Goodwin, D. W., and Reinhard, J., 1972, Disulfiramlike effects of trichomonacidal drugs, a review and double-blind study, *Q. J. Stud. Alc.,* 33:734–740.

Goodwin, D. W., Crane, J. B., and Guze, S. B., 1969, Alcoholic blackouts, *Am. J. Psychiat.,* 126:77–84.

Goodwin, D., and Guze, S. D., 1979, *Psychiatric Diagnosis,* Oxford University Press, New York.

Gould, L., Zahir, M., and DeMartino, A., Cardiac effects of a cocktail, *JAMA*, 218:1799–1802.

Guze, S. B., 1970, The need for toughmindedness in psychiatric thinking, *So. Med.*, 63:662–671.

Haglund, M. J., and Schuckit, M., 1982, The epidemiology of alcoholism, in *Alcoholism: Psychological and Physiological Basis* (N. Estes and E. Heinemann, eds.), C. V. Mosby Company, St. Louis.

Hakulinen, T., Lehtimak, L., and Lentonen, M., 1974, Cancer morbidity among two male cohorts, *Nat'l Canc. Inst.*, 52:1711–1717.

Hollister, L. E., 1973, *Clinical Use of Psychotherapeutic Drugs*, Charles C Thomas, Springfield, Ill.

Horwitz, L. D., 1975, Alcohol and heart disease, *JAMA*, 232:959–960.

Iber, F. L., 1971, Alcohol and the gastrointestinal tract, *New Eng. J. Med.*, 61:120–123.

Johnson, L. C., Burdick, J. A., and Smith, J., 1970, Sleep during alcohol intake and withdrawal in the chronic alcoholic, *Arch. Gen. Psychiat.*, 22:406–418.

Keeffe, E. B., and Smith, F. W., 1974, Disulfiram hypersensitivity hepatitis, *JAMA*, 230:435–436.

Kendell, R. E., and Staton, M. C., 1966, The fate of untreated alcoholics, *Q. J. Stud. Alc.*, 27:30–41.

Kissin, B., and Begleiter, H. (eds.), 1971a, *The Biology of Alcoholism, Physiology and Behavior*, vol. 2, Plenum Press, New York.

———, 1971b, *The Biology of Alcoholism, Clinical Pathology*, vol. 3, Plenum Press, New York.

Kitson, T. M., 1977, The disulfiram-ethanol reaction, a review, *J. Stud. Alc.*, 38:96–113.

Klatsky, A. L., Friedman, G. D., Siegelaub, A. B., and Gerard, M. J., 1977, Alcohol consumption and blood pressure, Kaiser-Permanente Multiphasic Health Examination Data, *New Eng. J. Med.*, 296:1194–1200.

Editorial, 1980, Screening tests for alcoholism? *Lancet*, 2:1117–1118.

Editorial, 1980, Alcoholic heart disease, *Lancet*, 1:961–962.

Editorial, 1981, Alcoholic brain damage, *Lancet*, 1:477–478.

Lemere, F., 1953, What happens to alcoholics, *Am. J. Psychiat.*, 109:674–676.

Lieber, C. S., 1973, Liver adaptation and injury in alcoholism, *New Eng. J. Med.*, 288:356–362.

———, 1975, Alcohol and malnutrition in the pathogenesis of liver disease, *JAMA*, 233:1077–1082.

Lindros, K. O., Stowell, A., Pikkarainen, P., and Salaspuro, M., 1981. The disulfiram (Antabuse)-alcohol reaction in male alcoholics: Its efficient management by 4-methylpyrazole, *Alcoholism: Clin. Exp. Res.*, 5:528–530.

Lishman, W. A., 1981, Cerebral disorder in alcoholism syndromes of impairment, *Brain*, 104:1–20.

Liu, Y., 1973, Leukopenia in alcoholics, *Am. J. Med.*, 54:605–606.

Lowry, W. S., 1975, Alcoholism in cancer of the head and neck, *Laryngoscope*, 85:1257–1280.

Ludwig, A. M., 1972, On and off the wagon, *Q. J. Stud. Alc.*, 33:91–96.

Ludwig, A. M., Levine, J., and Stark, L. H., 1970, *A Clinical Study of Treatment Efficacy*, Charles C Thomas, Springfield, Ill.

Lundy, J., Raaf, J. H., and Deakins, S., 1975, The acute and chronic effects of alcohol on the human immune system, *Surg. Gynec. Obstr.*, 141:212–218.

Merry, J., Reynolds, C. M., and Bailey, J., 1976, Prophylactic treatment of alcoholism by lithium carbonate, *Lancet,* 1:7984–7985.

Moore, R. A., 1971, The prevalence of alcoholism in a community general hospital, *Am. J. Psychiat.,* 128:130–131.

Morrison, J. R., 1974, Bipolar affective disorder and alcoholism, *Am. J. Psychiat.,* 131:1130–1134.

O., George, 1976, Alcoholics Anonymous, *JAMA,* 236:1505–1506.

Pader, E., 1973, Clinical heart disease and electrocardiographic abnormalities in alcoholics, *Q. J. Stud. Alc.,* 34:774–785.

Parker, B. M., 1974, The effects of ethyl alcohol on the heart, *JAMA,* 228:741–742.

Price, T. R. P., and Silberfarb, P. M., 1976, Disulfiram-induced convulsions without challenge by alcohol, *J. Stud. Alc.,* 37:980–982.

Rainey, J. M., Jr., 1977, Disulfiram toxicity and carbon disulfide poisoning, *Am. J. Psychiat.,* 134:371–378.

Robins, L. N., 1966, *Deviant Children Grown Up,* The Williams & Wilkins Company, Baltimore.

Ryan, C., 1982, Alcoholism and premature aging: A neuropsychological perspective, *Alcoholism: Clin. Exp. Res.,* 6:22–30.

Ryback, R. S., Eckhardt, M. J., and Pautler, C. P., 1980, Biochemical and hematological correlates of alcoholism, *Res. Com. Chem. Path. Pharmac.,* 27:533–550.

Schmidt, W., and deLing, J., 1972, Causes of death in alcoholics, *Q. J. Stud. Alc.,* 33:171–185.

Schuckit, M. A., 1972, Sexual disturbance in the woman alcoholic, *Human Sexual.,* 6:44–65.

———, 1973, Alcoholism and sociopathy: Diagnostic confusion, *Q. J. Stud. Alc.,* 34:157–164.

———, 1975, Drugs in combination with other therapies for alcoholics, in *Drugs in Combination With Other Therapies for Alcoholics* (M. Greenblatt, ed.), pp. 119–134, Grune & Stratton, Inc., New York.

———, 1977a, Alcoholism and depression: Diagnostic confusion, in *Proceedings of Alcoholism and Affective Disorder* (D. W. Goodwin and C. Erickson, eds.), Spectrum Publications, New York.

———, 1977b, Alcoholism: Natural history and outcome studies, presented at the Society for Epidemiologic Research Annual Meeting, June, 1977, Seattle, Wash.

———, 1977d, Geriatric alcoholism and drug abuse, *Gerontologist,* 17:168–174.

———, 1981a, Gamma glutamyl transferase and the diagnosis of alcoholism, *Advances in Alcoholism* II, 5, May.

———, 1981b, Disulfiram (Antabuse) and the treatment of alcoholic men, *Advances in Alcoholism,* II, 4, April.

———, 1983, Alcoholism and other psychiatric disorders, *Hosp. Com. Psychiat.,* 34:1022–1027.

———, 1984, *Drug and Alcohol Abuse: A Clinical Guide to Diagnosis and Treatment,* Plenum Publishing Company, New York.

Schuckit, M. A., and Morrissey, E. R., 1976, Alcoholism in women: Some clinical and social perspectives with an emphasis on possible subtypes, in *Alcohol Problems in Women and Children* (M. Greenblatt, and M. A. Schuckit, eds.), Grune & Stratton, Inc., New York.

Schuckit, M. A., and Winokur, G., 1972, A short term follow-up of women alcoholics, *Dis. Nerv. Syst.*, 33:672–678.

Schuckit, M. A., Pitts, F. N., Jr., Reich, T., King, L. J., and Winokur, G., 1969, Alcoholism, *Arch. Gen. Psychiat.*, 20:301–306.

Sellers, E. M., and Kalant, H., 1976, Alcohol intoxication and withdrawal, *New Eng. J. Med.*, 294:757–762.

Sundy, P., 1967, *Alcoholism and Mortality*, Universitetsforlaget, Oslo.

Tamerin, J. S., and Mendelson, J., 1970, Alcoholics expectancies and recall of experiences during intoxication, *Am. J. Psychiat.*, 126:1697–1704.

Tennant, F. S., Jr., 1977, Ambulatory alcohol detoxification, California Society for the Treatment of Alcoholism and Other Drug Dependencies, *Newsletter*, 4:1–3.

Viamontes, J. A., 1972, Review of drug effectiveness in the treatment of alcoholism, *Am. J. Psychiat.*, 128:120–121.

Victor, M., 1966, Treatment of alcoholic intoxication and the withdrawal syndrome, *Psychosom. Med.*, 28:636–649.

Victor, M., and Hope, J. M., 1955, The phenomenon of auditory hallucinations in chronic alcoholism, *Arch. Gen. Psychiat.*, 126:451–481.

Victor, M., Adams, R. D., and Mancall, E. L., 1959, Alcoholic cerebellar degeneration, *AMA Archives of Neurology*, 1:579–688.

Victor, M., Adams, R. D., and Collins, G. H., 1971, *The Wernicke-Korsakoff Syndrome*, F. A. Davis Co., Philadelphia.

Walker, D. W., Barnes, D. E., Riley, J. N., Hunter, B. E., Zornetzer, S. F., 1980, Neurotoxicity of chronic alcohol consumption: An animal model, in *Psychopharmacology of Alcohol* (M. Sandler, ed.), Raven Press, New York.

Warren, G. H., and Raynes, A. E., 1972, Mood changes during three conditions of alcohol intake, *Q. J. Stud. Alc.*, 33:979–989.

Whitefield, J. B., Hensley, W. J., Bryden, D., and Gallagher, H., 1978, Some laboratory correlates of drinking habits, *Ann. Clin. Biochem.*, 15:297–303.

Wilkinson, D. A., 1982, Examination of alcoholics by computed tomographic (CT) scans: A critical review, *Alcoholism: Clin. Exp. Res.* 6:31–44.

Wilson, A., Davidson, W. J., and Blanchard, R., 1980, Disulfiram implantation— A trial using placebo implants and two types of controls, *J. Stud. Alc.*, 41:429–436.

Wilson, A., 1975, Disulfiram implantation in alcoholism treatment, a review, *J. Stud. Alc.*, 36:555–565.

Wilson, A., Davidson, W. J., and White, J., 1976, Disulfiram implantation: Placebo, psychological deterrent, and pharmacological deterrent effects, *Br. J. Psychiat.*, 129:277–280.

Winokur, G., Clayton, P. J., and Reich, T., 1969, *Manic-Depressive Disease*, C. V. Mosby Company, St. Louis.

Winokur, G., Reich, T., Rimmer, J., and Pitts, F. N., 1970, Diagnosis and familial psychiatric illness in 259 alcoholic probands, III, Alcoholism, *Arch. Gen. Psychiat.*, 23:104–111.

Wu, C. F., Sudhakar, M., and Jaferi, G., 1976, Preclinical cardiomyopathy in chronic alcoholics: A sex difference, *Am. Heart J.*, 91:281–286.

Zelazowski, R., Golden, C. J., Graber, B., Blose, I. L., Bloch, S., Moses, Jr., J. A., Zatz, L. M., Stahl, S. M., Osmon, D. C., and Pfefferbaum, A., 1981, Relationship of cerebral ventricular size in alcoholics' performance on the Luria-Nebraska Neuropsychological Battery, *J. Stud. Alc.*, 42:749–756.

CHAPTER 7

Inpatient and Residential Approaches to the Treatment of Alcoholism

Marc A. Schuckit, M.D.
Professor of Psychiatry
University of California, San Diego, School of Medicine
Director of the Alcohol Treatment Program
Veterans Administration Medical Center
San Diego, California

I. INTRODUCTION

Inpatient and outpatient care are highly interrelated. Therefore, it is useful to deal with the two as somewhat separate but greatly overlapping aspects of care. This chapter assumes that the patient has already been identified and confronted and has agreed to enter treatment, as was discussed in detail in the previous chapter. The next stage is to determine if detoxification is needed, and, if so, whether the process will be handled on an inpatient (the safer way) or outpatient basis. The next question, whether you choose an inpatient or outpatient mode of rehabilitation, depends upon a variety of factors centering around the patient's needs, history of previous treatment, existing social supports and finances, and (unfortunately) the subjective bias of the health care deliverer.

NOTE: Supported by the Veterans Administration Medical Research Service, NIAAA grant #PHSAA04353, and Joan and Ray Kroc.

This chapter examines the rehabilitation process during the inpatient phase of treatment. Most inpatient programs begin with detoxification; because this is covered in detail in Chapters 2, 6, and 8, it will be noted only briefly here.

II. AN INTRODUCTION TO DETOXIFICATION

The treatment of alcoholic withdrawal is relatively simple and can be divided into three phases: identification of problems, general support, and active detoxification (detox). The first step involves the identification of medical disorders which may be present in the alcoholic. Because the depressant-abstinence syndrome is one of the most serious of any withdrawals (Sellers and Kalant, 1976), because alcohol does such serious damage to all body systems (Becker et al., 1974), and because the average alcoholic entering treatment is not young and healthy, it is important that each patient receive a good physical examination. The medical disorders that one can expect to find have been covered in Chapters 2 and 6. However, it should be noted that alcoholics present with elevated rates of heart disease (including cardiomyopathies), infections, bleeding disorders, electrolyte and glucose abnormalities, and neurologic damage. It is best to recognize and actively treat any serious medical problems immediately because of their potential dangers when added to a depressant-withdrawal syndrome.

General supportive modes for treating alcoholic withdrawal include such things as vitamins, rest, and adequate food and oral fluids. Intravenous (IV) fluids should usually be avoided because the average alcoholic tends to be overhydrated and not dehydrated (Knott and Beard, 1969). It is especially important to give thiamine: This vitamin is not stored well by the body, and alcohol may interfere with its absorption from the small intestine, with a resulting thiamine deficiency in most heavy drinkers, even the average well-nourished alcoholic (Becker et al., 1974). The usual dose is 100 mg intramuscularly or orally daily for three days, followed by oral multiple vitamins. Similar thiamine doses should be continued for two or more months in any patient continuing to show confusion, ataxia, cranial nerve dysfunction, or a peripheral neuropathy (Victor et al., 1971). Many treatment programs use other adjunctive approaches, including such things as exercise, establishment of a supportive milieu, beginning of counseling for alcoholism, etc.

These measures do not approach the physiologic aspects of depressant drug withdrawal. Even with the activities just enumerated, it can be expected that the averge patient will demonstrate autonomic nervous

Table 1
Detoxification

Symptoms	Treatment
Begin in hours, peak day 2 or 3, subside day 4 or 5 Anxiety Malaise ANS dysfunction Insomnia	Thiamine (100 mg IM × 3 days) Physical exam Multiple vitamins Food and rest
Convulsions OBS Hallucinations (visual or tactile)	Depressant drugs

system dysfunction (e.g., increased pulse and respirations and elevated temperature, as well as labile blood pressure), a coarse tremor, anxiety, and a series of other relatively mild somatic complaints (Sellers and Kalant, 1976). Somewhere between 5% and 15% of alcoholics going through withdrawal also demonstrate grand mal convulsions (not proven to be responsive to diphenylhydantoin (Dilantin)) (Schuckit, 1975; Gessner, 1974), an organic brain syndrome (confusion and disorientation), or hallucinations (usually visual or tactile). These problems peak in intensity on day two or three and last until day four or five (Sellers and Kalant, 1976).

Some treatment facilities choose to screen out patients with medical problems and those who appear to be headed for serious withdrawal and refer them to a hospital setting. This program is left with individuals at low risk for serious withdrawal who are then treated by the general supportive mechanisms outlined above and not given any specific type of depressant medication (Peterson, 1975). However, other programs choose to treat the entire picture of alcoholic withdrawal, including the anxiety and autonomic dysfunction. In order to do this, one must recognize the causes and treat the depressant withdrawal itself.

The paradigm for treatment is to administer a depressant drug (in this instance, either alcohol or a drug with cross-tolerance to ethanol—i.e., any other depressant medication, including all prescription hypnotics or antianxiety drugs (Schuckit, 1984) in high enough doses to abolish symptoms and then decrease the drug slowly, usually over five days. While any depressant drug, including alcohol, can be used (Schmitz, 1977), the most prevalent approach utilizes the antianxiety drugs such as chlordiazepoxide (Librium) or diazepam (Valium). These medications have relatively low rates of respiratory and blood pressure depression but do have long half-lives, and this allows for a smooth decrease in drug levels and a subsequent mild withdrawal. Most physicians use somewhere between

100 and 300 mg of Librium on the first day, with the specific dose adjusted for the individual patient depending upon his degree of addiction (which can be gauged by his autonomic nervous response) and his degree of alertness (Sellers and Kalant, 1976). After establishing the dose needed to abolish withdrawal symptoms on day one, the dose is usually decreased by about 20% of the original dose each day and depressant medications stopped on day four or five. This requires very careful patient management using the patient's degree of alertness and autonomic nervous system functioning (e.g., pulse and blood pressure) to avoid giving too much medication. The patient should never become intoxicated, very lethargic, or hypotensive.

Therefore it is important to withhold the medication if a patient is sleeping or shows a marked drop in blood pressure. For patients for whom accumulation of medication poses a particular problem (i.e., the elderly, those with kidney or liver disease, etc.), the shorter-acting benzodiazepines such as lorazepam (Ativan) and oxazepam (Serax) should be considered, although these require more frequent administration of medications and withdrawal might be less smooth (Greenblatt and Shader, 1978). Finally, some alcoholic patients will have a history of addiction to multiple drugs. For mixed depressant-opiate withdrawal, the more dangerous CNS depressant withdrawal should be treated first (holding the opiate dose constant if necessary). Where multiple depressants are involved, the longer-acting CNS depressant should be dealt with first—i.e., treat a mixture of alcohol and diazepam withdrawal as if diazepam were the only or major drug involved (Schuckit, 1984). Only after CNS depressant withdrawal has been completed should withdrawal from other drugs (e.g., opiates) be attempted (Schuckit, 1984).

III. A GENERAL INTRODUCTION TO INPATIENT TREATMENT

If you have read Chapter 6, you recognize that there are no magic cures for alcoholism. Our therapeutic manipulations are aimed at (1) maximizing physical and mental functioning by screening out serious medical and psychiatric disorders, (2) increasing motivation towards abstinence and keeping it as high as possible as long as possible, and (3) helping patients readjust to life without alcohol. For some individuals, treatment can be carried out solely in an outpatient mode, but others will require inpatient rehabilitation for detoxification and/or rehabilitation. This section briefly outlines the inpatient versus outpatient treatment choice and discusses aspects of patient heterogeneity. The next section reviews the steps which should be taken in your attempt to increase motivation (through outreach to the family, education, prescribing disulfiram, behavioral manipulations, etc.) and helping the patient to reestablish a life pattern without alcohol (through family and personal counseling, vocational rehabilitation, etc.).

A. Some Treatment Risks

No treatment maneuver is entirely benign, and it is important to recognize some potential dangers associated with inpatient care. By placing the alcoholic in an inpatient environment living in close contact with other patients, you expose him to *potential* risks for treatment-center-acquired infections (e.g., staphylococcus or tuberculosis) and to the potential of being harmed either physically or emotionally through the actions of other patients or staff members. On a more practical side, by being an inpatient the individual is kept away from his job with the subsequent loss of income, embarrassment in front of peers, and the possible loss of his livelihood. Similarly, by placing him in an inpatient environment he is being separated from his family which can precipitate a crisis of its own. Finally, in this less than exhaustive overview of potential dangers, the patient is being treated in a very artificial environment where lessons learned may not generalize in his mind to everyday living. Inpatient treatment has its place in alcoholic rehabilitation, but both the negative and positive aspects must be balanced before choosing this treatment mode for any individual.

B. Patient Heterogeneity

Of course, not all alcoholics are the same, and many people have different needs, as discussed by Dr. Pattison in Chapter 5. Sophisticated techniques are now being studied in attempts to stratify groups of patients so that we may understand more about their individual needs (Wanberg et al., 1977). However, at the present time it is not possible to apply a simple test and pigeonhole our patients into the best treatment. What is offered below are some *suggestions* about possible common-sense approaches to recognizing aspects of patient heterogeneity.

1. *Primary versus Secondary Alcoholism*

As discussed in Chapter 6, individuals meeting the criteria for alcoholism can be divided into those with no major preexisting disorders (primary alcoholism) and those demonstrating alcohol problems after the onset of another major psychiatric problem (secondary alcoholism). The distinction is important because secondary alcoholics are likely to run the course of their primary disorder, not that of alcoholism. The information in these two chapters deals mostly with primary alcoholism. For treatment of secondary alcoholism, you should probably add the usual regimen used for the primary illness to the regular alcohol program.

2. Potential Differences Based on Obvious Demographic Characteristics

Skid Row. While only about 3% of alcoholics come from skid row (Haglund and Schuckit, 1982), it is important to recognize these individuals because they have very special needs. These include an increased rate of serious medical problems (Brickner et al., 1972), the need for a realistic appraisal regarding the seriously compromised prognosis (Miller, 1975), and the establishment of realistic goals. You should note, however, that the middle-class working man and the housewife alcoholic represent the vast majority of alcoholic individuals undergoing treatment in the United States. Most of the treatment approaches discussed in this and the previous chapter apply to this group of middle Americans.

Women. It is also important to recognize the possible special treatment needs of women. Once one controls for socioeconomic class and primary (versus secondary) diagnosis, it does appear that the course of alcoholism in men and women is quite similar (Schuckit and Morrissey, 1976). However, counselors need to consider the effects of alcohol on moods as they relate to the menstrual cycle (Jones and Jones, 1976), the unique roles of women in the family (Polit et al., 1976) and in society (Wilsnack, 1976), and special child care needs (Streissguth, 1976; El-Guebaly and Offord, 1977). Program personnel should also recognize the woman alcoholic's possible preference to relate to female therapists and her special vocational opportunities once treatment is completed (Schuckit, 1977a).

A specific problem worthy of brief mention is the damage done "in utero" to the developing fetus from repeated high levels of ethanol. This Fetal Alcohol Syndrome can include a mixture of any of the problems including spontaneous abortion, a baby with low birthweight, levels of mental retardation ranging from very mild to moderately severe, cardiac ventricular septal defects, and malformations of the face and hands (Streissguth, 1978). Children born to heavy-drinking mothers may also go through mild to moderate abstinence syndromes resembling those seen with babies of narcotic addicts (a nervous infant with poor feeding and/or convulsions), but this picture is generally treated by supportive care.

Youth. Another special group is comprised of adolescents and young adults. "Alcoholics" is usually a misnomer as applied to this group, because many are multiple drug abusers and about 20% meet the criteria for the antisocial personality (Schuckit et al., 1977b). While these individuals need treatment, their polydrug background, their propensity toward antisocial behavior, and their youthful values and subculture raise many obvious special needs which should be taken into account (Schuckit, 1977b). Many of the same generalizations about inpatient treatment given below can be followed for the primary alcoholic young person, but one should add group meetings, education, and counseling on drugs, as well as group discussion of topics relevant to the adolescent world.

The Elderly. Another group with special needs is the elderly. It has been estimated that 10% of individuals over age 60 demonstrate serious problems, with the rate rising to as high as 20% to 30% among general medical or surgical inpatients or individuals residing in nursing homes (Schuckit and Miller, 1976). The actively drinking elderly alcoholic is less likely to drink daily, and tends to have fewer social problems but more medical (see Chapter 2 and the discussion in Chapter 6) and interpersonal difficulties related to their heavy drinking than the younger adult alcoholic. Adequate treatment probably requires additional referral to the special facilities available in the community to serve older citizens' medical and social needs (Schuckit, 1977c). Once again, the same general approach outlined below should be utilized, but special common-sense modifications should be added for dealing with elderly men and women, recognizing the greater necessity for supplying social welfare supports and dealing with the higher level of medical problems.

Minority Groups. Minority groups also have unique problems, but data in this area are seriously limited. Within these groups, especially among Native Americans (Westermeyer, 1972), drinking has a special meaning, and behavior while under the influence of alcohol must be understood within a social context. The same is true, but to a lesser extent, for Chicano and black Americans (Blane and Hewitt, 1976; Zimberg, 1974). While there are no good guidelines, a possible approach would utilize the same basic inpatient treatment principles given below but employ some understanding of the stresses for the specific population. One should consider using counselors of the relevant ethnic group and, in some instances, actual referral to an ethnically oriented facility.

The special characteristics regarding alcoholism for Native Americans, including both North American Indians and Eskimos, is worth further mention. While accurate statistics are difficult to obtain due to lack of adequate study, both direct and indirect indicators point to a high rate of alcohol morbidity and mortality within most such ethnic groups (Schaefer, 1981; Westermeyer, 1981). The causes of this high rate of alcohol-related pathology have not been determined, but theories include a response to recent (within the last 100 years) introduction to ethanol, cultural norms within Native American groups whereby alcohol is used for intoxication as part of social and religious ceremonies, and possible genetic influences. Whatever the reason, any health care practitioners dealing with Native Americans should be cognizant of these potential problems.

This discussion of special groups of alcoholics is far from exhaustive. What is important is to have a general treatment approach in mind and to recognize the relevant areas for possible modification for members of subgroups.

For these reasons, described in Chapter 6, outpatient care has both theoretical and cost-effectiveness advantages over inpatient alcohol rehabilitation. The criteria for choosing the inpatient mode are given on pages 312–314.

C. How to Refer to Established Programs

While physicians and other health care deliverers reading this chapter should be doing some inpatient alcoholism treatment on their own, some will prefer to use established alcohol programs. Choosing a good program to receive your referrals involves taking cognizance of some of the generalizations about treatment offered in this and the preceding chapter, especially the subsection on evaluation offered below.

You can gather information by asking colleagues, and, one hopes, by visiting a number of treatment programs. You will also be helped by observing the progress of patients you have referred—although for this it is frequently necessary to be aggressive in keeping active contact with the program so that you receive regular reports.

In general, the average "good" program uses common sense, offering treatment which does not appear to be potentially harmful but which has been demonstrated to be worth the cost. This requires a program that keeps good records and attempts to evaluate their efforts regularly through patient follow-up. Most good inpatient programs offer short-term inpatient therapy followed by long-term (at least six months and preferably a year) contact on an outpatient basis.

IV. DEVELOPING YOUR INPATIENT TREATMENT APPROACH

Most of the comments offered here assume that you are treating alcoholic inpatients as part of a more general practice. However, much of this information would apply equally well for establishing a formal program and for use in outpatient settings.

To review: After recognition, confrontation, and agreement regarding treatment, it is assumed that you recognized and carried out detoxification either on an outpatient, or, preferably, on an inpatient basis if needed. It is also assumed that the patient has been adequately evaluated medically and that any medical or surgical needs have been met. It is also assumed that you have probed to determine whether the patient is a polydrug user and that you have taken cognizance of this in planning withdrawal and rehabilitation.

In setting up your own treatment goals, it is important to recognize that the generalizations here can be used as a basis for planning therapy for *primary alcoholism*, but that modifications will, of course, be needed for individual patients, especially those in the relevant subgroups mentioned in the previous section. Secondary alcoholics will require additional active care for their primary psychiatric disorder, as noted briefly in Chapter 6.

A. Where to Do Treatment

Inpatient alcoholic rehabilitation can be carried out successfully in a variety of settings. You will use the facility which is most convenient to you and most appropriate regarding your training. No one approach is best.

It is possible to carry out good alcoholic detoxification and rehabilitation in a general medical hospital (Garber, 1972; West, 1976). The benefits of this approach are that it helps the physician stay within the medical model of treating his or her patient and may help the patient to accept treatment of a disorder which represents a serious threat to his health. Many patients may prefer being treated in a general medical hospital rather than going through any possible "stigma" of entering an alcohol or psychiatric facility. In this setting you can easily carry out good medical care or be sure that it is carried out for you. It is also an ideal place to do both detoxification (which, if carried out properly, will not disturb other patients) and rehabilitation. However, if any psychiatric emergency exists (e.g., severe depression or hallucinations), it will be important to get a psychiatric or psychological consultation. Also, before carrying out treatment in your general medical or surgical hospital it may be important for you to meet with the nursing and medical staff of that facility to acquaint them with what can be expected during alcoholic rehabilitation, as well as the usual good prognosis.

It is equally possible to carry out good inpatient alcoholic rehabilitation in a general psychiatric facility (Reding and Maguire, 1973). As is true in the medical hospital, this benefits the institution by boosting the census as much as 20% (Smith and Sommerfeld, 1968). With preparation of staff, one can easily carry out alcohol rehabilitation without an increase in patient problems over what would be expected for the general psychiatric inpatient (Smith and Sommerfeld, 1968). This facility is especially appropriate if the patient is suicidal or demonstrates an organic brain syndrome or alcoholic hallucinations or paranoia. One danger here is that the patient's medical needs might not be adequately met, although this is easily handled through consultation. An additional problem is the tendency to carry out more intensive psychotherapy with patients in this setting. The cost of this added treatment, however, may not be justified for the average alcoholic (Emrick, 1975).

Alcoholic rehabilitation can be carried out in almost any other type of facility. Of course, if you're already dealing with an alcohol rehabilitation program, your decisions are easy. However, if you are working in a specialized clinic (such as in prison) or with a special group of patients (such as drug abusers), you will utilize the same basic approach to alcoholic rehabilitation given below, using some common-sense modifications to meet your own client's needs.

B. The Use of All Available Resources

Patients enter treatment with a group of problems and assets. In dealing with their difficulties, it is advantageous to utilize all available resources.

The patient's family can be one of the most important assets. The spouse and/or older children should be included as part of therapy so that they can carry on the teaching and behavioral approaches in the home setting. Excluding them from treatment may result in their fear that the therapist and patient are blaming them for the alcoholic picture, and their consequent desire to undercut all therapeutic efforts. In addition, the family needs to understand that the "rules of behavior" which served them well when the patient was actively drinking may now change and roles may alter. Thus the alcoholic who years previously ruled the family with an "iron hand" may expect to reestablish the same pattern when sober, but the spouse, after taking major responsibility for the family for years, may be unwilling to relinquish control. These problems must be addressed during both patient and family counseling sessions (Steinglass, 1981). Family members and friends may find additional support from Alcoholics Anonymous (AA), affiliated groups aimed specifically at adults (e.g., Alanon), and those for teenagers (Alateen). The family may also give valuable information that will help the clinician to determine any special treatment needs and decide whether the problem is primary or secondary alcoholism.

The employer is another important resource (Greenleigh, 1975). Establishing contact when it seems relevant or asking the family or patient to inform the employer about the potential length of treatment and the fact that he will be returning to work soon (in one to three weeks) can help preserve a job and avoid a crisis which might have to be faced soon after discharge. Frequently, the employer is most concerned and willing to help. He can be very important in attempts to maximize the patient's motivation.

In a similar manner, those patients who come to you through the police or courts offer, indirectly, another asset with which to work (Gallant, 1971). An understanding judge can make probation contingent upon future therapy, which can emphasize how important treatment is in the patient's future. It also demonstrates how serious the problems are which will follow if the patient does not recover.

C. Be Sure You Know Your Goals

Specific definitions of problems and of treatment goals are required for good care. First, it is very important that secondary alcoholics be recognized because they often carry different prognoses and have different treatment needs. It is also important to establish realistic goals, which for the skid row alcoholic, for example, might be an improved medical condition and a chance to detoxify, with the hope that rehabilitation might become a viable alternative (Gallant, 1973). The goal for the average working alcoholic who has a family intact and a very limited police record would more realistically be total abolition of drinking problems.

This underscores the importance in defining recovery (Forrest, 1975, pp. 149–154). Most alcohol treatment programs recognize recovery as synonymous with abstinence. This is the safest and most easily measured goal, but abstinence should not be equated with total improvement of lifestyle; while the two are related, they are not necessarily the same (Pattison, 1976). Some clinicians and investigators feel that the alcoholic who refuses to accept abstinence can improve through learning "controlled" drinking (Pattison, 1976). This important topic is worthy of consideration and requires further testing, but at present it is the bias of this chapter that abstinence is the most viable goal in any alcohol treatment program.

Each patient comes to you with a variety of problems both directly and indirectly related to his drinking. When an individual enters therapy, it is important to recognize his level of functioning within the family, on the job, with the police, and with peers; his medical health and psychological problems are also important and should be monitored during recovery with special therapeutic efforts directed at them if necessary. Similarly, in carrying out evaluation of treatment success, progress in each of the above areas should be noted.

Related to the need to spell out multiple goals for each patient completely is the advisability of establishing a rough schedule for your "attack" on these problems and a rough gauge of what can be expected during patient recovery. It is also important to take cognizance of the limited number of hours of the day during the inpatient's stay and schedule his activities as completely as possible. This might include regular group therapy, educational sessions, and Alcoholics Anonymous meetings, but it might also require additional time for treatment of medical problems, family therapy sessions, and vocational rehabilitation. It is most efficient to make maximal use of the patient's time in the hospital, leaving only a limited amount of free time for him to sit and think. While reflection is important, *I feel* that alcoholics during inpatient recovery probably respond best to structure, and I am cognizant of the high inpatient costs and desirous of taking maximal advantage of the available time.

D. The Length of Inpatient Treatment

This section can be simply summarized as: Keep it short unless you've got *good* reasons to make it longer (Ravensborg and Hoffman, 1976; Williams et al., 1973; Edwards et al., 1977). Repeated comparison of short-term inpatient treatment (usually two weeks or less) with longer treatment (usually three to six weeks) reveals that the shorter treatment period is as effective as the longer. Of course, both types of treatment are combined with adequate outpatient follow-up (Pokorny et al, 1973). There is even a recent study done with a group of relatively good risk (i.e., married) patients that demonstrates that an intensive counseling session, with the option of future inpatient treatment if needed, may be as effective as routine inpatient care (Edwards et al., 1977). Nonetheless, considering the economic and personal costs of inpatient treatment, it is not possible to justify longer than two weeks for the average individual.

The data on exceptions to short-term hospitalization are much less solid. If an individual has serious medical problems that have not cleared after two weeks, is still demonstrating serious depressive symptoms (in which case he may have primary affective disorder and secondary alcoholism), or has impaired mental functioning as evidenced by confusion, then it makes sense to keep him in the hospital for a longer period of time. There is less "common-sense validation" for offering longer inpatient care for individuals who have not benefited from shorter-term treatment. There is no reason to assume that they'll do better with longer care than they would with another exposure to short-term inpatient treatment later, if needed, or to outpatient follow-up. Similar comments apply when one is faced with a group of inpatients about whom the counselor or therapist subjectively feels that longer treatment is needed.

The primary suggestion is that, as a general rule, one should keep inpatient treatment short. Before any exceptions are made one should take the costs involved in longer treatment and the lack of evidence of efficacy of longer-term treatment and balance this with individual subjective opinions in making the final decision.

E. The "Natural History" of the Recovery Process during Inpatient Care

In gauging the needs of a particular patient it is important to know what the literature suggests is the course of recovery for alcoholics. Also, aggressive efforts at gathering adequate information on past history to rule out preexisting psychiatric problems helps you make informed treatment decisions and know when serious problems are developing. Even after ruling out secondary alcoholism, a number of important clinical syndromes can be seen in the primary alcoholic. When these are present, psychiatric consultation can be used if you feel other primary problems must be ruled out.

1. Sadness

A picture of depression in apparent primary alcoholics should not be actively treated unless it persists for two weeks or more. Most alcoholics enter care with a pharmacologically induced deep, but transient, sadness which will clear spontaneously within days to a week (Gibson and Becker, 1973). The usual treatment should be counseling and observation. If symptoms don't improve in 7 to 10 days, antidepressant medications (e.g., desipramine) may be needed.

2. Psychosis

Alcoholic hallucinosis and paranoia are dramatic psychotic pictures which can be expected to clear within days or a week with general supportive care. Here the patient may demonstrate transitory auditory hallucinations or paranoid delusions which, viewed cross-sectionally, can look identical to schizophrenia. However, the psychotic picture can be expected to clear with two days to two weeks of abstinence and rarely requires antipsychotic medication. Thus, the treatment and prognosis are quite different from schizophrenia, a finding which underscores the potential importance of obtaining adequate psychiatric consultation on all alcoholic patients demonstrating such psychotic pictures (estimated to occur to a clinically significant degree in 5% or less of alcoholics).

3. Organic Brain Syndromes (Confusion)

Many alcoholics enter treatment in a state of confusion which should be carefully evaluated to rule out underlying medical disorders but which will probably improve or disappear rapidly with time. Patients usually begin to improve within days, but continued clearing of the mental state can be expected to occur slowly over a period of months.

The differential diagnosis is broad and includes vitamin deficiency syndromes which should respond to multivitamin (and especially thiamine) replacement, confusion associated with alcoholic withdrawal, CNS depressant intoxication in people with preexisting brain damage (e.g., the elderly), and nonspecific and usually clinically reversible brain damage associated with alcoholism (Schuckit, in press). Evaluation requires aggressive steps to rule out other treatable forms of confusion (e.g., Wernicke-Korsakov's syndrome, subdural hematomas, infections, bleeds, etc.).

4. Insomnia

Impaired sleep (both initial and terminal insomnia) is to be expected during active abuse and withdrawal from any depressant drug. Even though this might persist for several months (Johnson, 1970; Gross and Hostey, 1976), hypnotics should not be used because they cause more problems than they cure (Kales et al., 1974). Insomnia might best be handled through offering careful guidance on sleeping patterns, as discussed elsewhere in these two chapters.

It is not wise to prescribe a drug which may be associated with a rebound insomnia and which may lose effectiveness after two to four weeks to an individual who may demonstrate sleep problems for three or more months (Schuckit, 1981). It is better to explain to the patient how his sleep difficulties are related to his drug withdrawal, share the ways in which using hypnotics would tend to make the picture worse within several weeks, and prescribe some behavioral manipulations which may help him cope with the sleep problem. Most patients can place themselves on a rigid sleep/wake cycle, going to bed at the same time every night, reading or watching television if they cannot fall asleep, and awakening at the same time every morning (even if they have only had 15 minutes sleep). There should be no naps during the day and no caffeinated beverages after the evening meal. On such a regimen most patients will revert to a more normalizing sleep pattern fairly quickly.

5. Anxiety

Feelings of nervousness and anxiety are to be expected during withdrawal and for several months thereafter. Antianxiety drugs have no place in the treatment of this syndrome other than care for the immediate acute withdrawal syndrome. Patients can be counseled on recognizing anxiety symptoms and given some alternatives (e.g., talking, exercise, biofeedback, medication, a hobby) to help handle the symptoms.

One major difficulty is that many patients attempt to ignore the signs and symptoms of increasing anxiety until they are ready to "explode," and these individuals may be helped by pointing out early signs of tension such as "butterflies in the stomach," a mild tremor, sweating, etc. Once the anxiety symptoms are spotted by the patient, you can then work with him to find which of the alternate modes of handling tension (e.g., exercise, reading, meditation) appear to help most. In a manner similar to that described for insomnia, explaining to the patient that you recognize the problems but that the pharmacological difficulties cannot be adequately reversed by using another drug does seem to help patients to cope.

There is less known about the recovery process from alcoholism itself. In dealing with the average alcoholic one must recognize the natural history of going "on and off the wagon" (Ludwig, 1972) and the propensity towards "spontaneous" cure (Schuckit, 1984; Smart, 1976). It is also important to note that recovery may be a long process. Sometimes the individual enters therapy only to end up in trouble later; but eventually he may reenter treatment and reach the final goal. Therefore, in treating the alcoholic it is best to try to help him go through his recovery process by giving him good medical care, a place to talk, and help in dealing with life problems involving family, peers, and work. If an effort at rehabilitation doesn't "take," I attempt to maintain contact with the hope that the next time, either inpatient or outpatient counseling will have a more significant effect.

F. Psychotherapy: What Type Is Best?

Psychotherapy is being used in a relatively "loose" manner here to mean the interaction between patient and physician, counselor, etc., within an established goal-oriented framework. Thus, many interactions in the therapeutic setting can be subsumed under the term psychotherapy.

The therapist will probably use the approach he finds most comfortable, and this often reflects where he has been trained. However, there are some general rules to be kept in mind (Berger, 1983). Once again, it is best to follow the dictum of keeping it simple (Costello et al., 1976) because there is no evidence that treatments aimed at finding deep psychological meanings or those which require high levels of therapist training are any more effective than simple "day-to-day" discussions (Emrick, 1975; Armour et al., 1976). From the standpoint of the need to justify costs in training therapists, the average "good" treatment program probably utilizes discussions that deal with the patient's attempts to stop his alcohol-related difficulties, his "new" interactions with his family, the difficulties on the job, his self-concept, his physiological problems during the recovery, etc. These sessions are also used to educate the patient about his "disease" and give him some idea of continued risks he runs by a return to drinking.

The average counseling session requires a leader with knowledge about alcoholism and a level of sensitivity, but counseling may not need to be limited to those with advanced training in psychotherapy. During this "typical" session, the counselor can help the patient or group of patients to focus on the problems of the "here-and-now." Topics can include stresses at work and at home which tend to increase a desire to drink and possible mechanisms for dealing with these stresses, learning how to "say no" when offered alcohol, hints on ways of interacting with friends who expect the patient to drink, how to establish a new cadre of friends for whom alcohol is not important, the best manner of filling in the large amounts of free time that are generated by abstinence, vocational hints for finding work where alcohol is not so tempting, etc.

Comparisons of group and individual psychotherapy routinely reveal that group treatment is effective for the patient and it costs less than individual psychotherapy (Emrick, 1975). While some authors feel that group therapy has specific advantages (Forrest, 1975, pp. 93–100) because it allows the patient to share his feelings with a number of other people with similar problems and teaches social skills, etc., there is little hard evidence to back this up. For a basic introduction to group methods, the reader can review the excellent paper by Brown and Yalom (1977) and works by several other authors (Forrest, 1975, pp. 93–100; Fahr, 1976, pp. 637–653; Berger, 1983).

Group therapy sessions are an excellent place for an interdisciplinary treatment approach (Brown and Yalom, 1977). The physician's time might best be spent in supervision and in dealing with more seriously medically and psychologically ill patients, while the group can be effectively run by nurses, social workers, and paraprofessionals. The private physician in a small community might utilize a local counselor, a nurse, or a clergyman to help establish such a group.

Among the many special types of psychotherapy that can be used, two have been felt to be of specific help to the alcoholic: psychodrama (Davies, 1976) and transactional analysis (Gorad et al., 1971). While role-playing in front of the group, an example of the former, and learning about various aspects of communication and stereotyped behavior, an example of the latter, can be beneficial, there is no evidence that they are required as part of alcoholism therapy.

Individual psychotherapy, either alone or as part of the group, is also an important tool in dealing with the alcoholic. The general caveats for group therapy apply as well here, including the lack of data indicating that highly trained therapists are required. A specific model for individual psychotherapy in alcoholics has been offered elsewhere (Forrest, 1975, pp. 77–100).

One "special" case of alcoholism treatment is behavior modification (Briddell and Nathan, 1976). Such behavior approaches include mechanisms briefly alluded to above for handling insomnia and anxiety. Some programs have incorporated an adjunct to the usual counseling and outreach by giving the patient an additional edge when the desire to drink becomes strong (Weins et al., 1976). This form of *aversive conditioning* requires a series of sessions (often three times a week for two or three weeks) during which the patient is given an injection which makes him feel nauseated and the nausea is then coupled with the smell and taste of alcoholic beverages. As a result, the next time he sees, smells, or tastes alcohol, he is likely to feel nauseated and even vomit. In order to be maximally effective, these more formal types of behavior modification should be followed by a series of "refreshers" in which the patient undergoes an additional short series of aversive sessions every three months or so over the following year. Using this approach, the patient who very much wants to return to drinking can do so by gulping down alcohol quickly enough until nausea is no longer experienced. On the other hand, the individual who wishes to stop drinking can use the nausea as a reminder and a motivation builder which might add to his chance for abstinence.

While it is possible that a specific type of patient responds especially well to this mode of therapy, no reliable methods have yet been devised for choosing those particular patients. As things stand, this promising mode of treatment is a viable alternative for patients who prefer to receive the behavioral approach. This topic is mentioned here to note its potential importance in alcoholism treatment, but the reader is referred to the fine chapter by Dr. Nathan for a more substantial discussion.

In summary, the "psychotherapies" in alcoholic rehabilitation are general helping mechanisms. There is no proof that one approach is better than another, and the therapist is wise to take advantage of his prior training. However, it is advisable to keep the approach relatively simple because there is no evidence that dealing with "intrapsychic conflicts" is beneficial to the patient or cost-effective. Most therapists looking to maximize the treatment dollar use group therapy, emphasizing day-to-day life adjustment through discussions with an interdisciplinary therapeutic team ranging from paraprofessionals to physicians. Education is an important part of most rehabilitation efforts, and most programs recognize the importance of dealing with the patient and his family together.

G. Alcoholics Anonymous

Alcoholic rehabilitation has many components. It includes good medical care, thorough evaluation of prior medical and psychiatric problems, and a common-sense approach to psychotherapy or the utilization of behavior modification techniques. Most programs also choose to utilize Alcoholics Anonymous (AA) as part of a "broad brush" approach to treatment. Patients can begin attending meetings either at the treatment facility or by being issued passes to AA meetings in their neighborhood. This treatment component has been described in greater detail in Chapter 6.

H. Education

It is usually assumed that patients will do better if they (and their families) learn more about the causes, clinical course, and problems (medical, psychological, and social) of alcoholism. Education is usually given as group lecture/discussions which are offered daily. Although almost universally applied in inpatient settings and offering little or no patient risks, it is difficult to prove that these sessions actually enhance chances for recovery (Uecker and Boutilier, 1976).

It's possible to develop a "typical" series of lectures. These usually include several didactic and discussion sections dealing with the effect of alcohol on body systems, one or more sessions dealing with alcohol's effects on family functioning including sexual problems, one or several sessions introducing the patient to Alcoholics Anonymous—its goals as well as its assets and liabilities. Recovering alcoholics in your community can be very helpful in establishing this series, and a number of educational movies are available.

I. Vocational Training

Occupational adjustment is a very important part of aftercare. There is insufficient space to discuss this important topic here, but most clinicians should recognize and use hospital or government-based vocational programs for their patients.

J. Medications

This important topic is discussed in Chapters 6 and 8 and is mentioned only briefly here. The high rate of serious medical problems in alcoholics necessitates a variety of medications utilized for a specific problem for a limited period of time (Chapter 2). In addition, the minority of alcoholics demonstrating a primary psychiatric disorder with secondary alcoholism may require antidepressants, lithium, or antipsychotic medications to treat their primary illness.

Psychotropic medication *cannot* be justified for the average alcoholic (Rosenberg, 1974). After the initial withdrawal is completed, there is almost no indication for the use of hypnotics or antianxiety drugs in the alcoholic (Viamontes, 1972; Schuckit, 1975). Nor are there good controlled studies to demonstrate that the average alcoholic should be receiving drugs such as lithium, propranolol, or most other drugs, with the possible exception of disulfiram as discussed in Chapter 6.

One specific drug worthy of greater discussion is disulfiram, or Antabuse. This is primarily an "outpatient" approach inasmuch as it attempts to help the patient in the community to avoid returning to drinking on the spur of the moment. It can be used for the patient who enters outpatient care or during aftercare following an inpatient rehabilitation program. When given to patients with good medical functioning who have none of the contraindications to its use (as outlined in Chapter 6) it can probably be continued at 250 mg per day for 6 to 12 months. The data proving the efficacy of disulfiram is not exceedingly strong, but at least anecdotally, it does seem to help. Antabuse treatment is not a good mode of aversive conditioning, however, because the nausea reaction follows an unpredictable time course.

This has not been an exhaustive overview of inpatient treatment of alcoholism. It is, rather, a general summary of what is felt to be some of the most relevant material in aiding the clinician in establishing an inpatient alcohol treatment regimen. Because there are individuals who disagree with the generalizations presented here, the reader is advised to review some of the referenced texts and papers and to make up their own minds. The most important information can be summarized this way: It is the bias of this chapter that any deviation from the simplest helping approach must be justified by offering proof that the treatment is not causing more trouble than it is worth. In the field of alcoholism where there is a huge public need and a limited amount of money, any treatment that adds to the cost without increasing the benefits does damage.

V. SOME SPECIAL TREATMENT PROBLEMS

Up to this point this chapter has presented a general treatment approach to alcoholism in outpatient and inpatient settings. In addition to guidelines which apply to the majority of primary alcoholic patients, some special cases have been noted, including the needs of youth, the elderly, women, and minorities. This chapter has also covered what can be expected in the course of recovery from heavy drinking and the associated problems of sadness, insomnia, and confusion. It is not possible in a text of this length to treat exhaustively all therapeutic options, but a limited number of additional topics require emphasis.

A. Suicide

It has been estimated that 10% to 15% of alcoholics commit suicide, and many more attempt it (Goodwin and Guze, 1979; Goodwin, 1973). Thus suicide must be considered as a potential danger in dealing with any alcoholic. Suicide attempts probably fall into two categories—those that occur in an individual with primary affective disorder who is drinking heavily, and those that occur as a complication of the pharmacologic effects of alcohol in primary alcoholics (Mayfield and Montgomery, 1972).

The disorder in psychiatry with the highest suicide completion rate is the persistent sadness which occurs along with changes in body and mind functioning in the absence of a preexisting psychiatric disorder which is labeled primary affective disorder (Goodwin and Guze 1979). In one approach to this diagnosis, individuals are labeled either unipolar (i.e., they have only depressions and no manias) or bipolar (in which case they have both manias and depressions) (Winokur et al., 1969). Individuals with primary affective disorder and secondary alcoholism are at especially high rates for suicide, and you should be more likely to hospitalize them. If you are not a psychiatrist, be *certain* to get a psychiatric consultation for these patients. They will almost certainly require antidepressants such as trazadone (Desyrel), or nortriptyline (Pamilar), or lithium for unipolar and bipolar disorders respectively, as discussed briefly in Chapter 6.

Primary alcoholics also complete suicide (probably at a rate of around 10%) (Miles, 1977), usually in the midst of heavy drinking bouts.

Alcohol causes serious depression which tends to lift within days of the achievement of abstinence (Gibson and Becker, 1973). However, while drinking, the depression is real and quite dangerous. When a primary alcoholic presents with serious sadness and suicidal thoughts you should hospitalize him, recognizing that the depression and suicidal ideation will probably clear rapidly after which point a decision can be made regarding the necessity for hospitalization as part of alcoholic rehabilitation. Hospitalization for the primary alcoholic thinking about suicide is especially important if he does not have someone to watch over him during the next 12 hours when the suicidal propensity might be especially strong.

B. The Revolving-Door Alcoholic

Those physicians and other health care specialists who think they have only one or two alcoholic patients in their case load are probably referring to the skid row or revolving-door alcoholic (Gallant et al., 1973). In fact, because the average alcoholic is a blue-collar or white-collar worker presenting to health care specialists with medical or emotional problems, the physician is overlooking the 20% to 30% of his patients who have serious alcohol-related problems (Moore, 1971). However, the revolving-door type of alcoholic is a special case and worthy of comment.

At least 10% of the revolving-door population (so named because they tend to repeatedly walk out and back in the door of the treatment center) do achieve abstinence. However, this population tends to have acute medical care needs and should be offered the occasional opportunity to "dry out." In dealing with the revolving-door alcoholic one can keep the need for abstinence in mind, but do not gauge your success or failure solely by how many of these patients stop drinking. His "disease" is severe and almost out of control, and he often comes for help to be able to survive physically. You can hope your interactions lay the groundwork for future efforts at rehabilitation and do all you can to keep the door open to him; concentrate on his medical and personal needs.

C. Handling the VIP

In all aspects of medicine the Very Important Person who expects special treatment is, unfortunately, likely to receive inferior care. This is especially true in alcoholism where it is important for the health care specialist to sincerely confront the patient's behavior and educate the individual about his future problems. It is not possible to do this and "pull your punches." This brief note is included as a warning that when alcoholism reaches into the upper socioeconomic strata to physicians, bank vice-presidents, famous entertainers, and the like—as it frequently does—you must use the same general approach to the VIP that you use for the "average" middle-class primary alcoholic.

VI. AFTERCARE

A. General Aftercare

Alcohol problems have probably been going on for at least 10 years before the patient is confronted (Schuckit, 1984). Treatment aims at offering good general help, and, unfortunately, we have no magic cures. Therefore, it is not surprising that the recovery process from alcoholism tends to occur over a relatively long and difficult period. The patient may be easily detoxified if that is required and should be able to participate in a rehabilitation program, but he may relapse into serious drinking problems when facing real-life situations. Therefore, it makes good sense that outpatient aftercare must be an integral part of any inpatient treatment program.

The general approach to an extended interaction with the patient after discharge has been outlined for you in the previous chapter. From the moment you first see the patient, recognize that once detoxification and inpatient care (if required) are completed, you should continue to see that individual and members of the family for six months to a year.

During follow-up, the material to be handled with the primary alcoholic centers on general day-to-day life adjustment and deals with crises and situations that arouse a strong drive to return to drinking. At first the patient should probably be seen in group therapy once a week which, with continued abstinence (or only rare brief slips), would be decreased after several months to once every other week, then after several more months to once a month, followed by once every other month, which is then followed by infrequent contact over the subsequent second year. Before ending regular counseling sessions, the patient and family should be told that you are available by phone or through their attendance in a group, if necessary. They should also be encouraged to attend AA, and Alanon and Alateen where appropriate, regularly. If the patient has been medically screened and has agreed to take disulfiram, that medication is probably going to be continued for the first year (if you feel that the potential dangers do not negate its use).

B. Nursing Homes

Some individuals are not ready to return to "the real world" after their short-term inpatient treatment. If inpatient care is being offered in a hospital setting (either general medical or psychiatric), an extended stay in such a facility is usually prohibitively expensive. In such instances, a separate long-term program should be considered. For those with serious medical problems, a nursing home should be chosen on the same basis used for any medical convalescence. Those primary alcoholics still showing signs of confusion or disorientation should also be placed in a sheltered environment using the same general guidelines you would use for any organically impaired individual. However, continued confusion in an alcoholic does not necessarily mean a permanent organic brain syndrome because, with good nutrition and vitamin supplementation, some mentation might return.

C. Halfway Houses

Many states have established a network of halfway houses to serve alcoholics who have completed their formal rehabilitation but are not yet ready to return to the community. The reasons for continued care might be a lack of available resources, a very severe life crisis, or long-term persistent alcoholism that has not responded to inpatient care in the past. A halfway house usually offers continued group meetings, general supervised support for medication or for dealing with emotional problems and crises, and an exposure to AA. During their stay in a halfway house, patients usually continue in the outpatient rehabilitation phase of their inpatient treatment programs. Many of these facilities are excellent, but it is a good idea to visit the program and evaluate the staff and facilities carefully (Baker et al., 1974).

VII. EVALUATION

In alcoholism, the high rate of temporary improvement, the substantial proportion of patients with "spontaneous remission," and the history of fads in treatment programs has resulted in a number of touted "cures" which were only later discovered to be doing potential harm (Schuckit, 1977; Schuckit and Cahalan, 1976). We serve our patients best by doing all we can to remain objective in looking at our own efforts, constantly questioning whether we are giving the most benefit with the least harm. The very simplest treatments may turn out to be the best because they cost less and expose the patient to shorter treatment time and fewer dangers (Edwards et al., 1977).

Evaluation can be done (1) to monitor the progress of patients *or* (2) to determine if the program is *responsible* for the improvements or cures being seen. The former, monitoring treatment efforts, requires only tha you record good data about background and level of functioning when patients enter treatment and then follow up *all* patients who enter the program (Schuckit and Cahalan, 1976). This is a natural outgrowth of your commitment to maintain contact with the patient, even those who drop out of treatment.

Most programs do not evaluate the second option, program effectiveness. This would require a *random* assignment of all eligible patients to your regular program or to a waiting list (or at most a minimum treatment effort). However, it is relatively easy to evaluate the effectiveness of any changes added to your usual treatment efforts. Here, all eligible patients should be randomly assigned to your usual program or to the new procedure. After six months or a year you can do a follow-up study to evaluate the outcome of the two groups of patients and decide if the new therapy is worth keeping. Guidelines for this are presented in detail in another text (Schuckit and Cahalan, 1976).

In summary, evaluation is synonymous with good patient care. You can *monitor* your results by keeping goals and definitions clearly in mind and following up your patients. This is not an *evaluation* of whether your program is causing success because it does not tell you if your treatment was better than any other treatment or no formal care. While it would be delightful if you could engage in true evaluation of your efforts by doing controlled studies, the administrators of most treatment programs find themselves limited to utilizing controlled evaluations to help them decide whether they are going to *add* a new therapeutic mode to their already existing program.

VIII. ESTABLISHING A FORMAL TREATMENT PROGRAM—A SUMMARY

The discussion to this point has assumed that you are a health care deliverer (usually a physician) integrating treatment of the alcoholic into other treatment concerns with other patients. If you wish to establish a formal inpatient program for alcoholics, you should use the basic approaches outlined in this chapter to set up your goals and therapeutic regimen.

You should begin by being sure how you define alcoholism, reviewing various treatment resources available in your area, and establishing yourself in a facility (the choice will probably be based upon the practicalities of where you are and what your training is). You will probably select a staff which, to be cost-effective, utilizes individuals without degrees, or paraprofessionals (Armour et al., 1976; Canto, 1977; Rosenberg et al., 1976). Make every effort to establish an atmosphere of concern and questioning, avoiding therapists or counselors who are so overly committed to their approach that they cannot be effective. The necessity for evaluation, at least for monitoring outcomes, should be considered from the very beginning—this will require good intake records and follow-up procedures.

Patients will probably enter your two-week inpatient program after receiving an initial screening to rule out or recognize other psychiatric disorders and to allow you to treat any medical problems (of which there may be many). The patients' families should take part in the initial screening, where they are taught about the program and educated about what is to be expected during the process of recovery.

The alcoholic then undergoes detoxification, if necessary, and embarks upon his inpatient treatment program with the full understanding that this is just the beginning of his care and that outpatient follow-up is of great importance. He is usually placed in a fairly highly structured environment where his day is broken into group therapy sessions (usually led by paraprofessionals who in turn are supervised by a trained psychologist or psychiatrist), educational sessions about alcoholism, family group discussions, and Alcoholics Anonymous. Some programs may vary this by utilizing behavior modification techniques as the core of the treatment program. In addition, ancillary treatment modes, including psychodrama, recreational therapy, vocational counseling, and so on, can be used. If the patient has a primary psychiatric disorder other than alcoholism, appropriate referral is made.

During the patient's stay, the interdisciplinary staff will probably meet once or twice a week to discuss his progress. At discharge he will be introduced to his major therapist for his outpatient group sessions, which will be established for the patient (and, if necessary, for the family) beginning on a weekly basis, followed by decreasing frequency of therapy sessions over the subsequent year or two. With the exception of any medications needed for his or her medical disorders, the patient will probably be discharged on no other drugs, with the possible exception of disulfiram.

This simplistic overview reflects what has been outlined in this chapter. Don't assume that you can jump right in and establish a program. You must be sure that you are knowledgeable about alcoholism, that you have made adequae contacts within your community to be sure there is a need for an additional program, that you have visited other treatment programs, and that your training gives you the degree of competence necessary to do alcoholism treatment.

IX. IN CONCLUSION

Treating the alcoholic is both simple and highly complex. We have a responsibility to ensure that we are doing our best for our patients, and this includes keeping an open mind to be certain that our own emotions about what is "best" do not interfere with our ability to reevaluate our efforts constantly.

There are no magic cures in alcoholic rehabilitation. What this chapter has outlined for you, based upon the available literature and clinical experience, are some basic rules for inpatient care. These include a relatively simple program emphasizing outpatient care with inpatient rehabilitation when needed, employing nondegreed health care deliverers as well as professionals as a multidisciplinary team, emphasizing *helping* the patient to go through recovery, utilizing group therapy sessions, reaching out to both the patient and his or her family, and recognizing the special needs of some subgroup alcoholics.

REFERENCES

Armour, D. J., Polich, J. M., and Stambul, H. B., 1976, *Alcoholism and Treatment,* prepared for NIAAA, Report R-1739-NIAAA, Washington, D.C.

Baker, T. B., Sobell, M. B., Sobell, L. C., and Cannon, D. S., 1976, Halfway houses for alcoholics: A review, analysis and comparison with other halfway house facilities, *Int. J. Soc. Psychiat.,* 22:1–7.

Becker, C. E., Roe, R. L., and Scott, R. A., 1974, *Alcohol as a Drug. A Curriculum on Pharmacology, Neurology and Toxicology,* The Williams & Wilkins Company, Baltimore.

Berger, F., 1983, Alcoholism rehabilitation, *Hosp. Comm. Psychiat.,* 34:1040–1043.

Blane, H. T., and Hewitt, L. E., 1976, *Alcohol and Youth: An Analysis of the Literature 1960–1975,* Report for the NIAAA, contact ADM-281-75-0026, Washington, D.C.

Brickner, P. W., Greenbaum, D., Kaufman, A., O'Donnell, F., O'Brian, J. T., Scalice, R., Scandizzo, J., and Sullivan, T., 1972, A clinic for male derelicts, a welfare hotel project, *Ann. Int. Med.,* 77:565–569.

Briddell, D. W., and Nathan, P. E., 1976, Behavior assessment and modification with alcoholics: current status and future trends, in *Progress in Behavior Modification,* vol. 2 (M. Hersen, R. Eisler, and P. Miller, eds.), Academic Press, New York.

Brown, S., and Yalom, I. D., 1977, International group therapy with alcoholics, *J. Stud. Alc.,* 38:426–456.

Cantor, J. M., 1977, Alcohol drug counselors in the Veterans Administration—Five years experience, presented at the National Council on Alcoholism Eighth Annual Medical-Scientific Conference, May, 1977, San Diego, Calif.

Costello, R. M., Biever, P., and Baillargoon, J. G., 1976, Alcoholism treatment programming: Historical trends and modern approaches, presented at the

National Council on Alcoholism Seventh Annual Medical-Scientific Conference, May, 1976, Washington, D.C.

Davies, M. H., 1976, The origins and practice of psychodrama, *Br. J. Psychiat.*, 129:201–206.

Edwards, G., Orford, J., Egert, S., Guthrie, S., Hawker, A., Hensman, C., Mitcheson, M., Oppenheimer, E., and Taylor, C., 1977, Alcoholism: A controlled trial of "treatment" and "advice," *J. Stud. Alc.*, 38:1004–1031.

El-Guebaly, N., and Offord, D. R., 1977, The offspring of alcoholics, *Am. J. Psychiat.*, 134:357–365.

Emrick, C. D., 1975, A review of psychologically oriented treatment of alcoholism, II, *J. Stud. Alc.*, 36:88–108.

Fehr, D. H., 1976, Psychotherapy, in *Alcoholism* (R. E. Tarter and A. A. Sugerman, eds.), pp. 637–653, Addison-Wesley Publishing Co., Reading, Mass.

Forrest, G. G., 1975, *The Diagnosis and Treatment of Alcoholism*, Charles C Thomas, Springfield, Ill.

Gallant, D. S., 1971, Evaluation of compulsory treatment of the alcoholic municipal court offender, in *Recent Advances in Studies of Alcoholism: An Interdisciplinary Symposium* (N. Mello and J. Mendelson, eds.), U.S. Government Printing Office, Washington, D.C.

Gallant, D. M., Bishop, M. P., Mouledoux, A., Faulkner, M. A., Brisolara, A., and Swanson, W. A., 1973, The revolving-door alcoholic, an impasse in the treatment of the chronic alcoholic, *Arch. Gen. Psychiat.*, 28:633–638.

Garber, J. J., 1972, The chronic alcoholic in a small community hospital, *Minn. Med.*, 55:665–667.

Gessner, P. K., 1974, Failure of diphenylhydantoin to prevent alcohol withdrawal convulsions in mice, *Euro. J. Pharm.*, 27:120–129.

Gibson, S., and Becker, J., 1973, Alcoholism and depression, *Q. J. Stud. Alc.*, 34:400–408.

Goodwin, D. W., 1973, Alcohol in suicide and homicide, *Q. J. Alc.*, 34:144–156.

Goodwin, D., and Guze, S. D., 1979, *Psychiatric Diagnosis*, Oxford University Press, New York.

Gorad, S. L., McCourt, W. F., and Cobb, J. C., 1971, A communication approach to alcoholism, *Q. J. Stud. Alc.*, 32:651–668.

Greenblatt, D. J., and Shader, R. I., 1978, Prazepam and lorazepam, *New Eng. J. Med.*, 299:1342–1344.

Greenleigh Associates, Inc., 1975, *A Survey and Study of the Alcoholism Programs of Major Corporations Headquartered in New York City*, Executive Summary for the Corporate Headquarters Alcoholism Project, August, 1975.

Gross, M. M., and Hostey, J. M., 1976, Sleep disturbances in alcoholism, in *Alcoholism* (R. E. Tarter and A. A. Sugerman, eds.), pp. 257–308, Addison-Wesley Publishing Co., Reading, Mass.

Haglund, R. M. J., and Schuckit, M. A., 1977, The epidemiology of alcoholism, in *Alcoholism: Development, Consequences, and Interventions* (N. Estes and E. Heinemann, eds.), C. V. Mosby Company, St. Louis.

Janzen, C., 1977, Families in the treatment of alcoholism, *J. Stud. Alc.*, 38:114–130.

Johnson, L. C., 1970, Sleep during alcohol intake and withdrawal in the chronic alcoholic, *Arch. Gen. Psychiat.*, 22:406–418.

Jones, B. M., and Jones, M. K., 1976, Women and alcohol, in *Alcohol Problems* in *Women and Children* (M. Greenblatt and M. A. Schuckit, eds.), Grune & Stratton, Inc., New York.

Kales, A., Bixler, E. O., Tan, T., Scharf, M. B., and Kales, J. D., 1974, Chronic hypnotic-drug use, ineffectiveness, drug-withdrawal insomnia, and dependence, *JAMA*, 227:513–517.

Kitson, T. M., 1977, The disulfiram-methanol reaction, *J. Stud. Alc.*, 38:96–113.

Knott, D. H., and Beard, J. D., 1969, A diuretic approach to acute withdrawal from alcohol, *South. Med. J.*, 62:485–489.

Ludwig, A. M., 1972, On and off the wagon, *Q. J. Stud. Alc.*, 33:91–96.

Mayfield, D. G., and Montgomery, D., 1972, Alcoholism, alcohol intoxication, and suicide attempts, *Arch. Gen. Psychiat.*, 27:349–353.

Miles, D. P., 1977, Conditions predisposing to suicide, a review, *J. Nerv. Men. Dis.*, 164:231–246.

Miller, P. M., 1975, An analysis of chronic drunkenness offenders with implications for behavioral intervention, *Int. J. Addic.*, 10:995–1005.

Moore, R. A., 1971, The prevalence of alcoholism in a community general hospital, *Am. J. Psychiat.*, 128:638–640.

Pattison, E. M., 1976, Nonabstinent drinking goals in the treatment of alcoholism, *Arch. Gen. Psychiat.*, 33:923–930.

Peterson, W., 1975, A medical evaluation of the safety of nonhospital detoxification, presented at the National Council on Alcoholism Sixth Annual Medical-Scientific Conference, May, 1975, Milwaukee, Wisc.

Pokorny, A. D., Miller, B. A., Kanas, T., and Valles, J., 1973, Effectiveness of extended aftercare in the treatment of alcoholism, *Q. J. Stud. Alc.*, 34:435–443.

Polit, D. M., Nuttall, R. L., and Hunter, J. B., 1976, Women and drugs, *Urb. Soc. Change Rev.*, 9:9–16.

Ravensborg, M. R., and Hoffmann, J., 1975–1976, Program versus time: Length of stay patterns in alcoholism, *Drug Alc. Depend.*, 1:51–56.

Reding, G. R., and Maguire, B., 1973, Nonsegregated acute psychiatric admissions to general hospitals—continuity of care within the community hospital, *New Eng. J. Med.*, 289:185–189.

Rosenberg, C. M., 1974, Drug maintenance in the outpatient treatment of chronic alcoholism, *Arch. Gen. Psychiat.*, 30:373–377.

Rosenberg, C. M., Gerrein, J. R., Manohar, V., and Liftik, J., 1976, Evaluation of training of alcoholism counselors, *J. Stud. Alc.*, 37:1236–1246.

Schaefer, J. M., 1981, Firewater myths revisited, review of findings and some new directions, *J. Stud. Alc.*, Suppl. 9:99–117.

Schmitz, R., 1977, Alcohol in the withdrawal of the alcoholic, presented at the National Council on Alcoholism Eighth Medical-Scientific Conference, May, 1977, San Diego, Calif.

Schuckit, M. A., 1975, Drugs in combination with other therapies for alcoholics, in *Drugs in Combination with Other Therapies* (M. Greenblatt, ed.), pp. 119–134, Grune & Stratton, Inc., New York.

———, 1977a, *Alcoholism in Women: A Report to the President's Commission on Mental Health,* submitted for consideration to the President's Commission on Mental Health, August, 1977.

———, 1977b, *Alcohol and Youth: A Report to the President's Commission on Mental Health,* submitted for consideration to the President's Commission on Mental Health, August, 1977.

————, 1977c, Geriatric alcoholism and drug abuse, *Gerontologist*, 17:168–174.

————, 1977d, Alcoholism: Natural history and outcome studies, presented at the Society for Epidemiologic Research Annual Meeting, June, 1977, Seattle, Wash., ADAI Report No. 77-18.

————, 1981, Current therapeutic options in the management of typical anxiety, *J. Clin. Psychiat.*, 42:15–24.

————, 1982, The history of psychotic symptoms in alcoholics, *J. Clin. Psychiat.*, 43:53–57.

————, 1983, Alcoholism and other psychiatric disorders, *Hosp. and Com. Psychiat.*, 34:1022–1027.

————, 1984, *Drug and Alcohol Abuse: A Clinical Guide to Diagnosis and Treatment*, Plenum Publishing Company, New York.

Schuckit, M. A., and Cahalan, D., 1976, Evaluation of alcoholism treatment programs, in *Alcohol and Alcohol Problems: New Thinking and New Directions* (W. J. Filstead, J. J. Rossi, and M. Keller, eds.), Ballinger Publishing Co., Cambridge, Mass.

Schuckit, M. A., and Miller, P. L., 1976, Alcoholism in elderly men: A survey of a general medical ward, *Ann. New York Aca. Sci.*, 273:558–571.

Schuckit, M. A., and Morrissey, E. R., 1976, Alcoholism in women: Some clinical and social perspectives with an emphasis on possible subtypes, in *Alcoholism Problems in Women and Children* (M. Greenblatt and M. A. Schuckit, eds.), pp. 5–35, Grune & Stratton, Inc., New York.

Schuckit, M. A., Morrissey, E. R., Lewis, N. J. and Buck, W. T., 1977, Adolescent problem drinkers, in *Currents in Alcoholism*, vol. 2 (F. A. Seixas, ed.), pp. 325–355, Grune & Stratton, Inc., New York.

Sellers, E. M., and Kalant, H., 1976, Alcohol intoxication and withdrawal, *New Eng. J. Med.*, 294:757–762.

Smart, R. G., 1976, Spontaneous recovery in alcoholics, *Drug and Alc. Depend.*, 1:277–285.

Smith, C. M., and Sommerfeld, E. J., 1968, Managing alcoholics on an open psychiatric ward, *Q. J. Stud. Alc.*, 29:703–708.

Steinglass, P., 1981, The alcoholic family at home. Patterns of interaction in dry, wet, and transitional stages of alcoholism, *Arch. Gen. Psychiat.*, 38:578–584.

Streissguth, A. P., 1976, Maternal alcoholism and the outcome of pregnancy, in *Alcohol Problems in Women and Children* (M. Greenblatt and M. A. Schuckit, eds.), Grune & Stratton, Inc., New York.

Streissguth, A. P., 1978, Fetal alcohol syndrome: An epidemiologic perspective, *Am. J. Epidemiol.*, 107:467–478.

Uecker, A. E., and Boutilier, L. R., 1976, Alcohol education for alcoholics, relations to attitude changes and post-treatment abstinence, *J. Stud. Alc.*, 37:965–975.

Viamontes, J. A., 1972, Review of drug effectiveness in the treatment of alcoholism, *Am. J. Psychiat.*, 128:120–121.

Victor, M., Adams, R. D., and Collins, G. H., 1971, *The Wernicke-Korsakoff Syndrome*, F. A. Davis, Philadelphia.

Wanberg, K. W., Horn, J. L. and Foster, F. M., 1977, A differential assessment model for alcoholism, the scales of the alcohol use inventory, *J. Stud. Alc.*, 38:512–543.

West, J. W., 1976, The general hospital as a primary setting for the treatment of alcoholism, presented at the National Council on Alcoholism Seventh Annual Medical-Scientific Conference, May, 1976, Washir ̣ton, D.C.

Westermeyer, J., 1981, Research on treatment of drinking problems. Importance of cultural factors, *J. Stud. Alc.*, Suppl. 9:44–59.

Westermeyer, J., 1972, Options regarding alcohol use among the Chippewa, *Am. J. Orthopsychiat.*, 42:398–403.

Willems, P. J. A., Letemendia, F. J. J., and Arroyave, F., 1973, A two-year follow-up study comparing short with long stay in-patient treatment of alcoholics, *Br. J. Psychiat.*, 122:637–648.

Wilsnack, C. S., 1976, The impact of sex roles and women's alcohol use and abuse, in *Alcohol Problems in Women and Children* (M. Greenblatt and M. A. Schuckit, eds.), Grune & Stratton, Inc., New York.

Winokur, G., Clayton, P. J. and Reich, T., 1969, *Manic-Depressive Disease*, C. V. Mosby Company, St. Louis.

Woodruff, R. A., Jr., Clayton, P. J. and Guze, S. B., Suicide attempts and psychiatric diagnosis, *Dis. Nerv. Sys.*, 33:617–621.

Woodruff, R. A., Jr., Guze, S. B., Clayton, P. J. and Carr, D., 1973, Alcoholism and depression, *Arch. Gen. Psychiat.*, 28:97–100.

Zimberg, S., 1974, Evaluation of alcoholism treatment in Harlem, *Q. J. Stud. Alc.*, 35:550–557.

CHAPTER 8

Drugs Used in the Treatment of Alcoholism

Jerome H. Jaffe, M.D.
Professor of Psychiatry
University of Connecticut School of Medicine, Farmington
Director, Addiction Research Center
National Institute on Drug Abuse
Baltimore, Maryland

Domenic A. Ciraulo, M.D.
Assistant Professor of Psychiatry
Tufts University School of Medicine
Staff Psychiatrist
Veterans Administration Medical Center
Boston, Massachusetts

I. INTRODUCTION

The use of drugs in the treatment of alcoholism evokes feelings that go beyond the usual concerns about safety and efficacy. In the United States, and in some other countries as well, ex-alcoholic laymen, clergy, and nonmedical health professionals all play prominent roles in the treatment and rehabilitation of the alcoholic patient. In general, such groups believe that the alcoholic's central problem is the use of the drug (alcohol) to manage feelings, and that learning to cope with life while abstaining from alcohol (and other drugs) is the essence of treatment and the only acceptable goal of treatment. Such groups are understandably skeptical

NOTE: Preparation of this chapter was supported in part by NIAAA grant #AA03510, Center for the Study of Alcoholism, Department of Psychiatry, University of Connecticut School of Medicine, Farmington, Connecticut. Faith Jaffe and Ari Jaffe provided invaluable assistance in preparation and typing of the manuscript.

about the value of any treatment for alcoholism requiring a drug. There is a special concern about drugs with actions on the CNS, and not merely because the alcoholic is viewed as one who can easily become dependent on drugs other than alcohol. Ex-alcoholic counselors may feel that the very act of taking a drug tends to undermine the basic notion of abstinence. One exception is made for drugs such as disulfiram, where the act of taking the drug represents a decision not to drink. Furthermore, quite apart from this general bias against the use of psychoactive drugs, there is little solid evidence (except in the case of treatment of withdrawal syndromes) that pharmacologically based treatments are effective for the many problems facing the alcoholic patient. Despite the limited evidence, a number of drugs are widely used by physicians in treating alcoholics. These drugs, the evidence for their efficacy, and the way they are used are reviewed in this chapter. The writing of this chapter was greatly facilitated by several excellent and extensive reviews of similar material (Sellers and Kalant, 1976; Smith, 1978; Gessner, 1979; Behar and Winokur, 1979; Rada and Kellner, 1979; Sellers et al., 1981; Hoyumpa and Schenker, 1982; Sellers and Busto, 1982). Because of space limitations, in many places the reader is referred to one of these reviews rather than to the original publications.

II. DRUGS FOR ACUTE ALCOHOLIC INTOXICATION

A. Amethystic Agents

There are many situations in which it would be useful to have an *amethystic* agent, a drug that would counteract or antagonize the acute effects of alcohol. These situations range from the treatment of serious life-threatening overdoses and the calming of the combative, bellicose inebriate to the sobering up of the temporarily overindulgent. Unfortunately, there are, at present, no drugs which can be considered ethanol antagonists. According to several clinical reports, patients with high blood alcohol levels who are severely intoxicated or comatose may show arousal when given the opioid antagonist naloxone (0.4 mg to several mg) even when laboratory data indicate no recent narcotic use. However, naloxone does not significantly improve lesser degrees of alcohol intoxication. A recent review by Dole et al. (1982) of the effects of naloxone in alcoholic intoxication concluded that it was unlikely that the antidotal effect seen in comatose patients was due to any direct antagonism of the effects of alcohol. Instead, it seemed likely that, when naloxone was effective, it was because it was acting on endogenous opiates that were aggravating the basic pathology causing the coma. There is good experimental evidence that opioids, endogenous or exogenous, play an aggravating role in circulatory failure from many causes and in cerebral ischemia. There have also been clinical reports that naloxone is beneficial in treating shock due to sepsis, cerebral infarction, myocardial infarction, hemorrhage, and barbiturate overdose. In these situations, naloxone use resulted in improved circulatory status. Dole and coworkers (1982) interpreted the available data as supporting, although very tentatively, a beneficial role for naloxone in those cases of alcoholic coma in which ischemia and/or circulatory compromise are significant contributory factors.

Beyond this one interesting development, pharmacotherapy has little to offer in the practical management of acute alcoholic intoxication. The time-honored use of caffeine, usually in the form of copious amounts of black coffee, has little demonstrable antidotal effect (Nuotto et al., 1982). It is not yet certain whether giving large quantities of caffeine to alcohol-intoxicated people produces adverse effects, such as cardiac arrhythmias (Dobmeyer et al., 1983). Other drugs which have not proven to be of practical benefit in the treatment of intoxication include thyroid, thyroxine, B vitamins, pyruvate, amino acids, propranolol, amantadine, and fenmetozole (Sellers and Kalant, 1976; Rada and Kellner, 1979).

B. Altering Metabolism and Managing Overdose

Some agents, such as fructose, can produce a modest increase in the rate of metabolism of alcohol. Intravenous infusions can increase the rate by about 25%, but large doses may cause increased serum uric acid, lactic acidosis, and osmotic diuresis (Sellers and Kalant, 1976; Rada and Kellner, 1979). Oral administration of fructose can also increase the rate of ethanol metabolism, but is associated with gastrointestinal side effects. In general, fructose has not proven to be of any practical value in the management of acute intoxication.

The degree of alcohol intoxication depends on several factors: the blood alcohol concentration, the rapidity of the rise in blood levels, the period of time the blood alcohol level is maintained, the individual's degree of tolerance, and the presence of other drugs. The rapidity of rise in blood level after alcohol consumption depends in turn on the pattern of drinking, the state of the absorptive surface of the stomach and gastrointestinal tract, and the effects of food on gastrointestinal functioning.

The major focus of the treatment of acute intoxication depends on its severity. By itself, alcohol rarely causes coma. Death may occur at 400 mg %, but survival has been reported at 700 mg % (Sellers and Kalant, 1976). However, alcohol is frequently ingested along with other drugs. In the United States, alcohol in combination with other drugs (usually opiates or sedative/anxiolytics) is the leading cause of drug-induced deaths seen by medical examiners, exceeding deaths due to any other individual drug (ADAMHA, 1981). Fatalities have been reported with nonlethal levels of barbiturates combined with levels of alcohol that would ordinarily produce only intoxication. Other reasons for the wide variability in lethal levels of alcohol are differences in inherent and acquired tolerance and the presence of other injuries. With severe intoxication, the most important concern should be the support of respiration and the prevention of aspiration. The usual treatment involves good airway maintenance and time to allow the body's metabolic pathways to remove the alcohol. An average-size person can usually metabolize between 7 and 10 grams of alcohol per hour (equivalent to two-thirds of an ounce of 90-proof spirits or 8 to 12 ounces of beer) (Sellers and Kalant, 1976). This will ordinarily reduce blood levels by about 20 mg % each hour. The presence of other drugs or impaired hepatic function may alter these estimates.

Alcohol is so readily absorbed that gastric lavage, administration of charcoal, or induction of emesis are rarely indicated if the patient is seen more than two hours after alcohol ingestion. Such procedures may be useful if other drugs have also been ingested. Alcohol blood levels above 600 mg % or levels of 400 mg % accompanied by pH of less than 7.0, or the concurrent presence of a dialyzable drug may be an indication for dialysis. Stimulants, cold showers, and forced exercise have no useful role.

Some patients may have impaired mental functioning because the alcoholic intoxication is aggravated by low blood glucose levels. In any case of severe intoxication, blood glucose should be measured. Hypoglycemia, if present, should be treated. Intoxication disproportionate to the blood alcohol level (e.g., coma at levels below 400 mg %) suggests the presence of other drugs, head injury, or hepatic dysfunction. Administration of vitamins, especially thiamine, represents good prophylactic care, even though there is no evidence that they affect the level of intoxication.

Alcohol, like urea, has ready access to intracellular space and can cause major changes in intracellular osmolality. Indeed, excessive alcohol is the most common cause of a hyperosmolar state. For every 150 mg % of blood alcohol, plasma osmolality may increase by 30 osmol/kg of water. However, unless there has been severe vomiting, efforts to hydrate an intoxicated patient are ill-advised.

The bellicose "fighting drunk" continues to be a difficult management problem. The patient must be protected from himself/herself and from injuring others. Practical experience suggests that the presence of numerous *trained* personnel (at least one for each limb) is the most effective and least hazardous way to convince the acutely belligerent patient that it is pointless to resist judicious restraint. Conversely, token attempts at restraint with insufficient force may exacerbate belligerency. Staff members should remove sharp objects, eyeglasses, and dangling clothing before attempting to suppress a "fighting drunk." Because the patient may vomit and aspirate, patients for whom restraints are required must be monitored. A quiet comfortable environment is appropriate.

III. THE MANAGEMENT OF ALCOHOL WITHDRAWAL SYNDROMES

A. Hangover

The syndrome experienced the morning after a bout of heavy drinking (the hangover) may represent a very mild form of alcohol withdrawal, hence its partial suppression by additional alcohol ("hair of the dog"). Other etiological factors that have been postulated include toxic congeners and other chemicals in the alcoholic beverages, accumulation of acetaldehyde, disturbances of fluid balance, and gastrointestinal irritation and effects of smoke and noise. Some investigators have emphasized the role of psychological factors, including guilt and negative attitudes about alcohol use and intoxication. There has been one report of a double-blind study in which pyritinol (a derivative of pyridoxine) reduced hangover symptoms (Rada and Kellner, 1979).

B. Withdrawal

Chronic ingestion of ethanol leads to adaptive changes in the nervous system which tend to reduce the effects of ethanol on neural function (Mendelson and Mello, 1979). When ethanol ingestion is discontinued, or when the blood levels are sharply lowered for any reason, a variety of signs and symptoms—the withdrawal syndome—occur. The severity of this syndrome varies greatly. In very mild withdrawal, there may be no more than slight tremulousness, irritability, and insomnia appearing a few hours after blood levels decline and lasting about 48 hours. At the other extreme, the tremulousness, insomnia, mild gastrointestinal symptoms, anxiety, and irritability of the mild syndrome may progress further to include sweating, tachycardia, nausea, vomiting, fever, hallucinations, delusions, fluctuating levels of confusion and cognitive functioning, disorientation, and grand mal seizure. The time course of withdrawal phenomena is illustrated in Figure 1. Although the severity of withdrawal is generally proportional to the duration of the preceding alcohol exposure,

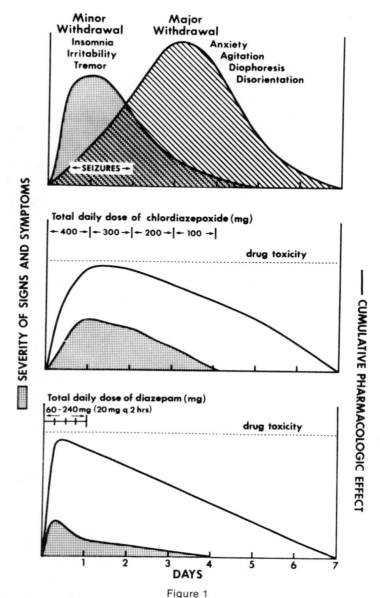

Figure 1

Effect of Chlordiazepoxide or Diazepam on Clinical Course of Withdrawal Reaction. (Modified from Sellers and Kalant, 1976.)

Upper panel shows the typical time course of untreated alcohol withdrawal. Represented are the two typical clinical presentations of alcoholic withdrawal. Middle panel indicates the cumulative pharmacologic effect of chlordiazepoxide and its active metabolite, desmethyl-chlordiazepoxide, during daily administration of decreasing doses of chlordiazepoxide during alcohol withdrawal. Since chlordiazepoxide and its metabolites have long half-lives they would accumulate over 5 to 7 days if they were given at the same dosage leading to maximum effects when such effects are no longer needed. With declining dosage such excess effects are avoided. Lower panel depicts the effect on withdrawal severity and body levels of benzodiazepine when 20 mg doses of diazepam are given every 2 hrs and titrated against withdrawal symptoms to produce a loading dose effect.

other factors are involved. Patients who have had withdrawal symptoms in the past appear to develop dependence more rapidly with subsequent exposure. Concurrent medical illness, such as trauma, pneumonia, or gastritis may act as precipitants of withdrawal or increase its severity. Such illnesses usually require specific therapy in addition to appropriate treatment of alcohol withdrawal.

Generally, if seizures occur, they do so within the first 24 hours. Seizures occurring more than 48 hours after blood levels fall should stimulate search for other causes, the most common of which is dependence on other longer-acting drugs such as benzodiazepines.

C. Outpatient versus Hospital Treatment

Most episodes of alcohol withdrawal are relatively mild and do not require hospital treatment. If patients are medically screened so that those with serious complications or illnesses are referred for hospital care, the overwhelming majority of the remaining cases can be safely managed on an ambulatory basis or in a nonhospital-based detoxification center (Feldman et al., 1975; Whitfield, 1980). Patients not suited for such care are those with coma, signs of trauma, acute abdominal pain, signs of pneumonia, or history of other types of drug abuse. Among patients without such complications, the incidence of fully developed delirium tremens is less than 1%, although for a small percentage of patients, other withdrawal problems (seizures, suicidal ideation, and hallucinations) may require transfer to a more intensive treatment setting. While some clinicians believe a previous history of seizures is not an absolute contraindication to nonhospital management (Whitfield, 1980), others have far more stringent criteria and would recommend hospitalization for all alcoholics with seizures, severe malnutrition or dehydration, severe tremulousness or hallucinosis, as well as those with a history of episodes of withdrawal that progressed to delirium or psychosis when untreated (Greenblatt and Shader, 1975). There is no clear consensus on the use of pharmacological agents in the ambulatory or nonhospital-based detoxification centers. Some clinicians take pride in avoiding use of any sedatives, relying solely on vitamins, nutrition, and good nursing care (Whitfield, 1980). Others emphasize the use of the same drugs and vitamins used in treatment of hospitalized alcoholics (Feldman et al., 1975; Rada and Kellner, 1979).

D. Pharmacotherapy of Withdrawal

While there is little doubt that careful nursing care alone can reduce the severity of the alcohol withdrawal syndrome (Frecker et al., 1982;

Naranjo et al., 1983; Sellers et al., 1983), judicious use of drugs for treatment of withdrawal, as well as better supportive care and treatment of medical and surgical complications, are all factors responsible for the present low rate of delirium tremens and mortality from alcohol withdrawal in most developed countries.

Among the general procedures now considered essential in treatment of withdrawal are the use of nutritional supplements and prompt attention to the manifestations of the complications of illnesses. Thiamine, 50 to 100 mg IM or IV, should always be given on admission. The routine use of daily multivitamins by injection or orally is also commonly recommended.

Many alcoholics appear to be dehydrated, but these appearances can be deceptive. During withdrawal, tissue water levels are higher than normal in most alcoholics (Besson et al., 1981; Eisenhofer et al., 1982), and routine use of parenteral fluids is not appropriate. On the other hand, alcoholics commonly have electrolyte imbalances. Most alcoholics are magnesium depleted regardless of serum concentrations. Since hypomagnesemia can contribute to lethargy, weakness, and decreased seizure threshold, some clinicians recommend magnesium supplementation. However, the apparent depletion may be a distribution phenomenon because levels return to normal after withdrawal without special attention to replacement (Gessner, 1979). Potassium deficiency is probably even more common, and since potassium is largely an intracellular ion, serum levels will not reflect the full degree of deficiency. Potassium deficiency can contribute to muscle weakness, fatigue, and cardiac arrhythmias, and it is especially problematic in patients taking cardiac glycosides. Potassium chloride is the supplement of choice; it is not needed once oral intake of food resumes (Sellers and Kalant, 1976; Shader and Greenblatt, 1975).

The major objectives of specific pharmacological treatment of the alcohol withdrawal syndrome are prevention of seizures, delirium, and arrhythmias. Suppression of anxiety and insomnia increase the likelihood that the patient will complete detoxification and facilitate treatment of other medical problems; however, complete suppression of all symptoms of withdrawal is not necessary. Mild withdrawal requires no pharmacological intervention, but it is not always possible to know which cases of mild withdrawal will progress to more serious stages; some authorities state that seizures and delirium sometimes appear abruptly without preceding milder manifestations (Shader and Greenblatt, 1975).

Well over a hundred different drugs and drug combinations have been described for the treatment of alcohol withdrawal. Yet, such is the state of the art that after reviewing the therapeutic trials published in English since 1954, covering 81 trials and 6808 patients, Moskowitz and coworkers (1983) concluded that "no definitive conclusions about the treatment of alcohol withdrawal other than the efficacy of benzodiazepines, can be ascertained." Other reviewers, perhaps using somewhat less stringent criteria, have drawn several conclusions from this same literature. Drugs that show cross-dependence with alcohol or raise brain GABA levels are consistently more effective than placebo in suppressing alcohol withdrawal. Alcohol itself is certainly the most widely used substance for suppressing withdrawal, but not generally in the context of treatment. Certain phenothiazines and dopaminergic blockers seem more effective than placebo, but these may have other drawbacks that weigh against their use (Gessner, 1979; Sellers and Kalant, 1976; Shaw, 1982).

E. Benzodiazepines

More than 20 benzodiazepines have been used clinically worldwide. At least 12 are marketed in the United States, and most have been shown to be effective in suppressing the symptoms of alcohol withdrawal, including anxiety, restlessness, insomnia, tremor, seizures, and the development of delirium. Because they all act at the same receptors (Braestrup, 1982; Tallman et al., 1980), theoretically all benzodiazepines should be equally effective if due consideration is given to differences in potency and rates of metabolism. There is no empirical evidence to suggest that any one benzodiazepine is significantly superior to another, but most of the clinical studies comparing benzodiazepines to placebo and to other drugs have been done with chlordiazepoxide and diazepam.

Benzodiazepines have also been compared to older drugs, such as paradelhyde, chloral hydrate, and barbiturates, and to various phenothiazines and dopaminergic blockers. The benzodiazepines are superior to the phenothiazines in preventing seizures and are probably as effective as older sedatives when given in adequate dosage (Gessner, 1979; Sellers and Kalant, 1976).

Available benzodiazepines now vary greatly in duration of action and complexity of the metabolic transformations which take place. The most commonly used benzodiazepines, chlordiazepoxide and diazepam, are converted by demethylation and hydroxylation into several active metabolites. At least one of these, desmethyldiazepam, has a half-life of 50 to 100 hours (Greenblatt and Shader, 1974). When given repeatedly, these benzodiazepines and their metabolites will accumulate and after several days may produce excessive sedation, confusion, and ataxia, especially in elderly alcoholics who clear desmethyldiazepam more slowly and who are more sensitive to its CNS depressant effects. Prazepam, clorazepate, and halazepam are also converted to desmethyldiazepam. Oxazepam, lorazepam, and temazepam form glucuronides directly and they are shorter acting; cumulation is not ordinarily a problem, and the elderly should clear them about as well as younger patients (Kraus et al., 1978).

The basic principle involved in using benzodiazepines to treat alcohol withdrawal is the rapid substitution of a drug that suppresses withdrawal, followed by a gradual tapering of drug levels over several days. Thus, the longer acting drugs are probably better choices than the very rapid-acting ones. The latter have the advantage of rapid onset of action and easier initial titration, but require more attention to the phase of dose reduction, sometimes leading to too much physician-patient interaction around the issue of dosage and frequency. With the longer-acting drugs, the effects cumulate, but once suppression of withdrawal is achieved they can be given infrequently or discontinued.

Figure 1 illustrates two suggested approaches to control of alcohol withdrawal with benzodiazepines. In one approach, chlordiazepoxide is given in relatively generous dosage the first day and is then gradually tapered over several days, but the maximum sedative effect is still seen during the second day because of the cumulative effect of longer-acting metabolites. In the second (loading dose) approach, shown in the lower panel, diazepam in 20 mg doses is used to provide rapid onset of action; additional dosage is given every two hours if needed, based on a standardized technique for assessing withdrawal. Once withdrawal is suppressed, little further additional medication is required, since the long-acting metabolites are largely self-tapering (Sellers et al., 1983).

Severity of withdrawal and dosage of benzodiazepines required both vary greatly. Rigid standing orders for benzodiazepine dosage or for parenteral fluids are not appropriate. If suppression of withdrawal is delayed and hallucinosis develops, dopaminergic blockers may be required in addition to benzodiazepines. Chlordiazepoxide and diazepam are slowly and inconsistently absorbed from intramuscular sites. If patients are unable to take drugs by mouth, these drugs should be given intravenously (Greenblatt and Shader, 1974). Lorazepam (Atavan) is promptly and predictably absorbed after IM administration. It has the additional advantage of being metabolized primarily by glucuronidation and its duration of action ($t\frac{1}{2}\beta$ about 12 hours) is less likely to be affected by liver disease (Kraus et al., 1978). In patients with cirrhosis or impaired liver function, free fractions of drug may be higher and the clearance of longer-acting benzodiazepines will be prolonged, so appropriate adjustments of dosage are required (Sellers and Kalant, 1976).

F. Phenothiazines and Dopaminergic Blockers

While phenothiazines appear to be better than placebo in treating unselected cases of alcohol withdrawal in general, in more severe withdrawal syndromes they are neither as safe nor as effective as the benzodiazepines and other drugs that exhibit cross-dependence with alcohol. Some phenothiazines, especially those with aliphatic side chains, have potentially serious side effects which outweigh their benefits: these include adrenergic blocking actions that can cause severe hypotension and lowering of seizure thresholds. Despite these shortcomings, the more potent phenothiazines or haloperidol, which cause less sedation and hypotension, are still often used for control of hallucinations once the period of risk for seizures has passed. Typical dosage of haloperidol is 0.5 to 2.0 mg IM every two hours until symptoms are controlled or five doses have been given (Gessner, 1979; Sellers and Kalant, 1976; Shaw, 1982).

G. Paraldehyde, Chloral Hydrate and Barbiturates

These older sedatives have demonstrable efficacy in suppressing alcohol withdrawal in both animals and man. They are probably not more effective than adequate doses of benzodiazepines. Although some paraldehyde is eliminated unchanged through the lungs (giving the breath a strong odor), most is still metabolized by the liver. Because of its relative toxicity paraldehyde should be considered obsolete. Chloral hydrate has no significant advantages over the benzodiazepines. Barbiturates are still preferred in some European countries and are believed to be more effective in severe withdrawal. They are occasionally still used in the United States for treatment of the rare patient refractory to benzodiazepines or in patients with combined alcohol-sedative dependence (Gessner, 1979).

H. Chlormethiazole (Heminevrin)

This derivative of the thiazol moiety of thiamine is a sedative-hypnotic with anticonvulsant activity. While it is not available in the United States, it is currently one of the most commonly used agents in Great Britain and Europe. It is demonstrably effective in suppressing withdrawal. It has a rapid onset of action, but a relatively shorter duration of action than the usual benzodiazepines. Dosage, therefore, is higher for the first few days and is then tapered. As with other sedatives, cases of abuse and overdosage have been reported (Gessner, 1979; Shaw, 1982).

I. Anticonvulsants

Seizures, when they occur during ethanol withdrawal, are most likely to develop between 21 and 48 hours after the last drink. Typically, seizures are grand mal and nonfocal. Usually one or two seizures are seen. Convulsions occurring late in the withdrawal period should raise the possibility of preexisting convulsive disorder or dependence on sedative-anxiolytics as well as alcohol (Sellers and Kalant, 1976). Phenytoin (diphenylhydantoin) is sometimes used as part of the treatment of alcohol withdrawal, although there is no strong evidence that it is routinely necessary or that it is the most appropriate anticonvulsant. Phenytoin does not suppress alcohol withdrawal seizures in animal models (Gessner, 1979); it is poorly absorbed from intramuscular sites, and when given orally at the usual maintenance dose (300 to 400 mg/day) it requires four to five days to reach therapeutically optimal effective serum levels (10 to 20 μg/ml). Sampliner and Iber (1974) reported that in alcoholic patients *who had a previous history of seizures not necessarily due to alcohol withdrawal,* 300 mg/day of phenytoin combined with up to 400 mg/day of chlordiazepoxide was superior to chlordiazepoxide plus placebo, even though the phenytoin serum levels reached with this dosing schedule were only 3 to 5 μg/ml.

For patients without a history of an underlying seizure disorder, the benzodiazepines or sedative-hypnotics usually used for treatment of withdrawal have adequate anticonvulsant activity to minimize the likelihood of seizures. Phenytoin may be indicated in alcoholics with known underlying seizure disorder. In such patients, if phenytoin maintenance had been stopped for more than five days prior to admission, a loading dose should be given. The dose usually recommended is one gram mixed with 250 to 500 ml of 5% dextrose in water infused slowly (no faster than 50 mg/min) over 1 to 4 hours. Maintenance should be started the next day (Greenblatt and Shader, 1975). On theoretical grounds, other anticonvulsants are more rational choices for use in alcohol withdrawal. In animal models of alcohol withdrawal, mephenytoin, phenacemide, and paramethadione do suppress seizures. In man, primidone has been reported to be more effective than phenytoin. Valproic acid, an anticonvulsant that may act in part by raising brain GABA, is effective in suppressing alcohol withdrawal seizures in animal models and has been used in Europe and Australia with favorable results in the treatment of alcohol withdrawal (Gessner, 1979; Shaw, 1982). However, in the United States, the manufacturer warns against its use in patients with hepatic dysfunction, a condition not uncommon among newly admitted alcoholics. Further, it produces CNS depression synergistically with barbiturates without altering plasma levels. Carbamazepine (Tegretol) has also been reported to be useful as primary treatment of withdrawal (Poutanen, 1979).

J. Miscellaneous Agents for Withdrawal: Propranolol, Lithium, Antihistamines

Propranolol, a beta-adrenergic blocker, decreases tremor and tachycardia during alcoholic withdrawal, but since it does not effectively suppress the more serious manifestations of withdrawal (e.g., delusions, seizures), its place in treatment is uncertain. It is contraindicated in heart failure, asthma, and diabetes, and probably adds little to the effects of benzodiazepines (Gessner, 1979; Sellers and Kalant, 1976; Shaw, 1982). Some clinicians believe that beta blockers are contraindicated precisely because they mask tremor and cardiovascular cues to the severity of withdrawal (Whitfield, 1980).

Lithium carbonate may decrease some subjective symptoms of withdrawal. At present, it has no practical place in the treatment of this phase of alcoholism (Gessner, 1979) but may be of some interest in prevention of relapse (see below). Hydroxyzine, an antihistamine with sedative effects, has not been found to be consistently superior to placebo in the treatment of alcohol withdrawal. At higher dosage its anticholinergic effects may cause dry mouth, urinary retention, and confusion and delirium, especially in older patients (Gessner, 1979; Sellers and Kalant, 1976).

IV. DRUGS USED IN THE POSTWITHDRAWAL PHASE TO DETER ALCOHOL CONSUMPTION

Among the major challenges in the months after cessation of drinking are the prevention of relapse to excessive alcohol use and the management of persistent emotional and physiological disturbances.

Pharmacological agents can be used to deter alcohol consumption in two basic ways. (1) Some drugs make the ingestion of alcohol aversive or hazardous (alcohol sensitizing drugs). (2) Other drugs themselves produce unpleasant toxic effects (conditioning agents), and can be given concurrently with small doses of alcohol in order to produce a conditioned response. Thereafter, the idea of ingesting alcohol evokes aversive feelings, and the drugs used for the conditioning need not be given on a regular basis.

A. Alcohol Sensitizing Agents

Many drugs which alter the body's response to alcohol make its ingestion unpleasant or toxic (see below), but only two of these, disulfiram and carbimide, are used in the treatment of alcoholism. Both of these drugs inhibit aldehyde oxidoreductase (ALDH, aldehyde dehydrogenase), the enzyme that catalyzes the oxidation of acetaldehyde to acetic acid. If alcohol is ingested after this enzyme is inhibited, blood acetaldehyde levels will rise, causing a syndrome that varies in intensity from mildly unpleasant to fatal, the severity varying with the dose of the sensitizing drug and the amount of alcohol ingested. In its mild form, when the amount of alcohol ingested is small (e.g., about an ounce of 80 proof whiskey), the face feels warm and the skin, especially of the upper chest and face, becomes flushed and red; the heart beats faster, there is pounding in the chest, and the blood pressure drops. There may also be nausea, vomiting, shortness of breath, sweating, dizziness, blurred vision, and confusion. The reaction lasts about 30 minutes. Most reactions are self-limited, but occasionally they may be life-threatening, even after relatively small amounts of alcohol (see below). The reactions after carbimide are generally milder than those after disulfiram, and the two agents differ significantly in their metabolism and in the onset and duration of the ALDH-inhibiting effects.

1. Disulfiram (Antabuse)

Disulfiram is almost completely absorbed after oral administration. It is rapidly metabolized to diethyldithiocarbamate (DDC), itself a substance that inhibits enzyme systems by chelating trace metals. DDC is in turn further degraded to diethylamine and several other substances, including carbon disulfide. Within the first day, about half of the drug and its metabolites is eliminated in the urine and feces. Enough carbon disulfide is eliminated in the breath to produce an unpleasant odor and to be detectable for purposes of measuring compliance. The inhibition of aldehyde dehydrogenase is irreversible, and renewed enzyme activity is a function of protein synthesis. Thus, the effects of disulfiram may outlast the sojourn of the drug in the body (Fried, 1980; Sellers et al., 1981).

Adverse Effects. Adverse effects from disulfiram are common. In addition to acetaldehyde oxidoreductase (acetaldehyde dehydrogenase), disulfiram inhibits a variety of other enzymes including dopamine beta-hydroxylase, xanthene oxidase, hexokinase, 3-phosphoglyceraldehyde dehydrogenase, beta-hydroxybutyrate dehydrogenase, and d-amino acid oxidase. It also inhibits hepatic microsomal drug-metabolizing enzymes such as the mixed function oxidase system (Fried, 1980; MacLeod et al., 1978). Thus, in addition to the toxicity of the disulfiram-ethanol reaction caused by the accumulation of acetaldehyde, adverse effects can occur as a result of multiple drug interactions, alterations in levels of normal body constituents and neurotransmitters, as well as from other toxic effects of disulfiram or its metabolites.

The disulfiram-ethanol reaction (DER) can sometimes be quite severe, including marked tachycardia, electrocardiographic changes, myocardial infarction, cerebrovascular hemorrhage, and cerebral infarction. Hypotension is sometimes accompanied by bradycardia, or even cardiac arrest secondary to vagal stimulation associated with retching or vomiting. Cardiovascular collapse, congestive failure, and convulsions have also been reported. While severe reactions are usually associated with high-dosage disulfiram (over 500 mg/day) and more than two ounces of alcohol, deaths have occurred with lower dosage and after a single drink (Lindros et al., 1981; Peachey et al., 1981a, 1981b; Sellers et al., 1981).

Most DERs are self-limited, and conservative measures to handle hypotension (modified Trendelenburg position) are usually adequate. Vagal-induced bradycardia may require cholinergic blockers. No demonstrably effective treatments for the DER are available. Although vitamins and antihistamines are often used, there is no evidence for their efficacy. In volunteers pretreated with disulfiram or carbimide, the drug 4-methylpyrazol which inhibits the metabolism of alcohol to acetaldehyde produced a prompt fall in blood acetaldehyde levels and an associated decrease in symptoms. Penicillamine is said to bind to acetaldehyde and has lowered blood levels in rats (Lindros et al., 1981).

In addition to the risks of the DER, the use of disulfiram is associated with numerous side effects and toxicities including drowsiness, lethargy, peripheral neuropathy, hepatotoxicity, and hypertension. Disulfiram and DDC inhibit dopamine beta-hydroxylase resulting in decreased brain norepinephrine levels and increased dopamine levels. The exacerbation of schizophrenic symptoms in schizophrenics and occasionally their appearance in nonschizophrenics, as well as the development of depression, may be linked to these actions. Alcoholics with low cerebrospinal fluid DBH activity are more likely to develop dysphoric or psychotic symptoms (Major et al., 1979; Sellers et al., 1981). (The adverse effects stemming from the interference of disulfiram with the metabolism and actions of other drugs is discussed below.)

Efficacy and Clinical Use. Although disulfiram has been used in the treatment of alcoholism for almost 35 years, problems in designing an adequate experiment make it difficult to say just how useful it is. Controlled studies are few, and in those which have been carried out the differences between subjects taking disulfiram and those given placebo are minimal. One problem is that patients may easily determine just what they are taking; until recently, another problem has been checking on compliance. In the most carefully controlled study to date, patients given 1 mg of disulfiram per day were compared to patients given therapeutic doses of 250 mg/day and an equally motivated control group that knew that they were not receiving disulfiram. A life-table analysis revealed that over the course of the year the two groups of patients receiving disulfiram did better in terms of abstinence than the control group, but a less complex analysis revealed little difference at the one-year point. There was no important difference between the two drug groups (Fuller and Roth, 1979; Fuller and Williford, 1981). From these findings, one might conclude that the therapeutic effects of disulfiram are due more to psychological than pharmacological factors. However, it is unlikely that these psychological factors could persist if, looming in the background, there were not the possibility that alcohol use would cause serious adverse reactions in those taking therapeutic doses of the drug.

Disulfiram is usually given orally. In the past, the daily dosage prescribed has been as high as 500 mg/day, but recent practice suggests that, compared to doses of 250 mg, the higher dosage increases side effects and toxic hazards without increasing therapeutic benefits. Disulfiram has also been used by subcutaneous implantation of 100 mg tablets (Esperal) in the abdominal wall (Wilson et al., 1980). Blood levels of disulfiram and DDC after implantation are probably too low in most cases to exert alcohol sensitizing effects for a period long enough to justify the implant, and benefits seen after such implantations are due primarily to psychological factors (Bergstrom et al., 1982; Sellers et al., 1981).

Patients should be carefully warned about the hazards of disulfiram, including the need to avoid over-the-counter preparations with alcohol and drugs that interact adversely with disulfiram (see below). There is some controversy about the ethics of prescribing disulfiram to anyone except those who want to use it, seek abstinence, and have no psychological or medical contraindications. But, disulfiram has been incorporated into court-related programs where its use is mandatory, and it is reported that in some countries the drug is given to excessive drinkers surreptitiously by family members (Fried, 1980). Sellers and coworkers (1981, 1982) set fairly stringent exclusionary criteria for using disulfiram, as well as rules for monitoring its safety, and for discontinuing its use in the event of noncompliance. Contraindications include myocardial disease; severe pulmonary insufficiency; severe liver dysfunction; chronic renal failure; organic mental disturbances; neuropathy; psychosis; difficulties in impulse control or recurrent suicidal ideation; the need for treatment with vasodilators, beta-adrenergic antagonists, monoamine oxidase inhibitors, tricyclic antidepressants or antipsychotic agents; pregnancy; and unwillingness to attend monthly meetings for medical and psychosocial assessment. Sellers et al. also recommend an initial complete mental and physical exam, including a laboratory screen and electrocardiogram as well as psychosocial assessment. This is followed by a monthly repeat of mental and physical exams, a quarterly repeat of selected laboratory work, and seminannual repeat of all initial exams. Some clinicians believe that such stringent criteria and routine exams may largely preclude the use of disulfiram in most alcoholics, or raise the cost of its use to prohibitive levels (Graff, 1982). Others find no contraindication to combining disulfiram with tricyclic antidepressants, provided that allowances are made for alterations in metabolism of the latter.

2. Calcium Carbimide

Calcium carbimide (citrated calcium carbimide, calcium cyanamide, Temposil), like disulfiram, inhibits aldehyde dehydrogenase. It is hydrolyzed in the gut to carbimide (cyanamide) and then rapidly absorbed. Unlike disulfiram, the enzyme inhibition is reversible, so that duration of action is short (less than one day). The usual dose of 50 mg must ordinarily be given twice a day to ensure continued alcohol sensitizing effects. As with disulfiram, the intensity of the carbimide-ethanol reaction (CER) is related to both dose of drug and dose of alcohol, but there is interindividual variability as well as variability in the same individual on different occasions.

Calcium carbimide does not inhibit the same wide range of enzyme systems inhibited for disulfiram; it does not cause as many adverse drug interactions; and it does not usually cause psychosis, drowsiness, or lethargy (Sellers et al., 1981).

The evidence for the efficacy of calcium carbimide in reducing relapse in alcoholics is no more solid than that of disulfiram. When alcoholics taking carbimide do drink small doses of ethanol, they find that after a delay of a few hours each subsequent dose of ethanol produces a progressively less distressing reaction, a phenomenon referred to as "burning off" the drug (Peachey et al., 1981a; Sellers et al., 1981). A similar phenomenon has been noted with disulfiram (Peachey et al., 1981c). Calcium carbimide is not available for clinical use in the United States.

3. Other Alcohol Sensitizing Drugs

In addition to the two agents currently used therapeutically to treat alcoholism, a number of other natural materials and clinically useful drugs also cause altered sensitivity and adverse responses to ethanol. Included here are monoamine oxidase inhibitors such as pargyline, antibiotics (the beta lactam cephalosporins, moxalactam, cefamandol, cefoperazone) (Elenbaas et al., 1982), and metronidazole (Flagyl). The latter was tried but found ineffective in treatment of alcoholism. In certain susceptible individuals taking oral hypoglycemic agents, chlorpropamide and tolbutamide, alcohol ingestion can produce a flushing reaction associated with modest rises in blood acetaldehyde levels (Barnett et al., 1981; Capretti et al., 1981). Other sensitizing substances include hydrogen sulfide, tetraethyl lead, pyrogallol, 4-bromopyrazole, and coprine (1-aminocyclopropranolol), the active ingredient in the inky-cap mushroom (*Coprinus atramentorius*) (Fried, 1980; Sellers et al., 1981).

B. Drugs Used to Create Conditioned Aversion to Alcohol

Three approaches have been used to create conditioned aversion to alcohol. Alcohol ingestion has been paired with electric shocks, with succinylcholine to produce transient but terrifying respiratory paralysis, and with drugs which induce nausea and vomiting. The two most popular drugs for producing the latter effect are emetine and apomorphine.

Despite skepticism about the degree to which conditioned aversion can carry over to real-life situations, chemical aversion has been used as the mainstay of a chain of proprietary hospitals specializing in the treatment of alcoholism. Although controls are lacking, and not all treated patients were followed, the proponents report three-year abstinence rates of 50% overall, with even higher rates among patients who were married, employed, or both (Neubuerger et al., 1981).

V. DRUGS IN THE TREATMENT OF POSTWITHDRAWAL AFFECTIVE DISTURBANCES

After a few days, the anxiety, insomnia, and general distress of the acute withdrawal syndrome merge imperceptibly into a postwithdrawal state that may last for weeks or months. While many alcoholics feel considerably better after a week or two, a substantial number continue to experience insomnia and symptoms of anxiety and depression. The frequency with which these symptoms are noted varies with the techniques used to measure them. If self-rating instruments for depression are used, such as the Beck, the Zung, or the SCL-90, the majority of alcoholics will report scores in the depressed range at the beginning of withdrawal; about half of these improve substantially fairly quickly. From 15% to 30%, however, continue to report high levels of anxiety and depression. There is some controversy about the clinical significance of such findings and whether intervention apart from efforts to prevent relapse are required (Keeler et al, 1979; Pottenger et al., 1978; Schuckit, 1979; Shaw et al., 1975; Nakamura et al., 1983).

To appreciate the difficulty in evaluating the efficacy of drugs in treating postwithdrawal disturbances, one need only consider the multiplicity of factors that could theoretically play some causal role. Figure 2 shows in a very schematic way the multiple interactions among (1) excessive alcohol intake; (2) acute and protracted withdrawal; (3) alcohol-induced CNS damage; (4) CNS damage from indirect effects of alcohol; (5) social, economic, and interpersonal losses; (6) antecedent psychiatric disorders; and (7) a cluster of signs and symptoms shown in Figure 2 as the "defeat/depression/hypophoria cluster." It is obvious from this complex figure that the emotional disturbances in the postwithdrawal period are unlikely to be homogeneous in origin, and that without careful attention to defining the patient populations, it would be difficult to obtain consistent findings from one study to another. This is indeed the case. Most of the drug studies from which inferences of efficacy must be drawn were carried out before the full extent of this diagnostic heterogeneity was fully recognized. Treatment was usually directed at target symptoms of depression and anxiety in unselected groups of detoxified alcoholics. Thus, unless the populations were unusually homogeneous by chance or the drug in question worked powerfully across diagnostic and etiological categories, positive findings would be unlikely.

There is now renewed interest in identifying the incidence and prevalence of psychiatric disturbances (in addition to alcohol abuse and dependence) among patients seeking treatment for alcohol problems. Similar studies have now been done among individuals in the community who drink to excess but do not seek treatment (Weissman and Myers, 1980). What emerges is that the majority of alcoholics who seek treatment have diagnosable disorders in addition to alcoholism (based on a lifetime diagnosis). Among the more common are major and minor depression, bipolar depression, depressive personality, antisocial personality, drug dependence, borderline personality, agoraphobia with panic episodes, and attention deficit disorder, residual type (hyperactivity syndrome) (Behar and Winokur, 1979; Hesselbrock et al., 1983; Mullaney and Trippett, 1979; Nace et al., 1982; Wood et al., 1983). Most of these diagnoses are associated with affective disturbances (usually depression, dysphoria, or hypophoria) that might have been manifest even in the absence of excessive alcohol intake.

Even if future drug studies were to attempt to control for this diag-

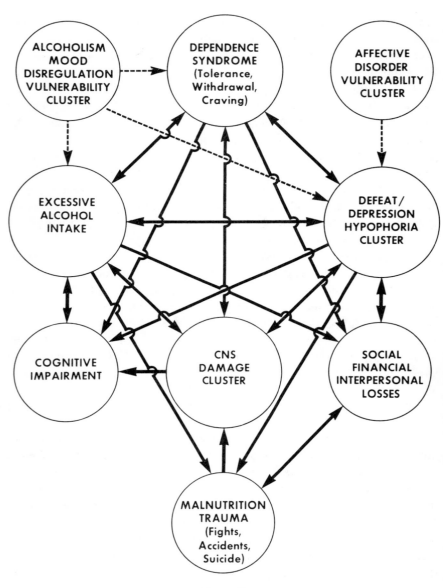

Figure 2
Postwithdrawal Disturbances.

nostic heterogeneity, it would still prove difficult to control for the variable degree to which protracted abstinence contributes to persistent emotional difficulties. It would be equally difficult to tease apart the role of brain damage (as revealed by CAT scans and tests of cognitive impairment) now recognized to be exceedingly common among excessive drinkers (Brandt et al., 1983; Porjesz and Begleiter, 1982; Wilkinson, 1982). It would indeed be surprising if the neural systems subserving mood could entirely escape damage, and in the individual case, the contribution of such damage to emotional difficulties cannot be determined with present methods.

Depressions requiring pharmacological intervention can sometimes be detected by the dexamethasone suppression test. Although both liver disease and withdrawal stress cause false positive responses to a 1 to 2 mg dose of dexamethasone, after about three weeks of abstinence, the incidence of escape from dexamethasone suppression is not greater among nondepressed alcoholics (i.e., about 5%) than among normal controls (Dackis et al., 1983; Khan et al., 1983).

Among the drugs that have been used or proposed as treatment for anxiety and depression in the postwithdrawal state are tricyclic antidepressants, monoamine oxidase inhibitors, benzodiazepines and other sedatives, phenothiazines and other dopaminergic blockers, dopaminergic agonists, lithium, and propranolol.

A. Tricyclic Antidepressants

After the benzodiazepines and neuroleptics, the tricyclic antidepressants are the most frequently prescribed drugs for treating alcoholic patients. However, because patients with alcoholism are routinely excluded from trials of antidepressants, there is little firm evidence of their efficacy, even in "primary depressives" with alcoholism. Controlled trials of the tricyclics have been conducted in more heterogeneous groups of alcoholics, and reviewers are generally negative in their assessments (Schuckit, 1979; Pattison, 1979). But, nonefficacy has not been proven. Failure to differentiate subtypes of depression among alcoholics, to measure plasma levels to assure adequate dosage and compliance, or to measure changes in depression as well as in drinking patterns are among the methodological problems that have complicated interpretation of available studies (Ciraulo and Jaffe, 1981). In addition, most studies began treatment immediately after withdrawal, when any drug-related improvement would be obscured by the rapid spontaneous improvement that usually occurs. Furthermore, most studies used therapeutically inadequate doses, and did not adjust for the fact that both cigarette smoking and alcoholism can stimulate liver enzymes that metabolize imipramine. Ciraulo et al. (1982) have reported that the intrinsic clearance of imipramine in alcoholics is 2.5 times that of controls, and after the standard 150 mg dose of imipramine, alcoholics have steady-state concentrations of imipramine and its metabolites significantly lower than levels considered therapeutic. The effects of alcoholism and smoking on the pharmacokinetics of other tricyclic antidepressants is less clear, as is the relationship between drug plasma levels and clinical response. The studies of doxepin and amitriptyline in alcoholics used doses that would now be considered barely adequate for nonalcoholic depressed patients. Despite these limitations, one study of doxepin and one of amitriptyline in unselected alcoholics showed some positive effects on mood (Ciraulo and Jaffe, 1981).

Imipramine and amitriptyline are now considered to be effective antianxiety and antipanic agents in nonalcoholic patients; and it is argued that the antipanic actions may be distinct from the antidepressant action (Ravaris et al., 1980; Zitrin et al., 1980). Although the older studies did, in fact, find that the tricyclics reduced anxiety in recently detoxified alcoholics, there have been no specific studies of tricyclics in detoxified alcoholics with diagnoses of panic disorder or generalized anxiety. Such studies are needed. It is worth noting that antipanic actions are not found with all drugs that have antidepressant actions (Sheehan et al., 1983).

Even if one accepts the view that most instances of postwithdrawal depression and "blues" will show spontaneous recovery within a few days to several weeks (Shuckit, 1983), there will still be some patients, either primary depressives with alcoholism as a secondary diagnosis, or a few primary alcoholics with secondary depression, whose severe and persistent depression requires treatment. In these cases, tricyclics should be employed with an awareness that both smoking and alcohol use accelerate the metabolism of the drugs used, and that alcoholics may not be compliant with respect to recommended dosage. Monitoring of plasma levels seems appropriate when response is not satisfactory.

B. Monoamine Oxidase Inhibitors

The "atypical depressions" for which MAO inhibitors seem to be particularly effective have some features in common with the syndromes seen in many alcoholic patients in the weeks and months following detoxification—e.g., dysphoria and anxiety without the classic endogenous vegetative signs. Because they have demonstrated antianxiety and antipanic effects (Quitkin et al., 1979; Ravaris et al., 1980), the MAO inhibitors would appear to be logical candidates for therapeutic trials in recovering alcoholics, many of whom experience panic episodes, often in association with depressive features (Mullaney and Trippett, 1979). However, at present these drugs have no demonstrated role in the rehabilitation of the alcoholic patient. Concerns about the need for careful compliance with dietary restrictions and about liver toxicity limit their use. However, the need to warn patients about the possible disulfiram-like effects if they drink ethanol should not be a drawback.

C. Benzodiazepines and Other Sedatives

The benzodiazepines are widely used in the treatment of alcohol syndromes, and they are effective in reducing the anxiety and insomnia associated with withdrawal. They have largely replaced other sedative agents in the treatment of postwithdrawal anxiety (Kissin, 1977). Since anxiety, depression, and sleep disturbances can persist for weeks or months following withdrawal, it is never clear where withdrawal ends and other causes of anxiety and disturbed sleep should be assumed. Most nonmedical personnel involved in the treatment of alcoholism have a bias against the use of any psychoactive agents to alleviate anxiety, and have particular antipathy toward the use of drugs than can induce any variety of dependence. There is little doubt that alcoholics are vulnerable to developing dependence on the benzodiazepines, although the probability of abuse and dependence may be lower than is generally believed (Bliding, 1978; Marks, 1978).

Some experts believe that there is an important place for benzodiazepines, judiciously prescribed. In some groups of alcoholics, the drop-out rate from treatment following brief withdrawal may be as high as 90%, often as a result of return to alcohol use. To the degree that early relapse is a result of continuing withdrawal-related affective disturbance (anxiety, depression, insomnia) that can be suppressed by low doses of benzodiazepines, retention in treatment will be enhanced (Kissin, 1977). This important benefit must be weighed against the risk of benzodiazepine dependence. There are probably some alcoholics who find benzodiazepines helpful in stopping alcohol use without becoming dependent on them, and still others who stop alcohol but substitute benzodiazepines. Some may derive no benefit at all. In one controlled study of prazepam in anxious patients, nonalcoholics did significantly better on prazepam, 10 mg three times a day, and anxious alcoholics did as well on placebo (Weir, 1978). Combining alcohol with benzodiazepines generally causes additive or synergistic increases in sedative effects and psychomotor impairment, and Schuckit (1983) suggests that combined dependence may increase the incidence of depressive symptoms. Combined dependence may be more difficult to treat and prognosis seems poorer than for pure alcoholism (Sokolow et al., 1981).

It can be argued that even if benzodiazepine dependence develops, it is less damaging than continued excessive use of alcohol, at least in terms of the effects on the liver. It has been reported that benzodiazepine use and dependence is less likely than alcohol dependence to induce cerebral atrophy as measured by CAT scans (Poser et al., 1983); if confirmed, this would be an important finding.

The benzodiazepines currently available for clinical use differ substantially in terms of pharmacokinetics, lipid solubility, acute subjective effects after oral doses, and frequency of reported dependence. It is likely, therefore, that not all benzodiazepines have the same potential for abuse. Kissin (1977) believes that chlordiazepoxide may be the benzodiazepine of choice. Bliding (1978) reported low levels of abuse with oxazepam. More recently, Jaffe et al. (1983) reported that halazepam produces minimal euphoria even at supratherapeutic doses. The problem of benzodiazepine dependence among alcoholics cannot be ignored; but neither should we ignore the possibility that, for some patients, benzodiazepine dependence, if it does occur, may be a more benign dependence than alcoholism.

D. Phenothiazines and other Dopaminergic Blockers

This group of drugs is of obvious importance in the treatment of alcoholics with schizophrenia. Several studies have compared dopaminergic blockers with placebo on target symptoms of anxiety, tension, or depression during the postwithdrawal phase (Behar and Winokur, 1979; Rada and Kellner, 1979; Smith, 1978). As with the studies of tricyclic antidepressants, patients on placebo showed substantial improvement, and differences in favor of the drugs were not great. In one study, low dosage of thioridazine was superior to placebo in reducing tension and insomnia, but the placebo group did better in terms of work and activity (Hague et al., 1976). As with the tricyclics, issues of design (dosage, criteria, timing) were biased against positive findings for dopamine blockers. For several reasons, however, a reassessment seems less urgent. The frequency with which tardive dyskinesia is seen with this group of drugs suggests that they are far less benign than was previously appreciated. Although these drugs have no abuse potential, there is reason to suspect that they are fundamentally dysphoric and therefore unlikely to be of significant help in the kinds of affective disorders encountered among nonschizophrenic alcoholics.

E. Dopaminergic Agonists

As noted previously, apomorphine has been used to induce vomiting in aversive conditioning treatment of alcoholism for many years. It has also been used for almost as long to reduce tension and craving, and while controlled studies are lacking, clinicians who have used it remain enthusiastic about its apparent capacity to reduce relapse (Feldmann, 1983; Smith, 1978). It is now recognized that apomorphine is a dopaminergic agonist. In Parkinsonism, dopaminergic deficiency produces depression as well as the characteristic motor signs, both of which are alleviated by l-dopa. It would not be surprising if dopaminergic agonists had some therapeutic value in some post-alcohol-withdrawal states.

F. Lithium

Several controlled studies comparing lithium to placebo in alcoholic patients have been reported. They have the following features in common. They began with recently detoxified alcoholics; in each, the dropout rate was high, with the percentage completing the trial period ranging from only 17% to 53%; and the measures of effectiveness included episodes of pathological drinking as well as measures of depression. The studies also differed in important ways. The initial study of Kline et al. (1974) involved 73 male veterans who had high scores on the Zung Self-Rating Scale for Depression. Thus, all subjects were depressed by this criterion, but those with unipolar and bipolar depression were excluded. The double-blind phase of the study lasted 48 weeks. At the end of this period, 16 lithium and 14 placebo patients were still in the study. The Zung scores for those remaining on lithium were comparable to those on placebo, but lithium patients had experienced significantly fewer days of pathological drinking and hospitalization for alcoholism.

The study of Merry et al. (1976) began with 60 men and 11 women; 48% of these patients had scores above 15 on the Beck Depression Inventory and were considered depressed. At the end of an average of 41 weeks of treatment, Beck scores improved for both groups, with those in the lithium group doing somewhat better than those in the placebo group. Among those categorized as depressed at the start of treatment, those on lithium had significantly fewer days spent drinking and fewer days of incapacitating drinking as compared to those on placebo. This conclusion was based on nine "depressed" patients on lithium and seven "depressed" patients on placebo.

A study by Pond et al. (1981) involved 47 patients and used MMPI profiles to assess depression. It was designed as a three-month cross-over in which the maximum period on lithium was three months. Nineteen subjects completed the study. No significant differences between conditions in terms of MMPI scores or drinking patterns were shown, but the investigators consider their own design to be inadequate to test the hypothesis.

Lithium has also been studied in institutionalized young delinquents with histories of aggressive behavior and in prisoners who had histories of recurrent patterns of violent behavior with minimal provocation. In these studies, violent, angry behavior decreased, while other forms of sociopathic behavior did not (Kellner and Rada, 1979). To the degree that alcoholism is particularly prevalent among these groups, and that among these groups the alcoholism has a particularly poor prognosis, these studies of lithium on prisoners and delinquents may have relevance for treatment.

Among the drugs that are potentially available for treatment, lithium has two major advantages. The plasma levels that produce therapeutic effects are generally agreed upon, and there are readily available methods for monitoring these levels and compliance. Its safety range, however, is narrow, and the potential side effects are many. At present, however, there is little evidence that alcoholics who do not have bipolar disorder or who after detoxification show few signs of depression as measured on either Beck or Zung rating scales will benefit from lithium. There also is little evidence that those who do benefit would not have done as well or better on some other medication.

G. Propranolol

Propranolol, a beta-adrenergic blocker, is superior to placebo in reducing tension, with or without depression, in recently detoxified alcoholics (Rada and Kellner, 1979), and it appeared to be superior to diazepam in a two week cross-over study (Carlsson and Fasth, 1976). While there is little likelihood of dependence, propranolol is known to produce confusion and other cognitive impairments, and other data on efficacy are not as positive (Sellers et al., 1981).

H. Amphetamines, Opiates, and Miscellaneous

It has been proposed that mood disregulation and alcoholism may be linked in some alcoholics to persistent minimal brain dysfunction (attention deficit disorder, hyperactivity). However, even the proponents of this hypothesis concede that the abuse potential of amphetamines and related drugs probably rules out their use in this population (Wood et al., 1983).

A century ago, some physicians viewed chronic opiate use as a far less socially and physically destructive form of dependence than alcoholism and noted that some alcoholics stopped drinking when they began using opiates (Terry and Pellens, 1928). With the discovery of opioid receptors and endogenous ligands for these receptors, there is renewed interest in the role of opioids in mental illness and particularly in alcoholism (Verebey, 1982). The advent of programs using methadone permits a reassessment of the impact of opioids on alcoholism. The consistent finding is that opioid addicts who have alcohol problems tend to reduce alcohol intake while using heroin. However, when heroin addicts are treated with stable doses of methadone, alcohol problems reemerge, and sometimes emerge de novo (Green and Jaffe, 1977).

Buspirone is an antianxiety agent with efficacy comparable to that of diazepam in neurotic outpatients. Unlike lorazepam, its sedative properties in normal volunteers were not accentuated by combination with alcohol (Seppälä et al., 1982); drug abusers do not find its acute effects reinforcing, and its abuse potential should be lower than that of benzodiazepines (Cole, 1983).

VI. SOME ALTERED DRUG REACTIONS OF CLINICAL IMPORTANCE IN ALCOHOLISM

Three general areas of altered drug actions are of concern to clinicians working with alcoholic patients. These are (1) those which occur when alcohol is ingested along with another prescribed drug (e.g., disulfiram or tricyclic antidepressants); (2) those which occur when several therapeutic drugs (e.g., disulfiram and benzodiazepines) interact with each other; and (3) those which are due to changes in the body caused by prolonged ingestion of alcohol (e.g., increased liver enzyme activity or decreased liver function due to cirrhosis). These areas have been reviewed recently by Hoyumpa and Schenker (1982) and by Sellers and Busto (1982). The following condensed presentation includes only a few of many potential interactions of clinical interest.

Drug interactions are commonly classified as either pharmacokinetic or pharmacodynamic, depending upon the mechanisms involved. Pharmacokinetic interactions include alterations in bioavailability, rate of absorption and/or distribution, hepatic clearance, and plasma protein binding. Pharmacodynamic interactions are those that affect the actions of the drug at biologically active sites, such as changes in receptor density or binding affinity, resulting in additive, synergistic, or antagonistic effects.

Clinical effects of *ethanol-drug interactions* are difficult to predict despite a voluminous literature on the subject. Pharmacokinetic interactions are the easiest to study in the laboratory, but they are often clinically less important than the pharmacodynamic effects. Ethanol-drug interactions are unique in that exposure to alcohol in our society is ubiquitous, allowing for a number of situations and conditions under which a drug may knowingly or unknowingly be given to someone who has ingested alcohol either on an acute or chronic basis.

Alcohol-Sedative-Anxiolytic Combinations. Published studies vary in the route, dosage, and concentration of alcohol administered, the use of alcoholic or normal subjects, accuracy of pharmacokinetic data interpretations (e.g., early studies often used the terms "half-life" and "clearance" interchangeably), and the degree to which study design approximates real-life situations or addresses clinically significant issues.

Despite the extensive and more easily studied kinetic interactions, which in general find that ethanol ingestion increases blood levels of benzodiazepines, it is the net effect of the drug combination in producing effects on mood and on cognitive, psychomotor, and vital functions that is socially and clinically significant. In this area, making inferences about the practical implications of alcohol-sedative combinations is fraught with even greater difficulties. Most studies of cognitive and psychomotor effects are carried out in normal volunteers or in well-nourished and healthy abstinent alcoholics. But in the real clinical situation, alcoholics are often neither abstinent nor well-nourished, and they are often quite tolerant to the effects of alcohol and anxiolytics.

Most studies have found either additive or synergistic increases in the sedative actions and psychomotor impairment. In any given situation, more than one mechanism may be responsible for the additive effects. Acutely, ethanol raises plasma levels of benzodiazepines, especially those transformed by N-demethylation and hydroxylation, by reducing clearance, resulting in higher levels at brain receptor sites (Sellers and Busto, 1982); there is some suggestion that ethanol may also enhance receptor binding of diazepines (Davis and Ticku, 1981).

Tricyclic Antidepressants. Alcohol accentuates the sedative and psychomotor impairing effects of tricyclic antidepressants in nonalcoholic subjects (Seppälä et al., 1975), and all patients need to be warned about hazards of such combinations while driving. Also of clinical relevance is the observation that both smoking and alcohol use may accelerate the clearance of tricyclic antidepressants so that depressed alcoholics being treated with these agents may not achieve expected blood levels with the usual dosage (Ciraulo et al., 1982).

Monoamine Oxidase Inhibitors. As mentioned above, some mono-amine oxidase inhibitors produce disulfiram-like effects. In addition, some alcoholic beverages (dark beer and red wines) may contain tyramine and will produce hypertensive episodes in patients taking MAOIs.

Oral Hypoglycemic Agents. Patients taking oral hypoglycemic agents (e.g., chlorpropamide, tolbutamide) may experience significant decreases in blood sugar levels if they ingest alcohol. This is so despite the observation that chronic ingestion results in more rapid metabolism of tolbutamide (Hoyumpa and Schenker, 1982). The alcohol sensitizing effects of oral hypoglycemics have been mentioned.

Acetaminophen. While acute alcohol ingestion decreases the rate of degradation of acetaminophen, the rate is increased after chronic administration; alcoholics may be more susceptible to acetaminophen induced hepatoxicity.

Salicylates and Aspirin. Ethanol enhances the tendency of salicylates to cause gastrointestinal bleeding.

Anticoagulants. Chronic drinkers metabolize warfarin more rapidly.

Disulfiram. The interaction of ethanol and disulfiram has already been described. Because disulfiram inhibits several enzyme systems in addition to ALDH, it alters the metabolism of a number of commonly used drugs. Disulfiram reduces clearance rates of chlordiazepoxide and diazepam, but those of oxazepam and lorazepam, drugs which are already hydroxylated and are metabolized primarily by glucuronide formation, are not altered. The clearance of phenytoin is also reduced, and dosage adjustments are required to avoid toxic accumulation; this is also true of the anticoagulant, warfarin, and the antibiotic agent, rifamipin (Hoyumpa and Schenker, 1982; Sellers et al., 1981).

VII. A PLEA FOR PERSPECTIVE

It bears repeated mention that even drugs which clearly influence pathological affective states (whether these be panic, depression, or several types of dysphoria) will not necessarily produce changes in alcohol use once a significant degree of dependence develops. This is so even if the pathological affective states were initially important causes of the excess drinking. Once the CNS changes and the complex learning that constitutes the dependence syndrome occur, alcohol dependence becomes a disorder in its own right (Edwards and Gross, 1976; Wikler 1980), and it does not resolve automatically simply because one significant major contributing factor is brought under control. Efforts to change pathological drug-use patterns must accompany any drug treatment aimed at control of pathological affective states.

Only two drugs come close to having any demonstrable role as deterrents to continued drinking—disulfiram and carbimide—and these require a supportive treatment program to be safe and effective. Fortunately, abstinence-oriented groups see the alcohol sensitizing agents as supportive of their goal of abstinence and are willing to work with physicians around the issue of proper dosage, compliance, and early detection of side effects. Programs such as Alcoholics Anonymous are often able to help an individual gain some control over drinking, although depressive, dysphoric, and panic symptoms may persist. It is important for those interested in the treatment of alcoholic patients to try to communicate the potential, if not the current value of pharmacological treatments of associated or alcohol-induced affective disturbances. Effective pharmacological treatments and abstinence-oriented change and support systems are complementary and not competitive.

REFERENCES

Alcohol, Drug Abuse, and Mental Health Administration, 1981, Data from the Drug Abuse Warning Network (DAWN), National Institute on Drug Abuse Statistical Series, Series I, Number I, U.S. Department of Health and Human Services, U.S. Public Health Service, ADAMHA, Rockville, Md.

Barnett, A. H., Gonzalez-Auvert, C., Pyke, D. A., Saunders, J. B., Williams, R., Dickenson, C. J., and Rawlins, M. D., 1981, Blood concentrations of acetaldehyde during chlorpropamide-alcohol flush, Br. Med. J., 283:939–941.

Behar, D., and Winokur, G., 1979, Research in alcoholism and depression. A two way street under construction, in Psychiatric Factors in Drug Abuse (R. W. Pickens and L. L. Heston, eds.), pp. 125–152, Grune & Stratton, Inc., New York.

Bergstrom, B., Ohlin, H., Lindblom, P. E., and Wadstein, J., 1982, Is disulfiram implantation effective?, Lancet, 1:49–50.

Besson, J. A. O., Glen, A. I. M., Foreman, E. I., MacDonald, A., Smith, F. W., Hutchison, J. M. S., Mallard, J. R., and Ashcroft, G. W., 1981, Nuclear magnetic resonance observations in alcoholic cerebral disorder and the role of vasopressin, Lancet, 2:923–924.

Bliding, A., 1978, The abuse potential of benzodiazepines with special reference to oxazepam, Acta Psychiat. Scand., Suppl. 24:111–116.

Braestrup, C., 1982, Neurotransmitters and disease, Lancet, 2:1030–1034.

Brandt, J., Butters, N., Ryan, C., and Bayog, R., 1983, Cognitive loss and recovery in long-term alcohol abusers, Arch. Gen. Psychiat., 40:435–442.

Brien, J. F., Peachey, J. E., and Loomis, C. W., 1980, Calcium carbimide-ethanol interaction, *Clin. Pharmacol. Ther.*, 27:426–433.

Capretti, L., Speroni, C., Girone, M., Coscelli, C., Butturini, U., and Rocca, G., 1981, Chlorpropamide—and tolbutamide—alcohol flushing in non-insulin-dependent diabetics, *Br. Med. J.*, 283:1361–1362.

Carlsson, C., and Fasth, B. G., 1976, A comparison of the effects of propranolol and diazepam in alcoholics, *Br. J. Addict.*, 71:321–326.

Ciraulo, D. A., and Jaffe, J. H., 1981, Tricyclic antidepressants in the treatment of depression associated with alcoholism, *J. Clin. Psychopharmacol.*, 1:146–150.

Ciraulo, D. A., Alderson, L. M., Chapron, D. J., Jaffe, J. H., Subbarao, B., and Kramer, P. A., 1982, Imipramine disposition in alcoholics, *J. Clin. Psychopharmacol.*, 2:2–7.

Cole, J., 1984, in press, Beta-blockers and buspirone, in *Psychiatry Update* (L. Grinspoon, ed.), American Psychiatric Press, Washington, D.C.

Dackis, C. A., Bailey, J., Pottash, A. L. C., Stuckey, R. F., Gold, M. S., 1983, Accuracy of dexamethasone suppression test in alcoholics (letter), *Archs. Gen. Psychiat.*, 40:586–587.

Davis, W. C., and Ticku, M. K., 1981, Ethanol enhances (3H) diazepam binding at the benzodiazepine-gamma-aminobutyric acid receptor-ionophore complex, *Molec. Pharmacol.*, 20:287–294.

Dobmeyer, D. J., Stine, R. A., Leier, C. V., Greenberg, R., and Schaal, S. F., 1983, The arrhythmogenic effects of caffeine in human beings, *New Engl. J. Med.*, 308:814–816.

Dole, V. P., Fishman, J., Goldfrank, L., Khanna, J. and McGivern, R. F., 1982, Arousal of ethanol-intoxicated comatose patients with naloxone, *Alcoholism: Clin. Exper. Res.*, 6:275–279.

Edwards, G., and Gross, M. M., 1976, Alcohol dependence: Provisional description of a clinical syndrome, *Br. Med. J.*, 1:1058–1061.

Eisenhofer, G., Whiteside, E., Lambie, D., and Johnson, R., 1982, Brain water during alcohol withdrawal, *Lancet*, 1:50.

Elenbaas, R. M., Ryan, J. L., Robinson, W. A., Singsank, M. J., Harvey, M. J., and Klaassen, D. C., 1982, On the disulfiram-like activity of moxalactam, *Clin. Pharm. Ther.*, 32:347–355.

Feldman, D. J., Pattison, E. M., Sobell, L. C., Graham T., and Sobell, M. B., 1975, Outpatient alcohol detoxification: Initial findings on 564 patients, *Am. J. Psychiat.*, 132:407–412.

Feldmann, H., 1983, Apomorphine in the treatment of alcohol addiction: neurophysiological and therapeutic aspects, *Psychiatr. J. Univ. Ottawa*, 8:30–37.

Frecher, R. C., Shaw, J. M., Zilm, D. H., Jacob, M. S., Sellers, E. M., and Degani, N., 1982, Nonpharmacological supportive care compared to chlormethiazole infusion in the management of severe acute alcohol withdrawal, *J. Clin. Psychopharmacol.*, 2:277–280.

Fried, R., 1980, Biochemical actions of anti-alcoholic agents, *Substance and Alc. Actions/Misuse*, 1:5–27.

Fuller, R. K., and Roth, H. P., 1979, Disulfiram for the treatment of alcoholism: An evaluation in 128 men, *Ann. Intern. Med.*, 90:901–904.

Fuller, R. K., and Williford, W. O., 1980, Life-table analysis of abstinence in a study evaluating the efficacy of disulfiram, *Alcoholism: Clin. Exp. Res.*, 4:298–301.

Gessner, P. K., 1979, Drug therapy of the alcohol withdrawal syndrome, in *The Biochemistry and Pharmacology of Ethanol* (E. Majchrowicz and E. Noble, eds.), 375–434, Plenum Press, New York.

Gragg, D. M., 1982, Drugs to decrease alcohol consumption, *New Engl. J. Med.*, 306:747.

Green, J., and Jaffe, J. H., 1977, Alcohol and opiate dependence: A review, *J. Stud. Alc.*, 38:1274–1293.

Greenblatt, D. S., and Shader, R. I., 1974, Benzodiazepines, *New Engl. J. Med.*, 291:1011–1015.

————, 1975, Treatment of the alcohol withdrawal syndrome, in *Manual of Psychiatric Therapeutics* (R. I. Shader, ed.), pp. 211–235, Little, Brown and Company, Boston.

Hague, W. H., Wilson, L. G., Dudley, D. L., and Cannon, D. S., 1976, Post-detoxification drug treatment of anxiety and depression in alcoholic addicts, *J. Nerv. Ment. Dis.*, 162:354–359.

Hesselbrock, M. N., Hesselbrock, V. M., Tennen, H., Meyer, R. E., and Workman, K. L., 1983, Measurement of depression in alcoholics, *J. Clin. Consult. Psychol.*, 51:399–405.

Hoyumpa, A. M., and Schenker, S., 1982, Major drug interactions: Effect of liver disease, alcohol, and malnutrition, *Ann. Rev. Med.*, 33:113–149.

Jaffe, J. H., Ciraulo, D. A., Nies, A., Dixon, R., and Monroe, L., 1983, Abuse potential of halazepam and diazepam in patients recently treated for acute alcohol withdrawal, *Clin. Pharmacol. Ther.*, 34:623–630.

Keeler, M. H., Taylor, I., and Miller, W. C., 1979, Are all recently detoxified alcoholics depressed? *Am. J. Psychiatr.*, 136, 586–588.

Kellner, R., and Rada, R. T., 1979, Pharmacotherapy of personality disorders, in *Psychopharmacology Update: New and Neglected Areas* (J. M. Davis and D. Greenblatt, eds.), pp. 29–63, Grune & Stratton, Inc., New York.

Khan, A., Ciraulo, D., Nelson, W., Becker, J., Nies, A., and Jaffe, J. H., 1984, Dexamethasone suppression test in recently detoxified alcoholics, *J. Clin. Psychopharmacol.*, 4:4–9.

Kissin, B., 1977, Medical management of the alcoholic patient, in *The Biology of Alcoholism - Volume 5. Treatment and Rehabilitation of the Chronic Alcoholic* (B. Kissin and H. Begleiter, eds.), pp. 55–103, Plenum Press, New York.

Kline, N. S., Wren, J. C., Cooper, T. B., Varga, E., and Canal, O., 1974, Evaluation of lithium therapy in chronic and periodic alcoholism, *Am. J. Med. Sci.*, 268:15–22.

Kraus, J. W., Desmond, P. V., Marshall, J. P., Johnson, R. F., Schenker, S., and Wilkinson, G. R., 1978, Effects of aging and liver disease on disposition of lorazepam, *Clin. Pharmacol. Ther.*, 24:411–419.

Lindros, K. O., Stowell, A., Pikkarainen, P., and Salaspuro, M., 1981, The disulfiram (Antabuse)-alcohol reaction in male alcoholics: Its efficient management by 4-methylpyrazole, *Alcoholism: Clin. Exp. Res.*, 5:528–530.

Major, L. F., Lerner, P., Ballenger, J. K., Brown, G. L., Goodwin, F. K., and Lovenberg, W., 1979. Dopamine beta-hydroxylase in the cerbrospinal fluid: Relationship to disulfiram induced psychosis, *Biol. Psychiat.*, 14:337–344.

Marks, J., 1978, *The Benzodiazepines: Use, Misuse, Abuse.* MTP Press, Ltd., Lancaster, England.

Mendelson, J. H., and Mello, N. K., 1979, Biological concomitants of alcoholism, *New Engl. J. Med.,* 301:912–21.

Merry, J., Reynolds, C. M., Bailey, J., and Coppen, A., 1976, Prophylactic treatment of alcoholism by lithium carbonate, *Lancet,* 2:481–482.

Moskowitz, G., Chalmers, T. C., Sacks, H. S., Fagerstrom, R. M., and Smith, H., 1983, Deficiencies of clinical trials of alcohol withdrawal, *Alcoholism: Clin. Exper. Res.* 7:42–46.

Mullaney, J. A., and Trippett, C. J., 1979, Alcohol dependence and phobias: Clinical description and relevance, *Psychiatry,* 135:565–573.

Nace, E. P., Saxon, J. J., and Shore, N., 1983, A comparison of borderline and nonborderline alcoholic patients, *Archs. Gen. Psychiat.,* 40:54–56.

Nakamura, M. M., Overall, J. E., Hollister, L. E. and Radcliffe, E., 1983, Factors affecting outcome of depressive symptoms in alcoholics, *Alcoholism Clin. Exp. Res.,* 7:188–193.

Naranjo, C. A., Sellers, E. M., Chater, K., Iversen, P., Roach, C., and Sykora, K., 1983, Non-pharmacological interventions in acute alcohol withdrawal, *Clin. Pharmacol. Ther.,* 34:214–219.

Neubuerger, O. W., Hasha, N., Matarazzo, J. D., Schmitz, R. E., and Pratt, H. H., 1981, Behavioral-chemical treatment of alcoholism: An outcome replication, *J. Stud. Alc.,* 42:806–810.

Nuotto, E., Mattila, M. J., Seppälä, T., and Konno, K., 1982, Coffee and caffeine and alcohol effects on psychomotor function, *Clin. Pharmacol. Ther.,* 31:68–76.

Pattison, E. M., 1979, The selection of treatment modalities for the alcoholic patient, in *The Diagnosis and Treatment of Alcoholism* (J. H. Mendelson and N. K. Mello, eds.), pp. 229–255, McGraw-Hill Book Company, New York.

Peachey, J. E., Brien, J. F., Roach, C. A., and Loomis, C. W., 1981a, A comparative review of the pharmacological and toxicological properties of disulfiram and calcium carbimide, *J. Clin. Psychopharmacol.,* 1:21–26.

Peachey, J. E., Maglana, S., Robinson, G. M., Hemy, M., and Brien, J. F., 1981b, Cardiovascular changes during the calcium carbimide-ethanol interaction, *Clin. Pharmacol. Ther.,* 29:40–46.

Peachey, J. E., Zilm, D. J., and Cappell, H., 1981c, "Burning off the antabuse": Fact or fiction?, *Lancet,* 1:943–944.

Pond, S. M., Becker, C. E., Vandervoort, R., Phillips, M., Bowler, R. M., and Peck, C. C., 1981, An evaluation of the effects of lithium in the treatment of chronic alcoholism. I. Clinical results, *Alcoholism: Clin. Exp. Res.,* 5:247–251.

Porjesz, B., and Begleiter, H., 1982, Evoked brain potential deficits in alcoholism and aging, *Alcoholism: Clin. Exp. Res.,* 6:53–63.

Poser, W., Poser, S., Roscher, D., and Argyrakis, A., 1983, Do benzodiazepines cause cerebral atrophy? (letter), *Lancet,* March 26, 1983, 715.

Pottenger, M., McKernon, J., Patrie, J. E., Weissman, M. M., Ruben, H. L., and Newberry, P., 1978, The frequency and persistence of depressive symptoms in the alcohol abuser, *J. Nerv. Ment. Dis.,* 166, 562–570.

Poutanen, P., 1979, Experience with carbamazepine in the treatment of withdrawal symptoms in alcohol abusers, *Br. J. Addict.,* 74:201–204.

Quitkin, F., Rifkin, A., and Klein, D. F., 1979, Monoamine oxidase inhibitors: A review of antidepressant effectiveness, *Arch. Gen. Psychiat.,* 36:749–760.

Rada, R. R., and Kellner, R., 1979, Drug treatment in alcoholism, in *Psychopharmacology Update: New and Neglected Areas* (J. M. Davis and D. Greenblatt, eds.), pp. 105–144, Grune & Stratton, Inc., New York.

Ravaris, C. L., Robinson, D. S., Ives, J. O., Nies, A., and Bartlett, D., 1980, Phenelzine and amitriptyline in the treatment of depression, *Arch. Gen. Psychiat.*, 37:1075–1080.

Sampliner, R., and Iber, F. L., 1974, Diphenylhydantoin control of alcohol withdrawal seizures: Results of a controlled study, *JAMA*, 230:1430–1432.

Schuckit, M., 1979, Alcoholism and affective disorder: Diagnostic confusion, in *Alcoholism and Affective Disorders* (D. W. Goodwin and C. K. Erickson, eds.), pp. 9–19, Spectrum Publications, Inc., New York.

Schuckit, M., 1983, Alcoholic patients with secondary depression, *Am. J. Psychiat.*, 140:711–714.

Sellers, E. M., and Busto, U., 1982, Benzodiazepines and ethanol: Assessment of the effects and consequences of psychotropic drug interactions, *J. Clin. Psychopharmacol.*, 2:249–262.

Sellers, E. M., and Kalant, H., 1976, Alcohol intoxication and withdrawal, *New Engl. J. Med.*, 294:757–762.

Sellers, E. M., Naranjo, C. A., Harrison, M., Devenyi, P., Roach, C., and Sykora, K., 1983, Diazepam loading: Simplified treatment of alcohol withdrawal, *Clin. Pharmacol. Ther.*, 34:822–826.

Sellers, E. M., Naranjo, C. A., and Peachey, J. E., 1981, Drugs to decrease alcohol consumption, *New Engl. J. Med.*, 305:1255–1262.

Sellers, E. M., Naranjo, C. A., and Peachey, J. E., 1982, letter, *New Engl. J. Med.*, 306:748.

Seppälä, T., Aranko, K., Mattila, M. J., and Shrotriya, R. C., 1982, Effects of alcohol on buspirone and lorazepam actions, *Clin. Pharmacol. Ther.*, 32:201–204.

Seppälä, T., Linnoila, M., Elonen, E., Mattila, M. J., and Maki, M., 1975, Effect of tricyclic antidepressants and alcohol on psychomotor skills related to driving, *Clin. Pharmacol. Ther.*, 17:515–522.

Shaw, G. K., 1982, Alcohol dependence and withdrawal, *Br. Med. Bull.*, 38:99–102.

Shaw, J. A., Donley, P., Morgan, D. W., and Robinson, J. A., 1975, Treatment of depression in alcoholics, *Am. J. Psychiat.*, 132:641–644.

Sheehan, D. V., Davidson, J., Manschreck, T., Van Wyck Fleet, J., 1983, Lack of efficacy of a new antidepressant (bupropion) in the treatment of panic disorder with phobias, *J. Clin. Psychopharmacol.*, 3:28–31.

Smith, C. M., 1978, *Alcoholism: Treatment*, Eden Press Ltd., Montreal.

Sokolow, L., Welte, J., Hynes, G., and Lyons, J., 1981, Multiple substance use by alcoholics, *Br. J. Addict.*, 76:147–158.

Tallman, J. F., Paul, S. M., Skolnick, P., and Gallager, D., 1980, Receptors for the age of anxiety: Pharmacology of the benzodiazepines, *Science*, 207:274–281.

Terry, C. E., and Pellens, M., 1928, *The Opium Problem*, Bureau of Social Hygiene, Inc., New York.

Verebey, K. (ed.), 1982, *Opioids in Mental Illness: Theories, Clinical Observations, and Treatment Possibilities*, The New York Academy of Sciences, New York.

Weir, J. H., 1978, Prazepam in the treatment of anxiety: A placebo-controlled multicenter evaluation, *J. Clin. Psychiat.*, 39:841–847.

Weissman, M. M., and Myers, J. K., 1980, Clinical depression in alcoholism, *Am. J. Psychiat.*, 137:372–373.

Whitfield, C., 1980, Nondrug detoxification, in *Phenomenology and Treatment of Alcoholism* (W. E. Fann, I. Karacan, A. D. Pokorny, and R. Williams, eds.), pp. 305–320, Spectrum Publications, Inc., New York.

Wikler, A., 1980, *Opioid Dependence*, Plenum Press, New York.

Wilkinson, D. A., 1982, Examination of alcoholics by computed tomographic (CT) scans: A critical review, *Alcoholism: Clin. Exp. Res.*, 6:31–45.

Wilson, A., Davidson, W. J., and Blanchard, R., 1980, Disulfiram implantation: A trial using placebo implants and two types of controls, *J. Stud. Alc.*, 41:429–436.

Wood, D., Wender, P. H., and Reimherr, F. W., 1983, The prevalence of attention deficit disorder, residual type, or minimal brain dysfunction, in a population of male alcoholic patients, *Am. J. Psychiat.*, 140:95–98.

Zitrin, C. M., Klein, D. F., and Woerner, M. G., 1980, Treatment of agoraphobia with group exposure in vivo and imipramine, *Arch. Gen. Psychiat.*, 37:63–72.

CHAPTER 9

Behavioral Assessment and Treatment of Alcoholism

Peter E. Nathan, Ph.D.
Henry and Anna Starr Professor of Psychology
Director, Center of Alcohol Studies
Rutgers University
New Brunswick, New Jersey

Raymond S. Niaura, B.A.
Research Associate, Alcohol Behavior Research Laboratory
Rutgers University
New Brunswick, New Jersey

Behavioral theorists, researchers, and clinicians differ on many issues; they are far from monolithic on matters of research, assessment, and treatment. On two matters, though, behavioral theorists, researchers, and clinicians agree. The first is that most human behavior is acquired according to the three principal modes of learning—classical, or Pavlovian conditioning, operant, or Skinnerian conditioning, and modeling, or vicarious conditioning. Accordingly, the prevailing behavioral view is that much of the behavior of alcoholics is learned. The second matter on which behavioral workers agree is the respect they accord empirical data, the scientific method, and the accepted rules of scientific enquiry. Theory, clinical experience, or consensus are not seen as adequate substitutes for empirical validation or confirmation. In contrast to many alcoholism workers, then, the behavioral clinician tends to insist on research findings that confirm the efficacy of an intervention technique or the helpfulness of an assessment method, rather than to accept theory or practice based upon some other standard of proof. This reliance on empirical validation has special relevance to the current behavioral view, for example, of the efficacy of controlled drinking treatment for alcoholism. A promising treatment approach when it was initially proposed, in the mid-1970s, controlled drinking treatment for alcoholics became much less appealing when further empirical research failed to confirm earlier promise. It is not now a treatment of choice for chronic alcoholics.

I. AN HISTORICAL PERSPECTIVE ON BEHAVIORAL THEORY AND PRACTICE

Even though a Soviet physician, Kantorovich, treated a group of chronic alcoholics with electrical aversion more than 50 years ago (with apparent success), it was not until the 1960s that electrical aversion and a few other behavioral procedures (e.g., systematic desensitization, covert sensitization, and chemical aversion) began to find widespread application. In fact, the only continuing use of behavioral methods to treat alcoholics during the roughly 30 years separating Kantorovich's demonstration and the 1960s was at the Shadel Sanatorium in Seattle during the 1940s and 1950s (Lemere and Voegtlin, 1950) where chemical aversion was employed to induce conditioned aversion to alcohol. That program, which appears to have met with success, is evaluated below.

Intensive clinical application of behavioral methods began in the early and middle 1960s and extended well beyond alcoholism to virtually the full range of psychopathology: from normal children in classroom settings, to individuals and families with no more than the usual "problems in living," to the psychotic, demented, criminal, and retarded. In the beginning, behavioral psychologists—some clinically trained, some trained in experimental laboratories, all immersed in learning theory and behavioral research—moved into clinical research settings. There they began to explore the utility of operant behavioral programs for chronic schizophrenics living in the bypassed back wards of state mental hospitals. Basic researchers like Lindsley and others demonstrated that the behavior of schizophrenics predictably adheres to the laws of conditioning and learning (Lindsley, 1950); and clinical researchers like Azrin, Ayllon, and others showed that behavior change methods derived from laboratory research on learning could be employed successfully to modify even the most deviant psychotic behaviors (Ayllon, 1963; Ayllon and Azrin, 1965). Their latter-day successors have extended this technology to token economy and other behavioral modification programs that are now an integral part of group treatment and educational programs throughout the country.

At about the same time a South African psychiatrist, Joseph Wolpe, and a countryman trained in clinical psychology, Arnold A. Lazarus, laid down a framework for development of individual behavior therapy procedures (Wolpe and Lazarus, 1966). Initially these centered on systematic desensitization, assertion training, and deep muscle relaxation, procedures that are effective in reducing the omnipresent anxiety of neurotic patients. Individual behavior therapy procedures now encompass such diverse treatment strategies as cognitive restructuring and reeducation, symbolic and participant modeling, self-monitoring, self-control training, and multimodal therapy. For readers who would like an overview of the current status of behavior therapy and behavior modification, several excellent surveys of the field have recently been published: the *Annual Review of Behavior Therapy: Theory and Practice* (Franks and Wilson, 1973–1980); *Behavior Modification* (Craighead, Kazdin, and Mahoney, 1981); and *Handbook of Clinical Behavior Therapy* (Turner, Calhoun, and Adams, 1981).

As behavior therapists continued to expand their armamentarium, in the middle and late 1960s, to confront an ever-expanding diversity of psychopathology, more and more persons began to focus their efforts on alcoholism. At first, these efforts began where Kantorovich left off—in the attempt to induce conditioned aversion to alcohol, usually by electrical aversion conditioning. These relatively unsophisticated efforts failed in large measure because they confronted only the alcoholic's uncontrolled drinking and not the associated behavioral deficits and excesses that maintain and are maintained by that drinking. Gradually, however, more comprehensive and sophisticated behavioral treatment programs came to the fore. It is on these latter programs that we focus later in this chapter.

The unidimensional behavioral treatment methods initially applied to the problem of alcoholism reflected an equally uncomplex view of etiology. Early behavioral theorists believed that alcoholics drink abusively because they have learned that alcohol is an effective means of reducing conditioned anxiety. Empirical support for this view derived from the animal laboratory (Conger, 1951, 1956), and clinical support came from the conviction that alcohol eases prevailing high levels of anxiety in alcoholics. Behavioral research with humans suggesting just the opposite (Mello, 1972; Nathan and O'Brien, 1971; Okulitch and Marlatt, 1972), however, weakened support for this unidimensional view of alcoholism etiology. In its place, multidimensional theories of etiology were proposed. One of the first stressed the influence of peer pressure on excessive early drinking by adolescents (Jessor, Collins, and Jessor, 1972); another early theory (Miller and Eisler, 1975) pointed to modeling of adult behavior—including parental alcoholism—as a factor in the disorder.

Etiologic theories of alcoholism from the behavioral perspective have grown both more numerous and more complex. As with behavioral theory generally, behavioral views on alcoholism have added cognitive elements—as mediating variables—to the learning factors considered responsible for development of abusive drinking. Nonetheless, even though cognitive social-learning theories predominate, unidimensional theories are still proposed [e.g., Tucker, Vuchinich, and Sobell (1981) see alcohol consumption as a "self-handicapping" strategy, while Hull (1981) proposes that alcohol serves to decrease self-awareness; both self-handicapping and decreased self-awareness are seen as reinforcing to some individuals]. Marlatt, active in the development of cognitive social-learning conceptualizations of alcoholism, portrays this view of alcoholism in the following words:

> Problem drinking is viewed as a multiply determined, learned behavioral disorder. It can be understood best through the empirically derived principles of social learning, cognitive psychology, and behavior therapies. . . . Particular attention is paid to the determinants of drinking behavior. These include situational and environmental antecedents, the individual's past learning history, prior experiences with alcohol, and cognitive processes and expectations about the effects of alcohol. Such factors serve as antecedent cues that often precipitate excessive alcohol use. An equal emphasis is placed on the consequences of drinking, which serve to maintain the behavior. . . . Also included in this class of variables are the social and interpersonal reactions experienced by the drinker (Marlatt and Donovan, 1982, p. 561).

A similar cognitive social-learning view of alcoholism etiology is proposed by Miller and Foy (1981, pp. 192–193).

Acceptance of contemporary social-learning views of alcoholism does not require rejection of other etiologic factors, including sociocultural (Cahalan and Room, 1974; Vaillant and Milofsky, 1982) and genetic/physiological ones (Goodwin and Guze, 1974). The behavioral position, instead, presumes that while learning may play a prepotent role in the alcoholism of some individuals, it does not necessarily do so in all persons. Examples of this interactional view of etiology include both our own theory of etiology, discussed in detail later in this chapter, which draws both on genetic and our own own behavioral research findings, and Tarter's view (1982), which accords responsibility for the behavioral stigmata of alcoholism in some persons to the impact of physiologically produced hyperactivity, expressed first during childhood.

II. BEHAVIORAL ASSESSMENT AND TREATMENT IN THE MANAGEMENT OF THE CHRONIC ALCOHOLIC

It is entirely possible to assess and treat chronic alcoholism within a consistent behavioral framework; many of the comprehensive treatment programs described below operate from that position. However, it is also possible to incorporate behavioral methods within a treatment regimen relying on a medical orientation to the disorder or on the peer-focused approach of Alcoholics Anonymous.

What do those who have developed behavioral assessment instruments and procedures have to offer the nonbehavioral clinician? To begin with, they have developed detailed drinking history protocols (e.g., Marlatt, 1975, 1981) which focus on a person's drinking pattern over time as it relates to decisions to remain sober, to resume drinking after a period of sobriety, or to continue to drink during a lengthy drinking episode. Though every clinician strives to uncover this information during the course of treatment in his or her own way, behavioral assessment procedures focus on accurate, reliable specification of drinking pattern and on identification of the environmental setting and circumstances within which drinking takes place. Accordingly, even for the clinician who operates from a nonbehavioral perspective, information of the kind provided by these methods can prove of value.

Similarly, behavioral clinicians require baseline (pretreatment) assessment of drinking behavior and associated behavioral and interpersonal problems, followed ultimately by similar posttreatment assessment. Any clinician will find this data valuable in determining the extent to which his or her interventions have an impact on patients' drinking behavior. A product of the empirical bent of the behavioral clinician, pre- and posttreatment assessment is the only way to amass empirical data attesting to the value of what we do for our patients.

It is also unnecessary to adopt a consistently behavioral approach to intervention in order to employ behavioral treatment procedures usefully. If treatment is to focus on the unconscious conflicts that cause a person to drink to excess, but this treatment approach is difficult to employ as long as the patient continues to drink, behavioral techniques that directly attack the excessive drinking (e.g., chemical aversion or contingency contracting) might be most useful. If AA is the treatment of choice—as it is for many alcoholics—a preliminary period of behavioral intervention designed to equip the patient with some of the social skills necessary to deal with the necessarily intensive interpersonal interaction attendant upon AA treatment might also be most helpful. Or, if the patient drinks to deal with omnipresent anxiety, perhaps a dual course of antianxiety medication and systematic desensitization therapy might work better than either alone.

A. Behavioral Assessment of Alcoholism

Until recently, most clinicians, strongly influenced by psychoanalytic theory, took the trait approach to assessment. Because psychoanalytic theory posits that personality structures laid down early in life determine later psychopathology, the psychoanalytic assessor sought to identify dynamic traits responsible for an individual's psychopathology. The assumption was that persons sharing a particular kind of psychopathology (e.g., alcoholism) also shared common psychopathologic traits or dynamics. In our judgment, the quest for a personality structure unique to and explanatory of alcoholism has not borne fruit: Unique alcoholic personality types have not been found (Costello, 1981; Hoffman, 1976; Partington and Johnson, 1969).

The behavioral view of assessment, by contrast, derives from the assumption that both maladaptive and adaptive behavior are learned and, hence, are subject to continual alteration and modification by past and present enviromental circumstances. Many of those who assess psychopathology from the behavioral perspective focus on five crucial assessment elements. As outlined by Tharp and Wetzel (1969), these include the following:

1. *The target behavior itself—its frequency, intensity, and pattern.* Both excessive drinking and the behavioral deficits and excesses which typically accompany it are target behaviors for alcoholics.
2. *Antecedent events—the "setting events" for the individual's maladaptive behavior.* Alcoholics typically point to stress, anxiety, depression, marital discord, job dissatisfaction, and interpersonal inadequacy as factors which lead them to uncontrolled drinking.
3. *Maintaining stimuli—the environmental factors which reinforce the target behaviors.* For alcoholics, maintaining stimuli include the physical or psychological removal from the "setting event" that results from continued intoxication ("I drink to forget everything") as well as sympathetic or nurturant behaviors—which reinforce the target behavior—from spouse or employer in the face of the alcohol problem.
4. *Reinforcement hierarchy—the range of factors in the environment which reinforce both target and nontarget behaviors.* Many alcoholics claim that "the only thing I have left is alcohol," even though behavioral researchers have identified a variety of other

reinforcers, environmental and personal, capable of modifying their behavior.

5. *Potentials for remediation in the environment.* As noted above, behavioral researchers and clinicians have identified a variety of reinforcers in the environment of alcoholics other than alcohol which are capable of effecting behavior change, including modification or elimination of their maladaptive drinking.

1. Assessment of the Target Behavior and its Antecedents

Assessment in the Laboratory. The first actual laboratory measures of "the target behavior" of alcoholism—drinking by chronic alcoholics—permitted Mello and Mendelson (1965, 1966) and Nathan and his colleagues (1970, 1971) to describe the drinking patterns of "skid row" alcoholics. Using an operant conditioning paradigm, these researchers established that many of their subjects drank in excess of a quart of beverage alcohol a day while demonstrating a biphasic pattern of drinking: a weeklong "spree" followed by a much lengthier period of "maintenance" drinking. Nathan and O'Brien (1971) also observed that most skid row alcoholics appear to be social isolates before, during, and after drinking, though later research by Bigelow, Griffiths, and their coworkers (1974, 1975) suggests that alcoholics who are less deteriorated socially do not show this degree of social isolation when they drink. When the drinking behavior of women was examined within the same paradigm (Tracey, Karlin, and Nathan, 1976), women alcoholics showed only a "maintenance" pattern of drinking; in that way they more closely resembled heavy-drinking males who were not alcoholics.

Another laboratory-based behavioral assessment strategy, the "taste test," requires subjects to consume alcoholic and nonalcoholic beverages in order to rate them along several taste dimensions "for research purposes." The real purpose of the procedure, though, is to measure alcohol consumption covertly. Marlatt used an "alcohol taste rating task" to explore the effects on consumption of a range of antecedent events: provocation to anger and opportunity for retaliation [social drinkers who were provoked to anger and could express it by retaliating against a confederate drank significantly less than provoked subjects who could not retaliate (Marlatt, Kosturn, and Lang, 1975)], threat of interpersonal stress [heavy-social-drinking males expecting to be evaluated by a group of women drank significantly more than subjects who did not expect to be evaluated (Higgins and Marlatt, 1975)], threat of impersonal stress [the threat of painful electric shock had no effect on drinking rate by alcoholics or nonalcoholics (Higgins and Marlatt, 1973)], and modeling [a heavy-drinking model increased drinking rate of heavy-social-drinking college students (Caudill and Marlatt, 1975)].

Other investigators have continued efforts to clarify relationships between environmental stressors and abusive drinking with the taste test. This work reflects, in part, continued interest in the tension-reduction hypothesis of alcoholism. Despite its problems, the tension-reduction model maintains appeal because it is virtually the only psychological/ behavioral theory to emphasize this very real (albeit short-lived) pharmacologic consequence of ethanol ingestion. As with prior efforts to find consistency in studies of this relationship, the current group of projects is in conflict. While two studies, one of college women, the other of college men, found that exposure to frustrating, tension-inducing intellectual tasks led to increased alcohol consumption (Noel and Lisman, 1980; Tucker et al., 1980), two others (of college males) did not find such an association (Gabel et al., 1980; Rohsenow, 1982). While the latter studies employed fear-inducing stimuli, and the former, frustrating intellectual tasks, this difference in tension-arousing stimuli doesn't seem sufficient to account for this conflict in results. A better explanation may be that subjects in the four studies maintained conflicting expectations about their purposes, expectations which influenced their drinking behavior to a greater extent than the tension-inducing stimuli themselves. This explanation suggests, in turn, that the tension-reduction motive, at least in social drinkers, may be a less robust determinant of drinking than some have believed.

Assessment of target behavior in the laboratory has also taken place in experimental bar settings. In one of the first such studies, Schaefer and his colleagues (1971) reported alcoholic and nonalcoholic subjects to drink in very different ways: Alcoholics tended to gulp straight drinks without ice while nonalcoholics preferred to sip mixed drinks, to which they usually added ice. Williams and Brown (1974) extended this research by reporting that New Zealand alcoholics differed from New Zealand nonalcoholics along precisely the same behavioral dimensions. In a replication and extension of this study by its second author (Brown, 1981), all 25 problem drinker subjects and six of 15 convicted drinking drivers, all New Zealanders, drank like the hospitalized alcoholics studied in 1974, while nine of 15 drinking drivers fell between the alcoholic and problem drinking groups and a group of normal drinkers in drinking pattern.

While investigations of the impact of social setting and group process on drinking have taken place in the natural environment, a recent investigation of these drinking antecedents (Tomaszewski, Strickler, and Maxwell, 1980) was undertaken in an experimental laboratory setting which permitted better controls over setting and social stimuli. College-age social drinker subjects consumed more when in group drinking settings, consonant with findings for social drinkers in a natural environment (e.g., Rosenbluth, Lawson, and Nathan, 1977) and divergent from findings for alcoholics in an experimental laboratory setting (Foy and Simon, 1978). Alcoholics and nonalcoholics may differ in the extent to which drinking environment influences their drinking behavior.

The most ambitious recent laboratory study of drinking utilized both an operant measurement system (to quantify the amount of "work" subjects were willing to emit to earn beverage alcohol) and an experimental bar setting. The study, by pioneering operant researcher Jack Mendelson and three colleagues (Babor et al., 1980), was designed to establish temporal and consumption parameters associated with a daily experimental bar "happy hour"; the "happy hour" involved a discount drink policy akin to "happy hours" in bars and taverns in the real world. The experimental bar "happy hour" was associated with a marked increase in consumption by both heavy- and casual-drinking subjects; interestingly, heavy drinkers increased their drinking more than casual drinkers, suggesting that discount policies adopted by bars and taverns may accelerate alcohol consumption by problem drinkers, a conclusion with important public policy implications.

Assessment in the Natural Environment. The laboratory measures of drinking reviewed above have one important limitation: All require actual consumption of alcohol. This means that alcoholics in or following treatment cannot be assessed by these methods. Consumption is most commonly assessed in the natural environment by the Michigan Alcoholism Screening Test (MAST: Selzer, 1971) and the Oates and McCoy (1973) and Cahalan, Cisin, and Crossley (1969) questionnaires. All three instruments are designed to elicit data on quantity and frequency of alcohol consumption, along with information on behavioral problems associated with that consumption. More behavioral is Marlatt's 19-page Drinking Profile Questionnaire (1976, 1981) which taps data on all five of Tharp and Wetzel's behavioral assessment elements. Along with the Drinking Profile, Marlatt recommends the following additional assessment procedures:

> . . . a personal biography (describing the history and development of the drinking problem); ongoing written accounts of the person's current drinking behavior and associated urges to drink in a daily diary format (self-monitoring); a detailed analysis of the client's ability to cope with a number of "high risk situations" associated with potential relapse (for instance, coping with feelings of anger, social pressures to resume drinking); direct observation of the client's drinking behavior in either analog drinking tasks (the

taste-rating task) or in seminaturalistic environments (the simulated bar setting); and an in-depth description of the person's general lifestyle (other persistent habits, exercise patterns, social support systems, work patterns, stress-management activities) (Marlatt, 1981, p. 30).

While syndromal rather than behavioral, in the sense that both describe the array of signs and symptoms that cohere frequently enough to constitute a syndrome, the syndromes of alcohol dependence and alcohol abuse of the third edition of the *Diagnostic and Statistical Manual of Mental Disorders* (1980) and the alcohol dependence syndrome proposed by Edwards and Gross (1976) and investigated by Skinner and Allen (1982) deserve brief mention here. Both seem likely to be integrated into behavioral assessment approaches to alcoholism because both rely most heavily on observed behavioral deficits and excesses rather than on the presumed or hypothesized sequelae of abusive consumption.

Nathan (1980) and Robins (1981) have recognized the problems of diagnosis of alcoholism, the unreliability of pre-DSM-III diagnostic criteria, and the resultant lack of agreement among clinicians that often prevented diagnostic consensus. Both have also recorded their admiration for the syndromally based distinctions between alcoholism and problem drinking that are reflected in DSM-III's operational criteria, which will permit reliable, widespread differentiation of Alcohol Dependence and Alcohol Abuse syndromes for the first time.

Skinner and Allen (1982) developed an Alcohol Dependence Scale of 29 items from Edwards and Gross's earlier (1976) description of an alcohol dependence syndrome. The 1982 study, designed to validate this syndrome and its scale in 225 alcohol abusers, revealed the following: (1) The scale exhibited substantial internal consistency reliability (.92); (2) higher levels of alcohol dependence (reflected by the scale) were associated with social consequences from drinking as well as with greater quantities of alcohol consumed; (3) as alcohol dependence increased, clients were less likely to appear for initial treatment sessions; and (4) degree of alcohol dependence was directly related to psychopathology as well as to physical symptoms of the nervous, cardiovascular, and digestive systems. The apparent reliabilty and validity of the Alcohol Dependence Scale suggests that it may have utility for treatment planning and diagnostic purposes. Moreover, the established psychometric properties of the scale may permit research relating degree of alcohol dependence with a range of correlated and causally linked variables for the first time.

The major problem for behavioral assessment in the natural environment is tracking the behavior of subjects whose participation in treatment or follow-up is irregular and unpredictable. This problem is especially troublesome when the assessment is a follow-up of therapy. Assessment for follow-up purposes requires both reliability of the assessment and evaluation of substantial numbers of treated patients. Given the chaotic nature of the lives of many alcoholics, how does one keep in contact with persons whose residences, jobs, and lives may change a great deal over a very short period of time?

Following extensive experience in designing and carrying out follow-ups of comparative treatment studies, L. C. Sobell has proposed the following criteria for alcoholism treatment outcome evaluations (1981, 1982):

1. *Plan evaluation prior to the study* (which maximizes the likelihood that assessment measures are maximally useful and subjects can be located for follow-up).

2. *Operationally define subject populations, treatments, and outcome measures* (so that the study can be replicated and its findings can be generalized).

3. *Obtain representative assessments of pretreatment functioning* (for posttreatment comparisons).

4. *Obtain comprehensive follow-up tracking information* (so that as few subjects as possible are lost to follow-up).

5. *Use outcome measures of known reliability and validity* (so that outcome data will reflect actual behavior rather than psychometric distortion).

6. *Use multiple measures of treatment outcome that are continuous and quantifiable whenever possible* (because single outcome measures may not adequately reflect prevailing behavior patterns).

7. *Use multiple information sources to verify subjects' self-reports* (because neither self-reports nor single information sources may adequately reflect behavior).

8. *Only interview subjects when they are alcohol-free* (because drunken subjects do not always provide reliable data).

9. *Use multiple follow-up contacts* (because reliance on a single follow-up contact increases the possibility of unrepresentative data).

10. *Use a minimum 12- to 18-month follow-up interval* (because drinking behavior over a shorter time-period is not predictive of long-term treatment effects).

11. *Use appropriate statistical analyses* (to control for pretreatment differences and to analyze for predictors of treatment outcomes).

Sobell has also examined the reliability of self-reports of drinking by alcoholics and problem drinkers (e.g., Maisto, Sobell, and Sobell, 1982; Sobell et al., 1979; Sobell, Sobell, and VanderSpek, 1979). These studies have established that, in the absence of sanctions or aversive contingencies for accurate reports of drinking, alcoholics and problem drinkers can be relied on to give accurate reports of drinking. This finding has been replicated by other investigators, including Michael Polich (1982), one of the authors of the two Rand surveys of clients of federally funded alcoholism treatment centers (Armor, Polich, and Stambul, 1978; Polich, Armor, and Braiker, 1981). A controversial design feature of those well-known surveys (reviewed below) was heavy reliance on clients' self-reports of drinking following treatment.

Follow-up workers have generally assumed that subjects who are most difficult to locate for follow-up purposes are most likely to have resumed drinking. However, a recent study of treatment outcome as a function of follow-up difficulty (LaPorte et al., 1981) revealed essentially no differences, in a sample of 142 subjects followed after treatment, between alcoholics and drug abusers who were readily located and those who required extraordinary efforts to locate. These data call into question the routine research-design decision to consider subjects who cannot be located for follow-up purposes as treatment failures, in the absence of definite proof of that status.

Other behavioral researchers working in the natural environment have developed and studied unobtrusive methods for recording detailed consumption data by patrons of commercial drinking establishments. Cutler and Storm (1975), Kessler and Gomberg (1975), Reid (1977), and Storm and Cutler (1981) gathered normative data on usual patterns of consumption in neighborhood bars. Rosenbluth, Lawson, and Nathan (1977) observed the drinking behavior of college students in a university-sponsored beer parlor, reporting differences among patrons' consumption rates as a function of sex (males drank more than females), group size (subjects drank more in groups than in dyads), and group composition (subjects drank more in opposite-sex than same-sex groups). Babor et al. (1980) compared drinking behavior by 16 regular bar patrons (eight men, eight women) during "happy hour" and non-"happy hour" periods in order to confirm observations made of 34 men in an experimental bar setting during conditions designed to replicate "happy hour" conditions in the natural environment. Under both experimental and natural conditions, the reduced costs of consumption led drinkers to increase their drinking substantially.

2. Assessment of Maintaining Stimuli

Most behavioral assessment efforts have focused on patterns of drinking, first in laboratory settings, more recently in natural environments. This emphasis on how alcoholics drink—including how much—stemmed from a surprising paucity of data on drinking by alcoholics. As this early behavioral assessment research developed in the late 1960s and early 1970s, the impact of specific environmental factors (stress and social interaction were two of the most common) on consumption rate and pattern began to be explored. So growth in efforts to assess antecedents of drinking ran almost parallel to development of procedures for assessment of the drinking itself.

Until recently, much less attention was paid to coordinated efforts to identify stimuli typically maintaining alcoholism, reinforcement hierarchies with the potential for reinforcing changes in alcoholic drinking, and environmental potentials for remediation of maladaptive drinking.

Speculation about stimuli which maintain alcoholism has led, over the years, to a variety of questionnaire and interview studies of drinkers' views on why they continue to drink. In their review of this research, Nathan and Lisman (1976) had the following to say about the three determinants of drinking behavior that researchers had explored most fully to that time:

> (*Social interaction factors*) . . . From research reviewed here, we now conclude that social interaction facilitates alcohol consumption in most alcoholics and has little or no effect on others. . . . It seems certain that the reciprocal reinforcement value alcohol and social interaction have for each other might well account for much of the marked resistance of the disorder to remediation (p. 506).
>
> (*Interpersonal anxiety and social stress*) . . . The tension-reduction model of alcohol consumption does not receive overwhelming support from the bulk of the experimental literature. . . . The results of studies which favor the model . . . seem more like isolated findings deriving from special stress conditions (e.g., isolated stress, interpersonal stress, retaliative stress) than from conditions which play important tension-inducing roles in the alcoholic's real life beyond the laboratory (p. 511).
>
> (*"Set" and social influence*) [Studies reviewed provide] initial and tentative confirmation for the long-held view that alcoholics as children may in fact have modeled heavy parental drinking behavior (just as alcoholics as adults model the drinking behavior of drinking companions) (p. 514).

Since this 1976 review, which reflected the paucity to that time of programmatic research on stimuli that maintain abusive drinking patterns, two such research programs have developed. The impact on drinking behavior of (1) expectations about alcohol's effects on behavior and (2) behavioral tolerance to alcohol's effects have been studied intensively in recent years.

Alcohol and Expectancies. In their move away from the tension-reduction model of alcoholism to the multidimensional, cognitive social-learning view of the disorder that now prevails, behavioral workers have invested heavily in research on the relative contributions to intoxicated behavior made by alcohol (1) as a drug and (2) as the focus of diverse, sometimes conflicting, expectations.

Marlatt, one of the central figures in the development of cognitive social-learning explanations of alcoholism, puts this line of research in the following perspective:

> Early behavioral studies of drinking and alcoholism were based on a tension-reduction hypothesis. This position assumed that alcohol has physiologically mediated tension- or drive-reducing properties, and that drinking in stressful situations would increase the probability of subsequent drinking in similar settings through the process of negative reinforcement. . . . More recent reviews have suggested that an individual's cognitive expectancies concerning the effects of alcohol may exert a greater degree of control over drinking and subsequent behavior than the pharmacological effects of the drug. . . . A number of specific expectations concerning alcohol appear to have developed through peer and parental modeling, past direct and indirect experiences with drinking and exposure to advertising media. . . . The first concerns the relationship between mood and alcohol consumption: alcohol is expected to reduce tension and eliminate or minimize negative affective states. . . . While the anticipated mood-altering effects of alcohol appear to motivate much drinking, how an individual expects to feel under the influence of alcohol does not always correspond to actual affective states while intoxicated. . . . Another specific expectancy is that alcohol will enhance social interaction and an individual's perception of personal control or power. . . . A final set of expectancies concerning drinking appears to have derived from assumptions of more traditional models of alcoholism, and are more applicable to alcoholics than to social drinkers. Problem drinkers who have internalized the belief system of such traditional models, particularly as espoused by Alcoholics Anonymous, expect to feel intermittent sensations of craving which may compel them to drink, with a resultant loss of control (Donovan and Marlatt, 1980, pp. 1159–1161).

Development of the "balanced placebo design," which permits an unencumbered view of alcohol's pharmacologic and expectancy-induced effects (Marlatt, Deming, and Reid, 1973; Wilson, 1981), has led to a diverse set of studies on the impact of expectations or beliefs about having consumed alcohol on subsequent drinking in alcoholics (Marlatt, Demming, and Reid, 1973), social anxiety (Wilson and Abrams, 1977), sexual responsiveness (Lansky and Wilson, 1981; Wilson and Lawson, 1976), aggression (Heermans and Nathan, 1982; Pihl et al., 1981), delay of gratification (Abrams and Wilson, 1980), mood states (McCollam et al., 1980), motor abilities (Vuchinich and Sobell, 1978), assertiveness (Parker, Gilbert, and Speltz, 1981), and cognitive processes such as attention and recognition memory (Lansky and Wilson, 1981). Generalizations from this research are difficult: Sometimes expectations about the impact of alcohol on behavior diverge from its actual effects (e.g., with regard to sexual responsiveness and mood), while at other times the two converge (e.g., vis-à-vis assertiveness and social anxiety). Convergence or divergence of expectations and drug effects, moreover, may vary as a function of subject sex, research setting, or experimental design. The unpredictability of findings on alcohol expectancies has led researchers in recent years away from efforts simply to identify additional behaviors affected by alcohol expectations and toward more active consideration of methodologic issues and more consistent attention to the clinical significance of expectancy phenomena.

Recent methodologic inquiries have concluded that (1) "cognitive labeling"(expectancy) explanations of alcohol effects may not exert as strong an influence on behavior as many have thought, due to the unduly narrow focus of some of the research on expectancies (e.g., only negative mood states rather than both negative and positive ones have been examined for expectancy effects) (Vuchinich and Tucker, 1980); (2) expectancy research (and the impact of expectancies on behavior) is limited by the amount of alcohol that can be given a subject before he/she will no longer subscribe to the experimental deception necessary for the study of this variable (Bradlyn, Stickler, and Maxwell, 1981); and (3) some studies using the balanced placebo have been faulty, rendering results uninterpretable, because (a) the credibility of the expectancy manipulation was not assessed, (b) the method of beverage presentation was not designed to heighten the credibility of the deception, and (c) subject variables affecting the deception were not taken into account (Rohsenow and Marlatt, 1981). These three papers highlight the emerging consensus that expectancies about the impact of alcohol on behavior are not so robust that they can be studied (or experienced) irrespective of crucial design shortcomings.

A related line of research involves exploration of alcohol expectancies by diverse groups of drinkers; these expectancies, presumably, influence decisions on when, where, and how much one drinks. One program of research (Brown et al., 1980; Christiansen and Goldman, 1983; Christiansen, Goldman, and Inn, 1982) identified six expectancy factors influencing problem and nonproblem drinking by both sexes across a wide age-range. The factors included physical tension reduction, diversion from worry, increased interpersonal power, magical transformation of experiences, enhanced pleasure, and modification of social-emotional behavior. While these findings are not surprising (the impact of all six expectancies has been explored empirically), the fact that these expectancies transcend age and sex differences and differentiate nonproblem and problem drinking adolescents as well is notable. Another recent survey of alcohol-related expectancies (Southwick et al., Lindell, 1981) also found differences between light and heavy drinkers in certain expectations about alcohol's effects: Heavy drinkers anticipated greater stimulation and pleasure from moderate drinking than lighter drinkers. A related, tantalizing finding that demands clarification is the report by a group of Norwegian investigators (Berg et al., 1981) that the drinking-related behavior of a group of 12 alcoholics, in an experimental drinking situation, was more heavily influenced by "instruction-induced expectancies" than was the behavior of a group of 12 social drinkers. Is alcoholic drinking a partial function of expectancies?

Alcohol, Blood Alcohol Level Discrimination Ability, and Tolerance. The conviction that tolerance to alcohol may be linked to development and maintenance of abusive consumption patterns is not a new one. Tolerance clearly influences drinking in two ways: It reduces the negative consequences of heavy drinking, especially in the young drinker, permitting heavier drinking than would otherwise be possible, and it lessens the positive consequences of drinking, motivating heavier drinking so that these desired consequences of drinking can be achieved.

Despite the apparent role tolerance plays in abusive drinking and, perhaps, even in the etiology of abusive drinking, the phenomenon has only recently been studied in human beings, both because its exploration requires actual alcohol administration and because reliable indices of human tolerance have been slow to develop. Most of the research described below developed from an initial interest in the disparate ability of alcoholics and nonalcoholics to discriminate their own levels of intoxication. [Actually, interest in discrimination capability derived from its possible role as a treatment method; only as the research progressed did it become clear that (1) blood alcohol level discrimination training had little therapeutic value and (2) it offered an approach to fuller understanding of human alcohol tolerance.]

Lovibond and Caddy (1970) were the first to explore blood alcohol level (BAL) discrimination training as a treatment for alcoholism. Two groups of their alcoholic subjects underwent BAL discrimination training during a single, two-hour session; the experimental group then received aversive shock conditioning designed to inhibit alcohol consumption at BAL's above 65 mg/%. Over the course of 6 to 12 sessions, given the opportunity to consume alcohol with instructions to maintain BAL below 65 mg/%, the experimental group received painful electric shock whenever they drank above the prescribed level while control subjects received random shock. At four months post-treatment, the experimental group was maintaining greater control over its drinking than the control group. Lovibond and Caddy attributed responsibility for this result to the

BAL discrimination skills and subsequent discriminated aversion they had effected.

Silverstein, Nathan, and Taylor (1974) decided to replicate and extend Lovibond and Caddy's study in order to examine the level of alcoholics' existing discrimination skills as well as factors involved in learning to monitor BAL. In the first, 10-day phase of their study, four male chronic alcoholics were given doses of alcohol during five, 2-day cycles sufficient to raise individual BALs on the first day of the cycle to 150 mg/%; by the end of the second day, to zero. During the first 2-day cycle, subjects estimated BALs eight times a day without receiving any feedback on the accuracy of their estimates. During the next three 2-day cycles, subjects were continuously alerted to the emotional and physical correlates of changing BAL while receiving accurate feedback after each estimate and positive reinforcement contingent on accurate BAL estimation for 50% of the trials. Training, feedback, and contingent reinforcement were withdrawn during the final 2-day cycle, in a return to baseline conditions. During the second phase of the study (lasting 26 days), three of the four alcoholics were trained successfully to reach and maintain a BAL of 80 mg/%.

Results from both phases of the study pointed to the external feedback on accuracy provided subjects after their own BAL estimates as the single most important factor influencing BAL estimation accuracy. Estimation error scores decreased substantially (from the first baseline session) during the training cycles (when feedback was provided) and increased again nearly to baseline levels when feedback was removed (during the second baseline session). Subjects were able to maintain BALs within prescribed limits during the second phase of the study only so long as accurate feedback was provided. Lovibond and Caddy's (1970) conclusion that their alcoholic subjects had learned to monitor internal cues of intoxication was called into question by these data (Lovibond and Caddy never actually directly assessed this ability, pre- or posttraining). As a consequence, Silverstein, Nathan, and Taylor (1974) concluded their report by suggesting that inability to monitor internal cues to intoxication may be an essential characteristic of alcoholic populations.

In a related study, Bois and Vogel-Sprott (1974) reported modest success training social drinkers to estimate BAL and, subsequently, to use the estimates to self-titrate alcohol intake. Nine male social drinkers estimated BAL without feedback on accuracy during an initial session, did so again with feedback during a second session, and then did so once again without feedback during a final session. Estimation accuracy, which improved from the first to the second sessions, remained high during the third session, despite the removal of feedback, suggesting that these social drinkers, unlike Silverstein, Nathan, and Taylor's alcoholics, could acquire and maintain the ability to estimate BAL on the basis of internal cues. (However, since programmed drink consumption was identical across sessions, subjects may also have linked these external cues to the feedback provided in the second session.)

Huber, Karlin, and Nathan (1976) next focused directly on whether nonalcoholics could acquire and maintain discrimination ability on the basis either of internal or external cues. After measures of pretraining estimation accuracy were obtained, 36 social drinkers were divided into three training groups, which received (a) internal training only, (b) external training only, or (c) both internal and external training. Internal training focused on changes in mood and bodily sensations as a basis for reflecting changes in BAL. External training relied on a programmed booklet designed to teach subjects relationships between amount and frequency of alcohol intake and changes in BAL. All subjects were provided feedback on accuracy after each estimate during this session.

Subjects gave all estimates without any feedback during the third, and final, test session. Half the subjects in each of the three training groups were told the actual alcohol content of their drinks; half were not. All subjects significantly improved BAL estimation accuracy during the second, training, session and then maintained this level of accuracy during the third, test, session, independent of the kind of training received and whether or not they had known the alcohol content of their test session drinks. These results raised, again, the possibility that a major difference between alcoholics and social drinkers may be the ability to monitor the internal consequences of drinking. However, since Silverstein, Nathan, and Taylor's study had not controlled for timing, knowledge of drink content, and other possible external cues to intoxication during drink administration, the question whether alcoholics could learn to discriminate BAL on the basis of internal cues remained open.

Accordingly, Lansky, Nathan, and Lawson (1978) replicated the study of social drinkers by Huber, Karlin, and Nathan (1976) with two groups of alcoholics, one receiving internal cue training, the other, external cue training. Unlike the social drinkers Huber and his colleagues studied, none of the alcoholic subjects could discriminate BAL when they depended on internal feelings and sensations for this purpose, although they could do so when using external cues.

At about the same time, Lansky et al. (1978) analyzed data from all subjects of BAL discrimination accuracy studies at Rutgers' Alcohol Behavior Research Laboratory to that time. They reported significant *baseline* discrimination ability differences between alcoholics and social drinkers: Social drinkers were better able to discriminate BAL before training than alcoholics. This finding suggested again that the inability to monitor the internal consequences of alcohol consumption may be a characteristic feature of chronic alcoholism.

The next step in the research program at the Rutgers Laboratory was investigation of the determinants of this difference between alcoholics and nonalcoholics. Environmental (drinking pattern), hereditary (familial alcoholism), and combined environmental-hereditary (tolerance level) factors were chosen for study. Accordingly, Lipscomb and Nathan (1980) divided a group of 24 undergraduate males into four experimental groups on the basis of drinking pattern (heavy versus light) and familial alcoholism (presence or absence of alcoholism in a parent). The subjects participated in a three-session BAL discrimination training and test procedure comparable to that used by Huber, Karlin, and Nathan (1976) and Lansky, Nathan, and Lawson (1978), but utilizing only internal cue training. No differences in BAL discrimination accuracy on the basis of drinking history or familial alcoholism were found. But when subjects were grouped according to performance on a standing-steadiness measure of tolerance, significant BAL discrimination accuracy differences were observed. Subjects with minimal sober-intoxicated body sway difference scores (defined as high tolerant) were significantly less accurate at BAL discrimination than those whose sober-intoxicated difference scores were maximal (defined as low tolerant).

Lipscomb and Nathan's failure to find a relationship linking familial alcoholism and tolerance conflicts with recent data reported by Schuckit and his colleagues (Schuckit, 1980; Schuckit et al., 1981). Male undergraduates and nonacademic staff with a positive family history of alcoholism were matched with a control group according to drinking history, race, and height-to-weight ratio. None of the matched subjects had parents or siblings diagnosed as alcoholic, and none fulfilled criteria for alcoholism. Measures of blood acetaldehyde levels, subjective intoxication, and EMG were taken at 30-minute intervals after ethanol was ingested by subjects in both groups. Positive family history subjects consistently demonstrated less subjective intoxication during the course of the experiment, suggesting greater tolerance to the behavioral effects of alcohol.

The disparity between the two studies in the strength of the link between family history of alcoholism and tolerance, observed by Schuckit and his co-workers but not by Nathan and his colleagues, may be best explained by referring to the interaction of the effects of family history and drinking history. Specifically, it is possible that family history of alcoholism is associated with predisposition to develop early, rapid tolerance to alcohol *which is only realized when sustained alcohol consumption occurs.* In other words, only by heavy drinking would family history influence tolerance development. In this regard, the subjects in Schuckit's study may have been drinking longer and more heavily than those in Lipscomb and Nathan's study (though differences in drinking history measures between the two studies make a direct comparison impossible). Differences in criteria used to select subjects with a positive family history of alcoholism may also have played a role in this disparity. While Lipscomb and Nathan (1980) required subjects claiming a family history of alcoholism to point to a parent who had sought or received treatment for alcohol abuse, Schuckit looked for major life problems related to alcohol, including marital separation or divorce, multiple arrests, physical evidence that alcohol had harmed health, or a job loss or layoff related to drinking. Perhaps Schuckit's criteria yielded subjects whose parents or siblings were more likely to have been diagnosed as primary alcoholics and who may have also consumed larger quantities of alcohol throughout their lifetimes. Again, between-study comparisons are difficult because detailed information on the drinking histories of parents and siblings is not available.

Research currently under way at Rutgers' Alcohol Behavior Research Laboratory aims to elucidate the process and mechanisms of tolerance development in persons all the way along the social-drinker–alcoholic continuum. At this time, drinking history and expectancy and classical conditioning effects are being studied in order to begin exploration of the manner in which tolerance may manifest itself across levels and patterns of alcohol consumption, as well as to identify factors responsible for development of tolerance in both the short- and long-term.

An early study in this program investigates relationships between drinking history—prior exposure to alcohol—and tolerance development. As mentioned previously, the negative findings in the Lipscomb and Nathan study (1980) may have been due, in part, to measurement problems surrounding the assessment of drinking histories. Accordingly, the study explores measures and models of alcohol consumption and drinking history most predictive of tolerance development. In recognition of the striking paucity of data on the time course of development, maintenance, and dissipation of tolerance in humans, the study investigates conflicting theories, derived from the animal literature, linking time, consumption, and degree of behavioral tolerance. Among questions for which answers are sought are (1) how long it takes tolerance to develop in a heavy-drinking person, (2) whether prior heavy drinking, followed by a period of abstention, affects subsequent development of tolerance, (3) whether, and to what extent, tolerance is characteristic of social-drinking—as against heavy-drinking—populations, and (4) to what extent acute and chronic tolerance are related.

Young social drinkers have been recruited to participate in a five-session tolerance induction and assessment study. Males between the ages of 19 and 25 have been divided by drinking patterns (heavy and light) and whether they have been drinking at their present level of consumption for less or more than three years. Drinking histories are assessed by an interview designed to provide an accurate picture of alcohol consumption over the last year and an exhaustive description of the immediate past nine weeks of drinking [Armor and Polich's interview format (1982) is used, in part, for this purpose].

Each subject participates in a single-session, alcohol-free training and habituation period, in which all tolerance measures are administered repeatedly. This step is designed to bring performance to a stable baseline and to control for practice effects during the subsequent tolerance induction and testing phases of the study. During the next experimental session, subjects are tested for initial levels of tolerance three times—once while sober, and twice after consuming 1 gm/kg absolute ethanol in a 1 to 4 solution of tonic water. The pre-post alcohol test sequences are timed so that ascending and descending limb comparisons can be made at the same average BAL, yielding a measure of acute tolerance. Prior to the next (third) session, all subjects refrain from consuming alcohol for two weeks to allow tolerance to dissipate. This design feature allows a "carry-over" effect to be demonstrated, should one exist. Subjects are then tested three more times; each session is separated by one alcohol-free day, to induce further tolerance.

A battery of sensory-perceptual, psychomotor, and cognitive measures of tolerance are administered to determine whether and how tolerance may generalize across functions. A system of incentives for good test performance is utilized to minimize variability due to motivational differences and to maximize chances of observing a tolerance effect.

Increasing evidence has accumulated to suggest that environmental cues present at the time of drug and alcohol intake may be important in the development of tolerance (Hinson and Siegel, 1980; LePoulos and Cappell, 1979; Siegel, 1975). This body of evidence supports a classical conditioning model of tolerance in which environmental cues associated with prior drug intake are seen to elicit conditioned compensatory reactions which attenuate the systemic effects of the drug. The conditioned stimuli (CS) are the cues associated with drug administration. The unconditioned stimulus (UCS) is drug consumption. The conditioned response is demonstrated by presenting the usual cues for drug administration (CS) in the absence of the drug itself (UCS). According to classical conditioning theory, the CR should then mimic the UCR. However, evidence to suggest that the CR is often opposite in direction to the UCR (perhaps to prepare the organism for the unconditioned effect of the drug) has been reported. As a consequence of the repeated pairings of stimuli related to drug intake with the systemic effects of the drug, the conditioned compensatory reaction often increases in magnitude. As the compensatory CR increases in magnitude, the effect of the drug decreases, producing tolerance.

This view of tolerance development is strongly supported in the animal literature, but no direct study of conditioning processes involving humans has yet been attempted. In order to test the validity of the hypothesis in human subjects, they should appear tolerant only when they are tested in the presence of the environmental cues associated with drug administration. This "discriminative control of tolerance" design (Siegel, 1975) was employed in a study recently completed at the Alcohol Behavior Research Laboratory.

After pretest and habituation to all measures, two groups of subjects participated in a 10-session tolerance development program. Both groups received an equal number of administrations of alcohol and a nonalcoholic substance on an alternating schedule during the first phase of the experiment. The only difference between the groups was with respect to the environmental cues associated with ingestion. One group consistently received alcohol in a "home" environment, a small bedroom with comfortable features, while the nonalcoholic beverage was consumed in a "distinct" environment, a large testing room containing physiological recording equipment. The other group was treated in the same fashion except that the consumption of beverages was reversed between the "home" and "distinct" environments. In addition, the taste cues for each beverage were disguised with colors and flavors so that subjects could not associate a particular beverage with a certain environment. After the tolerance induction phase of the study was completed, each subject was tested twice more: once in the tolerance test phase when all subjects consumed alcohol in the "distinct" environment, and once in the compensatory test phase when all subjects received a nonalcoholic beverage to drink, also in the "distinct" environment. Cognitive, psychomotor, mood, and physiological tests of tolerance were administered throughout.

Expected findings include that (1) subjects who expected alcohol (who drank alcohol in the "distinct" environment) will display greater evidence of tolerance than subjects who did not expect alcohol during the tolerance test phase of the experiment, and (2) subjects who expected alcohol will display compensatory responses opposite in direction to the unconditioned effects of alcohol when they were tested in the "distinct" environment, while subjects who did not expect alcohol will not change relative to their nonalcohol baseline during the compensatory response phase of the experiment.

Research in the planning stage includes a study of early experiences with alcohol by alcoholics and nonalcoholics to test the hypothesis that alcoholics experienced greater levels of tolerance early in their drinking, and studies determining whether tolerance and the cognitive dysfunctions associated with chronic alcohol ingestion share more than a similar time-course.

3. Assessment of Reinforcement Hierarchies and Potentials for Remediation

Interest in reinforcement hierarchies by behavior therapists has been longstanding. Shortly after individual behavior change techniques began to be developed, behavior therapists felt the need to construct questionnaires and checklists on which patients could indicate the specific kinds of behaviors they found most and least reinforcing. Even though reinforcement checklists suffered from the same shortcomings of other self-report instruments, they did provide therapists some information on the kinds of reinforcers that might be used to induce behavior change.

Cohen, Bigelow, Griffiths, Liebson, and their colleagues at the Baltimore City Hospitals went well beyond dependence on self-report instruments in their systematic exploration of environmental reinforcers capable of modifying maladaptive drinking (e.g., Bigelow et al., 1972; Bigelow et al., 1981; Bigelow et al., Griffiths, 1976). Among their findings are the following: (1) An enriched—more comfortable, more interesting—living environment was preferred over an impoverished one to the extent that consumption was reduced when "moderate" drinking led to access to the enriched environment. (2) Drinking was also reduced when a brief period of contingent social isolation followed consumption of 1-ounce drinks of beverage alcohol. (3) Opportunity to earn a weekend pass to visit friends or family similarly resulted in reduced drinking when the passes were contingent upon moderate drinking.

Explicit behavioral exploration of potentials for remediation in the environment have taken a variety of forms. They are discussed below in our review of behavioral treatment methods effective in the natural environment.

B. Behavioral Treatment of Alcoholism

1. Goals of Treatment

Until the decade of the 1970s, virtually every alcoholism worker accepted but one treatment goal: total, complete, and absolute abstinence. Choice of this goal was based upon the widely held conviction that alcoholism is a physical disease characterized by craving for alcohol during periods of sobriety, loss of control over drinking during periods of intoxication, and associated neurologic, gastrointestinal, cardiac, and hematologic disorders secondary to the disease of alcoholism.

There are several other good reasons for maintaining abstinence as the sole criterion of successful treatment for alcoholism. Adoption of the disease model of alcoholism—concluding that alcoholism is a physical disease—both removes the moral stigma from which alcoholics have long suffered and justifies the abstinence criterion because one cannot, obviously, provide a sick person with the agent which has caused his/her sickness. Further, abstinence is the easiest of all treatment goals to define and monitor. One is either abstinent or one is not; there are no degrees of abstinence. In addition, abstinence is a goal appropriate for all alcoholics: One would certainly not want one's alcoholic taxi driver, pilot, surgeon, or accountant to aspire to anything else. Finally, for those alcoholics whose alcoholism has been accompanied by serious physical sequelae, a treatment goal that does not center on abstinence is life-threatening.

Given this weight of public and professional opinion, why has another treatment goal—that of controlled social drinking—engendered so much public support—and public controversy? In our judgment, the concept of controlled social drinking achieved viability because of the following:

1. Some alcoholics drink normally, in controlled fashion, either spontaneously or following treatment, for substantial periods of time.
2. Abstinence, apparently, is not always a component of successful treatment for alcoholism. In fact, some alcoholics report far greater personal distress during periods of abstinence than during periods of moderate alcohol consumption.
3. The disease model of alcoholism—and its corollaries, loss of control and craving—does not seem to have firm basis in empirical fact.

There is now a substantial literature, appearing mostly during the last 15 years, which suggests that some abusive drinkers—the precise number and kind remain uncertain—adopt patterns of controlled social drinking either spontaneously or following treatment (Miller and Caddy, 1977). While many alcoholics maintain such a pattern for only a brief time before lapsing again into uncontrolled consumption, the voluminous literature attesting to controlled drinking by alcoholics (dating from publication in 1962 of Davies' follow-up of 93 recovered "alcohol addicts") is nonetheless impressive. However, as reviewers of this literature (Brownell, 1982; Emrick, 1975, 1982; Hamburg, 1975; Nathan, 1981; Nathan and Lansky, 1978) acknowledge, many of these studies share conceptual and methodologic shortcomings. Among these problems are small sample size, too-brief follow-up, inadequate assessment of drinking behavior during follow-up, inaccurate initial diagnosis of alcoholism, and imprecise definition of "controlled drinking" posttreatment.

Many of the same criticisms have been voiced of the "Rand Reports" (Armor, Polich, and Stambul, 1978; Polich, Armor, and Braiker, 1981), a national survey of approximately 14,000 clients of 44 federally funded Alcoholism Treatment Centers. The major finding offered in the 1978 report—that some 70% of clients completing treatment showed improvement in drinking behavior at 6- and 18-month follow-ups—received surprisingly little attention compared to the following secondary finding:

> While this improvement rate is impressive, it is important to stress that the improved clients include only a relatively small number who are long-term abstainers. About one-fourth of the clients interviewed at 18 months have abstained for at least six months. . . . The majority of improved clients are either drinking moderate amounts of alcohol—but at levels far below what could be described as alcoholic drinking—or engaging in alternating periods of drinking and abstention (Armor et al., p. v).

Among the findings of the four-year report (Polich, Armor, and Braiker, 1981) were that (1) roughly one in five of patients followed through the four-year period who were both alive and could be interviewed at the four-year mark were judged to be drinking without problems, (2) nonproblem drinkers were no more likely than abstainers to manifest concurrent psychiatric symptoms, and (3) nonproblem drinkers did not appear more likely than abstainers to relapse into problem drinking.

Despite the fact that these findings are not relevant to the question of nonproblem drinking treatment goals because none of the treatment programs surveyed maintained such goals, critics of the Rand reports have chided their authors for advocating controlled-drinking treatment over abstinence-oriented treatment. While the Rand Reports are irrelevant to the arguments surrounding choice of goals of treatment, they do provide additional proof that some alcoholics, during some of their lives, drink without problems—just as, during other periods of their lives, they remain abstinent. A relatively small number of alcoholics appear capable of maintaining nonproblem drinking patterns for lengthy time periods; those who do are generally younger and less deteriorated physically, psychologically, and socially.

As problematic as it is to use data from the Rand Studies to enlighten oneself on the controversial matter of treatment goals, it is as difficult to evaluate their methodology to determine the validity of their findings. An assessment of the 18-month study's design and procedures in the first edition of this book remains helpful:

Most of the follow-up assessments were based on patients' self-reports of changes in drinking behavior and in vocational and familial adjustment. Self-reports have been criticized by many as unreliable and self-serving. Further, improvement in psychological functioning, job performance, family adjustment, and drinking behavior was not measured directly. . . . Finally, much more emphasis was placed on the significance of improvements in drinking as a measure of therapeutic efficacy than improvements in other important areas of life functioning, a decision which has been questioned. . . . But the Rand Study also had important strengths. It surveyed a very large group of geographically and demographically diverse clients with relatively sophisticated sampling procedures designed to ensure the representativeness of the sample. It developed survey instruments which sampled a broad range of behaviors relevant to alcoholism. It followed subjects for longer than the usual follow-up interval and succeeded in reaching over 2000 of them at the 6-month mark and over 600 at 18 months. Finally, the study was designed to permit pre- and post-treatment comparisons of subjects' level of functioning in a variety of spheres. . . . In short, the survey could be considered a representative model of modern survey methodology (Nathan and Lipscomb, 1979, pp. 318–319).

In terms of subject numbers, design scope, and follow-up intervals as well as sampling methods and procedures, the four-year Rand Study continues at the state-of-the-art of survey research. In fact, the four-year study was improved considerably over its predecessor. It incorporated a number of positive changes in follow-up and self-report procedures: Multiple collateral measures absent in the 18-month report were added; the follow-up "hit" rate was increased from 60% at 18 months to 85% at four years, decreasing the possibility of nonresponse bias; the lengthening of the drinking assessment period from 30 days to 6 months resulted in the reclassification of short-term abstainers in the 18-month study and a subsequent reduction in the percentage of remission from 67% to 54%. In addition, the criteria used for determining alcohol problems at four years were made more stringent. Taken together, these methodological changes strengthen the four-year report. However, limitations inherent in the study's original design remain. These include (1) the absence of a noncontract control group, along with insufficient data to determine if the contract group was equivalent to other groups at baseline, a group without which it is impossible to determine if improvement is related to treatment, to regression to the mean, or to spontaneous remission; (2) the absence of multiple samples on all measures across the four-year follow-up period; and (3) discrepancies in operational definitions of dependent variables between the 18-month and four-year studies.

The two Rand reports lend support to the controversial conclusions, cited above, that (1) some alcoholics drink normally, in controlled fashion; (2) abstinence does not always have to be a part of successful alcoholism treatment; and (3) craving and loss of control are not invariable accompaniments of alcoholism. The reports do not, however, add anything to the issue of the viability of controlled social drinking treatment.

A variety of explicit behavioral attempts to induce controlled drinking have been reported over the past several years. Most of these therapeutic approaches have claimed that their techniques change abusive drinking into controlled social drinking in some subjects for some length of time. Unfortunately, like the literature on spontaneous return to controlled drinking, this literature cannot answer the crucial questions: How many alcoholics? For how long a time? Our own analysis of these studies is that, with one exception (the well-known study by Mark and Linda Sobell, discussed in detail below), outcome data on controlled drinking treatment of chronic alcoholics has not been encouraging. We conclude that sufficient data do not exist to justify widespread application of controlled drinking treatment to groups of alcoholic clients. By contrast, more recent research on controlled drinking treatment for problem drinkers (also reviewed below) is more promising. It suggests that these methods may be useful to persons who have not yet developed alcohol dependence. Very recent studies also indicate that nonproblem-drinking methods may comprise an effective prevention strategy for persons at risk to develop drinking problems, suggesting another avenue for exploration of these procedures.

The traditional view that craving and loss of control invariably accompany abusive drinking, in that way proving that alcoholism is a physical disease, has also been questioned on empirical grounds. To this end, research indicates both that alcohol given to sober alcoholics in disguised form often fails to induce craving for the subtance (e.g., Cutter, Schwaab, and Nathan, 1970; Marlatt, Demming, and Reid, 1973; Merry, 1966) and that many alcoholics who have been drinking in uncontrolled fashion can modify their drinking on being given appropriate contingent reinforcement for doing so (Gottheil, Crawford, and Cornelison, 1973; Marlatt, 1978; Nathan and O'Brien, 1971; Strickler et al., 1976). If craving and loss of control are not universal phenomena, does this not raise the question of the general validity of the physical disease model of alcoholism?

Another traditional view, that the alcoholic who achieves abstinence will also demonstrate improvement in other areas of functioning, has also been challenged by Miller and Caddy (1977) and Pattison (1976), both of whom cite an impressive number of studies which show that

. . . the use of total abstinence as the outcome criterion of alcoholism treatment is misleading. It may be associated with improvement, no change, or deterioration in other critical areas of total life health (Pattison, 1976, p. 180).

In fact, data from the four-year Rand Study (Polich, Armor, and Braiker, 1981) suggested that certain groups of nonproblem drinkers had a better prognosis for an enhanced quality of life than some groups of abstainers (this relationship, valid for younger nonproblem drinkers, did not hold for older ones).

Given these data—and the strongly held views of those who hold divergent opinions on the question of treatment goals, we offer the following guidelines for choice of treatment goals, subject to change as more data illuminate the issue.

1. For a variety of reasons, abstinence ought to be the goal of treatment for alcoholism. These reasons include the accepted notions that most of us function better when we are sober, that abstinence-oriented treatment works for many persons while the success rate of controlled-drinking treatment, especially for alcoholics, is problematic, and that death follows the decision of many chronic alcoholics to resume or continue drinking.

2. Alcoholics who have achieved sobriety must not be led to believe that they can ever drink in controlled fashion; no available data suggest that we have the means to enable alcoholics to achieve that goal.

3. Alcoholics who have repeatedly tried and failed to achieve abstinence, who despair of ever doing so, who remain physically able to drink moderately, and who are sufficiently intact intellectually to understand the hazards of drinking moderately and the consequences of failing to do so can be considered candidates for controlled drinking treatment—but only as a last resort. The reason? A pattern of controlled social drinking, less desirable than abstinence, is nonetheless more desirable than uncontrolled social drinking.

4. Problem drinkers and those at risk for problems with alcohol now appear to be the "clients of choice" for controlled drinking treatment and prevention. Whether controlled drinking treatment is the treatment of choice for these individuals, however, remains to be seen. Hence, clinicians should exercise great care in choosing this treatment goal for these clients.

5. What is needed most, before rational decisions on treatment goals can be made for anyone, is additional comparative research on the applicability, efficacy, and permanence of the results both of abstinence-oriented and controlled-drinking-oriented treatment of alcoholics, problem drinkers, and those at risk for either or both.

2. Behavioral Treatment Procedures That Focus on Abusive Drinking

Electrical Aversion. It is ironic that the behavior therapy procedure most closely linked with both behavior therapy and alcoholism—electrical aversion—is almost certainly ineffective.

One of the major reasons that electrical aversion has been associated through the years with both behavior therapy and the behavioral treatment of alcoholism was the reported success of Soviet physician N. V. Kantorovich's use of electrical aversion more than 50 years ago. Pairing the sight, taste, and smell of beverage alcohol with painful electric shock, Kantorovich reported that 70% of his small group of subjects had remained abstinent during follow-up periods ranging from 3 weeks to 20 months. Control subjects given hypnotic suggestion or medication did not do nearly so well.

Despite these early findings, it was not until the 1960s that investigators began concurrent exploration of the efficacy of electrical aversion as treatment for both homosexual and alcoholic behavior. Though most researchers, including McGuire and Vallance (1964), Blake (1965, 1967), MacCulloch, Feldman, and Orford (1966), and Sandler (1969), reported varying degrees of "success," critical evaluation of their research reveals small numbers of subjects, short follow-up periods, relatively small proportions of patients maintaining abstinence, and the absence of direct efforts to assess development of actual conditioned aversion to ethanol. That none of these studies incorporated a control group or offered a "standard" treatment for comparative purposes adds to our skepticism concerning these results.

The late 1960s and 1970s signaled the advent of more adequate research on electrical aversion: Control groups began to be employed, more subjects were chosen for each study, better measures of outcome were used, and electrical aversion was more often embedded in more comprehensive treatment packages than before. To this end, Vogler and his colleagues (1970, 1971) reported encouraging short-term abstinence data but disproportionate losses of subjects from electrical aversion treatment groups. Miller and his co-workers (1973) found no difference in consumption between experimental and control subjects on Miller's "taste test." And after Hedberg and Campbell (1974) compared four separate behavioral treatment approaches (behavioral family counseling, systematic desensitization, covert sensitization, and electrical aversion), they reported that electrical aversion, unlike the other three treatment methods, had absolutely no impact on drinking by alcoholic subjects.

Perhaps the most convincing demonstration of the ineffectiveness of electrical aversion as a treatment for alcoholism was that by Wilson, Leaf, and Nathan (1975). After receiving a very large number of aversion conditioning trials extending over several days, their alcoholic subjects were permitted to drink *ad libitum* in a laboratory setting which neither encouraged nor discouraged consumption. Results were that subjects drank with undiminished enthusiasm, just as they had during a compara-ble *ad libitum* period pretreatment; Wilson and his coworkers concluded that conditioned aversion had not been established by the aversion condi-tioning procedure.

We conclude, then, that electrical aversion conditioning does not induce conditioned aversion to ethanol and, for that reason, does not merit further consideration as a treatment for alcoholism.

Covert Sensitization. Covert sensitization is an aversion technique that has been used to diminish a variety of "approach disorders," includ-ing smoking, obesity, sexual deviance, and alcoholism. Developed by Cautela (1966, 1970), covert sensitization aims to induce aversion by verbal means; the aversive goal is, usually, nausea. Anant (1967) strengthened the reach of covert sensitization for alcoholics by emphasiz-ing the (imagined) taste of the target beverage in the process of verbal induction of nausea, in order to pair taste and nausea to establish a con-ditioned aversion. A more detailed review of covert sensitization is pro-vided by Elkins (1975).

Despite strong evidence that humans do acquire genuine taste aver-sions and that this capacity can be exploited to treat alcoholism (see, for example, the following section reviewing chemical aversion treatment for alcoholics), covert sensitization has not heretofore been considered effec-tive, largely because treatment studies reported on small numbers of sub-jects, followed for brief periods of time and assessed by weak outcome measures.

However, a recent report on use of covert sensitization as a principal alcoholism treatment modality (Elkins, 1980) is much more adequate methodologically and much more convincing clinically. Of 57 chronic alcoholic subjects (one of whom was female) who entered treatment, 52 remained in treatment for at least six covert sensitization sessions. A variety of physiological correlates of nausea (including respiratory and GSR changes) confirmed nausea induction in 45 subjects. Of this group, 29 developed "conditioned nausea," which means that an association was established between alcohol cues (e.g., sight, smell, taste, and swal-lowing) and the experience of nausea. Mean total abstinence after dis-charge for this group of subjects was 13.74 months; the other subjects were abstinent, on average, for fewer than 5 months.

While these data neither establish the superiority of this treatment technique over other methods nor assess the method's cost-effectiveness, they do suggest the need for modification of the prevailing view that covert sensitization is no more useful than electrical aversion in the treat-ment of alcoholism—subject, of course, to extensive additional con-firmatory findings.

Response Prevention. Response prevention, proven effective for phobic and compulsive disorders (Nathan, Witte, and Langenbucher, 1983), is aptly named. Phobic patients are prevented from escaping from situations in which they are phobic; compulsive patients are prevented from emitting the ritualized behavior they believe necessary to avoid the anxiety they anticipate in its absence.

A similar treatment method has recently been tested on a small group (N = 6) of Scottish alcoholics (Blakey and Baker, 1980). After a thorough behavioral assessment, which yielded comprehensive data on patients' drinking antecedents and consequences, all six subjects were first exposed to the actual stimuli most strongly associated with their drinking, and then prevented from drinking. Thus,

A 42-year old married man, whose second marriage had recently broken up, had been a heavy drinker for many years and suffered slight liver damage. Prior to his in-patient admission he was drinking beer at every available opportunity. He was seen as an in-patient. The assessment of his drinking indicated that opening times and being in pubs were important antecedent stimuli. Also, general periods of stress, and nagging and arguments with his wife led to his drowning his sorrows in a big way. The treatment involved patient and therapist going to pubs together, at first in "easy" ones (where he knew few people) with the plan of progressing to his well-known pubs . . . the therapist and patient drank soft drinks whilst in the pub. Two sessions were conducted in different pubs, both of which the patient previously dreaded, predicting that he would not be able to cope. However, they proved far less difficult than he predicted. He had been trying to trace his wife, who was at that stage located and he decided to leave the area. He felt he had sufficiently mastered his drinking to totally abstain . . . (Blakey and Baker, 1980, p. 322).

Given the promise of response prevention with other behavioral disorders and the fact that five of six chronic alcoholics treated in this study remained abstinent at follow-up intervals up to nine months, response prevention appears to hold considerable appeal, especially in a multifaceted program designed to confront not simply the client's excessive drinking but other associated behavioral excesses and deficits as well.

Chemical Aversion. In the 1940s and 1950s, Voegtlin, Lemere, and their colleagues at the Shadel Hospital in Seattle published a series of reports on the successful use of chemical aversion to treat alcoholism. Until a few recent publications by Wiens, Neubuerger, and their colleagues at Raleigh Hills hospitals in Portland, Oregon, and Sacramento, California, appeared, reports on chemical aversion were conspicuously lacking from the literature. This surprising lack of interest in a treatment with as extensive and as promising an early history as chemical aversion derived in large part from much stronger, long-lived (and, it now seems, misplaced) interest among behavioral clinicians in electric shock as a stimulus for conditioning aversion to ethanol.

In partial explanation of the apparent success of chemical aversion and failure of electrical aversion to establish conditioned aversion to ethanol, Wilson and Davison (1969) and Garcia, Hankins, and Rusiniak (1974) suggest that nausea is "biologically appropriate" to alcohol while electric shock is not: Many people have experienced nausea, few, electric shock, after drinking. For this reason alcoholics are more likely to develop and maintain an association between alcohol and nausea than between alcohol and shock. Baker and his colleagues (Baker and Cannon, 1982; Crawford and Baker, 1982) offer another empirically based explanation: Taste-mediated learning is a principal means by which animals make judgments, often after only one trial, on the wholesomeness of food; hence, when taste-mediated learning involves the pairing of a nausea-inducing drug with the strong taste of beverage alcohol, it is likely to be acquired, and to persist, by animal and human being.

The procedures followed at the Shadel Hospital were described by Voegtlin (1940) and Lemere and Voegtlin (1950). In brief, patients were hospitalized for approximately 10 days; the five treatment sessions were spaced on alternate days. Treatment sessions were held in rooms specially designed to minimize distractions and maximize visibility of a large array of alcoholic beverages. An emetine-pilocarpine-ephedrine mixture was administered intravenously, producing nausea within 2 to 8 minutes. Immediately prior to initial signs of nausea, the patient was given a drink of his/her preferred beverage to smell, then to taste. Further drinks were given over a 30-minute to 1-hour period, as nausea and vomiting persisted.

"Booster" reconditioning sessions were generally offered to all patients at any time they felt the urge to drink, or, routinely, 6 to 12 months after inpatient treatment.

With some variation, essentially the same treatment sequence continues to be followed at the Shadel Hospital as well as at the several Raleigh Hills hospitals which also offer chemical aversion as the cornerstone of their alcoholism treatment efforts.

Results of the first 13 years of treatment at the Shadel Hospital were based on follow-up data from 4096 of 4468 patients treated, a most impressive follow-up of 92%. Forty-four percent of these patients had remained totally abstinent over 2 to 13 years, while another 7% had relapsed and been successfully retreated. Of patients followed up, 60% had been abstinent for one year, 51% for 2 years, 38% for 5 years, and 23% for 10 years.

These outcome data are remarkably similar to those reported more recently by other facilities offering chemical aversion treatment. Wiens et al. (1976) reported that 63% of 261 alcoholic patients treated by emetine conditioning at Raleigh Hills Hospital in Portland were abstinent after one year, results strikingly similar to the one-year figure of 60% cited by Lemere and Voegtlin. This figure is even more impressive since the Portland group considered patients who could not be located for follow-up as treatment failures. The Portland Hospital has also examined outcomes for a subgroup of 78 persons treated during the years 1978–1979 who were 65 years or older on admission (Wiens et al., 1983). The expectation was that these clients would benefit less from treatment than younger clients, on the assumption that they have fewer personal and familial resources on which to base posttreatment sobriety. Surprisingly, follow-up revealed that 65.4% of these clients had maintained continuous sobriety over a 12-month follow-up period.

Two reports from another Raleigh Hills hospital, located in Sacramento, California, add to the conviction that chemical aversion, in the context of the multidimensional program provided at these hospitals, is an effective treatment for alcoholism (Neubuerger et al., 1981; Neubuerger et al., 1982). Surveying patients treated at the hospital between 1976–1979, the authors report one-year abstinence rates averaging 54% (ranging from a low of 36% for patients who were younger than 62 years of age, disabled, unemployed, and on Medicare, to a high of 73% for patients who were married and employed).

Why do these outcome data appear to be so much better than those from other approaches to alcoholism? One answer is that alcoholics undergoing chemical aversion treatment now, as in the 1940s, probably enter treatment with better prognoses than those who enter most other kinds of treatment. To begin with, patients entering chemical aversion programs (which are costly) must have substantial private financial resources or health insurance, both of which would require them to be either recently or still employed. Recent or current employment suggests a modicum of ability to function adequately in the world. Further, these patients also differ in educational and socioeconomic level from alcoholics treated elsewhere, additional indications of their superior treatment potential. Finally, patients who complete a chemical aversion treatment sequence must be highly motivated to change their drinking behavior because the treatment is both expensive and extremely unpleasant. It is well accepted, of course, that positive treatment motivation is one of the most important predictors of successful treatment.

It is also worth noting that abstinence rates for "graduates" of the Shadel program were positively related to the number of booster sessions patients attended, while 67% of Raleigh Hills patients abstinent for one year had attended an average of six reconditioning sessions. Periodic booster reconditioning sessions clearly are important in maintaining the effectiveness of this treatment mode, a conclusion echoed by other behavior therapists (e.g., Sobell and Sobell, 1973; Vogler et al., 1975).

Chemical aversion is not the only therapeutic modality available to patients at the Shadel and Raleigh Hills facilities. Rehabilitation and personal counseling, family therapy, a variety of behavioral self-control methods, and access to local Alcoholics Anonymous groups, all provided in a supportive atmosphere, are regular components of the therapy package offered at these facilities.

Research exploring whether pairing chemically induced nausea with alcohol produces a reliable aversion to alcohol in humans has recently been reported. Cannon and Baker (1981) randomly assigned 20 male alcoholic volunteers to a chemical aversion conditioning group (N = 7), an electrical shock aversion conditioning group (N = 7), and a nontreatment control group (N = 6). Only subjects in the chemical aversion group acquired conditioned aversion to alcohol; the aversion was reflected in attitudinal, behavioral, and psychophysiological changes. Cannon, Baker, and Wehl (1981) followed up these 20 subjects, reporting that chemical aversion subjects were drinking somewhat less than subjects in the other two groups at the six-month follow-up mark, but that the three groups did not differ in drinking outcomes at the one-year mark. Clearly, much more research on both the nature and extent of aversion consequent to chemical aversion conditioning, as well as its relationship to changes in drinking behavior, are called for.

We conclude that chemical aversion can be effective in the context of a carefully orchestrated treatment program accompanied by adjunctive counseling and attention to social support systems and followed by booster sessions.

3. Behavioral Treatment Procedures That Focus on Antecedents and Consequences of Drinking

Contingency Contracting. The phrase "contingency contracting" describes a behavior modification procedure familiar to every parent: the making of a prior agreement with a child that performance of a desired behavior or modification or elimination of an unwanted behavior will produce a consequence that is reinforcing both to child and parent.

Contingencies have always been a part of both formal and informal treatment for alcoholism. The alcoholic whose wife refuses to talk to him, have sex with him, or cook for him if his drinking continues is being subjected to a punishment contingency, as is the saleswoman who is told that she will lose her job if she continues to drink. Professionals with limited experience with alcoholics often marvel at the dramatic ineffectiveness of these powerful contingencies—at the fact that alcoholics continue to drink in the face of such dire consequences. The behavioral explanation of this paradox is twofold: (1) What may be punishing to an observer may be reinforcing—or at least not punishing—to the alcoholic. And (2) a contingency is effective only when it is based on mutual agreement, carefully observed, and consistently carried out; spouses and employers rarely adhere to contingency contracts as rigorously as they should for maximum effectiveness.

In a very real sense, Alcoholics Anonymous involves the contingent management of alcoholics. Among AA's most effective sources of therapeutic effectiveness are the social sanctions attached to membership in the group. The longer the alcoholic remains dry and a member of AA, the more severe the ultimate punishing contingency for drinking again: disapproval by sponsor and fellow members who have become increasingly important to the now-dry alcoholic. Why is this contingency more effective for many alcoholics than the threat of losing family, friends, and job? Because AA membership, often a last resort for those who have lost all other reason to live, is shared with men and women whose fellowship is based upon common experience and common tragedy. To lose their friendship or to let them down is truly to give up on oneself and them— once and for all.

Contingency management, to be most effective, must draw upon individuals and settings in the alcoholic's life situation which have the potential to support or maintain beneficial change in drinking behavior. As such, these potentials for remediation in the environment have presumably already been identified by the contingency manager in his/her initial behavioral assessment of the alcoholic.

"Community Reinforcement Counseling." A contingency management approach that successfully enlisted a wide range of community support systems was the "community reinforcement counseling" program developed by Hunt and Azrin (1973) and later modified by Azrin (1976). The program was designed to provide chronic alcoholic inpatients with focused behavioral training to improve vocational, interpersonal, and familial problems of long standing. Once family, job, and friends began to be experienced as more reinforcing by the alcoholics (because they were successful in dealing with them), these new-found reinforcers could be incorporated into a contingency management program in which the patients, now living outside the hospital, were permitted continued access to them contingent on sobriety. At a six-month follow-up, the eight alcoholics who had received community reinforcement counseling had spent significantly less time drinking, unemployed, away from home, or in-

stitutionalized than eight other alcoholics provided only the hospital's standard therapy program.

A subsequent modification of the community reinforcement counseling method, reported by Azrin (1976), yielded outcome data that were just as positive. The same basic contingency format was employed, along with the following modifications: (1) Disulfiram was given all experimental clients in order to reduce the likelihood that impulsive drinking would reduce the effectiveness of the contingency contract. (2) A regular reporting system, which relied on clients, family, friends, and employers, was instituted to provide counselors with immediate "early warning" of clients' drinking or other problems. (3) A neighborhood "buddy," who offered himself as a source of continuing social support both before and after formal professional counseling stopped, was selected and trained for peer advisement. (4) Group counseling, to reduce the amount of expensive professional time required for individual counseling, was begun. With these changes, instituted to enhance the effectiveness of community reinforcement counseling, to extend its therapeutic impact beyond its formal termination date, and to reduce its cost, the 10 patients in the modified program showed significant improvement along a variety of dimensions over 10 control-group patients.

Why do so few alcoholics provided traditional therapy and so many of Azrin's patients change their drinking patterns, given that both strive for improvements in family and job functioning? Two factors probably account for the relative success of community reinforcement counseling. The first is its focus on specific reeducation techniques and procedure for heightening effectiveness in family and vocational spheres; too often, traditional therapy concentrates on achievement of insight into behavioral problems or focuses on attempts to "improve communication" between family members without doing anything about fundamental gaps in knowledge about how to behave in the family and on the job. Second, there is understandable reluctance on the part of many therapists to go to great lengths to improve family or job functioning, then to withhold access to them when the patient drinks. To do so, however, is to emphasize to the patient that they are more important (and can be more reinforcing) than alcohol.

Contingency Contracting with "Public Drunkenness Offenders." Selecting 20 chronic alcoholic men from among a group of "public drunkenness offenders" interviewed in the Jackson, Mississippi, city jail, Miller (1975) contracted with 10 of these men to provide them a broad range of goods and services in exchange for "demonstrated attempts to control their drinking" upon their release from jail. The other 10 men were control subjects who received the same goods and services whether or not they drank. Miller (1975, p. 916) reports:

> Housing was arranged through an agreement with the Salvation Army. Normally, this agency will only allow sober individuals to board two days. Under a special agreement, any of the subjects could be housed or fed, or both, at this agency for the duration of the program. . . . Employment was obtained primarily through Manpower and the Mississippi State Employment Service. . . . If a subject were in need of medical assistance, arrangements were made with either the Veterans Administration Hospital or the University Hospital to treat him. . . . Clothing was obtained via the Salvation Army Store, Goodwill Industry Store, or donations to the program. Subjects eligible for veterans assistance could be provided with canteen booklets exchangeable for cigarettes, meals, or clothing at the Veterans Administration Hospital. . . . Subjects also received counseling sessions geared toward advising them on numerous practical problems in life, such as money management.

The 10 experimental subjects were deprived of access to these reinforcers for five days whenever their blood alcohol levels, assessed at unpredictable intervals, exceeded 10 mg/100 ml during the two months this contingency was in force. Results were that subjects who were provided these material reinforcers contingently significantly decreased in mean number of arrests and rate of drinking and significantly increased in mean number of hours employed per week posttreatment; the 10 control subjects showed essentially no changes in any of these behaviors.

Contingency Contracting at the Baltimore City Hospitals. Finer-grained analysis of the effects of contingent reinforcement and punishment has been a consistent goal of a research group at the Baltimore City Hospitals. Among the first of the group's efforts to use natural contingencies in this way was Bigelow's successful effort to induce abstinence in four Baltimore City Hospitals' employees in danger of being fired for drinking on the job (Bigelow, Liebson, and Lawrence, 1973). Required by contingency contract to report daily to the hospital's Alcoholism Treatment Unit for Antabuse therapy, the four were told that failure to report would result in no work and no pay. The contingency produced striking improvements in all employees' job performance and attendance. In like fashion, Liebson and his coworkers (1973) drew up contracts with nine heroin addicts who were simultaneously abusing alcohol. The contracts specified that each man would be maintained on methadone (a potent reinforcer) so long as he continued to ingest Antabuse and to maintain abstinence from alcohol. The treatment was a rousing success with a group of patients notoriously difficult to treat: Drinking took place on only 1.4% of patient days when methadone maintenance was contingent on disulfiram ingestion, but on 19.2% of days when it was not.

Laboratory studies by the same group (Cohen et al., 1971; Bigelow, Liebson, and Griffiths, 1973, 1974) have also demonstrated that chronic alcoholic inpatients will voluntarily moderate their alcohol intake (for example, by drinking no more than 5 to 7 ounces of beverage alcohol a day when up to 24 ounces are available) when doing so results in reinforcement and not doing so results either in punishment or loss of reinforcement. Among the reinforcers and punishers explored in this context have been enriched versus impoverished ward-living environments, weekend passes and special ward privileges versus no passes and limited privileges, moderate alcohol on a subsequent drinking day versus no alcohol on that day, and usual socialization privileges versus brief periods of interpersonal isolation.

Overall Evaluation of Contingency Contracting. We conclude that contingency contracting has shown real promise as a means to manage effectively the behavior of alcoholics in outpatient settings. So long as reinforcement for continued sobriety is more powerful than alcohol itself—and a surprisingly large number of things in the natural environment seem to be—the alcoholic can be helped to moderate his/her drinking or to terminate it.

Social-Skills Training. Behavioral clinicians have developed a variety of social-skills training programs for alcoholics in the belief that deficits in interpersonal skills lead to failure in interpersonal situations, and that consistent failure in interpersonal settings increases the likelihood that sober alcoholics will return to abusive drinking to escape from the experience of interpersonal failure.

Oei and Jackson (1980) reported 3-, 6-, and 12-month follow-up data for four groups of eight chronic alcoholics each. The groups received (1) group social-skills training, (2) individual social-skills training, (3) group traditional supportive treatment, or (4) individual traditional supportive treatment. Over a period of three weeks, social-skills training subjects attended 12 sessions of two hours each. They focused, successively, on (1) nonverbal expression (e.g., eye contact), (2) refusing unreasonable requests, (3) making difficult requests, (4) expressing and receiving positive feelings, (5) replying to criticism, and (6) initiating conversations. Modeling of these skills by therapists was followed by therapist-client role-playing; videotapes of role-playing permitted corrective feedback and behavior modification. Between-session homework assignments were given and completed. Group social-skills training subjects listened to a brief lecture, watched a therapist model a social skill, then participated in individual therapist-client role-playing and videotape feedback. Individual social-skills training subjects received 15 minutes of individual skill training each session, then viewed the videotape of the group session. Traditional supportive treatment subjects discussed, individually or in a group, "general practical problems (e.g., marital, monetary) clients were facing."

Social-skills training subjects improved significantly more than subjects receiving traditional supportive treatment on social skills, alcohol intake, and assertiveness measures; group social-skills training subjects scored consistently better than individual social-skills training subjects on all measures except alcohol intake. We conclude, with the authors, that targeted social-skills training offers promise (though not in isolation from treatment methods which focus on consumption as well), and that group treatment may work somewhat better than individual treatment because of the opportunity for social support, feedback, and practice it provides. A recent report on the successful application of a similar social-skills training program, included in a broadly behavioral treatment program for hospitalized chronic alcoholics (Jones, Kanfer, and Lanyon, 1982) did not, however, find the social-skills training group superior to a traditional discussion control group. This study, in turn, was a replication of an earlier study (Chaney, O'Leary, and Marlatt, 1978) which had found social-skills training to be superior to other components of a broad-spectrum behavioral treatment program. These data, taken together, encourage further exploration of social-skills training for alcoholics, but they do not provide unequivocal support for the treatment method.

Oei and Jackson also reported, more recently, on a comparative study of the social-skills training package described in their 1980 paper alone and combined with cognitive restructuring, a newly popular behavioral treatment procedure (1982). The cognitive restructuring focused on irrational beliefs about drinking practices, causes of drinking, and treatments for abusive drinking, as well as on other irrational beliefs about drinking. The 32 patients selected for this comparative study were divided into four groups: (1) social-skills training, (2) cognitive restructuring, (3) a combination of cognitive restructuring and social-skills training, and (4) traditional supportive therapy. Cognitive restructuring, alone and in combination with social-skills training, turned out to be more effective in producing lasting social-skill increments and decreased alcohol consumption over a 12-month follow-up. These results validate inclusion of cognitive restructuring in broad-spectrum behavioral treatment programs, but leave open the question of inclusion of the social skills component of those programs.

Cognitive restructuring is but one element of what some have come to call behavioral self-control treatment strategies. Recent years have seen a decided increase in use of these techniques by behavioral clinicians, and not simply with alcoholics, in recognition of data which suggest that they have greater "staying power" than treatment methods which do not address the thoughts and feelings that clients have about their disabilities and their chances for successfully modifying them. Marlatt, whose cognitive social-learning views on etiology have previously been cited, has the following to say about necessary elements of behavioral self-control treatment programs:

> The ideal self-control program should prove itself to be effective in maintaining behavior change for clinically significant periods of time following initial treatment (as demonstrated by long-term follow-up) compared to the best available alternative programs. . . . The ideal should enhance and maintain an individual's compliance and adherence to program requirements such as the continuation of required techniques such as record-keeping, relaxation training, and rehearsal of new skills. . . . The ideal program should consist of a mixture of both specific behavioral techniques (e.g., skill training, exercise, etc.) and cognitive intervention procedures (e.g., cognitive restructuring, increased attention to covert ideation such as rationalization and denial, use of coping imagery, etc.). . . . In addition to teaching cognitive strategies and behavioral coping skills, the ideal program should also facilitate the development of motivation and decision-making skills as applied to ongoing changes that occur during the maintenance phase of therapy (Marlatt and Parks, 1982, pp. 453–454).

Other elements of Marlatt's ideal program include replacement of maladaptive behavior patterns by adaptive ones that are nonetheless as reinforcing as the maladaptive ones, and inclusion of techniques to enable the client (1) to cope effectively with problem situations with the potential to cause relapse, (2) to deal more effectively with failure experiences more generally, and (3) to increase the client's sense of self-efficacy in specific problem situations.

If the nonbehavioral reader experiences a sense of *deja vu* on reading of the inclusion of cognitive elements in alcoholism treatment, it may be because these treatment procedures have much in common with traditional psychotherapy, although their focus on specific problem areas and their expectation of targeted behavioral changes are different.

4. Broad-Spectrum Behavioral Treatment Procedures

A lesson that clinicians working with alcoholics from other theoretical perspectives know well has more recently been learned by behavior therapists. That lesson is that alcoholism is a multifaceted disorder with physical, psychological, and interpersonal sequelae; it is not simply a disorder of excessive alcohol consumption or of disordered antecedents to or consequences of drinking. Accordingly, its successful treatment cannot focus on but one of these behaviors; instead, all must be confronted.

Almost 15 years ago, at a time when virtually all behavioral approaches to alcoholism focused solely on the maladaptive drinking response itself, Arnold Lazarus, then and now an influential behavior therapist, suggested instead that a "broad-spectrum" approach to alcoholism might work better (1965). Among the separate elements of Lazarus's treatment package were: (1) medical attention to alcohol-related physical problems; (2) aversion conditioning, to modify or eliminate abusive drinking; (3) behavioral assessment, to identify "specific stimulus antecedents of anxiety preparatory to systematic desensitization"; (4) assertiveness training, to equip the patient better to respond more appropriately to interpersonally stressful social situations; (5) behavioral rehearsal, to develop more effective interpersonal skills; (6) hypnosis, "to countercondition anxiety-response habits"; and (7) marital therapy, to help the patient's spouse modify the spouse's central role in the patient's alcoholism. The broad-spectrum behavior therapy packages described below, developed years after Lazarus's conceptual paper, correspond closely to his suggestions.

Although a variety of broad-spectrum behavioral treatment packages have been evaluated in recent years, only a few are reviewed here. The first of these programs, developed by Sobell and Sobell (1973a, 1973b, 1976), is reviewed because it was the first broad-spectrum package designed specifically to explore the efficacy of controlled drinking treatment, because the follow-up procedures it employed were innovative and comprehensive, and because the study and its authors have recently been attacked for incomplete reporting of data and duplicity. Evaluation of the second package, by Vogler and his colleagues (1975, 1977a, 1977b) is instructive because the efficacy of a treatment package offered both to alcoholics and to problem drinkers is compared. The third broad-spectrum approach reviewed here (Pomerleau, 1976, 1978) represented the first behavioral effort to identify and treat middle- and upper-middle-class alcoholics, a group previously ignored by behavior therapists involved in alcoholism treatment. The final broad-spectrum treatment package to be reviewed (Sanchez-Craig, 1980; Sanchez-Craig and Annis, 1982) is notable because it appears to offer to problem drinkers and those at risk for problem drinking a promising prevention opportunity. Because effective prevention programs have been rare (Nathan, 1983), especially for these groups, this work is especially encouraging.

The IBTA Study. Psychologists Mark and Linda Sobell evolved a broad-spectrum behavioral treatment package they called "individualized behavior therapy for alcoholics (IBTA)" in 1970. The treatment evaluation study of IBTA they subsequently carried out at the Patton (California) State Hospital has become extremely well-known—and very controversial—for two reasons: because it revealed that, regardless of assigned treatment goal (abstinence or controlled drinking), experimental patients (those receiving IBTA) one and two years posttreatment were drinking in controlled fashion significantly more frequently than control patients, and because two other psychologists (Pendery and Maltzman, 1982) have raised questions about the adequacy of the study's design and follow-up methodology and, by implication, about the integrity of its authors. Specifics of IBTA included the following (M. B. Sobell, 1978, pp. 158–159):

> Irrespective of a subject's assigned treatment goal, all experimental treatment sessions focused directly on drinking behavior, tailoring the treatment as specifically as possible to meet each individual's needs, and emphasizing helping the subject identify the functions of excessive drinking and develop alternative, more beneficial ways of dealing with those situations. . . . The only explicit difference in treatment between the non-drinker and controlled drinker experimental groups was that the controlled drinker subjects were trained in methods of non-problem drinking and allowed to practice these behaviors during sessions. . . . The vast majority of IBTA treatment sessions can most accurately be termed "behavior change training sessions." The sequence of these sessions incorporated a four-stage process: (1) Problem Identification—Subjects were trained to identify the specific circumstances which had in the past and were likely in the future to result in drinking that would have adverse consequences for the individual; (2) Identification of Alternative Responses to Drinking—Subjects were assisted in generating a series of behavioral options to be used when confronted with problem situations; (3) Evaluation of Alternatives—Subjects were taught how to evaluate each of these behavioral options in terms of their short-term and, especially, long-term effects; (4) Preparation to Engage in the Best Behavioral Alternative—Subjects then practiced the alternative responses which could reasonably be expected to incur the least self-damaging long-term consequences in each instance. Various procedures and behavioral techniques, specific to each individual case, were used to accomplish this objective.

First-year outcome data, reported in 1973 (Sobell and Sobell, 1973b), revealed that both experimental treatment groups (nondrinkers and controlled drinkers) achieved levels of functioning, including levels of alcohol ingestion, superior to their respective control groups. These data were based on follow-up information from 69 of the study's original 70 subjects, an impressive follow-up retention rate. At the end of the second follow-up year, experimental subjects with the assigned treatment goal of controlled drinking were continuing to function better than their controls, while the experimental, nondrinker subjects were doing better, but not significantly better, than their controls (Sobell and Sobell, 1976). Unexpectedly, subjects in the controlled drinker experimental group reported significantly more abstinent days than nondrinker experimental subjects—for whom abstinence was the sole treatment goal.

The study's experimental design, conceptual basis, and fundamental aims were both roundly criticized and widely lauded through the decade of the 1970s. Those who criticized questioned the ethics of controlled drinking treatment in the absence of data attesting to its efficacy, the dual status of the lone follow-up worker (L. C. Sobell) as coinvestigator, and reliance on patient self-reports as principal sources of follow-up information. Those who lauded the study point to the unusually large number of alcoholic subjects selected, treated, and followed to the end of the two-year follow-up mark, the innovative nature of the behavioral treatment program that was employed, and the courage of two young investigators in choosing to study as controversial a subject as controlled drinking. Greater detail in criticism of this study is provided by Emrick (1975), Hamburg (1975), and Nathan and Briddell (1977).

Publication in *Science,* the prestigious journal of the American Association for the Advancement of Science, of a follow-up study of the 20 experimental, controlled drinker subjects treated by the Sobells more than ten years before by psychologists Mary Pendery and Irving Maltzman (Pendery and Maltzman, 1982) shocked many alcoholism workers when the authors of the follow-up reported that only one of the 20 subjects had successfully controlled his drinking over several years and that most of the 20 had experienced a high incidence of rehospitalization, alcohol-related arrests, and heavy-drinking bouts. It is unfortunate that Pendery and Maltzman failed to report on a parallel follow-up of control subjects; the absence of data on control subjects makes valid conclusions from their data on experimental subjects impossible. Even though most of the experimental subjects, 10 years later, were doing badly, it is possible that the control subjects had done even worse. Without comparative data, valid conclusions on the efficacy of the treatment provided the experimental subjects cannot be reached. An unpublished version of the paper by Pendery and Maltzman, and media interviews of the two, raised additional questions, including the initial random assignment of subjects to experimental and control groups, the frequency of subject follow-up, and the integrity of the Sobells' reports of design, procedures, and outcome.

The seriousness of these charges led the Addiction Research Foundation of Toronto, the Sobells' employer, to appoint a four-person committee of enquiry to look into these allegations. After a lengthy, very thorough consideration of all available documentation from the Sobells' original study, including raw data, tape-recorded interviews conducted by the Sobells with experimental and control subjects, and sworn affidavits from research assistants who had taken part in the study, but without the cooperation of Pendery and Maltzman who refused to furnish data from their own follow-up, the committee concluded that the Sobells had carried out the research in the way they reported, and that they had not misrepresented the results. By design, however, the committee did not evaluate a central issue raised by Pendery and Maltzman: whether alcoholics can be taught to moderate their drinking.

Our own view of this matter is that there is only one proper forum for questions about scientific data and the integrity of scientists: the scientific journals. We do not believe that the media are an appropriate place for such charges since the media's standards of proof have little or nothing to do with those of science. It is ironic, of course, that these charges were brought at this time, well after responsible clinicians had concluded that the available data do not justify continued use of controlled drinking treatment with alcoholics (Brownell, 1983; Nathan, 1981; Nathan and Lipscomb, 1979).

Integrated Behavior Change Techniques for Problem Drinkers and Alcoholics. Three reports (Vogler, Compton, and Weissbach, 1975; Vogler, Weissbach, and Compton, 1977; Vogler et al., 1977) described the same set of "integrated behavior change techniques" used to treat groups of alcoholics and problem drinkers. One of the most interesting aspects of this work is that a set of procedures first applied to a group of inpatient alcoholics (Vogler et al., 1975) was then used to modify the drinking behavior of a group of problem drinkers. In principal, the Vogler studies make an additional important contribution; their "unpackaging" research design was to permit assessment of the relative contribution to treatment success of the several components of the total treatment package. In practice, however, the actual pattern of findings did not allow these planned comparisons.

Vogler's "integrated behavior change techniques" included video-taped self-confrontation of drunken behavior (to increase motivation for therapy); discrimination training for blood alcohol concentration (to enable subjects to judge with increased accuracy their level of intoxication, in order to maintain their drinking at more moderate levels); aversion training (to establish a conditioned aversion to alcohol); discriminated avoidance practice in which shocks were given for overconsumption (to sharpen the conditioned aversion to alcohol so that it became specific to overconsumption); alternatives training and behavioral counseling (to help patients develop alternative and incompatible responses to the setting events that previously occasioned overdrinking); and alcohol education. Most of these procedures were also components of the Sobells' IBTA (Vogler and the Sobells worked together for a time at the Patton State Hospital), although the manner in which the procedures were introduced into therapy and the sequencing of their introduction differed in the Sobell and Vogler studies.

In the first investigation of the efficacy of "integrated behavior change techniques" (Vogler et al., 1975), two matched groups of chronic hospitalized alcoholics were treated. One group of 23 men received the full treatment package over a period averaging 45 days; a second group of 19 men, whose treatment lasted an average of 22.5 days, received only alternatives training, behavioral counseling, and alcohol education. Subjects in both groups attended booster treatment sessions once a week during the month following treatment, then once a month for a year.

A gross measure of outcome—number of subjects who had maintained abstinence or were drinking in controlled fashion during each follow-up interval—failed to reveal differences between the two treatment groups (65% of patients in both groups met the criteria for success). A finer measure of outcome, however, revealed that patients in the first group had consumed significantly less ethanol, reflected in ounces per month, than those in the second group over the one-year follow-up period. Other outcome indices, including preferred beverage, preferred locus of consumption, and number of days lost from work pre- and posttreatment, failed to reveal additional differences between the two groups. Essentially the same pattern of group differences in outcome was observed at the 18-month follow-up mark (Vogler, Weissbach, and Compton, 1977).

Four groups of problem drinkers participated in a second trial of Vogler's integrated behavior change techniques (Vogler et al., and Martin, 1977). Referred by various community agencies or responding to newspaper advertisements, subjects were considered problem drinkers (but not alcoholics) if they had never been diagnosed alcoholic or been hospitalized for alcohol-related problems but had consumed alcohol in sufficient quantities to produce legal, marital, and/or vocational problems. From an original pool of 409 subjects, 80 were followed through to the one-year follow-up mark. Of these subjects, 23 received the full complement of integrated behavior change techniques (group 1), 19 were given blood alcohol level discrimination training, behavioral counseling, alternatives training, and alcohol education (group 2), 21 received only alcohol education (group 3), and 17 were provided behavioral counseling, alternatives training, and alcohol education (group 4).

The treatment goal for subjects in all groups was moderation. Fifty of the 80 subjects completing treatment and follow-up were considered moderate drinkers at the one-year follow-up mark; 3 additional subjects had maintained abstinence over the same period. Overall, subjects had decreased their consumption of absolute ethanol by between 50% and 65%. Unexpectedly, membership in treatment groups was not associated with differential outcomes. Vogler and his colleagues explain these findings by pointing to variability among subjects in pretreatment drinking rates and social characteristics, to dependence upon self-reports by subjects for most of the outcome data, and to the fact that subjects in all four groups were given a strong learning orientation to treatment which may have increased the motivation of all to change their drinking patterns. The latter explanation, in turn, calls into question whether the specialized behavioral treatment procedures provided subjects in groups 1 and 2 added anything to overall outcome; if not, one must ask whether it is necessary to maintain broad-spectrum treatment regimens since they are expensive and require skilled workers for their application. For that matter, one must also question the clinical viability of any set of treatment procedures associated with an 80% attrition rate at the one-year follow-up mark. One might also ask, in the same context, whether sufficient attention to the problems of maintaining subjects in treatment and active follow-up was paid, given the dramatic subject losses experienced over the course of the study. Nonetheless, one must also be impressed by the numbers of subjects in this study drinking more moderately at the one-year follow-up mark, even if many or most of them would never have progressed to alcoholism. Success in helping such individuals develop more moderate patterns of alcohol consumption is significant.

Broad-Spectrum Behavioral Treatment for Middle-Income Problem Drinkers. The problem drinkers to whom Pomerleau and his colleagues at the University of Pennsylvania School of Medicine offered broad-spectrum behavior therapy were as different from those treated by Vogler and his colleagues as Vogler's subjects were from the chronic alcoholics to whom the Sobells offered IBTA. Middle-class alcoholics, Pomerleau's patients were almost certainly more highly motivated for treatment, more intact intellectually, socially, and emotionally, and possessed of greater familial, vocational, and economic resources than other groups of broad-spectrum behavior therapy patients studied (Pomerleau et al., 1978).

Pomerleau's problem drinkers came to him via physician referrals and announcements in local media. Thirty-two subjects were ultimately selected for the first trial of the new treatment package. Of these problem drinkers, 18 were randomly assigned to behavioral treatment and 14 to "traditional" treatment. Treatment, behavioral and traditional, was conducted in groups of 3 to 7 problem drinkers for 90 minutes once a week for three months, then for five additional sessions programmed at increasing intervals for another nine months.

Behavioral treatment consisted of the following four overlapping phases:

1. *Baseline:* After an interview designed to elicit a detailed drinking history and to provide information on the treatment program, a treatment fee (on a sliding scale from $500 to $85, based on ability to pay) was collected. A "commitment fee" of up to $300 was also requested; this sum could be earned back if the subject followed all treatment instructions concerning record-keeping, regular treatment attendance, regular sobriety, performance of designated nondrinking activities, and commitment to follow-up contacts. At this time subjects were also instructed in how to keep a detailed record of consumption, drink by drink, as well as how to identify situations which characteristically led to excessive drinking; no effort was made to induce a change in normal drinking during this initial phase of the treatment program.

2. *Reduction in drinking:* Subjects designated daily quotas for a week's worth of drinking at a time, as well as final treatment goals. Emphasis was placed on gradual, steady improvement rather than abrupt, rapid change. Moderate drinking rather than abstinence was allowed if a subject requested it, if he had shown some control over his drinking during the recent past, and if there were no medical contraindications to continued drinking. For these subjects, the final goal of the reduction phase of the study was three days a week of abstinence and consumption of no more than 3 ounces of ethanol on days when drinking was permitted and no more than 10 ounces of ethanol a week overall. Subjects selecting abstinence set similar interim goals, but all aimed to reach abstinence within two weeks. Stimulus control and contingency management techniques were emphasized to enable subjects to identify appropriate and inappropriate drinking circumstances (e.g., drinking with family at dinner rather than with coworkers at a tavern after work), to delay or interfere with maladaptive drinking patterns (e.g., keeping a glass filled with a soft drink in one's hand at a social gathering), and to increase the likelihood of not drinking in designated situations (e.g., choosing to attend only those gatherings at which drinking will not take place).

3. *Behavior therapy for associated behavioral problems:* During this phase of the program emphasis was placed on identifying and altering associated behavioral problems with the capacity to affect

drinking behavior. Among the behavioral techniques employed to deal with such behaviors as anger, anxiety, depression, and marital and vocational dysfunction were assertion training, systematic desensitization, and deep muscle relaxation. Behavior rehearsal and modeling, along with family counseling, were also employed in this effort to confront problems associated with the patient's maladaptive drinking.

4. *Maintenance of therapeutic gain:* To help patients maintain gains in drinking behavior and in social and vocational spheres, they were encouraged to develop interests in activities (hobbies, physical exercise, academic work) which can be pursued alcohol-free. New friends, rather than old drinking companions, were recommended. Toward the end of this phase of formal treatment, contact with the therapist was gradually thinned in order to maintain the thrust of therapy for as long as possible.

The traditional treatment offered in this comparative study was designed to last as long and be as intensive as the behaviorally oriented treatment; scheduled to cost from $5 to $30 a session for 17 sessions, it did not require prepaid commitment fees nor were refunds available. Stages in this treatment included an introductory phase, lasting 3 sessions, devoted to development of group cohesion and mutual trust among group members. Total abstinence was strongly encouraged at the same time that denial patterns were identified. The second, confrontation phase of this therapy, lasting 6 or 7 sessions, also focused on denial patterns, as well as on development of insight into the nature of personal denial mechanisms. The third, resolution phase, lasting 2 or 3 sessions, undertook to channel the intense emotions generated in the preceding phase of treatment into productive, future-directed activity; during the same phase, adjunctive psychotherapy for depression, anxiety, family problems, etc. was provided. During the five remaining sessions of this treatment, supportive therapy for nondrinking continued.

Both traditional and behavioral treatment were provided by professionals experienced in the treatment mode they were offering. Of 18 patients treated by behavioral techniques, 16 remained in treatment throughout; by contrast, of 14 patients treated by traditional procedures, only 8 remained to the end of the treatment. Drinking rate decreased significantly from screening to the end of the follow-up year in both treatment groups. Significantly fewer behavioral participants dropped out of treatment.

These data suggest an advantage for behavioral over traditional treatment: Even though subjects in both groups decreased their drinking rate, more behavioral than traditional subjects stayed with treatment. On the other hand, it is impossible to identify the variable or variables in behavioral treatment responsible for this outcome difference because the two treatments differed so completely—extra treatment factors such as prepaid commitment fees and monetary penalty for dropping from treatment were not a part of traditional therapy, and subjects in the traditional group could only aspire to abstinence, while those in the behavioral group could aim either for abstinence or controlled drinking.

A Cognitive-Behavioral Program for Early-Stage Problem Drinkers. The three broad-spectrum behavior change programs reviewed to this point shared a comprehensive, multifaceted behavioral approach to alcoholic drinking and its associated behavioral deficits and excesses, the assumption that controlled drinking treatment might have important value for alcoholics and serious problem drinkers, and the conviction that an intensive program requires full-time, inpatient access to patients. Despite these notable efforts by the Sobells, Vogler and his colleagues, and Pomerleau and his colleagues, the successes of the latter two outcome studies were relatively modest, while the results of the Sobells' study, much more encouraging, nonetheless stand alone in their encouragement of controlled-drinking treatment for persons seriously abusing alcohol.

Martha Sanchez-Craig, a psychologist at the Addiction Research Foundation, Toronto, has developed a cognitive-behavioral program specifically designed for early-stage problem drinkers. Her cognitive-behavior therapy methods, aspects of her experimental design (e.g., a completely randomized assignment of patients to controlled-drinking or abstinence groups), and her design of treatment follow-up all reflect important lessons learned from the studies of the 1970s.

Subjects were 70 socially stable problem drinkers who met criteria which assured their good physical health and status as early-stage problem drinkers. Following thorough pretreatment assessment and unconstrained random assignment to a treatment goal of abstinence or controlled-drinking, subjects participated in one of the following treatment programs:

Abstinence Treatment	*Controlled-Drinking Treatment*
1. Notification of goal and introduction to treatment.	1. Notification of goal and introduction to treatment.
2. Teaching self-monitoring of drinking.	2. Teaching self-monitoring of drinking.

3. Teaching problem-solving and developing cognitive and behavioral coping.
4. Continuation of problem-solving and self-monitoring.

5. Continuation of problem-solving and self-monitoring.

6. Continuation of problem-solving and self-monitoring.

7. Termination of treatment.

3. Teaching problem-solving and developing cognitive and behavioral coping.
4. Reassessment of moderate drinking goal, and continuation of problem-solving and self-monitoring.
5. Setting rules and guidelines for moderate drinking, and continuation of problem-solving and self-monitoring.
6. Preparation for resumption of drinking, and continuation of problem-solving and self-monitoring.
7. Termination of treatment.

Treatment was by one of two therapists, each of whom taught controlled drinking to half the subjects assigned and abstinence to the remainder. Six weekly, individual sessions were required for treatment; each lasted less than 90 minutes.

A thorough description of the treatment program is provided by Sanchez-Craig (1979). During the first three weeks of treatment (Sanchez-Craig, 1980), subjects in the abstinence condition drank on a greater number of days (P > .05) and drank more heavily when drinking occurred (P < .01). Analysis of the acceptability of drinking goal to subjects indicated that the assigned goal was more frequently accepted by subjects in the controlled-drinking condition (P < .001). Six-month follow-up data on the 59 subjects who remained in treatment and could be located for follow-up (Sanchez-Craig and Annis, 1982) indicated no significant pretreatment-posttreatment differences between conditions in drinks consumed on drinking days, frequency of drinking, drinking style, percentage of abstinent, moderate, and heavy drinking days, or typical beverage consumed. Despite these data, the authors of the report conclude that controlled drinking is an appropriate goal for early-stage problem drinkers (1) because more of these subjects reacted favorably to a goal of moderate drinking than to a goal of abstinence, (2) because compliance to the assigned drinking goal during treatment was higher in the controlled-drinking group (e.g., 80% of controlled-drinker subjects drank moderately, while only 20% of abstinence subjects remained abstinent), and (3) because 67% of subjects in the abstinence group developed moderate drinking practices on their own through treatment. Sanchez-Craig and

Annis (1982) conclude that the abstinence goal is especially unacceptable to early-stage problem drinkers and that a moderate drinking treatment goal may be the only basis on which early prevention efforts may be offered—and accepted.

Essentially the same conclusion was drawn by the authors of two additional explorations of moderate drinking goals for young drinkers (Burish et al., Cooper, and Sobell, 1981; Strickler, Bradlyn, and Maxwell, 1981), as well as by many of the authors of case reports of behavioral treatment of alcoholics in a recent book bringing together a series of such reports (Hay and Nathan, 1982).

Predictors of Treatment Outcome. The question of whether selected demographic, personal and drinking history, and personality variables can predict response to behavioral treatment for alcoholism has been much discussed. In our chapter for the first edition of this book (Nathan and Lipscomb, 1979), for example, we emphasized the need to develop predictors of successful response to abstinence-oriented and controlled-drinking-oriented treatment. Three studies of outcome predictors merit mention here.

Upon analyzing predictors of success in the Sobells' individualized behavior therapy for alcoholism program, Maisto, Sobell, and Sobell (1980) reported that (1) drinking outcomes stabilized between one and two years following treatment, (2) drinking behavior during the six months preceding this criterion period was the best predictor of outcome, (3) a strong relationship between a controlled-drinking treatment goal and controlled-drinking outcomes was found while treatment goal was unrelated to abstinent treatment outcomes, and (4) total pretreatment alcohol-related hospitalizations were negatively related to controlled-drinking outcomes.

Sparked by four-year Rand Survey data to the effect that some groups of moderate drinkers had better prognoses for avoidance of relapse than some groups of abstainers, Finney and Moos (1981) studied 131 patients who returned to their families after treatment in one of five residential, abstinence-oriented treatment programs. Persons who began drinking moderately within six months after alcoholism treatment had a higher relapse rate at a two-year follow-up than did six-month abstainers, though the two groups did not differ on nondrinking outcome variables. Another perspective on the same issue—therapists' views on the criteria to use when assigning clients to abstinence or controlled-drinking goals— was explored in a survey of 62 alcoholism therapists at 22 alcoholism treatment facilities in Indiana (Perkins, Cox, and Levy, 1981). While sex of patient and sex of therapist played no role in projected assignment of patients to treatment goals, controlled drinking was more strongly recommended for alcoholics of higher social class, especially women, and for alcoholics with longer histories of controlled drinking, especially men.

Despite the fact that these three studies are among the first to provide empirical data on predictors of outcome, it is encouraging that the question is now considered an important one, and that efforts to answer it from data are being made. We await additional data before drawing firm conclusions on predictors of behavioral treatment outcome.

III. CURRENT STATUS AND FUTURE TRENDS IN BEHAVIORAL ASSESSMENT AND TREATMENT OF CHRONIC ALCOHOLISM

A. Current Status

Behavioral assessment and treatment of chronic alcoholism is now widely accepted as a viable alternative to traditional efforts to diagnose and treat chronic alcoholics.

Those who have developed procedures for behavioral assessment have led us to attend more closely to the environmental determinants—the "setting variables"—of maladaptive drinking as well as the consequences of that drinking. Further, the well-known behavioral devotion to precision in defining the parameters of maladaptive drinking has convinced us of the importance of objective assessment of changes in that behavior both following treatment and in its absence. The recent interest on the part of behavioral clinicians in empirical data to permit rational assignment of clients to treatment outcome goals is also a most encouraging development.

Contributions by those who have developed behavioral treatment methods include a treatment approach focused on abusive drinking which appears to work well with highly motivated individuals who wish to achieve and maintain abstinence (chemical aversion) as well as another promising abstinence-oriented but, as yet, unproven method directed to the target behavior (covert sensitization) and another promising but unproven set of procedures for modifying antecedents and consequences of drinking (social-skills–self-control training methods). The apparently slight value of electrical aversion as a behavioral technique for inducing abstinence, despite a lengthy history of efforts to use it for that purpose, has also been identified.

The men and women who have investigated behavioral treatment approaches to alcoholism have also proposed a variety of multifaceted behavioral treatment packages. What these packages offer over unidimensional treatment is attention both to the patient's maladaptive drinking and to the associated behavioral deficits and excesses which typically accompany his/her alcoholism. Some of these efforts have focused on controlled drinking treatment; results suggest, in our judgment, that nonabstinent treatment goals may be appropriate for problem drinkers, but are not so for chronic alcoholics. The potential value of these methods for prevention, with social drinkers and early-stage problem drinkers, has also recently been explored.

B. Future Trends

While no one has the prescience to anticipate the most important future trends in a field as diverse and dynamic as the one of which we have written in this chapter, we here hazard prediction of a few of the more likely directions.

1. *Exploration of cognitive mediating processes important to the maintenance of chronic alcoholism—along with procedures for their modification by behavioral means—will increase rapidly over the next few years.* The nature and influence of cognitive processes on other kinds of adaptive and maladaptive behavior have begun to be studied intensively by behavioral researchers outside the alcoholism arena (Bandura, 1977; Mahoney, 1974; Meichenbaum, 1977). In parallel with this thrust, alcohol researchers have begun to test out the role of such cognitive variables as imagery, verbal coding of information, and self-control processes in the behavior of chronic alcoholics (Marlatt, 1977; Wilson, 1977a). No longer will behavioral researchers, it now seems clear, be content to attribute responsibility for maladaptive drinking solely to external, environmental variables; the important additional impact of what alcoholics tell themselves about their drinking and its effects on them must be studied.

    One logical outcome of these basic research findings has been their application to broad-spectrum behavior therapy programs. The development of cognitive strategies for increased self-control and delay of gratification particularly recommend themselves in this context.

2. *Increasing attention will be paid to efforts to "unpackage" the separate components of broad-spectrum behavioral treatment programs.* To this time, only occasional efforts to identify the "active" ingredients of broad-spectrum behavioral treatment packages have been attempted, in large part because behavioral

researchers have been preoccupied with efforts to establish the comparability (and if possible, the superiority) of their treatment programs to older, more widely accepted ones.

Initial forays into the perils of "unpackaging" have been made by Lovibond and Caddy (1976) and Vogler and his colleagues (1975, 1977). In neither instance, however, did the "unpackaging" extend far enough to permit specification of the "active ingredients" of the overall treatment package.

3. *Systematic development of new components of broad-spectrum behavioral treatment programs will take place in order to expand the range of associated behavioral problems that can be confronted by these treatment packages.* It is not enough to introduce new elements into a comprehensive treatment package simply because they have face validity that makes them seem capable of confronting a behavioral problem typical of chronic alcoholics. Instead, efforts to establish the separate viability of these procedures vis-à-vis the problem behavior in question must take place first. Though this kind of research is of the high-risk variety because it does not guarantee the marked (and, hence, publishable) effects that can be achieved by multifaceted treatment packages, it is an absolute prerequisite for development of rational treatment packages resting on firm empirical foundations.

4. *More emphasis on primary and secondary prevention of alcohol problems and less emphasis on tertiary prevention will increasingly characterize the field.* As elsewhere, behavior therapists working with alcoholics have chosen to concentrate their efforts on the remediation of existing severe problems. Much less attention has been paid to adolescents at risk for alcoholism or to problem drinkers who might already have begun to acquire the behavioral stigma of alcoholism. Now that behavioral procedures have been shown to have demonstrable value for the treatment of chronic alcoholism, some clinicians have begun to recognize the wisdom of bringing to problem drinkers some of the benefits of methods available previously only to confirmed alcoholics. Our own analysis of past and present efforts to prevent alcoholism leads us to conclude that, despite the infusion of large sums of money for these programs, we have not developed the ways and means to prevent alcoholism in groups at risk (Nathan, 1983). It is for this reason that we are particularly enthusiastic about the efforts of Sanchez-Craig and her colleagues (Sanchez-Craig, 1980; Sanchez-Craig and Annis, 1982) to teach moderate drinking to early-stage problem drinkers. Perhaps this kind of "targeted" ef-

fort to work with this at-risk group at this targeted intervention level will yield outcomes superior to those achieved up to this time.

5. *The conceptual and political issues which have separated behavioral clinicians from other alcoholism workers will begin to break down.* While this prediction is, admittedly, more wish than reality, we do see early, tentative recognition of common problems that face all clinicians, as well as increased willingness to work together to solve them. The growing recognition by all that controlled drinking is not a viable treatment goal for alcoholics has increased willingness to work together to solve such problems. It has also increased the acceptability of other behavioral treatment procedures by nonbehavioral clinicians, as has the recognition by behavioral clinicians of the role of cognitive-mediators in behavior and behavior change. The reliance on empirical research and on careful pre- and posttreatment assessment by behavioral clinicians also seems to have been recognized as useful and to have been adopted more widely by nonbehavioral clinicians.

REFERENCES

Abrams, D. B., and Wilson, G. T., 1980, Self-control of delay of gratification, unpublished manuscript, Rutgers University, New Brunswick, N.J.

American Psychiatric Association, 1980, *Diagnostic and Statistical Manual of Mental Disorders,* Third Edition, American Psychiatric Association, Washington, D.C.

Anant, S. S., 1967, A note on the treatment of alcoholics by a verbal aversion technique, *Can. Psychol.,* 8:12–22.

Armor, D. J., and Polich, J. M., 1982, Measurement of alcohol consumption, in *Encyclopedic Handbook of Alcoholism* (E. M. Pattison and E. Kaufman, eds.), Gardner Press, New York.

Armor, D. J., Polich, J. M., and Stambul, H. B., 1978, *Alcoholism and Treatment,* John Wiley & Sons, New York.

Ayllon, T., 1963, Intensive treatment of psychotic behaviour by stimulus satiation and food reinforcement, *Behav. Res. Ther.,* 1:53–61.

Ayllon, T., and Azrin, N. H., 1965, The measurement and reinforcement of behavior of psychotics, *J. Exp. Anal. Behav.,* 8:357–383.

Azrin, N. H., 1976, Improvements in the community reinforcement approach to alcoholism, *Behav. Res. Ther.,* 14:339–348.

Babor, T. F., Mendelson, J. H., Uhly, B., and Souza, E., 1980, Drinking patterns in experimental and barroom settings, *J. Stud. Alc.,* 41:635–651.

Baker, T. B., and Cannon, D. S., 1982, Alcohol and taste-mediated learning, *Addict. Behav.,* 7:211–230.

Bandura, A., 1977, *Social Learning Theory,* Prentice-Hall, Inc., Englewood Cliffs, N.J.

Berg, G., Laberg, J. C., Skutle, A., and Öhman, A., 1981, Instructed versus pharmacological effects of alcohol in alcoholics and social drinkers, *Behav. Res. Ther.*, 19:55–66.

Bigelow, G., Cohen, M., Liebson, I., and Faillace, L., 1972, Abstinence or moderation? Choice by alcoholics, *Behav. Res. Ther.*, 10:209–214.

Bigelow, G., Liebson, I., and Griffiths, R. R., 1973, Experimental analysis of alcoholic drinking, Paper read at American Psychological Association, August, 1973.

Bigelow, G., Liebson, I., and Lawrence, C., 1973, Prevention of alcohol abuse by reinforcement of incompatible behavior, Paper presented at Association for Advancement of Behavior Therapy, December, 1973.

Bigelow, G., Liebson, I., and Griffiths, R. R., 1974, Alcohol drinking: Suppression by a behavioral time-out procedure, *Behav. Res. Ther.*, 12:107–115.

Bigelow, G. E., Stitzer, M. L., Griffiths, R. R., and Liebson, I. A., 1981, Contingency management approaches to drug self-administration and drug abuse: Efficacy and limitations, *Addict. Behav.*, 6:241–252.

Blake, B. C., 1965, The application of behaviour therapy to the treatment of alcoholism, *Behav. Res. Ther.*, 3:78–85.

Blake, B. G., 1967, A follow-up of alcoholics treated by behaviour therapy, *Behav. Res. Ther.*, 5:89–94.

Blakey, R., and Baker, R., 1980, An exposure approach to alcohol abuse, *Behav. Res. Ther.*, 18:319–325.

Bois, C., and Vogel-Sprott, M., Discrimination of low blood alcohol levels and self-titration skills in social drinking, *Q. J. Stud. Alc.*, 35:87–97.

Bradlyn, A. S., Strickler, D. P., and Maxwell, W. A., 1981, Alcohol, expectancy and stress: Methodological concerns with the expectancy design, *Addict. Behav.*, 6:1–8.

Brown, R. A., 1981, Measurement of baseline drinking behaviour in problem-drinking probationers, drinking drivers, and normal drinkers, *Addict. Behav.*, 6:15–22.

Brown, S. A., Goldman, M. S., Inn, A., and Anderson, L. R., 1980, Expectations of reinforcement from alcohol: Their domain and relation to drinking patterns, *J. Consult. Clin. Psychol.*, 48:419–426.

Brownell, K. D., 1982, The addictive disorders, in *Annual Review of Behavior Therapy* (C. M. Franks, G. T. Wilson, P. C. Kendall, and K. D. Brownell, eds.), The Guilford Press, New York.

——, 1983, The addictive disorders, in *Annual Review of Behavior Therapy* (C. M. Franks, G. T. Wilson, P. C. Kendall, and K. D. Brownell, eds.), The Guilford Press, New York.

Burish, T. G., Maisto, S. A., Cooper, A. M., and Sobell, M. B., 1981, Effects of voluntary short-term abstinence from alcohol on subsequent drinking patterns of college students, *J. Stud. Alc.*, 42:1013–1020.

Caddy, G., and Lovibond, S. H., 1976, Self-regulation and discriminated aversive conditioning in the modification of alcoholics' drinking behavior, *Behav. Ther.*, 7:223–230.

Cahalan, D., Cisin, I. H., and Crossley, H. M., 1969, *American Drinking Practices*, Rutgers Center of Alcohol Studies, New Brunswick, N.J.

Cahalan, D., and Room, R., 1974, *Problem Drinking among American Men*, Rutgers Center of Alcohol Studies, New Brunswick, N.J.

Cannon, D. S., and Baker, T. B., 1981, Emetic and electric shock alcohol aversion therapy: Assessment of conditioning, *J. Consult. Clin. Psychol.*, 49:20–33.

Cannon, D. S., Baker, T. B., and Wehl, C. K., 1981, Emetic and electric shock alcohol aversion therapy: Six- and twelve-month follow-up, *J. Consult. Clin. Psychol.*, 49:360–368.

Caudill, B. D., and Marlatt, G. A., 1975, Modeling influences in social drinking: An experimental analogue, *J. Consult. Clin. Psychol.*, 43:405–415.

Cautelà, J. R., 1966, Treatment of compulsive behavior by covert sensitization, *Psychol. Rep.*, 16:33–41.

Cautela, J. R., 1970, Covert reinforcement, *Behav. Ther.*, 1:33–50.

Chaney, E., O'Leary, M., and Marlatt, G. A., 1978, Skill training with alcoholics, *J. Consult. Clin. Psychol.*, 46:1092–1104.

Christiansen, B. A., and Goldman, M. S., 1983, Alcohol-related expectancies vs. demographic/background variables in the prediction of adolescent drinking, *J. Consult. Clin. Psychol.*, 51:249–257.

Christiansen, B. A., Goldman, M. S., and Inn, A., 1982, Development of alcohol-related expectancies in adolescents: Separating pharmacological from social-learning influences, *J. Consult. Clin. Psychol.*, 50:336–344.

Cohen, M., Liebson, I. A., Faillace, L. A., and Allen, R. P., 1971, Moderate drinking by chronic alcoholics, *J. Nerv. Ment. Dis.*, 153:434–444.

Conger, J. J., 1951, The effects of alcohol on conflict behavior in the albino rat, *Q. J. Stud. Alc.*, 12:1–29.

———, 1956, Alcoholism: Theory, problem and challenge, II, Reinforcement theory and the dynamics of alcoholism, *Q. J. Stud. Alc.*, 17:291–324.

Costello, R. M., 1981, Alcoholism and the "alcoholic" personality, in *Evaluation of the Alcoholic: Implications for Research, Theory, and Treatment*, NIAAA Research Monograph No. 5, NIAAA, Rockville, Md.

Craighead, W. E., Kazdin, A. E., and Mahoney, M. J. (eds.), 1981, *Behavior Modification*, Houghton Mifflin Company, Boston.

Crawford, D., and Baker, T. B., 1982, Alcohol dependence and taste-mediated learning in the rat, *Pharm. Biochem. Behav.*, 16:253–261.

Cutler, R. E., and Storm, T., 1975, Observational study of alcohol consumption in natural settings, *J. Stud. Alc.*, 36:1173–1183.

Cutter, H. S. G., Schwab, E. L., and Nathan, P. E., 1970, Effects of alcohol on its utility for alcoholics, *Q. J. Stud. Alc.*, 30:369–378.

Davies, D. L., 1962, Normal drinking by recovered alcohol addicts, *Q. J. Stud. Alc.*, 23:94–104.

Deardorff, C. M., Melges, F. T., Hout, C. N., and Savage, D. J., 1975, Situations related to drinking alcohol: A factor analysis of questionnaire responses. *J. Stud. Alc.*, 36:1184–1195.

Donovan, D. M., and Marlatt, G. A., 1980, Assessment of expectancies and behaviors associated with alcohol consumption: A cognitive-behavioral approach, *J. Stud. Alc.*, 41:1153–1185.

Edwards, G., and Gross, M. M., 1976, Alcohol dependence: Provisional description of a clinical syndrome, *Br. Med. J.*, 1:1058–1061.

Elkins, R. L., 1975, Aversion therapy for alcoholism: Chemical, electrical or verbal imagery?, *Internat. J. Addict.*, 10:157–209.

Elkins, R. L., 1980, Covert sensitization treatment of alcoholism: Contributions of successful conditioning to subsequent abstinence maintenance, *Addict. Behav.*, 5:67–89.

Emrick, C. D., 1975, A review of psychologically oriented treatment of alcoholism, *J. Stud. Alc.*, 367:88–108.

Emrick, C. D., 1982, Evaluation of alcoholism psychotherapy methods, in *Encyclopedic Handbook of Alcoholism* (E. M. Pattison, and E. Kaufman, eds.), Gardner Press, New York.

Finney, J. W., and Moos, R. H., 1981, Characteristics and prognoses of alcoholics who become moderate drinkers and abstainers after treatment, *J. Stud. Alc.*, 42:94–105.

Foy, D. W., and Simon, S. J., 1978, Alcoholic drinking topography as a function of solitary vs. social context, *Addict. Behav.*, 3:39–41.

Foy, D. W., Miller, P. M., Eisler, R. M., and O'Toole, D. H., 1976, Social skills training to teach alcoholics to refuse drinks effectively, *J. Stud. Alc.*, 37:1340–1345.

Franks, C. M., and Wilson, G. T., 1973, 1974, 1975, 1976, 1977, 1978, 1979, 1980, *Annual Review of Behavior Therapy*, Brunner/Mazel, New York.

Gabel, P. C., Noel, N. E., Keane, T. M., and Lisman, S. A., 1980, Effects of sexual versus fear arousal on alcohol consumption in college males, *Behav. Res. & Therapy*, 18:519–526.

Garcia, J., Hankins, W. G., and Rusiniak, K. W., 1974, Behavioral regulation of the milieu interne in man and rat, *Science*, 185:824–831.

Goodwin, D. W., and Guze, S. B., 1974, Heredity and alcoholism, in *The Biology of Alcoholism*, vol. 3 (B. Kissin and H. Begleiter, eds.), Plenum Press, New York.

Gottheil, E., Crawford, H., and Cornelison, F. S. Jr., 1973, The alcoholic's ability to resist available alcohol, *Dis. Nerv. Sys.*, 34:80–84.

Griffiths, R. R., Bigelow, G., and Liebson, I., 1974, Assessment of effects of ethanol self-administration on social interactions in alcoholics, *Psychopharmacologia*, 38:105–110.

———, 1975, Effects of ethanol self-administration on choice behavior: Money vs. socializing, *Pharmacol., Biochem. Behav.*, 3:443–446.

Hedberg, A. G., and Campbell, L., 1974, A comparison of four behavioral treatments of alcoholism, *J. Behav. Ther. Exp. Psychiat.*, 5:251–256.

Heermans, H. W., and Nathan, P. E., The effect of alcohol, arousal, and aggressive cues on human physical aggression in males, Unpublished manuscript, Rutgers University, New Brunswick, N.J.

Higgins, R. L., and Marlatt, G. A., 1973, The effects of anxiety arousal upon the consumption of alcohol by alcoholics and social drinkers, *J. Consult. Clin. Psychol.*, 41:426–433.

———, 1975, Fear of interpersonal evaluation as a determinant of alcohol consumption in male social drinkers, *J. Abnormal Psychol.*, 84:644–651.

Hinson, R. E., and Siegel, S., 1980, The contribution of Pavlovian conditioning to ethanol tolerance and dependence, in *Alcohol Tolerance and Dependence* (H. Rigter, and J. C. Crabbe, eds.), Elsevier, Amsterdam.

Hoffman, H., 1976, Personality measurement for the evaluation and prediction of alcoholism, in *Alcoholism: Interdisciplinary Approaches to an Enduring Problem* (R. E. Tarter and A. A. Sugerman, eds.), Addison-Wesley Publishing Co., Reading, Mass.

Hoffman, H., Jackson, D. N., and Skinner, H. A., 1975, Dimensions of psychopathology among alcoholic patients, *Q. J. Stud. Alc.*, 36:825–837.

Huber, H., Karlin, R., and Nathan, P. E., 1976, Blood alcohol level discrimination by nonalcoholics: The role of internal and external cues, *J. Stud. Alc.*, 37:27–39.

Hull, J. G., 1981, A self-awareness model of the causes and effects of alcohol consumption, *J. Abnormal. Psychol.*, 90:586–600.

Hunt, G. M., and Azrin, N. H., 1973, The community-reinforcement approach to alcoholism, *Behav. Res. Ther.*, 11:91–104.

Jessor, R., Collins, M. I., and Jessor, S. L., 1972, On becoming a drinker: Social-psychological aspects of an adolescent transition, *Ann. N.Y. Acad. of Sci.*, 197:199–213.

Jones, S. L., Kanfer, R., and Lanyon, R. I., 1982, Skill training with alcoholics: A clinical extension, *Addict. Behav.*, 7:285–290.

Kessler, M., and Gomberg, C., 1974, Observations of barroom drinking: Methodology and preliminary results, *Q. J. Stud. Alc.*, 35:1392–1396.

Lang, A. R., Goeckner, D. J., Adesso, V. J., and Marlatt, G. A., 1975, The effects of alcohol on aggression in male social drinkers, *J. Abnormal Psych.*, 84:508–518.

Lansky, D., Nathan, P. E., Ersner-Hershfield, S. M., and Lipscomb, T. R., 1978, Blood alcohol level discrimination: Pre-training monitoring accuracy of alcoholics and nonalcoholics, *Addict. Behav.*, 3:209–214.

Lansky, D., Nathan, P. E., and Lawson, D. M., 1978, Blood alcohol level discrimination by alcoholics: The role of internal and external cues, *J. Consult. Clin. Psychol.*, 46:953–960.

Lansky, D., and Wilson, G. T., 1981, Alcohol, expectations, and sexual arousal in males: An information processing analysis, *J. Abnorm. Psychol.*, 90:35–45.

LaPorte, D. J., McLellan, A. T., Erdlen, F. R., and Parente, R. J., 1981, Treatment outcome as a function of follow-up difficulty in substance abusers, *J. Consult. Clin. Psychol.*, 49:112–119.

Lazarus, A. A., 1965, Towards the understanding and effective treatment of alcoholism, *S. Afr. Med. J.*, 39:736–741.

Le, A. D., Poulos, C. X., and Cappell, H. D., 1979, Conditioned tolerance to the hypothermic effect of ethyl alcohol, *Science*, 206:1109–1110.

Lemere, F., and Voegtlin, W. L., 1950, An evaluation of the aversion treatment of alcoholism, *Q. J. Stud. Alc.*, 11:199–204.

Lemere, F., Voegtlin, W. L., Broz, W. R., and O'Halloren, P., 1942, Conditioned reflex treatment of alcohol addiction, V. Type of patient suitable for this treatment, *Northwestern Medicine, Seattle*, 4:88–89.

Liebson, I., Bigelow, G., and Flame R., 1973, Alcoholism among methadone patients: A specific treatment method, *Am. J. Psychiat.*, 130:483.

Lindsley, O. R., 1960, Characteristics of the behavior of chronic psychotics as revealed by free-operant conditioning methods, *Dis. Nerv. Sys.*, 21:66–78.

Lipscomb, T. R., and Nathan, P. E., 1980, The effects of drinking pattern, family history of alcoholism and tolerance to alcohol on blood alcohol level discrimination, using internal cues, *Arch. Gen. Psychiat.*, 37:571–576.

Lloyd, R. W., and Salzberg, S. C., 1975, Controlled social drinking: An alternative to abstinence as a treatment goal for some alcohol abusers, *Psych. Bull.*, 82:815–842.

Lovibond, S. H., and Caddy, G. R., 1970, Discriminated aversive control in the moderation of alcoholics' drinking behavior, *Behav. Ther.*, 1:437–444.

MacCulloch, M. J., Feldman, M. P., Orford, J. F., and MacCulloch, M. L., 1966, Anticipatory avoidance learning in the treatment of alcoholism: A record of therapeutic failure, *Behav. Res. Ther.*, 4:187.

Mahoney, M. J., 1974, *Cognition and Behavior Modification*, Ballinger, Cambridge, Mass.

Maisto, S. A., Sobell, M. B., and Sobell, L. C., 1980, Predictors of treatment outcome for alcoholics treated by individualized behavior therapy, *Addict. Behav.*, 5:259–264.

————, 1982, Reliability of self-reports of low ethanol consumption by problem drinkers over 18 months of follow-up, *Drug and Alc. Depend.*, 9:273–278.

Marlatt, G. A., 1976, The drinking profile: A questionnaire for the behavioral assessment of alcoholism, in *Behavior Therapy Assessment: Diagnosis, Design, and Evaluation* (E. J. Mash and L. G. Terdal, eds.), Springer, New York.

Marlatt, G. A., 1978, Craving for alcohol, loss of control, and relapse: A cognitive-behavioral analysis, in *Alcoholism: New Directions in Behavioral Research and Treatment* (P. E. Nathan and G. A. Marlatt, eds.), Plenum Press, New York.

Marlatt, G. A., 1981, The drinking history: Problems of validity and reliability, in *Evaluation of the Alcoholic: Implications for Research, Theory, and Treatment*, NIAAA Research Monograph No. 5, NIAAA, Rockville, Md.

Marlatt, G. A., Demming, B., and Reid, J. B., 1973, Loss of control drinking in alcoholics: An experimental analogue, *J. Abnormal Psychol.*, 81:233–241.

Marlatt, G. A., and Donovan, D. M., 1982, Behavioral psychology approaches to alcoholism, in *Encyclopedic Handbook of Alcoholism* (E. M. Pattison and E. Kaufman, eds.), Gardner Press, New York.

Marlatt, G. A., Kosturn, C. F., and Lang, A. R., 1975, Provocation to anger and opportunity for retaliation as determinants of alcohol consumption in social drinkers, *J. Abnormal Psych.*, 84:652–659.

Marlatt, G. A., and Parks, G. A., 1982, Self-management and interpersonal skills learning, in *Self Management and Behavior Change: From Theory to Practice* (P. Karoly and F. H. Kanfer, eds.), Pergamon Press, New York.

McCollam, J. B., Burish, T. G., Maisto, S., and Sobell, M., 1980, Alcohol's effects on physiological arousal and self-reported affect and sensations, *J. Abnormal. Psychol.*, 89:224–234.

McGuire, R. J., and Vallance, M., 1964, Aversion therapy by electric shock, a simple technique, *Br. Med. J.*, 1:151–152.

Meichenbaum, D. H., 1977, *Cognitive-Behavior Modification*, Plenum Press, New York.

Mello, N. K., 1972, Behavioral studies of alcoholism, in *The Biology of Alcoholism*, vol. 2 (B. Kissin and H. Begleiter, eds.), Plenum Press, New York.

Mello, N. K., and Mendelson, J. H., 1965, Operant analysis of drinking patterns of chronic alcoholics, *Nature*, 206:43–46.

Mendelson, J. H., and Mello, N. K., 1966, Experimental analysis of drinking behavior of chronic alcoholics, *Ann. N.Y. Acad. Sci.*, 133:828–845.

Merry, J., 1966, The "loss of control" myth, *Lancet*, 1:1267–1268.

Miller, P. M., 1975, A behavioral intervention program for chronic public drunkenness offenders, *Arch. Gen. Psychiat.*, 32:915–918.

————, 1976, *Behavioral Treatment of Alcoholism,* Pergamon Press, New York.

Miller, P. M., and Eisler, R. M., 1975, Alcohol and drug abuse, in *Behavior Modification Principles, Issues, and Applications* (W. E. Craighead, A. E. Kazdin, and M. J. Mahoney, eds.), Houghton Mifflin Company, Boston, Mass.

Miller, P. M., and Foy, D. W., 1981, Substance abuse, in *Handbook of Clinical Behavior Therapy* (S. M. Turner, K. S. Calhoun, and H. E. Adams, eds.), John Wiley & Sons, New York.

Miller, P. M., Hersen, M., Eisler, R., and Hemphill, D. P., 1973, Electrical aversion therapy with alcoholics: An analogue study, *Behav. Res. Ther.,* 11:491–497.

Miller, P. M., Becker, J. V., Foy, D. W., and Wooten, L. S., 1976, Instructional control of the components of alcoholic drinking behavior, *Behav. Ther.,* 7:472–480.

Miller, W. R., and Caddy, G. R., 1977, Abstinence and controlled drinking in the treatment of problem drinkers, *J. Stud. Alc.,* 38:986–1003.

Mills, K. C., Sobell, M. B., and Schaefer, H. H., 1971, Training social drinking as an alternative to abstinence for alcoholics, *Behav. Ther.,* 2:18–27.

Nathan, P. E., 1976, Alcoholism, in *Handbook of Behavior Modification* (H. Leitenberg, ed.), Appleton-Century-Crofts, Inc., New York.

————, 1980, Alcoholism and DSM III, *Advances in Alcoholism,* 1:15.

————, 1981, The data on controlled drinking treatments, *Advances in Alcoholism,* 2:13.

————, 1983, Failures in prevention: Why we can't prevent the devastating effect of alcoholism and drug abuse on American productivity, *Am. Psychol.,* 38:459–467.

Nathan, P. E., and Lansky, D., 1978, Management of the chronic alcoholic: A behavioral viewpoint, in *Controversy in Psychiatry* (J. P. Brady and H. K. H. Brodie, eds.), W. B. Saunders Company, Philadelphia, Pa.

Nathan, P. E., and Lipscomb, T. R., 1979, Behavior therapy and behavior modification in the treatment of alcoholism, in *The Diagnosis and Treatment of Alcoholism* (J. H. Mendelson, and N. K. Mello, eds.), McGraw-Hill Book Company, New York.

Nathan, P. E., and Lisman, S. A., 1976, Behavioral and motivational patterns of chronic alcoholics, in *Alcoholism: Interdisciplinary Approaches to an Enduring Problem* (R. E. Tarter and A. A. Sugerman, eds.), Addison-Wesley Publishing Company, Reading, Mass.

Nathan, P. E., and O'Brien, J. S., 1971, An experimental analysis of the behavior of alcoholics and nonalcoholics during prolonged experimental drinking, *Behav. Ther.,* 2:455–476.

Nathan, P. E., Titler, N. A., Lowenstein, L. M., Solomon, P., and Rossi, A. M., 1970, Behavioral analysis of chronic alcoholism, *Arch. Gen. Psychiat.,* 22:419–430.

Nathan, P. E., Witte, G., and Langenbucher, J. W., 1983, Behavior therapy and behavior modification, in *Clinical Methods in Psychology,* Second Edition (I. B. Weiner, ed.), Wiley-Interscience, New York.

Neubuerger, O. W., Hasha, N., Matarazzo, J. D., Schmitz, R. E., and Pratt, H. H., 1981, Behavioral-chemical treatment of alcoholism: An outcome replication, *J. Stud. Alc.,* 42:806–810.

Neubuerger, O. W., Miller, S. I., Schmitz, R. E., Matarazzo, J. D., Pratt, H., and

Hasha, N., 1982, Replicable abstinence rates in an alcoholism treatment program, *JAMA*, 248:960–963.

Noel, N. E., and Lisman, S. A., 1980, Alcohol consumption by college women following exposure to unsolvable problems: Learned helplessness or stress induced drinking? *Behav. Res. & Therapy*, 18:429–440.

Oates, J. F., and McCoy, R. T., 1973, *Laboratory Evaluation of Alcohol Safety Interlock Systems*, National Highway Traffic Safety Administration, U.S. Department of Transportation.

Oei, T. P. S., and Jackson, P., 1980, Long-term effects of group and individual social skills training with alcoholics, *Addict. Behav.*, 5:129–136.

————, 1982, Social skills and cognitive behavioral approaches to the treatment of problem drinking, *J. Stud. Alc.*, 43:532–547.

Ogborne, A. C., and Bornet, A., 1982, Abstinence and abusive drinking among affiliates of Alcoholics Anonymous: Are these the only alternatives?, *Addict. Behav.*, 7:199–202.

Okulitch, P. V., and Marlatt, G. A., 1972, Effects of varied extinction conditions with alcoholics and social drinkers, *J. Abnormal Psychol.*, 79:205–211.

O'Leary, D. E., O'Leary, M. R., and Donovan, D. M., 1976, Social skill acquisition and psycho-social development of alcoholics: A review, *Addict. Behav.*, 1:111–120.

Paredes, A., Jones, B. M., and Gregory, D., 1974a, An exercise to assist alcoholics to maintain prescribed levels of intoxication, *Alcohol Technical Reports*, 2:24–36.

Paredes, A., Gregory, D., and Jones, B. M., 1974b, Induced drinking and social adjustment in alcoholics, *Q. J. Stud. Alc.*, 35:1279–1293.

Parker, J. C., Gilbert, G., and Speltz, M. L., 1981, Expectations regarding the effects of alcohol on assertiveness: A comparison of alcoholics and social drinkers, *Addict. Behav.*, 6:29–33.

Partington, J. T., and Johnson, F. G., 1969, Personality types among alcoholics, *Q. J. Stud. Alc.*, 30:21–34.

Pattison, E. M., 1976, A conceptual approach to alcoholism treatment goals, *Addict. Behav.*, 1:177–192.

Pattison, E. M., Sobell, M. B., and Sobell, L. C. (eds.), 1977, *Emerging Concepts of Alcohol Dependence*, Springer, New York.

Pendery, M. L., and Maltzman, I. M., 1982, Controlled drinking by alcoholics? New findings and a reevaluation of a major affirmative study, *Science*, 217:169–175.

Perkins, D. V., Cox, W. M., and Levy, L. H., 1981, Therapists' recommendations of abstinence or controlled drinking as treatment goals, *J. Stud. Alc.*, 42:304–311.

Pihl, R. O., Zeichner, A., Niaura, R., Nagy, K., and Zacchia, C., 1981, Attribution and alcohol-mediated aggression, *J. Abnormal. Psychol.*, 90:468–475.

Polich, J. M., 1982, The validity of self-reports in alcoholism treatment, *Addict. Behav.*, 7:123–132.

Polich, J. M., Armor, D. J., and Braiker, H. B., 1981, *The Course of Alcoholism: Four Years After Treatment*, John Wiley & Sons, New York.

Pomerleau, O. F., Pertschuk, M., and Stinnett, J., 1976, A critical examination of some current assumptions in the treatment of alcoholism, *J. Stud. Alc.*, 37:849–867.

Pomerleau, O. F., Pertschuk, M., Adkins, D., and Brady, J. P., A comparison of behavioral and traditional treatment for middle-income problem drinkers, *J. Behav. Med.*, 1:187–200.

Reid, J. B., 1978, The study of drinking in natural settings, in *Behavioral Approaches to Assessment and Treatment of Alcoholism* (G. A. Marlatt and P. E. Nathan, eds.), Rutgers Center of Alcohol Studies, New Brunswick, N.J.

Robins, L. N., 1981, The diagnosis of alcoholism after DSM III, in *Evaluation of the Alcoholic: Implications for Research, Theory, and Treatment*, NIAAA Research Monograph No. 5, NIAAA, Rockville, Md.

Rohsenow, D. J., 1982, Control over interpersonal evaluation and alcohol consumption in male social drinkers, *Addict. Behav.*, 7:113–121.

Rohsenow, D. J., and Marlatt, G. A., 1981, The balanced placebo design: Methodological considerations, *Addict. Behav.*, 6:107–122.

Rosenbluth, J., Nathan, P. E., and Lawson, D. M., 1978, Environmental influences on drinking by college students in a college pub, *Addict. Behav.*, 3:117–121.

Sanchez-Craig, M., 1979, Reappraisal therapy: A self-control strategy for abstinence and controlled drinking, Paper at Taos International Conference on Treatment of Addictive Behaviors, Taos, N.M.

———, 1980, Random assignment to abstinence or controlled drinking in a cognitive-behavioral program: Short-term effects on drinking behavior, *Addict. Behav.*, 5:35–39.

Sanchez-Craig, M., and Annis, H. M., 1982, Initial evaluation of a program for early-stage problem drinkers randomization to abstinence and controlled drinking, American Psychological Association Annual Meeting, Washington, D.C., August, 1982.

Sandler, J., 1969, Three aversive control procedures with alcoholics: A preliminary report, Paper read at Southeastern Psychological Association, April, 1969.

Schaefer, H. H., Sobell, M. B., and Mills, K. C., 1971, Baseline drinking behavior in alcoholics and social drinkers: Kinds of drinks and sip magnitude, *Behav. Res. Ther.*, 9:23–27.

Schuckit, M. A., 1980, Self-rating of alcohol intoxication by young men with and without family histories of alcoholism, *J. Stud. Alc.*, 41:242–249.

Schuckit, M. A., Engstrom, D., Alpert, R., and Duby, J., 1981, Differences in muscle-tension response to ethanol in young men with and without family histories of alcoholism, *J. Stud. Alc.*, 42:918–924.

Selzer, M. L., 1971, The Michigan Alcoholism Screening Test: The quest for a new diagnostic instrument, *Am. J. Psychiat.*, 127:1653–1658.

Siegel, S., 1975, Evidence from rats that morphine tolerance is a learned response, *J. Comp. Physiol. Psychol.*, 89:498–506.

Silverstein, S. J., Nathan, P. E., and Taylor, H. A., 1974, Blood alcohol level estimation and controlled drinking by chronic alcoholics, *Behav. Ther.*, 5:1–15.

Skinner, H. A., and Allen, B. A., 1982, Alcohol dependence syndrome: Measurement and validation, *J. Abnormal Psychol.*, 91:199–209.

Sobell, L. C., Maisto, S. A., Sobell, M. B., and Cooper, A. M., 1979, Reliability of alcoholics' self-reports of drinking and related behaviors one year prior to treatment in an outpatient treatment program, *Behav. Res. Ther.*, 17:157–160.

Sobell, L. C., and Sobell, M. B., 1981, Outcome criteria and the assessment of alcohol treatment efficacy, in *Evaluation of the Alcoholic: Implications for Research, Theory, and Treatment*, NIAAA Research Monograph No. 5, NIAAA, Rockville, Md.

————, 1982, Alcoholism treatment outcome evaluation methodology, in *Prevention, Intervention and Treatment: Concerns and Models*, NIAAA Alcohol and Health Monograph No. 3, NIAAA, Rockville, Md.

Sobell, M. B., 1978, Empirically derived components of treatment for alcohol problems: Some issues and extensions, in *Behavioral Assessment and Treatment of Alcoholism* (G. A. Marlatt and P. E. Nathan, eds.), Rutgers Center of Alcohol Studies, New Brunswick, N.J.

Sobell, M. B., and Sobell, L. C., 1973a, Individualized behavior therapy for alcoholics, *Behav. Ther.*, 4:49–72.

————, 1973b, Alcoholics treated by individualized behavior therapy: One year treatment outcome, *Behav. Res. Ther.*, 11:599–618.

————, 1976, Second-year treatment outcome of alcoholics treated by individualized behavior therapy: Results, *Behav. Res. Ther.*, 14:195–215.

Sobell, M. B., Sobell, L. C., and VanderSpek, R., 1979, Relationships among clinical judgment, self-report and breath analysis measures of intoxication in alcoholics, *J. Consult. Clin. Psychol.*, 47:204–206.

Southwick, L., Steele, C., Marlatt, G. A., and Lindell, M., 1981, Alcohol-related expectancies: Defined by phase of intoxication and drinking experience, *J. Consult. Clin. Psychol.*, 49:713–721.

Storm, T., and Cutler, R. E., 1981, Observations of drinking in natural settings: Vancouver beer parlors and cocktail lounges, *J. Stud. Alc.*, 42:972–997.

Strickler, D., Bigelow, G., Lawrence, C., and Liebson, I., 1976, Moderate drinking as an alternative to alcohol abuse: A nonaversive procedure, *Behav. Res. Ther.*, 14:279–288.

Strickler, D. P., Bradlyn, A. S., and Maxwell, W. A., 1981, Teaching moderate drinking behaviors to young adult heavy drinkers: The effects of three training procedures, *Addict. Behav.*, 6:355–364.

Tarter, R. E., 1982, Experimental psychology and alcoholism: Assessment, contribution, and impact, in *Encyclopedic Handbook of Alcoholism* (E. M. Pattison and E. Kaufman, eds.), Gardner Press, New York.

Tharp, R. G., and Wetzel, R. J., 1969, *Behavior Modification in the Natural Environment*, Academic Press, New York.

Tomaszewski, R. J., Strickler, D. P., and Maxwell, W. A., 1980, Influence of social setting and social drinking stimuli on drinking behavior, *Addict. Behav.*, 5:235–240.

Tracey, D., Karlin, R., and Nathan, P. E., 1976, Experimental analysis of chronic alcoholism in four women, *J. Consult. Clin. Psychol.*, 44:832–842.

Tucker, J. A., Vuchinich, R. E., and Sobell, M. B., 1981, Alcohol consumption as a self-handicapping strategy, *J. Abnormal Psychol.*, 90:220–230.

Tucker, J. A., Vuchinich, R. E., Sobell, M. B., and Maisto, S. A., 1980, Normal drinkers' alcohol consumption as a function of conflicting motives induced by intellectual performance stress, *Addict. Behav.*, 5:171–178.

Turner, S. M., Calhoun, K. S., and Adams, H. E. (eds.), 1981, *Handbook of Clinical Behavior Therapy*, John Wiley & Sons, New York.

Vaillant, G. E., and Milofsky, E. S., 1982, The etiology of alcoholism, *Amer. Psychologist*, 37:494–503.

Voegtlin, W. L., 1940, The treatment of alcoholism by establishing a conditioned reflex, *Am. J. Med. Sci.*, 199:802–809.

Vogel-Sprott, M., 1975, Self-evaluation of performance and the ability to discriminate blood alcohol concentrations, *J. Stud. Alc.*, 36:1–10.

Vogler, R. E., Compton, J. V., and Weissbach, T. A., 1975, Integrated behavior
change techniques for alcoholics, *J. Consult. Clin. Psychol.*, 42:233–243.

Vogler, R. E., Lunde, S. E., Johnson, G. R., and Martin, P. L., 1970, Electrical
aversion conditioning with chronic alcoholics, *J. Consult. Clin. Psychol.*,
34:302–307.

Vogler, R. E., Lunde, S. E., and Martin, P. L., 1971, Electrical aversion conditioning with chronic alcoholics: Follow-up and suggestions for research, *J.
Consult. Clin. Psychol.*, 36:450.

Vogler, R. E., Weissbach, T. A., and Compton, J. V., 1977a, Learning techniques
for alcohol abuse, *Behav. Res. Ther.*, 15:31–38.

Vogler, R. E., Weissbach, T. A., Compton, J. V., and Martin, G. T., 1977b,
Integrated behavior change techniques for problem drinkers in the community, *J. Consult. Clin. Psychol.*, 45:267–279.

Vuchinich, R., and Sobell, M. B., 1978, Empirical separation of physiological and
expected effects of alcohol on complex motor performance, *Psychopharmacology*, 60:81–85.

Vuchinich, R. E., and Tucker, J. A., 1980, A critique of cognitive labeling explanations of the emotional and behavioral effects of alcohol, *Addict. Behav.*,
5:179–188.

Wiens, A. N., Menustik, C. E., Miller, S. I., and Schmitz, R. E., 1983, Medical-
behavioral treatment of the older alcoholic patient, Unpublished manuscript,
University of Oregon Health Sciences Center, Portland, Oregon.

Wiens, A. N., Montague, J. R., Manaugh, T. S., and English, C. J., 1976, Pharmacological aversive conditioning to alcohol in a private hospital: One year
follow-up, *J. Stud. Alc.*, 37:1320–1324.

Williams, R. J., and Brown, R. A., 1974, Differences in baseline drinking behavior
between New Zealand alcoholics and normal drinkers, *Behav. Res. Ther.*,
12:287–294.

Wilson, G. T., 1978, Booze, beliefs, and behavior: Cognitive processes in alcohol
use and abuse, in *Alcoholism: New Directions in Behavioral Research and
Treatment* (P. E. Nathan and G. A. Marlatt, eds.), Plenum Press, New York.

Wilson, G. T., 1981, Expectations and substance abuse: Does basic research
benefit clinical assessment and therapy?, *Addict. Behav.*, 6:221–231.

Wilson, G. T., and Abrams, D., Effects of alcohol on social anxiety and physiological arousal: Cognitive versus pharmacological processes, *Cog. Ther.
Res.*, 1:195–210.

Wilson, G. T., and Davison, G. C., 1969, Aversion techniques in behavior therapy: Some theoretical and metatheoretical considerations, *J. Consult. Clin.
Psychol.*, 33:327–329.

Wilson, G .T., and Franks, C. M. (eds.), 1982, *Contemporary Behavior Therapy*,
The Guilford Press, New York.

Wilson, G. T., and Lawson, D. M., 1976, Expectancies, alcohol, and sexual
arousal in male social drinkers, *J. Abn. Psychol.*, 85:489–497.

Wilson, G .T., Leaf, R., and Nathan, P. E., 1975, The aversive control of excessive drinking by chronic alcoholics in the laboratory setting, *J. Appl. Behav.
Anal.*, 8:13–26.

Wolpe, J., and Lazarus, A. A., 1966, *Behavior Therapy Techniques*, Pergamon
Press, London.

CHAPTER 10

The Role of
the Social Setting
in the Prevention
and Treatment
of Alcoholism

Norman E. Zinberg, M.D.
Clinical Professor of Psychiatry, Harvard Medical School
Director of Psychiatric Training
The Cambridge Hospital
Cambridge, Massachusetts

Kathleen M. Fraser, Ed.M.
Research Consultant, Department of Psychiatry
The Cambridge Hospital
Cambridge, Massachusetts

For many years students of the use of intoxicants believed that two variables—*drug* (the pharmacological action of the drug itself) and *set* (the user's attitudes about use and his personality)—were responsible for an individual's decision to use an intoxicant and for its effect upon him. Two events of the 1960s and 1970s in the arena of illicit drug use have pointed to the power and importance of a third variable, the physical and social *setting* in which use takes place (Zinberg and Robertson, 1972).

The first event was the noticeable change between the early 1960s and mid-1970s in the effect of LSD on its users (Zinberg, 1974). The second was the high incidence of heavy heroin use by American troops in Vietnam (Zinberg, 1972), followed by a drastic reduction in their use of the drug after returning to the United States. Neither of these phenomena could be explained in terms of drug and set alone. Both of them demonstrated that the setting variable was equally, if not more influential in determining the difference between drug use and drug abuse (Zinberg et al., 1978a).

Although considerable attention has been paid recently to the setting variable in relation to the use of illicit drugs (Zinberg et al., 1977), very little interest has been shown in the influence of setting upon the general social use of America's most popular intoxicant, alcohol (Straus, 1973). Less attention still has been paid to the effect of setting upon the treatment of alcoholism. It is true that certain aspects of setting, such as peer-group influence and the importance of ethnic background, are recognized sporadically as significant factors in the development of drinking patterns (Bacon, 1969), but they are not seen as reflections of the social sanctions and rituals[1] which most young people internalize during childhood and adolescence (Zinberg et al., 1975).

Because the physical and particularly the social setting are crucial factors in both the prevention and treatment of alcoholism, this chapter focuses on these two topics. One section is devoted to prevention, and two others to treatment.

In an historical approach to the subject of prevention, the whole range of American history is divided into five periods, each described in terms of drinking behavior and the social sanctions and rituals that operated to control it. This historical section demonstrates that when social controls were strong, alcohol was used in a moderate, responsible way by the general public, whereas the weakening or abrogation of such controls led to abuse. The prevention of alcoholism, or the responsible use of alcohol, seems to have been most evident in American life when the social mores supported controlled use, rather than when the deliberate attempt was made to prohibit all drinking through legislation.

The two sections on treatment of alcoholism deal with two relatively unsuccessful methods of treatment and one more successful approach. The section on the medical and psychiatric models, approaches which have not yet proved uniformly effective, is relatively short. The second and much longer section discusses the most successful treatment modality, the self-help organization called Alcoholics Anonymous. These two

---

[1]Social sanctions are the norms and beliefs concerning the ways in which a particular drug should be used, and also the ways in which the harmful physiological and psychological effects of the drug can be avoided. Rituals are stylized drug-using behaviors and practices which relate to the means by which the drug is obtained and administered, the physical setting chosen for use, the using circumstances and using companions selected, the activities in which the user engages when he is intoxicated, and any specific activities undertaken after intoxication which the user regards as part of the using process (Zinberg et al., 1978b).

sections on treatment illustrate the point that when the influence of social sanctions and rituals on alcohol use is recognized, and when these forms of social control are incorporated into treatment principles and methods, treatment achieves a high rate of success. But when the influence of setting is not recognized, treatment does not work well.

The brief concluding section sums up the ironies, paradoxes, and complexities that characterize the interrelationship between the setting variable and the prevention and treatment of alcoholism.

I. PREVENTION: A HISTORY OF THE SOCIAL CONTROL OF DRINKING IN AMERICA

A survey of the literature on alcohol use and alcoholism from Colonial times to the late twentieth century has failed to turn up any comprehensive history of alcohol use and abuse. Alcohol studies tend to be specific and problem-oriented, emphasizing when and where alcohol problems develop rather than dealing with the causes of drinking behavior. Hence they have a consistently negative ring which echoes the wary and ambivalent attitude toward alcohol that is characteristic of this country even today (Bacon, 1969; Straus, 1973).

Yet the consistent interest in alcohol use over the centuries cannot be denied, nor the powerful moral bias against such use. Interestingly enough, the evidence points to the existence of historical cycles in which control of use and lack of control alternate. These variations seem to be correlated with changing social factors, although this correlation is far more evident through hindsight than it could have been at the time.

A. Applicable Standards of Control

In describing and analyzing the changing patterns of alcohol use in America during the past three and a half centuries, it is difficult to single out the sociocultural factors that caused these changes. There was no intellectual inquiry into the ways in which moderate use of alcohol could be sustained, and therefore no theory of controlled use that included a set of standards to regulate behavior. As a consequence, we have been obliged to amalgamate a set of standards from the cross-cultural researchers (Chafetz and Demone, 1962; Lolli, 1970; Lolli et al., 1958; Wilkinson, 1973). The following five sociocultural standards, or cultural variables, appear to be directly correlated with controlled drinking behavior.

1. Group drinking is clearly differentiated from drunkenness and is associated with ritualistic or religious celebrations. For example,

the group may participate in the preparation of the alcoholic beverage to be consumed.

2. Drinking is associated with eating or ritualistic feasting, or the beverage is actually consumed with the food.

3. Both of the sexes, as well as different generations, are included in the drinking situation, whether they drink or not.

4. Drinking is divorced from the individual effort to escape personal anxiety or difficult (intolerable) social situations. Further, alcohol is not considered medicinally valuable.

5. Inappropriate behavior when drinking (violence, aggression, overt sexuality) is absolutely disapproved, and protection against such behavior is offered by the "sober" or the less intoxicated. This general acceptance of a concept of restraint usually indicates that drinking is only one of many activities and thus carries a low level of emotionalism, and also that drinking is not associated with a male or female "rite de passage" or any sense of superiority on the part of one sex or the other.

The cross-cultural data from which these five standards have emerged suggest that such socially generated customs, rituals, and social sanctions have a direct bearing upon the management (control) of alcohol use. When the changes in social drinking patterns in American history are examined in the light of these five standards, one fact stands out across three centuries. This culture, much more than others, has always behaved with great ambivalence toward the *idea* of alcohol use; but at the same time its historical record reveals numerous clearly identifiable and constantly changing rules and customs that deal with the reality of use.

B. The Colonial Period

The first century and a half (1620–1775) illustrates the typical American ambivalence toward alcohol use, but it was not a period of seriously problematic drinking. The American colonists firmly believed in, and were almost fanatical about, the medical and spiritual benefits of regular consumption. This belief was so widespread that for more than 30 years an abstainer had to pay an insurance rate that was 10% higher than that levied on a drinker (Kobler, 1973). Nevertheless, the colonists appear to have been deliberate and conservative in their prescriptions for consumption, and they also had powerful proscriptions concerning deportment. "Liquor was given to man for the benefit of the group, and not for the wasteful gratification of individual vision." Stringent penalties, progressively more severe, were applied to "flagrant abusers of nature's gifts" (Krout, 1925). Such prohibitory laws as the colonists enacted were intended to prevent drunkenness, not to eliminate alcohol, "the good creature of God" (Kobler, 1973).

The small, cohesive, religiously oriented, and homogeneous communities that made up most of America before the Revolution exercised stringent controls over the social behavior of members. And the incidence of serious problems with alcohol was reported to be low. This low level of alcohol problems did not necessarily represent a low rate of consumption, however. Our forebears did not limit themselves to a few beers. On the contrary, Colonial life was "verily soaked with alcohol," according to one chronicler (Mitchell, 1946). But this use was carefully ritualized. Colonial farmers avoided water in favor of gulping rum or cider, but they did it at specific times. For example, a jug of cider often awaited the farmer at the end of each cultivated row in his field. Children and merchants were released for rum or cider "10 o'clocks," and there was a 4 o'clock "beer break." Religious and political gatherings in particular were considered official occasions for the consumption of barrels of "spiritous," domestically produced beverages (Earle, 1902; Krout, 1925; Mitchell, 1946; Rublowsky, 1974).

Single families produced enormous quantities of alcohol. It has been recorded that as many as 500 to 1000 barrels of cider were produced for domestic use each year by most families, who also fermented untold quantities of various concoctions labeled "wine." These beverages were consumed with meals because the colonists were notoriously fearful of contaminated water. Certainly men and women drank together, not only during mealtimes but on other social occasions. Nor was there any inhibition against mixing of generations: the children drank along with their elders, and in these small homogeneous communities several generations were represented at the "groaning boards," and each consumed its share of the cider, wine, or rum. In fact, seventeenth-century New England infants were delivered in freezing cabins while their mothers were under the influence of "groaning beer," a potent beverage brewed sometime during the seventh month of gestation and consumed with dietary beer, wine, and cider for two months prior to, and a half-year following, delivery (Earle, 1902). Those toddlers and children who had not been claimed by baptism-day pneumonia were given each day "two to four small beers, and a glass or two of wine and cider" (Earle, 1902).

It seems remarkable that alcohol-related problems remained at such a low level when alcohol was considered so valuable nutritionally. It can only be conjectured that the Colonial ordinances, which reflected the social standards for acceptable rates of drinking, were sufficiently powerful to limit the extent to which alcohol was used and thus to deal with potentially difficult social situations.

For example, in the Connecticut and Massachusetts Bay colonies no man could drink over "one half pint of wine at a time, or tipple over half an hour, or drink at all after nine o'clock at night" (Earle, 1902). In Boston, "if a stranger called for more drink than the officer thought in his judgment he could soberly bear away, he would presently countermand it and appoint the proportion beyond which he could not get one drop" (Earle, 1902). One writer presented wry testimony to the success of early, locally controlled drinking behavior. "With ministers, constables, deacons, parsons, tithing men all watching the tavern door the Puritan had little chance to become a toper even an [if] he would" (Earle, 1902).

This preoccupation with deportment, with so many people overseeing every aspect of drinking, must have given strong support to the fifth standard of control mentioned above—the notion that inappropriate behavior when drinking was frowned upon. Certainly the sober or less intoxicated were more than willing to apply concepts of restraint if drinking behavior resulted in aggressive, violent, or sexually provocative behavior. Moreover, the complete acceptance of drinking in the colonies as well as the complete acceptance of the restrictions placed upon it indicates that drinking was accompanied by a low level of emotionalism. The Colonial American was concerned about appropriate and religiously defined behavior. The ordinances governing tavern drinking and possible "unseemly behavior" were strict indeed. Alcohol's status as both a beverage and a quasimedical potion may well have served to regularize and institutionalize it in such a way that it was not generally associated with excess emotionalism, with male or female *rites de passage,* or with any sense of superiority or personal mastery. The severe limits placed on the amount of alcohol used certainly would have made it difficult to regard the capacity to hold liquor as an index of male or female superiority.

Several sources mention the relative absence of alcohol-related problems in the colonies. Judge Samuel Sewall's journal and several of his letters refer to the "safe streets of Boston towne," where the good judge could "stumble home alone in the dark from his love-making without fear of molestation" (Earle, 1902). John Winthrop wrote "with great satisfaction" of a "great training" in Boston in 1641 when "200 men drilled for two days without one case of drunkenness being observed, although the supply of wine, small beer, and other liquors was abundant" (Krout, 1925). Colonial chroniclers, of course, compared the relative order of this continent with the fearful excesses described in England at the same time, where "residents feared to venture abroad after dark unless protected by armed retainers for gangs of drunken ruffians roamed the streets." There is little doubt that the colonists' concern with excessive drinking practices in part fulfilled their wish to differentiate themselves from the mother country (Krout, 1925).

During the Colonial period tavern-keeping was a highly respected political and moral occupation. The task of regulating drinking was a prestigious one; tavern-keepers were considered akin to ministers and were held responsible for the social order. Early records at Harvard College listed students according to the social prominence of their families, and until the late eighteenth century these records placed sons of tavern-keepers ahead of clergymen's sons (Krout, 1925).

C. The Revolutionary and Post-Revolutionary Periods

Changes in Colonial drinking habits had already begun to occur before the Revolution—changes that were to be fostered by that war and were to characterize America by the nineteenth century. Records indicate that excessive drinking and the ordinary use of "hard" liquor had become a social problem of some concern. This change in drinking habits appears to have resulted from the almost magical value of locally distilled spirits when exchanged for slaves, British dry goods, gold, and molasses in the African and West Indian Markets. Moreover, the colonists, initially loath to employ liquor in a one-sided barter with the Indians, eventually joined frontier tradesmen in pouring kegs of highly touted "ardent spirits" into troublesome or fur-wealthy tribes. Breweries became distilleries, whiskey and rum were soon more profitable commodities than corn and sugar, and the decline of the Northern slave trade was ameliorated by the mercantilists' heavy investment in intoxicants. Liquor sold on the Western frontiers was always sure to bring huge profits to the Southern colonies and the Caribbean settlements (Kobler, 1973; Krout, 1925).[2]

The most important changes in standards related to the running of taverns. The regulation of drinking now fell to eager businessmen, who infiltrated what had been a political, moral, and respected occupation. Soldiers returning from the Revolutionary War, as well as retiring politicians, invested in taverns and implored the legislators to protect their interests along with those of the newly wealthy distillery owners and bond merchants. The replacement of the domestic and medicinal use of alcohol by taverns which, while heavily patronized, were no longer morally respected indicated a shift in the attitude toward alcohol use and in the concept of controls. In this important shift in attitude, post-Revolutionary America seems to have begun to worship alcohol, to use it to excess, and to make its taverns places in which drinking became the main activity. The excesses of some Federal statesmen are well chronicled. For example, one-fourth of Washington's household expenses as President went

[2]The political use of alcohol in Indian management is immortalized in the name of a borough of the nation's largest city, if we are to believe those linguists who claim that the original form of "Manhattan" translates loosely as "the place where we all got high" (Kobler, 1973).

to meet his liquor bill. Jefferson spent nearly $11,000 on wine and was known for his fine taste in champagne (Kobler, 1973).

The increase in consumption which was to fire the imagination of early temperance advocates is documented by the following description of domestic alcohol production:

> In 1792, there were 2,579 registered distilleries in the colonies, which then had a population slightly above 4,000,000. Production, as reported to tax assessors, totaled 5,200,000 gallons, and consumption, counting imported spirits, came to 11,008,447 gallons, or an average of 2½ gallons for every man, woman and child in the country. Within the next eighteen years the number of distilleries increased to 14,191 and consumption tripled. This brought the per capita consumpion to 4½ gallons. If, moreover, the probable non-drinkers were omitted and the number of illicit stills estimated, the average annual intake of the actual drinkers appeared vastly greater—at least 12 gallons (Kobler, 1975).

Other writings appeared that criticized the inadequate enforcement of the antidrunkenness ordinances and issued a decidedly class-conscious warning concerning the probable results of allowing servants, slaves, Indians, and other commoners access to powerful intoxicants (Furnas, 1965).

In this new preoccupation with alcohol use, an increasing shift occurred between use at home and use in saloons and taverns. Further, the second standard of control—the association of drinking with eating—was weakened because most saloons and taverns were poorly equipped as restaurants. Very little food was served with alcohol, and its consumption became increasingly divorced from feasting in a ritual sense and even from ordinary food consumption. Food was not "promoted" by tavern-keepers and saloon-keepers because their profits depended upon the sale of alcohol (Ade, 1931; Kobler, 1973; Krout, 1925).

D. The Nineteenth Century

The nineteenth century witnessed three social developments which drastically affected the use of alcohol in this country: the Industrial Revolution; the proliferation of saloons and taverns; and the temperance movement.

One of the most distressing effects of the Industrial Revolution on society was the increasing separation between men and women in general, and of men from their families in particular. Earlier, on farms and in artisan shops, men had either worked in the home or very close to the home. Now, their work began to take them far from home, and as their ambitions and need for money increased, so did the amount of time that they spent away from their families. And "family" women had no place either in the frontier saloon or the urban tavern. In the same way, wives in the East had no place in early factories and mines, and the sharp differentiation of sexual stereotypes which left the woman as both the manager of the home and children and the moral arbiter of cultural norms served to increase the already existing American ambivalence toward alcohol use (Kobler, 1973; Krout, 1925; Sinclair, 1962).

When saloon drinking became segregated by sex and age, the American idea about drinking became more negative and, probably as a result of this new attitude, actual drinking behavior became more profligate. For one thing, strictures on consumption were relaxed. In large measure these ideals of daily consumption were affected by the experiences of Revolutionary soldiers who had received daily pints or more of "the best liquor" at training musters and who, when stores were low, had received much of their food rations in the form of a flask of brandy or a quart of cider because alcohol was portable and did not spoil readily. Wholesale merchants with military contracts had succeeded in convincing George Washington and his contemporaries that spirits were needed to maintain a high level of readiness among troops (Krout, 1925). A bottle of rum replaced the keg of cider near the scullery door at home, and visitors were expected to share the equivalent of several shots of liquor at even casual social events. The drunkard became an object of humor which found its way into literature. Citizens could recognize neighborhood soldiers in depictions of comical inebriates. Contemporary accounts began to speak of a "general moral decay," and ministers exhorted legislators to deal with "flippant, gambling, tippling youngsters who spend their time in frivolous pursuits." Street drinking was tolerated, and daylong sojourns in local grog shops were not interrupted by local officials. In the West, saloon customers were noted for their high spirits and aggressive and violent behavior. Frontiersmen escaped from long periods of solitude on the farm or of driving cattle and sought companionship and social release through drinking. In addition, the frontier saloon became a focal point of sexual activity, and the only women permitted were prostitutes (Furnas, 1965; Krout, 1925).

The excesses of the "olde tyme saloon" were not limited to the Western frontier. Such saloons were fixtures in all cities and villages. Tavern drinking by factory workers and young single men became the norm. The conditions favoring conviviality and emotional release were highly valued and connected with longings that were only secondarily dependent upon the consumption of alcohol, but this consumption under these social conditions became the basic social behavior. It soon became clear that "holding your liquor" was a mark of manliness and manhood, and the macho quality of alcohol use in this country undoubtedly became a powerful symbol at that time, further weakening the fifth standard of control. It should not be assumed that this drinking behavior was confined to the newly emerging urban laboring class and the Western frontiersmen. Those schooled at Yale, Harvard, and the other elite universities found that breweries and taverns adjoined school dining halls, and class meetings often boasted a decanter of brandy or flasks of rum (Lucia, 1963). During the eighteenth century, there had been proscriptions at Harvard and Yale against the use of "mixed or spiritous drinks without permission or adult sanction" (Warner, 1970). The prevalence of college-level education was obviously low, but the attention given to college drinking by the press seems to have been substantial. Newspaper accounts of riots, rampages, vandalism, and injury are legion. In terms of intensity and lack of control, the drinking of the young and wealthy scions of America's establishment resembled that of frontier ruffians rather than that of their Protestant forefathers. The standard of consumption became the bottle, and the standard of behavior certainly did not reflect the colonists' overriding concern with deportment. Accounts of the atmosphere of the nineteenth-century "bar" included not only idyllic portraits of joyful revelry by lonely and civilization-starved settlers, but also frightening descriptions of greedy violence perpetrated by soddenly inebriated near-barbarians. In these circumstances it is perhaps understandable that early temperance advocates endowed alcohol with exclusively destructive and dangerous qualities. The belief was commonly held that nobody who began to use alcohol would be able to control his use successfully (Ade, 1931; Maddox, 1970; Warner, 1970).

The excesses of the nineteenth century, complicated by the Industrial Revolution, led to an enormous growth in the temperance movement, which had begun to blossom toward the end of the 1700s. Now temperance advocates had at hand many examples of excesses to use in their descriptions of alcohol. Ironically, their vocal fury had already begun to constrain some of the drinking behavior that as "drys" they were so concerned about. There is evidence that before the First World War the "olde tyme saloon" evolved into a sort of working-class institution. Drinking abuses actually decreased in the Eastern cities as the saloons turned into homes away from home for the poorly housed working class, and also in the Midwest as communities coalesced into organized sociopolitical groups. As the West was won and male settlers were joined by the civilizing elements—women, families, and churchmen, as well as professionals in medicine, law, and business—the community aspect of alcohol use began to be more evident. Although the cohesive and church-centered village atmosphere of the early colonies may not have been replicated among the heterogeneous ethnic groups of the century's end, a workable system of social behavior seems to have developed.

The saloon may actually have helped to develop a better definition for alcohol use by strengthening the first, second, and third standards of control. It appears, first, that group drinking began again to be distinguished from drunkenness as drunkenness met increasing social disapproval. Second, saloons began to serve food. The free lunch—a spread of meat, bread, and boiled vegetables—which made its debut in the large Eastern cities, rapidly became popular in the Midwest. Saloons, taverns, and men's clubs began to act as restaurants in communities that needed them. And third, women began to accompany their husbands to neighborhood saloons in the East and increasingly in the Midwest. It soon became obvious that prostitutes were not the sole female patrons of local bars and taverns (Ade, 1931; Goode, 1972; Kobler, 1973; Krout, 1925; Sinclair, 1962).

There was still a great deal of social concern about alcohol use, however, and children were gradually excluded from the saloons. George Maddox (1970) claims that "Americans drink with a certain sadness," a kind of guilty confusion born out of their ambivalence toward alcohol, and during the period toward the end of the nineteenth century and before the First World War, that "sadness" seemed to characterize drinking behavior throughout the United States. Drinking was no longer the "answer" for those seeking to escape personal anxiety or intolerable social conditions. Nor was alcohol the universal panacea of medicine and nutrition.

The end of the nineteenth century also saw a sharp increase in popular concern with inappropriate behavior and therefore the strengthening of the fifth standard of control. The use of taverns for brawling and the release of high spirits dropped markedly both in the East and in the West as communities coalesced and became more concerned with a variety of proprieties. The rise of unionism in the United States is also credited with reducing uncontrolled drinking and violent behavior. As social conditions improved there was a greater capacity for a reasonable family life, and alcohol was used less as a relief from intolerable conditions. At the same time, the level of emotionalism attached to drinking, particularly the concept of machismo—male superiority shown in the capacity to hold liquor—began to drop.

E. The Prohibition Period

In spite of the apparent improvement in the way most of the population coped with alcohol, the temperance movement continued to gain strength. And ironically, as the community culture, particularly in the West, moved from unrestrained license to a more moderate drinking pattern with fewer claims of the medicinal value or resulting manliness of alcohol use, people found it harder to defend the occasional use of alcohol. The moralistic group in the temperance movement which saw total abstinence as the only goal became dominant, and as is common in political life, the moderates found it difficult to defend their middle-of-the-road position. Thus, at the very time when drinking problems began to abate and drinking behavior to improve, the Prohibition movement gained its greatest strength.

What is more, the Prohibition movement began to change its character. A deluge of shrill propaganda gradually replaced the more realistic and factual presentations of the problems that arose from alcohol excesses. Pamphlets, journal articles, and even traveling orators and stage companies all touted the dangers of alcohol. During this phase the Prohibition movement was so successful politically that by 1919 when the Volstead Act, which provided for federal enforcement of Prohibition, was finally passed by the United States Congress, 21 states were already dry (Furnas, 1965; Kobler, 1973; Sinclair, 1962).

Descriptions of drinking behavior written during Prohibition are almost always descriptions of excess. While the antisaloon leagues joyfully subscribed to the demographic evidence of a decline in the number of people using alcohol during the first six years of Prohibition, writers in both camps claimed that continuing drinkers were consuming inordinate amounts of liquor. After 1925 the increasingly prorepeal sentiment paralleled a substantial increase in the number of drinkers, although it is probable that user rates did not approach the levels of the 1970s until well after Utah ratified the 21st (Repeal) Amendment on December 5, 1933 (Kobler, 1973; Sinclair, 1962).

Certainly the years between 1920 and 1933 provided little opportunity for the development of control-oriented drinking customs. In the speakeasy perhaps even more than in the old-fashioned saloon, the first standard of control was absent. Drinking was not clearly differentiated from drunkenness, nor, obviously, was it associated with ritualistic or religious celebrations. People did not take the trouble to go to a speakeasy, present the password, and pay high prices for very poor quality alcohol simply to have a beer. When people went to speakeasies, they went to get drunk.

In addition, the second standard went by the board. With rare exceptions in the big cities of the East, speakeasies almost never served food. The presentation of alcohol itself was regarded as the special occasion, and food and social rituals were relegated to minor positions of importance.

As for the third standard, although a number of women went to speakeasies, and perhaps in even larger numbers than during the saloon era, illicit establishments were principally for men. The alcohol-centered, crime-permeated atmosphere of the Prohibition-time "joint" was considered "no place for a lady." Thus the monitoring of behavior that accompanied "family" drinking was lost, and cross-generational socializing was removed from the usual site of alcohol consumption.

The fourth standard of control was also lost because the atmosphere of the speakeasy alone exerted a tremendous pressure to drink heavily. The act of breaking the law just to go to such a place was sufficient to create a powerful emotional charge. The speakeasies quickly became places where people could retreat in order to deal with personal anxieties or difficult social situations.

Above all, the first standard was completely abandoned. Not only were the sanctions against drunkenness nonexistent in speakeasies, but the appeal of illicit behavior to those who had already broken the law by going to them was extremely powerful. Bouncers guarded the door of every speakeasy and ostensibly guarded the patrons, though their actual function was to protect the profits of bootleggers and help them deal with the law. Almost from the moment of entry the speakeasy customer passed into a situation where aggressive and even violent behavior was encouraged. The bouncers dealt with threats from the police and often from rival speakeasy owners; they did not monitor the deportment of customers. In such a situation neither parents nor responsible community leaders could encourage moderate drinking without condoning the breaking of the law. It is likely that during Prohibition the procuring and using of alcohol became a powerful facet of "coming of age" for many social groups (Kobler, 1973).

Thus speakeasies, along with that bedroom on wheels, the automobile, became the focus for other social upheavals of the 1920s, helping to change the norms of sexual propriety, female role-assumption, and cultural cohesiveness. The changes in mores characteristic of that decade were most evident in the speakeasy, and an increasing emphasis on sexualized relationships developed there. Even without overt violent or sexualized behavior, the speakeasies, in contrast to the saloons of the nineteenth century, stood for illicit behavior, law-breaking, and violence. The headlines at the time were full of gang wars and busts by police—almost a pitched battle among the police, gangsters, and to a certain extent, that section of the public which opposed the Volstead Act (Kobler, 1973).

Demographic data on the rates of abusive drinking are difficult to obtain. It is likely that physicians, law enforcement officers, and social service personnel were not always aware of alcohol's influence on their clients' problems, whether these were medical, legal, social, or psychological. It is possible too that many alcoholics and problem drinkers were reluctant to discuss their illicit consumption, that professionals did not report their clients' illegal behavior, and that reporting methods were inadequate.

Even without conclusive evidence, it is fair to say that Prohibition resulted in a decrease in the absolute numbers of drinkers. Those who were not committed drinkers could easily "do without." But those who remained drinkers may have constituted a pool of individuals with a higher-than-average potential for abuse, a potential encouraged by the "climate of excess" created by the spirit of condoned law-breaking.

What can be finally said about this last "experiment in abstinence" is that it failed. In a nation with an historical tradition of strong drink and high profits, the attempts to legislate a new social norm that forbade drinking could not work. Prohibition prevented the development of realistic public attitudes toward alcohol for at least one generation, and it may have curtailed the growth of the responsible drinking practices that had emerged during the 25 or so years preceding passage of the Volstead Act. Prohibition denied that alcohol was a controllable substance, and inadvertently elevated it to a position of almost magical importance—the source of enormous profits, pervasive corruption, and unpredictable pharmacological effects. Removing alcohol from the norms of everyday society increased drinking problems. Without well-known prescriptions for use and commonly held sanctions against abuse, Prohibition drinkers were left almost as defenseless as were the South American Indians in the face of Spanish rum and brandy (Chafetz and Demone, 1962).

F. After Repeal

The years that immediately followed the repeal of Prohibition in 1933 were by all accounts "wet." The women who joined men in bars, cocktail parties, and domestic drinking in general are held responsible for the now ubiquitous "mixed drinks." Adolescents resurrected the stamina-measuring college drinking customs of the eighteenth and nineteenth centuries and extended them to high school and the armed services. Advertising efforts paired drinking with sophistication and "good taste" and laid the groundwork for today's "champagne of bottled beer" and many other such appellations. Statistics show that per capita drinking unquestionably rose throughout the 1930s, interrupted only by the Second World War when alcohol was harder to come by and there seems to have been some reduction in its use. Following the Second World War the rate of drinking increased precipitously until 1965 when it began to decline (*Historical Statistics of the United States*, 1976; *Vital Statistics of the United States*, 1972).

At the same time, the first three standards that control drinking reappeared. Between the late 1950s and the early 1980s the emphasis on drunkenness has declined while the emphasis on moderate drinking has increased. Certainly in the early 1980s drinking is cross-sexual and cross-generational. Women's level of alcohol consumption may not yet equal that of men, but parity is being approached. Drinking is done routinely in the home at all class levels. The beer after work and the beer in front of the TV are as important as the cocktail and the martini before dinner. The increasing popularity of wine with dinner points to the normal association of drinking and eating.

As for the fourth standard, drinking as a release from intolerable personal anxiety or desperate social situations continues to exist actively in this culture, but the rate of such "escape drinking" has been either aggravated or ameliorated, depending on one's point of view, by the influx of other drugs and various illicit behavior patterns. Turning finally to the fifth standard, although association of alcohol with violence and aggressiveness has continued during these decades in a more moderate way than during our frontier past, it is promulgated far less by the culture per se. Certainly the late 1960s reflected a sharp decline in the belief that the capacity to hold liquor, to be drunk, indicated male superiority. Throughout the 1960s the emotionalism surrounding drinking focused on the conflict between "the juicers and the heads" (drinkers and illicit drug users). Moderate drinkers began to defend their alcohol use more readily and with less moral concern than had the moderates at the turn of the century (Kobler, 1973; Krout, 1925; Sinclair, 1962). The growing respectability of moderate intoxicant use is an interesting change which offers some promise for the future development of controlled use of alcohol and the prevention of alcoholism.

II. TREATMENT: MEDICAL AND PSYCHIATRIC EFFORTS

Not surprisingly, during the "wet" 1930s, when prevention of alcohol abuse had reached a low level due to the weakening of controlling social sanctions and rituals, medical doctors began to direct their efforts toward the treatment of alcoholism. For the first time physicians took alcoholism seriously as a medical condition and saw that the "disease" concept of alcoholism originally proposed by E. M. Jellinek (1960) actually referred to a medical entity (Glueck, 1942).

This view of alcoholism as a medical and sometimes a psychiatric phenomenon gradually removed drinking from the "vice" category. Although illness, like badness, is considered a form of deviancy in this culture (Parsons, 1951), it is one that carries less social opprobrium. Illness is widely equated with weakness, which is certainly more acceptable than badness in the late twentieth century. To characterize a condition as an illness implies an absolute standard of health and thus opens up the possibility of degrees of health, while defining a behavior as a vice precludes distinctions and degrees. In the case of drinking, the disease concept of alcoholism leaves moderate drinking free of taint.

For decades, if not centuries, medical men had known that alcohol affected liver and other bodily functions, but they had not paid much attention to these findings or made use of them in treatment. Now, in the 1930s, solid research began to be done on the effects of alcohol on the liver, heart, peripheral nerves, and brain, so that doctors could confidently warn patients of the consequences of their drinking (Hoff, 1962). These medical men expected that the weighty evidence against alcohol would enable patients to stand firm against their urges to drink. Doctors also began to prescribe nutritional supplements, and eventually an alcohol antagonist, called Antabuse, which had been developed in Sweden and which made it impossible for the patient to drink without becoming violently ill.

Also beginning in the 1930s, organized medicine began to take psychiatry seriously. During and after the Second World War this new field not only became important as a medical specialty, but it also assumed an increasingly powerful role as a social force. Psychiatric interest in alcoholism and other addictive syndromes led to the publication of such papers as those of Rado (1926, 1933, 1958), Abraham (1927), and others (Glover, 1932; Knight, 1937a, 1937b; Yorke, 1970), which correlated the eventual development of alcohol problems with unresolved early intrapsychic conflicts. The theory that associated alcoholism with primitive desires for greater oral satisfaction was so appealing that it has been difficult if not impossible to eradicate.

But neither the medical nor the psychiatric approach was especially successful in curbing alcoholism. The drug Antabuse did not fulfill its promise because antagonizing the effects of alcohol had little to do with stilling the basic and powerful urge to drink (Bennett et al., 1951; Bowman and Simon, 1955). Neither did the psychiatric interpretations of early conflict and the conscious linkage between the infant's bottle and the whiskey bottle quench the alcoholic's thirst. Gradually the realization began to dawn that alcoholism could not be viewed solely as a medical or as a psychiatric condition (Agrin, 1964; Armstrong, 1958; Chafetz, 1959; Feldmann, 1959; Hill and Blane, 1967; Riley and Marden, 1946; Szasz, 1967).

In recent years there have been some changes in the awareness by many psychiatrists of the problem of treating people in severe difficulty with alcohol. Most psychiatrists and most psychiatric installations still unconsciously hang out the sign characterized by George Vaillant (1983) as "Alcoholics Need Not Apply," and all too many of them still worry more about patients' complaints of depression following loss of a job or key people in their lives than about the drinking that caused such loss. But there is some change. More and more psychiatrists and other therapists see drinking as the key problem. They restrict their interventions to the inhibitions against the patient's (or the client's) view of the drinking as *the* primary issue. Their psychological discussions with these patients tend to focus more on the painful loss associated with cessation of drinking than on other losses. Preparing these drinkers for the disappointments attendant on sobriety is an important step. Sobriety can save their lives and give them the opportunity to reestablish a human existence, but it is not the hoped-for magical cure for all problems. They are still people who have to deal with many conflicts and the horrid legacies of bitterness and pain resulting from their drinking period.

As the more knowledgeable therapists point out to their patients, the powerful denial of the obvious difficulty with drinking comes at least in part from the sense that being unable to drink responsibly in a drinking culture represents a shameful belief that these patients are inherently defective, weak, bad, different from others, and that this "fact" must be concealed. By taking up this last issue, these therapists can point their patients toward Alcoholics Anonymous and can insist that this approach obviates any conflict between that organization and a therapy that agrees completely on the primacy of the cessation of drinking behavior rather than on other internal psychological difficulties (Zinberg, 1983).

III. TREATMENT: AA's USE OF RITUALS AND SOCIAL SANCTIONS TO PREVENT DRINKING

In the mid-1930s, when medicine and psychiatry were attempting to treat the disease of alcoholism, a completely different approach to the problem was offered by an organization called Alcoholics Anonymous (AA). Founded in 1935 by two alcoholics—Dr. Bob, a New York surgeon, and Bill W., a stockbroker—AA required its members to admit their powerlessness over alcohol, to vow abstinence, and to commit their lives to helping others similarly diseased to recover, that is, to maintain sobriety (*Alcoholics Anonymous,* 1939). AA's specific "prescription" for recovery was the "twelve steps" in behavior (*Twelve Steps and Twelve Tradi-*

tions, 1965),[3] which were seen as including every aspect of human functioning: spiritual, mental, emotional-communal, and physical.

AA presumed a disease concept of alcoholism which was quite different from the medical model but which carried the same implications. The alcoholic was considered to be in the grips of "disease" and therefore to be unable to deal with his drinking. This change in the popular judgment of the drinker made his "treatment" more acceptable socially and helped to alleviate his guilt. Though insisting that alcoholics had to become abstinent to recover from their disease, AA was not prohibitionist. It only prescribed abstinence for those who could not handle alcohol as most others could.

The growth of AA has been phenomenal. In 1955, 20 years after its founding, AA boasted 6000 groups with 150,000 members. For 1981, the AA General Service Office reported 24,293 groups with 455,505 members, not including those in hospitals and prisons. This is an impressive growth rate for any organization, but especially for one that is run entirely by volunteers. AA's rise to prominence is especially notable because of its documented rate of success in combating alcoholism without reliance on professionally developed intervention or technology. In large measure this success has resulted from the extreme subtlety of its basic principles (Zinberg, 1977).

Most observers of alcoholism agree that the alcoholic's denial of his problem is the greatest obstacle to recovery (Bailey and Leach, 1965). AA

---

[3]The twelve suggested steps of AA are the following (*Twelve Steps and Twelve Traditions,* 1955):

1. We admitted we were powerless over alcohol—that our lives had become unmanageable.
2. Came to believe that a Power greater than ourselves could restore us to sanity.
3. Made a decision to turn our will and our lives over to the care of God *as we understood Him.*
4. Made a searching and fearless moral inventory of ourselves.
5. Admitted to God, to ourselves, and to another human being the exact nature of our wrongs.
6. Were entirely ready to have God remove all these defects of character.
7. Humbly asked Him to remove our shortcomings.
8. Made a list of all persons we had harmed, and became willing to make amends to them all.
9. Made direct amends to such people wherever possible, except when to do so would injure them or others.
10. Continued to take personal inventory and when we were wrong, promptly admitted it.
11. Sought through prayer and meditation to improve our conscious contact with God *as we understood Him,* praying only for knowledge of His will for us and the power to carry that out.
12. Having had a spiritual awakening as the result of these steps, we tried to carry this message to alcoholics and to practice these principles in all our affairs.

has no magical approach to this psychological block. When a drinker contacts the organization, members work patiently to show him (or her) that his (or her) symptoms indeed indicate a disease called alcoholism. The "pigeon's" (new member's) acceptance of this fact takes the form of a confession which is absolutely indispensable. Once this basic inhibition against self-awareness has been breached, AA refuses to go further. It does not attempt to show how the same type of defense mechanism, which limits self-awareness, may be operating in other aspects of the individual's personality. Instead, it focuses on the one issue, alcoholism, and leaves the rest of the personality alone. AA recognizes, as many psychiatrists do not, that the one job of stopping alcohol intake is quite enough to handle.

As an organization AA offers the great benefit of fellowship to alcoholics, surely some of the loneliest people on earth (Trice, 1957). But because AA realizes that accepting the enormous help this fellowship provides might give the "pigeon" a sense of personal dependence and therefore a sense of guilt, it attempts to ensure that help is impersonal. Consequently, the program is arranged so that every time a member calls for help, a different person is likely to answer the telephone and take up the "twelve-step" work. The insistence that members remain in constant touch with the organization, even when they are traveling, answers their great need for company and thus minimizes their feelings of guilt. Perhaps even more important, twelve-step work provides a chance for those being gratified to gratify others. This not only relieves guilt; it also encourages self-esteem.

AA refers to itself as "the last house on the street." This means that alcoholics who judge themselves harshly and constantly and who correctly perceive that they are so judged by most of their peers have one place which will not turn them away, no matter how degraded or despairing they may appear. AA says that such people need never be without hope and that they will not be judged in that place no matter how often they succumb to their "disease." They can always turn into the "last house" and find acceptance from others.

A last tenet of AA, basic but little understood, is the view that an alcoholic is always recovering, never recovered. One is sober from minute to minute, from day to day; and because the next drink is always imminent, overconfidence is dangerous. An AA member may stay sober, but by a constant awareness of what must be overcome he or she is always potentially a drinker.

This is a remarkable insight. It rests upon the recognition that the alcoholic has two fears which are so strong as to be phobic: the fear of drunkenness and the fear of sobriety. These phobias continue to appear all the way from detoxification to the last stage of recovery. The alcoholic, despite all pleas that he or she likes to drink, that drinking makes one feel better and more able to exist in one's own skin as well as with other people, comes to loathe and fear his or her drunkenness. Will this person once more be compelled to defile and degrade himself or herself physically, emotionally, and socially by getting and staying drunk? But even in the depths of torment in a detoxification ward, the alcoholic will insist that some day he or she can become a controlled drinker. Whatever drink supplies, it is much prized; to an alcoholic the prospect of a life without drink is terrifying, even phobic (Zinberg, 1977).

AA's method is to "allow" the imminent danger of drinking to continue as a fantasy/fear. This leaves the AA member with an ongoing desire for whatever is obtained from drink as well as an awareness of the moment-by-moment conquest of the desire to drink. Thus the reality of sobriety, which at first seems so frighteningly gray, is balanced by the stimulating fantasy of drinking. Unfortunately for the alcoholic, this drinking fantasy fastens upon that one moment when the ethanol-engendered glow allowed him or her to feel like a king and screens out the sullen, surly, deteriorated aftermath, whereas the alcoholic's view of sobriety focuses upon the moment when he or she felt most inadequate. In time, however, the social and psychological advantages of sobriety tip the balance toward abstinence; the experience of being in control of oneself and able to interact with people directly rather than through a boozy haze becomes reinforcing. Unlike the members of the straight world, to whom the advantages of sobriety are self-evident, AA does not underestimate the alcoholic's fear of being sober. Instead, by insisting that the alcoholic is always recovering, never recovered, it keeps the possibility of drinking always at hand but still a hand's breadth away.

Over the years, AA has achieved remarkable success. In 1973 Barry Leach estimated that 20% of its members remain sober for five years or more. The organization's own figures are even more optimistic and become more so each year. But with success, the organization has assumed a position very different from its original intent. Rather than using its deep understanding to define the whole concept of alcoholism, to investigate the social determinants of abuse, and to deal with prevention as well as treatment, it has become the chief successful treatment modality. Because of the failure of the medical and psychiatric approaches, many community mental health centers have abandoned their efforts to treat alcoholics. Instead, they refer all clients with "drinking problems" to AA before their intake interviews are completed.

AA has succeeded so remarkably because its sound basic principles have evolved into powerful social sanctions which are supported by rituals. The primary sanction, of course, is that any continuation of drinking is equivalent to death. Though this knowledge alone is patently ineffective with most alcoholics, it forms an effectual part of AA's ritualized and institutionalized program. This program evokes a number of other sanctions which uphold the basic sanction against any drinking; for example, one saying warns that an alcoholic cannot afford resentment, excess ambition, or relaxation of the knowledge that "one drink is too many and a thousand too few." In addition, AA's rituals—the form of the meetings, getting a sponsor, speaking at meetings, the insistence on attending many meetings, the coffee and soft drinks that are served there—all directly reinforce the sanctions.

The rituals and sanctions of the AA community are reminiscent of those found in Colonial America, but at the same time there is a major difference. Whereas the AA proscriptions forbid any drinking at all, the Colonial standards of control were directed against excessive drinking or drunkenness.

For instance, the AA sanction against judging or condemning those who are ill with alcoholism parallels the colonists' ordinances which were intended to protect the individual from the embarrassment or harassment that might result from drinking too much. Again, like the colonists' association of drinking with eating, the food and soft beverages served at AA gatherings support the sense of community and of cross-sexual, cross-generational inclusion.

The underlying religious insistence of AA which asks members to turn to "God as you know Him to be" and invokes the help of a higher power suggests another parallel with the colonists. Although AA's "surrender to a higher power" is closer to Eastern ideas of spiritual relationship than to the rigid religiosity of the Colonial period, it too gives its community a powerful and binding outside authority. This rather vague religious insistence, which leaves specific ideas about God up to the individual, appeals even to those potential members who are nonbelievers.

Again, AA's terms of membership, or inclusion, depend upon factors more characteristic of Puritan America than of the heterogeneous society of the twentieth century. Like the early Calvinists, AA members agree to social sanctions which decree that they save themselves and support the community. These include an agreement to ask for specifically defined guidance and monitoring from their fellow members. The AA member contracts "for the rest of his [or her] life to atone for his [or her] failure—to combat his [or her] disease" (*Alcoholics Anonymous,* 1939; *Twelve Steps and Twelve Traditions,* 1955).

The AA member, like the Puritan, stands against the larger population; ill and different, he or she is obliged to attend meetings frequently and to perform twelve-step work to maintain sobriety. The Puritan settler had similar life-long responsibilities to perform, a similar sense of regular group attendance, and even a similar sense of religious difference. Deviations were not tolerated in the colonies, and the chief deviants—"witches"—were punished by exclusion.

AA's success in treating alcoholism raises the question: Could not, and should not, its methods be applied to the prevention of alcoholism? So far AA has focused on the *treatment* of an existing condition, not its *prevention*. But if the social sanctions and social rituals constitute the most effective means of preventing abuse—and they did in the Colonial period—could not AA's use of this form of social control to prevent *all* drinking be transferred to the prevention of excessive drinking?

The enormous growth of interest in self-help groups points to the possibility that AA, or an organization like it, will be asked to help controlled drinkers who do not want to get out of control. It has already been reported, in fact, that some people who are only moderately heavy drinkers have gone to AA meetings and become avid AA members.

Unfortunately, it seems that the same subtle dynamics which have made AA so effective in treating the alcoholic would not be effective in the prevention of alcoholism. Membership in AA depends—initially and forever—upon self-identification as an alcoholic. The members are deviants from the larger culture—people for whom the sanctions against immoderate drinking, the controls assumed by a social-drinking nation, have failed, and for whom abstinence is the only answer. Incipient, temporary, or marginal drinking problems are not in the organization's province.

AA has fostered the development of a cohesive subculture—a culture within a culture—and has evolved powerful social sanctions and rituals to govern it. Interestingly enough, these social controls are effective because the behavior required—abstinence—is not demanded by the larger culture, because the sanctions contradict what has already been taught and internalized, and because the population of the group sees itself as desperate, different, and ill. In twentieth-century America the cultural mores which support moderate drinking are so intrusive that they are hard to resist. To develop a new set of social sanctions and rituals that promote abstinence has required the development of a community within the larger community, which must go to great lengths to achieve and continue this separateness. AA has recognized this need and has insisted on anonymity, disregard of ambition, and rigidity about principles. These differences from the reigning cultural outlook are imaginary walls which separate its members from the larger community, at least as far as drinking is concerned.

Maintaining a restricted community without impervious walls is no easy task in this media-dominated society. If AA were to reach out and try to assert itself in the prevention of alcoholism, if it were to begin making fine distinctions between different kinds of drinking behavior, its capacity to treat alcoholism would be weakened. It could hardly hold to the abstinence line with drinkers who might argue that they were not out of control and therefore did not have to break with the general cultural mores. This likelihood explains why the Rand Report which suggested that alcoholics could become controlled drinkers was so threatening to AA (Armour et al., 1976).

The social principles underlying the prevention, rather than the treatment, of alcoholism condone drinking as such but define responsible, moderate drinking behavior (Zinberg et al., 1975). The social sanctions and social rituals that prevent alcohol abuse function by saying, "Know your limit," which means, "It's O.K. to drink up to your limit." This view is utterly opposed to the disease model of AA, to its insistence on abstinence, to the character and cohesiveness of its membership, and to its essential separation from the larger culture. If prevention of alcoholism were to be added to its already formidable tasks, not only would much of its effectiveness as a treatment modality be lost, but its methods would probably fail to work as preventive measures.

IV. IRONIES, PARADOXES, AND COMPLEXITIES

The topic considered in this chapter—the importance of the social setting variable in the prevention and treatment of alcoholism—is filled with ironies, paradoxes, and complexities.

Clearly the social setting with its ever-evolving sanctions and rituals is crucial, not only in the promotion of controlled drinking and therefore in the prevention of alcoholism, but also in the treatment of the alcoholic. But the development of these sanctions and rituals, as well as their application to both processes, is extremely complex, linked as they are to a number of other coexisting and interacting cultural and social factors which are constantly being affected by economic and political change.

It is paradoxical that the same set of social controls (sanctions and rituals) that work in treating alcoholism would probably not function to prevent it. This is because the goal of prevention is different from the goal of treatment. The goal of the most successful treatment modality is abstinence, whereas the goal of prevention is moderate use. Ironically, except in the case of the alcoholic, controls directed toward abstinence seem to lead to increasing drug use rather than responsible use (Zinberg et al.,

1975). Perhaps it is just as well that the goal of abstinence can only be achieved in a small, cohesive, and sometimes desperate community such as AA, which is controlled by definite social sanctions and rituals. It certainly cannot be achieved through legislation, such as the Volstead Act, imposed upon a modern, heterogeneous, pluralistic society.

AA is not the only small community to have achieved its goal, in this case abstinence, through evolved social controls. The Puritan colonies also used controls to achieve their particular goal, moderate use, or prevention of abuse. As long as this goal continued to be approved by society and was supported by social sanctions and rituals, moderate use of alcohol was maintained. But in a later period when attitudes and sanctions relaxed, the attempt to recreate them through peremptory legislation failed. However, reasonable legislation to establish standards that will coerce drinkers into AA or into the kinds of medical and psychiatric treatment described earlier can be a useful part of a changing social setting that sharply separates use from misuse.

The social setting has a crucial effect on the individual member of society and the likelihood that he or she will be able to use alcohol but avoid alcoholism. An individual living within a society or community (or ethnic group) which expects or condones excessive use of alcohol will naturally internalize that attitude. But if the social sanctions and rituals of a society press toward controlled use, the likelihood is that the individual will internalize them and become a moderate drinker.

It is interesting to note the national trend toward greater moderation. Figures from the Secretary of Health and Human Services in January of 1981 show that at that time more light wine and beer was consumed per capita than distilled spirits. As far as is known, this was the first time in the history of the United States that this had been true. Such a shift toward less powerful spirits continues and could well indicate the extent to which standards for moderation are being internalized (*Fourth Special Report to the U.S. Congress on Alcohol and Health,* 1981). If this internalization does not work for the moderate drinker, he or she will probably become a problem drinker. Then, because the medical and psychiatric approaches to treatment, which do not recognize the crucial influence of social controls, have not yet solved the problem of alcoholism, the problem drinker will probably have no choice but abstinence as a method of recovery.

REFERENCES

Abraham, K., 1927, The psychological relations between sexuality and alcoholism, in *Selected Papers on Psychoanalysis,* pp. 80–89, Hogarth Press, London.

Ade, G., 1931, *The Old Time Saloon: Not Wet—Not Dry, Just History,* Gale Research Corporation, Detroit.

Agrin, A., 1964, Who is qualified to treat alcoholism? *Q. J. Stud. Alc.,* 25:350–389.

Alcoholics Anonymous, 1939, Alcoholics Anonymous World Services, Inc., New York.

Armour, D. J., Ponch, J. M., and Stambul, H. B., 1976, *Rand Report—Alcoholism and Treatment,* The Rand Corporation, California.

Armstrong, J. D., 1958, The search for the alcoholic personality, *Ann. Am. Acad. Pol. & Soc. Sci.,* 315:40–47.

Bacon, S., 1969, Introduction, in D. Cahalan, I. H. Cisin, and H. M. Crossley, *American Drinking Practices: A National Survey of Behavior and Attitudes,* No. 6, Rutgers Center for Alcohol Studies, New Brunswick, N.J.

Bailey, M. B., and Leach, B., 1965, *Alcoholics Anonymous: Pathways to Recovery—A Study of 1058 Members of the A.A. Fellowship in New York City,* National Council on Alcoholism, New York.

Bennett, A. E., McKeever, C. G., and Turk, R. E., 1951, Psychotic reactions during tetraethylthiuram disulfide (Antabuse) therapy, *JAMA,* 145:483–484.

Bowman, A., and Simon, A., 1955, A clinical evaluation of tetraethylthiuram disulfide (Antabuse) in the treatment of the problem drinker, in *Management of Addiction* (E. Podolsky, ed.), Philosophical Library, New York.

Chafetz, M. E., 1959, Practical and theoretical considerations in the psychotherapy of alcoholism, *Q. J. Stud. Alc.,* 20:281–291.

Chafetz, M. E., and Demone, H. W., Jr., 1962, *Alcoholism and Society,* Oxford University Press, New York.

Earle, A. M., 1902, *Customs and Fashions in Old New England,* Charles Scribner's Sons, New York.

Feldmann, H., 1959, The ambulatory treatment of alcoholic addicts: A study of 250 cases, *Br. J. Addictions,* 55:121–127.

Fourth Special Report to the U.S. Congress on Alcohol and Health from the Secretary of Health and Human Services, January, 1981, U.S. Department of Health and Human Services, Public Health Service, ADAMHA, National Institute on Alcohol Abuse and Alcoholism, U.S. Government Printing Office, Washington, D.C.

Furnas, J. C., 1965, *The Life and Times of the Late Demon Rum,* G. P. Putnam's Sons, New York.

Glover, E., 1932, On the etiology of drug addiction, *Int. J. Psycho-Anal.,* 13:298–328.

Glueck, E., 1942, A critique of present-day methods and treatment of alcoholism, *Q. J. Stud. Alc.,* 3:79–91.

Goode, E., 1972, *Drugs in American Society,* Alfred A. Knopf, New York.

Hill, M. J., and Blane, H. T., 1967, Evaluation of psychotherapy with alcoholics: A critical review, *Q. J. Stud. Alc.,* 28:76–104.

Historical Statistics of the United States, Colonial Times to 1970, Part 1, 1976, U.S. Department of Commerce, Bureau of the Census, U.S. Government Printing Office, Washington, D.C.

Hoff, E. C., 1961, The use of pharmacological adjuncts in the psychotherapy of alcoholics, *Q. J. Stud. Alc.,* 28:76–104.

Jellinek, E. M., 1960, *The Disease Concept of Alcoholism,* College and University Press Services, Inc., New Haven, Conn.

Knight, R. P., 1937a, Dynamics and treatment of chronic alcohol addiction, *Bull. Menn. Clin.*, 1:233–250.

————, 1937b, The psychodynamics of chronic alcoholism, *J. Nerv. Ment. Dis.*, 86:538–548.

Kobler, J., 1973, *Ardent Spirits, The Rise and Fall of Prohibition*, G. P. Putnam's Sons, New York.

Krout, J. A., 1925, *The Origins of Prohibition*, Alfred A. Knopf, New York.

Leach, B., 1973, Does Alcoholics Anonymous really work? in *Alcoholism: Progress in Research and Treatment* (P. G. Bourne and R. Fox, eds.), pp. 245–284, Academic Press, New York.

Lolli, G., 1970, The cocktail hour: Physiological, psychological and social aspects, in *Alcohol and Civilization* (S. P. Lucia, ed.), McGraw-Hill Book Company, New York.

Lolli, G., Serrianni, E., Golder, G., and Luzatto-Fegiz, P., 1958, *Alcohol in Italian Culture*, The Free Press, Glencoe, Ill.

Lucia, S. P. (ed.), 1963, *Alcohol and Civilization*, McGraw-Hill Book Company, New York.

Maddox, G. L. (ed.), 1970, *The Domesticated Drug: Drinking among Collegians*, College and University Press Services, Inc., New Haven, Conn.

Mitchell, E. V., 1946, *It's an Old New England Custom*, Vanguard Press, New York.

Parsons, T., 1951, *The Social System*, The Free Press, Glencoe, Ill.

Rado, S., 1926, The psychic effect of intoxicants, *Int. J. Psycho-Anal.*, 7:396–413.

————, 1933, The psychoanalysis of pharmacothymia, *Psychoanal. Quart.*, 2:1–23.

————, 1958, Narcotic bondage, in *Problems of Addiction and Habituation* (P. H. Hock and J. Zubin, eds.), pp. 27–36, Grune & Stratton, Inc., New York.

Riley, J. W., Jr., and Marden, C. F., 1946, Changing concepts in the training of therapists for alcohol treatment, *Q. J. Stud. Alc.*, 7:240–270.

Rublowsky, J., 1974, *The Stoned Age: A History of Drugs in America*, G. P. Putnam's Sons, New York.

Sinclair, A., 1962, *Prohibition: The Era of Excess*, Little, Brown and Company, Boston, Toronto.

Straus, R., 1973, Alcohol and society, *Psychiatric Annals* reprint, Insight Communications, Inc., New York.

Szasz, T., 1967, Alcoholism: A socio-medical perspective, *Washington Law J.*, 6:255–268.

Trice, H. M., 1957, A study of the process of affiliation with Alcoholics Anonymous, *Q. J. Stud. Alc.*, 18:39–54.

Twelve Steps and Twelve Traditions, 1955, Alcoholics Anonymous World Service, Inc., New York.

Vaillant, G., 1983, *The Natural History of Alcoholism: Course, Patterns, and Paths to Recovery*, Harvard University Press, Cambridge, Mass.

Vital Statistics of the United States, 1972, U.S. National Center for Health Statistics, Washington, D.C.

Warner, H. S., 1970, Alcohol trends in college "life," in *The Domesticated Drug: Drinking among Collegians* (G. L. Maddox, ed.), College and University Press Services, Inc., New Haven, Conn.

Wilkinson, R., 1970, *The Prevention of Drinking Problems: Alcohol Control and Cultural Influences,* Oxford University Press, New York.

Yorke, C., 1970, A critical review of some psychoanalytic literature on drug addiction, *Br. J. Med. Psychol.,* 43:141–159.

Zinberg, N. E., 1972, Heroin use in Vietnam and the United States: A contrast and a critique, *Arch. Gen. Psychiat.,* 26:486–488.

————, 1974, *"High" States: A Beginning Study,* Drug Abuse Council Publication SS-3, Drug Abuse Council, Inc., Washington, D.C.

————, 1977, Alcoholics Anonymous and the treatment and prevention of alcoholism, *Alcoholism: Clin. Exp. Res.,* 1:91–101.

Zinberg, N. E., Harding, W. M., and Apsler, R., 1978a, What is drug abuse? *J. Drug Issues,* 8:9–35.

Zinberg, N. E., Harding, W. M., Stelmack, S. M., and Marblestone, R. A., 1978b, Patterns of heroin use, *Ann. N.Y. Acad. Sci.,* 311:10–24.

Zinberg, N. E., Harding, W. M., and Winkeller, M., 1977, A study of social regulatory mechanisms in controlled illicit drug users, *J. Drug Issues,* 7:117–133.

Zinberg, N. E., Jacobson, R. C., and Harding, W. M., 1975, Social sanctions and rituals as a basis for drug abuse prevention, *Am. J. Drug & Alc. Abuse,* 2:165–181.

Zinberg, N. E., and Robertson, J. A., 1972, *Drugs and the Public,* Simon and Schuster, New York.

CHAPTER 11

The Effectiveness and Cost of Alcoholism Treatment: A Public Policy Perspective

Leonard Saxe, Ph.D.
Associate Professor of Psychology, Boston University
Boston, Massachusetts

Denise Dougherty, M.A.
Office of Technology Assessment
Washington, D.C.

Katharine Esty, Ph.D.
Boston University
Boston, Massachusetts

In the U.S. Senate, the Committee on Finance has primary responsibility for Medicare legislation. The Finance Committee, in mid-1982, held hearings on Medicare reimbursement for alcoholism treatment (U.S. Senate,

NOTE: This chapter is based on a monograph prepared for the U.S. Congress, Office of Technology Assessment (OTA) and requested as part of the OTA project, "Assessment of Medical Technology and Costs of the Medicare Program." The authors wish to thank OTA staff, particularly Anne Burns, Cynthia King, Pamela Simerly, and Clyde Behney for their assistance. In addition, appreciation is expressed to Michelle Fine who worked with us on the original version. The opinions expressed in this chapter reflect those of the authors and not, necessarily, those of OTA. Denise Dougherty was affiliated with Boston University at the time this chapter was initially prepared.

1982). The specific impetus for the hearings was a series of news stories reporting fraud and abuse of Medicare funds in alcoholism treatment hospitals. The Committee had been struggling with how to contain health costs and use Medicare dollars most efficiently. Medicare regulations, with respect to alcoholism treatment, favor care delivered in hospitals under the supervision of medical personnel. In the course of its investigation, the Senate Finance Committee found a diversity of viewpoints concerning the advisability of continuing such Medicare coverage for alcoholism. Some experts argued that alcohol problems were best treated in inpatient settings; others argued that self-help groups, such as Alcoholics Anonymous (AA), and various outpatient and even nonmedical approaches work just as well.

Anyone involved in the diagnosis and treatment of alcoholism is aware of the complexities of the problem. Whether alcoholism is considered a physiological, psychological, or socially based problem, generalizations about effective treatment are difficult to make. Many different and conflicting claims, each with its own internal logic and research evidence, support the use of various forms of treatment. For policymakers, such as United States Senators, the array of treatments presents a confusing picture. Although it is clear that alcoholism is a major health problem, it is unclear to policy makers whether scarce resources can be profitably used to combat its effects.

This chapter describes a policy-oriented analysis of the current state of knowledge about alcoholism. A longer version of this review was originally prepared in response to Congressional concern about the effectiveness of alcoholism treatment (see Saxe et al., 1983).[1] The chapter focuses on treatment outcome research and its relationship to the costs of alcoholism. The goal is to place knowledge of alcoholism treatment into a perspective useful for decision-making about alternative policies. The present chapter includes, first, a brief overview of alcoholism as a public policy problem. Next, methodological issues in assessing treatment effectiveness research and the findings of research are summarized. The discussion then shifts to cost-effectiveness and cost-benefit analysis (CEA/CBA) and a review of the findings of CEA/CBA studies of alcoholism treatment. Finally, implications of the research for reimbursement policy are discussed.

---

[1]The report was requested by the Senate Finance Committee. They asked OTA, a Congressional agency which conducts assessments of scientific issues, to provide the review. The present authors assisted OTA in this task. As an OTA case study, this report was neither reviewed or approved by OTA's Congressional Board.

I. A PUBLIC POLICY PROBLEM

Alcoholism constitutes a vast syndrome of medical, economic, psychological, and social problems (Institute of Medicine, 1980). From 10 to 15 million Americans are believed to have serious problems directly related to the use of alcohol, and up to 35 million more individuals are estimated to be indirectly affected. Although estimates are imprecise, alcohol abuse has been implicated in half of all automobile accidents and homicides, as well as in one-quarter of all suicides (see Eckardt et al., 1981; NIAAA, 1981). The social and economic costs to society of alcoholism, particularly to the health care system, are staggering. Alcoholism may be responsible for up to 15% of the nation's health care costs and for significantly lowering the productivity of workers at all strata of the economic system.

Although from a public policy perspective monetary costs are very important, the primary costs of alcoholism to society in the United States may be more than economic. Alcoholism and alcohol abuse adversely affect the health, social relations, psychological well-being, and economic status of both those who abuse alcohol and many with whom alcoholics come into contact. The extent of these effects is difficult to determine because an alcoholic may create problems for many others, including family, friends, and coworkers. In addition, many of the impacts of alcoholism are difficult to detect and attribute to alcohol use. Such effects, for example, include medical complications, criminal behavior, and exacerbation of depression and other psychological conditions.

A. Alcohol Use

A substantial number of Americans use alcoholic beverages, at least occasionally. The Gallup poll, which began collecting data about alcohol use in 1939, reports relatively stable patterns in alcohol use over the past few decades. Consistently, about two-thirds of the adult population (slightly more men than women), report occasional or frequent use of alcoholic beverages. Per capita consumption has also remained stable at about 2.6 gallons per year. In the United States, however, about 10% of the population accounts for more than half the alcohol consumed; less than half is consumed by a large group of infrequent drinkers and a small group of regular moderate drinkers (Klerman, 1982).

Alcohol, especially when consumed in large quantities or habitually, is related to various health problems; most importantly, problems such as organ damage (particularly, to the liver), brain dysfunction, cardiovascular disease, and mental disorders have been linked to alcohol use (see Eckardt et al., 1981). It has a significant effect on mortality rates; in general, alcoholics' life expectancy is 10 to 12 years shorter than average. Cirrhosis of the liver, a direct result of long-term alcohol consumption, is currently the fourth leading fatal disease. When other effects of alcohol abuse are counted, alcoholism is an even more significant mortality factor. Alcoholics have significantly higher suicide rates than do nonalcoholics, as well as accident rates that are significantly greater than normal. Each of these factors results in a significant number of deaths for individuals who abuse alcohol at all age levels (Public Health Service, 1979). In terms of morbidity, it has been estimated that alcoholic patients comprise from 30% to 50% of all hospital admissions. Although these admissions are most often for other disorders, alcoholism inevitably complicates recovery.

Governmental recognition of the problems posed by alcohol abuse resulted in the establishment, over 10 years ago, of the National Institute on Alcoholism and Alcohol Abuse (NIAAA) and the requirement of periodic reports to Congress on progress in combating alcoholism (e.g., NIAAA, 1978, 1981). Health professionals and researchers are becoming more knowledgeable about alcoholism as more data about the problems posed by the effects of alcoholism become known (see Institute of Medicine, 1980). However, despite recognition of the range of problems caused by alcoholism and alcohol abuse, an estimated 85% of alcoholics and problem drinkers receive no treatment for their condition (NIAAA, 1981). Although approximately 1.6 million alcoholics and problem drinkers received treatment from private and public sources, and over 600,000 alcoholics participated in meetings of AA groups, at least 8 to 10 million other alcoholics and problem drinkers received no treatment.

B. Perspectives on Alcoholism

One reason that policy makers have been slow to take action with regard to the alcoholism problem is that although alcoholism and alcohol abuse are today acknowledged to be multifaceted problems, they have not always been viewed this way. Historically, alcohol abuse was either accepted as normal behavior or, in some cases, viewed as a moral problem and treated as criminal behavior (see Aaron and Musto, 1981). In the 1950s, though, both the World Health Organization and the American Medical Association gave formal recognition to alcoholism as a medical disease (see Jellinek, 1952, 1960).

Despite increasing emphasis on alcoholism as a medical rather than a criminal or moral problem, disagreement continues about what constitutes alcoholism, and there is probably no single best definition (Mendelson and Mello, 1979). Some definitions of alcoholism consider merely the quantity of alcohol consumed or the frequency of drunkenness. More recent definitions consider the degree to which serious medical or social dysfunctions result from alcohol use (Schuckit et al., 1969) and the degree of psychological dependence or physical addiction to alcohol (Sellers and Kalant, 1982). Whatever definition is employed, however, it is often difficult to obtain reliable diagnostic data (Goodwin et al., 1970). This compounds definitional problems and influences diagnostic decisions and treatment of alcohol abusers.

The determination of the underlying causes of alcoholism has been even more intensely debated than its definition. At least three major views of the etiology of alcoholism can be identified: (1) medical, (2) psychological, and (3) sociocultural. Each of these perspectives is associated with a particular set of treatment approaches. As described below, however, treatment is often based on several etiological perspectives, and practitioners often accept the view that alcoholism is based on multiple factors.

Each approach to the etiology of alcoholism has received some empirical support, and it is probably most reasonable to view alcoholism as multiple in origin and complex in development. Multivariant models of alcoholism have recently been proposed (Kissin and Hanson, 1982; Pattison et al., 1977). Pattison et al., for example, contend that alcohol dependence subsumes various syndromes defined by drinking patterns and the adverse consequences of such drinking. An individual's use of alcohol can be considered on a continuum from nonuse, through nonproblem drinking, to various degrees of deleterious drinking. The development of alcohol problems follows variable patterns over time, and, according to Pattison et al., abstinence bears no necessary relation to rehabilitation. Psychological dependence and physical dependence on alcohol are separate and sometimes unrelated phenomena, but continued drinking of large amounts of alcohol over an extended period of time is likely to initiate a process of physical dependence. Alcohol problems are typically interrelated with other life problems, especially when alcohol dependence is long established.

C. Populations: Incidence and Treatment

One feature of alcoholism that has increased the concern of public policy makers is that alcohol abuse problems are widespread among various demographic and social groups. Although alcoholism may manifest itself differently across groups, and treatment effectiveness may vary systematically across sociodemographic groups, there is little evidence that prevalence differs. Recent interest has focused on tailoring treatments to the diverse needs of subpopulations (Solomon, 1981). Like Pattison et al., Solomon argues that demographic characteristics such as gender, race, ethnicity, social class, and age critically influence both treatment selection and treatment effectiveness (Pattison, 1979, 1980).

Having a job, a stable income, and a reliable set of social and personal supports correlate positively with treatment outcomes (Baekeland, 1977). Men and women from lower socioeconomic classes—those most dependent on public resources, such as Medicaid and Medicare, for health services—appear to respond less well to traditional treatment services than do middle- and upper-class adults. Being working class or poor often involves unstable employment prospects and related disruptions of stable family relationships (Kasl and Colb, 1979; Stack, 1974; Valentine, 1978). Such a multiplicity of problems undermines simple or cheap interventions designed to reduce alcohol problems (NIAAA, 1981).

Specific groups differentially receive treatment. As an example of this variation, Table 1 compares the treatment population in NIAAA-funded treatment centers with the population as a whole (based on 1980 census data). As shown in Table 1, whereas women, for example, constitute over half of the population, they represent less than one-fifth of the NIAAA-funded treatment population. Whites, the elderly, and the young are also underrepresented. Males, blacks, youths, Hispanics and Native Americans, on the other hand, are overrepresented in terms of treatment.

The reasons for these variations are not clear. It has been postulated that overrepresentation may result from real need. For example, some populations may experience more culturally based stress than others, and respond to the stress with excessive drinking. Alternatively, the source of the data may be a cause of the variation. Some groups may be more likely to seek or be referred to treatment in publicly funded programs than in private ones. As is discussed below, private alcoholism treatment facilities attract male patients of higher socioeconomic status.

Likewise, underrepresentation may be a function either of less need or of a mismatch between patient needs and program characteristics. With the elderly, for example, studies have indicated both an overall decline in alcohol use with age (Armor et al., 1977), and a significant number of elderly with alcohol-related problems (see NIAAA, 1978a). With respect to treatment compatibility, it has been hypothesized that social service agencies treating the aged are not equipped to deal with alcoholism, and that alcoholism treatment centers are oriented to younger, rather than older, clientele. Similarly, women, who on the whole report less drinking (Gallup poll), experience greater problems with alcoholism when they do drink (Bourne and Light, 1979). As with the elderly, treatment centers are often not equipped to deal with the special needs of women (e.g., for child

Table 1
Comparison of Alcoholics in NIAAA-Funded Treatment Programs with the General Population

Characteristic	Alcoholics in NIAAA-Funded Treatment Programs with Characteristic	Characteristic	General Population with Characteristic
Age:			
18 and under	5.2%	Under 18[a]	28.1%
19–35	49.4	18–34	20.7
36–64	43.3	35–64	30.9
Over 64	2.0	Over 64	11.3
Mean age	36 years	Median age	30 years
Gender:			
Female	18.9%	Female	51.4%
Male	81.1	Male	48.6
Race/ethnicity:			
Black	17.4%	Black	11.7%
American Indian and Alaskan Native	5.9	American Indian and Alaskan Native	0.6
Hispanic	10.5	Hispanic	6.4[b]
White and other minorities	65.4	White and other minorities	87.7
Marital status:			
Married	25.0%	Married	65.7%
Single	34.5[c]	Single	20.1
Separated or divorced	33.0	Separated or divorced	6.2[d]
Widowed	3.7	Widowed	8.0
Education:			
Mean school years completed	10.8 years	Median school years completed	12.5 years

[a] NIAAA reporting categories and Census reporting categories are not equivalent.
[b] Persons of Spanish origin may be of any race; therefore, figures shown do not add to 100 percent.
[c] NIAAA category is "never married."
[d] Census category is "divorced."

SOURCE: National Institute on Alcohol Abuse and Alcoholism, Alcohol, Drug Abuse, and Mental Health Administration, Department of Health and Human Services, *National Drug and Alcoholism Treatment Utilization Survey* (Rockville, Md.: National Institute on Alcohol Abuse and Alcoholism, June 1981); and Bureau of the Census, Department of Commerce, *1980 Census of Population; 1980 Supplementary Reports*, Document No. PC 80-51-3 (Washington, D.C.: Department of Commerce, 1980).

care) (Beckman and Kocel, 1982). Drunk drivers and skid row alcoholics also constitute special subpopulations with particular needs (NIAAA, 1978, 1981).

Given the estimate that 85% of the alcohol-abusing population does not receive any treatment, arguments about whether specific subpopulations are underserved or overserved may pale by comparison. The important point for both treatment providers and policymakers may be to insure that facilities are available to treat the needs of all alcoholics. For researchers, the task is to uncover patterns of alcoholism and demographic variations that permit optimization of patient-treatment matches (see Bourne and Light, 1979; Donovan and Jessor, 1979; Johnson, 1982; Kane, 1981). Although a great deal of research has been conducted on various psychological factors in alcohol abuse, demographic indicators have proven to be more strongly predictive of treatment success (Solomon, 1981). Drinking behavior variables (periodic rather than daily drinking, absence of delirium tremens) have been shown to have even stronger predictive validity.

D. Treatment Settings and Providers

From a policy implementation point of view, although the etiology and prevalence of alcoholism represent important information, the nature of treatments is the central focus. Recently, a great deal of discussion has concerned the relation of treatment setting characteristics to outcome. The focus of these efforts is to discover effective treatment programs and appropriate patient-setting matches (see Beckman and Kocel, 1982; Bromet et al., 1976; Costello, 1975a, 1975b); yet, differentiating among various settings may be difficult. Whether inpatient or outpatient, or medical/nonmedical, settings often differ on several dimensions and are not easy to classify. Below, the most common treatment settings for alcoholism, as well as the providers who deliver alcoholism services, are described.

1. Inpatient Care

The distinguishing characteristic of inpatient care is overnight stay in a medical facility. Inpatient settings include: (1) alcoholism detoxification units and rehabilitation units in general hospitals, (2) alcoholism treatment units in state and private psychiatric hospitals, and (3) free-standing alcoholism rehabilitation facilities.

In addition to providing medical services to alcoholics not being treated primarily for their alcoholism, general hospitals have recently begun to provide services directly to alcoholics (Pattison, 1979). This practice represents a change in the long tradition of hospitals refusing to serve anyone with a primary diagnosis of alcoholism. General hospitals stress evaluation of medical status and frequently use pharmacotherapy (Diesenhaus, 1982). They tend to admit alcoholics who are socially stable and who have experienced fewer years of heavy drinking than other alcoholics. Third-party medical insurance coverage is typically provided for inpatient care in general hospitals and Medicare, for example, provides coverage for up to three weeks of combined detoxification and rehabilitation in an inpatient medical setting (Health Care Financing Administration, 1979).

Psychiatric hospitals also provide inpatient care, but, as Diesenhaus (1982) notes, there may be more stigma associated with "psychiatric" care than with "medical" care. Alcoholism treatment programs in state mental hospitals, in particular, have in the past been underfunded, accorded low status, staffed by untrained personnel (Cahn, 1970), and regarded as ineffective (Ludwig et al., 1970; Moore and Buchanan, 1966). Their patients have typically been lower-middle-class and relatively disabled, both socially and vocationally (Pattison, 1979).

The characteristics of state and private psychiatric hospital populations may be changing, however, as reimbursement for alcoholism treatment becomes more widely available. Private mental hospitals provide treatment to a substantial number of patients who abuse alcohol, although alcoholism may not be the primary diagnosis. Psychiatric hospitalization is believed to be indicated when a severe psychiatric condition exists, regardless of its relationship to a drinking problem. It is also indicated when an opportunity to interrupt a drinking pattern or to motivate a resistant patient is needed (American Medical Association, 1977; Moore, 1982).

Moore's analysis of a survey of private psychiatric hospitals found that the mainstay of these programs was a combination of individual and group psychotherapy, alcoholism education, AA, and Antabuse (Moore, 1977). As an example, the Alcoholic Recovery Program at the Menninger Hospital in Kansas uses a multivariant program that addresses the psychological, biological, spiritual, and social aspects of alcoholism (Fusillo and Skoch, 1981). The two-month treatment program consists of educational lectures, recreational activities under the direction of a leisure therapist, family sessions, group sessions, and nutritional advice, as well as restricted access to alcohol. Although physical evaluations are made, medical treatment is not a major focus. The Menninger program follows AA philosophy, but employs a treatment team of professionals and paraprofessionals (including psychiatrists, nurses, psychologists, social workers, alcoholism counselors, and medical internists).

Free-standing alcoholism rehabilitation units are often nonprofit organizations affiliated with, but not necessarily located in, hospitals that provide inpatient programs with a nonmedical orientation, although medical and psychiatric support is available (Pattison, 1979; Stuckey and Harrison, 1982). In these facilities, a therapeutic milieu is created in which alcoholic patients take some responsibility for program planning, activities, and ongoing maintenance. AA meetings are usually part of the community life, and family sessions are often a. part of the program. Treatment includes lectures, nonpsychodynamic group counseling, family sessions, and attendance at AA meetings (Pattison et al., 1969). Pattison characterizes these programs, of which the Hazelden Foundation in Minnesota is a prototype, as having a "sense of 'elan,' commitment, and surety of purpose." They typically serve a socially competent, middle-class working clientele in a treatment program that lasts from three to six weeks.

Another type of free-standing rehabilitation facility has been called an aversion-conditioning hospital (Pattison et al., 1969; Smith, 1982). Such facilities are often proprietary and offer residential treatment for from 10 to 14 days. Their programs tend to attract socially competent, upper-class patients, and, according to Pattison (1979), they have a strong medical orientation. Treatment consists first of detoxification, followed by emetine (chemical) aversion conditioning. Counseling, along with various forms of group therapy and education are also offered as part of such treatment programs (Smith, 1982; Tuchfeld et al., 1982). In most cases, hospitals provide follow-up and continuing programs. The Raleigh Hills and Schick-Shadel hospital systems are examples of facilities that include aversion conditioning as an important component of their inpatient treatment.

2. Outpatient Care

Services provided on an inpatient basis are most often compared to alcoholism services provided on an outpatient basis. In some cases, these services are medically based, while in other cases they are nonmedically based and provided in residential facilities or other settings. Outpatient facilities vary widely in the extent of their medical orientation. The more medically oriented outpatient facilities include: (1) private physicians' offices, (2) community mental health centers, and (3) some free-standing outpatient clinics. The less medically oriented include other free-standing outpatient clinics, as well as various nonhospital residential facilities.

Alcoholics who consult private physicians usually do not present with a primary complaint of alcoholism. Nonetheless, they reportedly comprise a substantial proportion of general physician and internist case loads (see, e.g., Dunn and Clay, 1971; *Medical Times*, 1975). Although general physicians do not typically refer patients to alcoholism treatment programs (perhaps because the patients they treat are less dysfunctional), they may provide other services. Such physicians may prescribe a program of Antabuse maintenance, treat acute intoxication and mild withdrawal symptoms, use the doctor-patient relationship to engage patients in a treatment program, and involve the spouse and family in helping patients deal with their problems (Pattison, 1977).

Community mental health centers (CMHCs) are institutions formerly operated under guidelines of the federal CMHC Act or under state or local legislation modeled after the Act. CMHCs provide a broad range of mental health services and treat alcoholism as only one of many problems presented by patients. For insurance reimbursement, guidelines distinguish between hospital- and nonhospital-based community mental health centers and free-standing outpatient clinics.

As defined by the NIAAA (1981), free-standing outpatient clinics are facilities that "one would enter only to receive alcoholism services." They provide a multiplicity of medical, psychological, and social services to a broad spectrum of patients. Treatment services may consist of outpatient individual, group, family, or marriage counseling; drug therapies; and vocational, social, and recreational services. Medicare coverage for free-standing outpatient clinic patients is provided for services such as drug therapy, psychotherapy, and patient education that are reasonable and necessary and provided incidentally to the physician's professional service (Health Care Financing Administration, 1982). Marital and family therapies, however, have been specifically excluded.

Day care is treatment provided by a facility in which the patient does not reside. The patient participates in a treatment program with or without medication, usually for five or more hours per day, five or more days per week. Some of these treatment facilities are especially geared to alcoholics, while others serve a general psychiatric population (NIAAA, 1981). Day hospitalization programs per se are not covered by Medicare, although individual services provided in these programs may be covered under outpatient guidelines. Meals, transportation, and recreational and social activities are not covered.

3. Intermediate Care

Residential programs that provide primarily rehabilitation services to patients can be considered intermediate care facilities (Armor et al., 1978). Many of the patients in such programs have formerly been treated in hospitals. Such facilities include halfway houses, quarterway houses, and recovery homes. Typically, intermediate care facilities are community based and peer-group-oriented residences. They attempt to provide food, shelter, and supportive services in a nondrinking atmosphere. Residents in these programs are considered recovering alcoholics. They are ambulatory and mentally competent. Typically, they are without spouse or immediate family. Such facilities provide psychological support and help with problems, such as reentry to the work force.

4. Other Settings

Alcoholism treatment services are provided to varying degrees by correctional facilities, courts [e.g., driving-while-intoxicated (DWI) programs], business and industry, and the so-called skid row system of agencies (Wiseman, 1970). Various federal and local government agencies support alcoholism treatment programs in correctional and military facilities, but the contribution of these programs to alcoholism treatment, as well as the contribution of employee assistance programs, has been relatively small. Most such programs serve only as referral sources to the kinds of programs discussed previously and do not provide direct treatment.

5. Utilization

Estimating the use of treatment settings is difficult because of multiple sources of data. There is also a tendency for patients to seek and receive treatment in several different settings, even over the course of a relatively short time period. The most reliable data are available for government-sponsored programs. Until recently, when authority for alcoholism treatment programs was given to states with federal assistance through block grants, each NIAAA-funded treatment center and each project were required to collect and report data on treatment utilization.

In 1980, 460 NIAAA-funded projects reported serving almost 250,000 people (NIAAA, 1982). The vast majority of patients in NIAAA-funded facilities received outpatient treatment, sometimes in conjunction with inpatient treatment. Of the patients who received 24-hour residential care (some of these patients also receive outpatient care), 3% were hospital inpatients and 23% were in other facilities. The most common inpatient treatment was either social or medical detoxification. The most common outpatient service was individual counseling, followed by group counseling and crisis intervention. Approximately one-quarter of the patients received follow-up or aftercare.

Estimates of the number of people receiving treatment for alcoholism in other than NIAAA-funded projects during 1976 and 1977 have been made by Vischi et al. (1980). According to these data, the largest population is served by AA programs. As noted above, however, data such as those of Vischi et al. are problematic because some patients may receive treatment through multiple sources (this is especially so for AA programs). Furthermore, to the extent that alcoholic patients are treated under other diagnoses, these figures underestimate the problem of alcoholism. Not known is the number of alcoholics who receive no treatment at all; as noted above, estimates are as high as 85% of the total population of alcoholics (NIAAA, 1981).

6. Treatment Providers

Another major issue in the treatment of alcoholism and provision for its coverage concerns which providers are most effective, and, more particularly, what degree of staff professionalization is required to maximize treatment effectiveness. The present reimbursement system favors medically trained personnel. Prior to the entry of psychiatry and psychology professionals in the 1970s, roles within the alcohol-treatment work force were not distinct. Most treatment took place in nonmedical settings where alcoholism counselors served as primary therapists, administrators, support staff, advocates, and outreach workers. The increased involvement of physicians and the entrance of professionally trained personnel diminished the role of alcoholism counselors. Physicians, psychiatrists, psychologists, and social workers took over both treatment and supervisory roles.

The National Drug and Alcoholism Treatment Utilization Survey (NDATUS) (see Camp and Kurtz, 1982) indicates that the three largest categories of workers in alcoholism treatment programs are administrative and support staff, counselors, and nurses. Counselors without professional degrees comprise the largest single category (17%) of direct service workers in "alcohol only" programs. Alcoholism counselors (degree unspecified) comprise 37% of the project staff in NIAAA-funded treatment centers (Ferguson and Kirk, 1979). Although alcoholism counselors dominate the field, their distribution varies greatly by treatment setting. Halfway houses and free-standing clinics employ proportionately more counselors without professional degrees than do community mental health centers. Hospital programs rely primarily on medical staff (Camp and Kurtz, 1982).

Alcoholism counselors have objected to the overprofessionalization of the treatment process, claiming that the "functional difference between them and professionals is unclear because both perform many of the same functions in the treatment process," although professionals get paid more (Camp and Kurtz, 1982). In addition, from the view of counselors many of whom are recovering alcoholics, professionalization threatens potential success of alcoholism services, the key ingredient of which is self-help. There is little empirical evidence, however, to assess the effectiveness of various treatment providers.

E. Conclusions

The treatments used for alcoholism are diverse, including medical and psychotherapeutic approaches, as well as various other approaches, such as self-help programs based on the AA model. Most treatment programs combine a number of techniques. Adding to this complexity is that settings where treatment is delivered differ from one another on a number of key dimensions, including outpatient versus inpatient treatments, staffing patterns, and the kinds of populations who choose or are chosen for the setting. Moreover, alcohol abuse is present in various population groups, although it may manifest itself differently and require different forms of treatment.

In comparing reviews and studies of alcohol treatment programs, the principal task of this chapter, this complexity of etiology, treatment, settings, and patients must be kept in mind. Many studies focus on a single aspect of treatment or explore a particular hypothesis, making comparisons between studies extremely difficult. Generalizable statements about treatment effectiveness are, thus, difficult to develop. Reflecting the complex realities of patients in need of treatment and the settings and modalities available, treatment research is plagued with a host of methodological problems. These problems are discussed in the next section.

II. METHODOLOGICAL CONSIDERATIONS

In order to answer policy questions about alcoholism treatment, it is clear that research evidence could potentially play an important role. Yet, the development of a body of research on alcoholism treatment is fairly recent and, at present, somewhat ill formed. The lack of a well-developed research base is probably not surprising, for until relatively recent times, treatment for alcoholism was more likely to be incarceration or custodial care than medical or psychological therapy (cf. Voegtlin and Lemere, 1942). A scientific research base has formed along with the development of treatments (Caddy, 1978; Crawford and Chalupsky, 1977; Hill and Blane, 1967; Sobell and Sobell, 1982). Research on alcoholism treatment is, however, difficult to conduct. Because of interactions among patient characteristics, treatment settings, services offered, and practitioner characteristics design and measurement problems abound. For treatment research to be valid, there must be clarity about what is being tested, what is being compared, which subject populations are involved in the research, and what is being measured. Operationally, these validity conditions refer to (1) treatment design, (2) research design, (3) sampling, and (4) outcome measures.

A. Treatment Design

Treatment design involves the extent to which clarity about the "active ingredients" of the program being tested can be achieved. Questions such as whether the program involves a single treatment, a combination of treatments, or a combination of treatment and nontreatment factors must be answered. Often, because alcoholism treatment programs are multivariant, resulting research is confounded by an inability to separate effects (Baekeland et al., 1975; Pattison, 1972; Tuchfeld et al., 1982). The extent to which the impact of any one component of the treatment can be measured is limited, of course, when all patients receive or have concurrent access to several treatment components. Clarity about what the program includes is essential to being able to attribute outcomes to particular treatments or packages of treatments. Lumping treatment programs under umbrella terms such as "inpatient" or "outpatient," without clarifying which specific services are offered or utilized, obscures differences among treatments. By lumping treatments, one is unable to decipher which treatment is effective, for whom, and under what conditions (cf. Solomon, 1981).

B. Research Design

A valid research design requires systematic comparison. At a minimum, such comparisons involve a single group of patients measured before treatment and after treatment. Optimally, they involve two or more randomly assigned groups (an experimental group and a comparison or control group) of patients tested before and after treatment (see Wortman and Saxe, 1982). The latter design is usually called a "true" experiment (Cook and Campbell, 1979; Saxe and Fine, 1981), or in health care research, a randomized clinical trial (RCT) (Cochrane, 1972). RCTs are considered the most definitive experimental method to evaluate treatment efficacy (Office of Technology Assessment, 1982). The advantage of such designs is that they allow differences in outcomes to be attributed more confidently to the treatment and not to preexisting differences in the samples tested. RCTs are, however, relatively rare in alcoholism research. Comparative data on treatment groups are typically not available, and most research merely "tracks" patients during and after treatment (Hill and Blane, 1967; Mandell, 1979; Sobell and Sobell, 1982).

Although the absence of comparative data is a fundamental deficit of the alcoholism treatment literature (Baekeland, 1977; Tuchfeld et al., 1982), there are additional methodological problems. Data are often presented in aggregate form, so that patient outcomes are often not differentiated by severity of initial symptoms or patient characteristics. Social class information may be lacking, and age, gender, and social-situation differences may be obscured. A related issue is that multivariate analyses which are useful for examining demographic factors are typically unavailable [for an exception, see the Rand studies (Armor et al., 1978; Polich et al., 1981)]. Such analyses require large patient groups and present difficulties both in data collection and analysis.

C. Sampling

An additional methodological problem in alcoholism research concerns sampling of research subjects. Issues of sampling concern (1) eligibility for treatment, (2) selection for participation in research, and (3) availability for follow-up research. If the general population of alcoholics is not represented in the research samples, or if certain groups (e.g., working-class adults, women) are underrepresented, the generalizability of research findings is limited.

Perhaps the most important sampling problem is that individuals who receive alcoholism treatment services are probably not a representative group of problem drinkers (Baekeland et al., 1975). Many programs explicitly exclude those patients who have poor prognoses for recovery— particularly those from lower income groups and the unemployed. Even without exclusion criteria, individuals who elect treatment undoubtedly differ from those who do not (Caddy, 1978; Hill and Blane, 1977). Relative to those alcoholics who do not receive treatment, those who receive treatment may be more visible (hence their referral to treatment), more socially connected (treatment seeking is encouraged), more motivated (and so seek treatment), and more confident of success (and willing to risk treatment). It is also possible that those who seek treatment see themselves as more helpless (and, thus, reliant on treatment) and in more trouble (and, perhaps, pushed into treatment). The absence of data on alcohol abusers who do not seek treatment limits generalizability and the establishment of realistic spontaneous remission rates (see Smart, 1976; Tuchfeld, 1981).

Sampling bias involves not only constitution of the treatment population, but who is available for and who is willing to be involved in research. Especially if research involves long-term follow-up, only a select group of alcoholics may agree to be involved (cf. Baekeland et al., 1975; Mandell, 1979). If there are systematic differences between dropouts and those alcoholics who remain in treatment (as is reasonable to expect), generalizations are limited. There is some evidence that those who are difficult to follow up have the poorest treatment outcomes (Moos and Bliss, 1978), although contrary evidence is also available (cf. Polich et al., 1981). In addition, because patients may receive different treatments based on their ability to pay or have insurance coverage, comparing outcomes of treatment settings is potentially confounded.

D. Outcome Measures

Finally, the way in which treatment outcomes are measured significantly affects the interpretation of alcoholism research. Self-reports on drinking behavior, interviews with spouses, supervisor-based job productivity reports, blood alcohol levels, psychological improvement, and attendance at a treatment center have been utilized as outcome measures. The degree to which different studies utilize different conceptual outcomes, operational outcomes, and measurement techniques limits comparisons that can be drawn across treatments.

The appropriateness of various measures of outcome is controversial. The criterion of abstinence from alcohol use has, traditionally, been used as the single measure of treatment effectiveness. Some studies have also measured various behaviors related to drinking; for example, frequency of drinking, number of ounces of ethanol ingested, number of binges, and days of abstinence. More recently, other outcome measures, such as job productivity, family adjustment, legal problems, psychological well-being, and continuation of treatment, have been utilized. Physical health has been another important criterion and is importantly related to cost-benefit analyses of treatment. Much of the debate about outcome measures has focused on self-reports, which are often believed to be low in accuracy (Emrick and Stilson, 1977). Despite sound reasons why self-reports should yield unreliable results, a number of studies report high concordance between self-reports of use and physiological measures (Gerard and Saenger, 1966; Polich et al., 1981). Ironically, even physiological measures themselves may be poor indicators of the extent of alcohol abuse (Justin, 1979).

Recent debate within the alcoholism field has focused on whether "controlled drinking" or "nonproblem drinking" can be considered a successful outcome of alcohol treatment (see Heather and Robertson, 1981). It is both an important methodological issue and one with numerous policy implications. Sobell and Sobell (1971) have been the most prominent advocators of controlled drinking. Their view challenges the idea of alcoholism as a unitary syndrome with the treatment goal of abstinence (cf. Pattison et al., 1977; Pendery et al., 1982). They argue that the exclusive use of abstinence as the outcome obscures partial improvement, neglects improvements in other areas of life functioning, is difficult to validate, and represents a narrow understanding of the multifaceted alcoholism syndrome (Sobell and Sobell, 1978). Pattison (1966), and Gerard et al. (1962) present data indicating that abstinence does not necessarily result in improvement ,in an alcoholic's problems. In some cases, once abstinence is achieved, problems in other areas increase. The solution of these methodological problems would seem to be multidimensional measurements of outcome. Indeed, such a recommendation is strongly encouraged by several recent reviews (Caddy, 1978; Foster et al., 1972; Moos et al., 1982; Sobell and Sobell, 1982). Although the primary goal of alcohol treatment is elimination of drinking, treatment efficacy can best be evaluated by multidimensional outcome measures. Most available studies, however, do not take this approach.

E. Conclusion

Conducting outcome evaluation research on alcoholism treatments is undoubtedly difficult. Since these difficulties are reflected in current evaluations, many presently urgent policy questions can probably not be answered by available research. Much research is flawed by problems in design, sampling, or outcome measurement. Nevertheless, the "whole" of available research on alcoholism is probably greater than the sum of its constituent parts. By carefully considering the results of individual studies, each of which handles somewhat different methodological problems, it may be possible to draw conclusions from the substantial body of valuable literature. The following section's review of this literature attempts not to dismiss any body of research, but to utilize all available information. Where necessary, limitations and inherent inferential problems are noted.

III. EFFECTIVENESS RESEARCH

Despite the lack of well-controlled and generalizable research on the efficacy and effectiveness of treatments for alcoholism, a vast literature describes and analyzes treatment effects. Below, several of the principal literature reviews are described and analyzed in terms of their public policy implications. These reviews cover much of the research available and summarize current research-based wisdom about alcoholism treatments. In addition, specific studies related to particular treatment settings and modalities are analyzed.

A. Reviews

In the earliest comprehensive review of treatment effectiveness, Voegtlin and Lemere (1942) considered over 100 studies that appeared in the literature between 1909 and 1940. Voegtlin and Lemere concluded that poor "statistical" evidence existed and that none of the treatments then available for alcoholism had proven effective. In a systematic review of each treatment modality, however, it was suggested that some techniques showed good effects and appeared promising. Among these were treatments such as inpatient psychotherapy and certain drug therapies. What seems clear from Voegtlin and Lemere's review, and has been partially supported by later reviews, is that treatments for alcoholism are differentially effective for particular populations and that treatments offered in combination seem more effective.

1. Emrick

Emrick's (1974, 1975, 1979) reviews of treatment effectiveness research, although not the first to appear subsequent to Voegtlin and Lemere's review, are important because of their emphases on methodologically acceptable studies. Hill and Blane's earlier review on psychotherapeutic methods of treating alcoholics found that only 2 out of 49 available studies met minimum methodological standards (Hill and Blane, 1967). In 1974, Emrick reviewed 271 reports found in the alcoholism literature published between 1952 and 1971. Sixty-seven percent of the almost 14,000 patients in these studies either improved or were abstinent at follow-up. Emrick's conclusion was that "once an alcoholic has decided to do something about his drinking and accepts help, he stands a good chance of improving." Emrick cautioned, however, that no evidence documents that one treatment modality is more effective than another. Although Emrick seemed to indicate that many alcoholics can stop drinking with minimal or no treatment, and that abstinence rates do not differ between untreated and minimally treated alcoholics, he also maintained that rate of improvement correlates positively with amount of treatment received: Forty-two percent improved with little or no treatment, and 63% improved with treatment.

An update of Emrick's original review (1975) added 126 studies of "psychologically oriented" treatments for alcoholism to those studies previously reviewed. The focus of this review was primarily on the effects of treatment versus those of no treatment. The results, however, are difficult to interpret because there were relatively few studies with no-treatment conditions and because patient characteristics were not controlled. Emrick also included a group of studies with minimal treatments. No significant differences were found in either abstinence or improvement rates between the no- and minimal-treatment studies: 13% and 21% were abstinent, respectively, and 41% and 43% at least somewhat improved, respectively. Emrick did, however, find that more than minimal treatment had an effect on abstinence and improvement rates. Of those with more than minimal treatment, 28% were abstinent and 63% were improved after six months or more.

A later Emrick (1979) review focused exclusively on alcoholism RCTs. Such studies deal with the most significant confounding factor in alcoholism research—the inferential biases that result from patient self-selection of treatment modality. Emrick documented 90 studies that used random assignment of patients to two or more treatments. Almost all of these studies compared treatments to one another rather than to "no treatment." In general, Emrick was able to distinguish few differences. There seemed to be more evidence of the efficacy of behavioral approaches. For nonbehavioral approaches, brief interventions were as successful as longer ones. Although it might be concluded that treatment for alcoholism is not effective, the limits of the research considered in Emrick's analyses should be recognized. In particular, the review of RCTs is limited by the fact that the studies tended to be behavioral studies with very specific objectives.

2. Baekeland, Lundwall, and Kissin

Following Emrick's initial work, Baekeland et al. (1975) reviewed the state of knowledge about the effectiveness of particular treatments for alcoholism. Their substantive conclusions are difficult to summarize. For each of the settings and treatment modalities, some evidence of successful outcome was found. For example, their analysis of 30 studies of inpatient treatment indicated improvement rates of almost 50%. When corrected for attrition from the study sample and spontaneous remission, however, the improvement rates were lower, approximately 30%. In comparing inpatient treatment with outpatient care, Baekeland et al. concluded, as did Emrick, that although methodological caveats apply, research does not demonstrate that inpatient care offers greater likelihood of successful treatment. One problem identified was that characteristics of the patient, rather than the treatment, seemed to affect outcome significantly. The issue is complex because one of the central differences between patients may be their persistence in continuing treatment. Patients with stable marital and occupational status and higher socioeconomic status have better outcomes in that they are more likely to continue treatment.

It is also clear from the review by Baekeland et al. that there are considerable differences as to who receives particular treatments. One example is AA. According to Baekeland et al., the large membership AA has attracted is not representative of alcoholics. For various reasons, there are many alcoholics for whom the program is not a good option. The question, then, is to what extent AA's reported effectiveness is a function of self-selection by potential members with the best prognoses.

3. Costello

Another set of systematic reviews of the alcoholism treatment and evaluation literature appeared in 1975 by Costello (1975a, 1975b). In his first report, Costello analyzed the results of 58 treatment evaluations published between 1951 and 1973. A follow-up report (Costello, 1975b) separately analyzed 23 of these studies that had the longest-term follow-up (two years). In a 1977 updating of this data base, 22 additional studies representing more recent approaches were located and compared to the original set (Costello et al., 1977). Costello's reviews rated studies according to outcome and tried to determine if differences in the characteristics of the treatment programs were related to the outcomes. Studies were grouped in five categories, from best to poorest, on the basis of both the percentage of successful abstainers and the percentage of problem drinkers. The average percentages, in Costello's initial analysis, varied from 12% successes and 60% problems to 45% successes and 44% problems.

The findings for the initial samples indicated that small programs using various intensive techniques (inpatient care, drugs, psychotherapy) were most successful. The findings were ambiguous, however, as it was also the case that programs that used patient selection criteria were most successful. Although it might be inferred that the research was designed to achieve the best outcomes, this finding may also demonstrate the value of providing intensive therapy only when it has a reasonable chance of success. Like other reviewers, Costello found that patients with characteristics such as stable marital and occupational status were more likely to benefit from treatment.

Costello's (1977) update of his initial work validated the original conclusions. Although a very small overall increase in successful outcomes and reduction in problem drinking can be detected, the range of outcomes is about the same. His analysis suggests that approximately 45% of patients in good treatment programs can be expected to be without significant problems, and an almost similar rate of patients can be expected to have relapses. It is difficult to know how to interpret these rates. Compared with treatment success rates for some terminal illnesses, the success rates are good; when viewed against spontaneous remission rates of perhaps 30%, they appear less promising. The key question is to what extent the outcome of treatment for alcoholism is determined by patient characteristics.

4. Rand Studies

The so-called Rand Studies (Armor et al., 1978; Polich et al., 1981), which first appeared in 1976 and have been a focal point of debate and policy for alcoholism treatment, are not actually reviews of the alcoholism literature. The studies represent follow-ups at 6 and 18 months and 4 years of patients treated at NIAAA-funded Alcoholism Treatment Centers (ATCs). The importance of the Rand Studies is that this work systematically assesses outcomes of a large sample of alcoholic patients who received a wide variety of treatments.

In the initial study, Armor et al. considered data from almost 2000 patients treated at eight ATCs. The investigators analyzed data at 6 and 18 months after treatment. At the 6-month followup, 68% of patients completing treatment showed improvements in their drinking behavior. At the 18-month follow-up, the results were similar: 67% showed improvement, 24% had been abstinent for at least 6 months, 21% had been abstinent for 1 month, and the remaining 22% were characterized as normal drinkers. Patients were considered to be in remission if they either abstained from drinking or engaged in normal drinking (moderate quantities without signs of impairment). By this criterion, 68% of patients were in remission at 6 months and 67% at 18 months; furthermore, relapse rates did not seem related to ability to abstain. Fifty-three percent of those who made only a single contact (the "untreated" population) with an ATC were in remission.

In a follow-up to the initial survey, Polich et al. (1981) collected and analyzed data from a random sample of over 900 patients who had periodical data for the first study. Interview data were obtained from 85% of the sample. The principal finding of the Rand analyses was that although a large percentage of alcoholics go into remission for periods of time, a substantial proportion relapse and reenter treatment. Only 7% of the total sample abstained throughout the entire four-year period, and nearly 15% died (mortality was 2.5 times what would have been expected). Nonetheless, there was a significant decrease in the percentage of individuals with very serious alcoholism problems. At the time of initial treatment, over 90% were drinking with serious problems; after four years, however, only 54% were drinking with serious problems. The significance of this reduction is difficult to determine. The results may be due to individuals entering treatment at the worst phase of their problem (for these individuals, some improvement would be expected). Improvement may also not be directly attributable to treatment. No particular treatment method seemed to achieve consistently positive results.

B. Treatment Settings

These reviews suggest that alcoholism treatment has demonstrable positive effects, although evidence on the superiority of particular treatments is lacking. The important policy issue of the extent to which alcoholism treatment should be supported is thus only partially addressed.

The question of which treatments have the best demonstrated effectiveness under particular conditions for which patients also remains unanswered. Below, additional evaluative research on a number of specific treatments and settings is reviewed. Both the setting of treatment and the use of treatment modalities such as psychotherapy, drugs, and self-help treatments are considered. Although not comprehensive, the discussion covers treatments that are the most frequently employed and are the current focal points of discussion about alcoholism treatment.

Perhaps, as noted earlier, the most controversial treatment issue concerns the use of inpatient versus outpatient treatment settings. The necessity for hospitalizing alcoholics to provide treatment above that necessary for detoxification or dealing with other medical complications is both a substantive problem (relating to treatment goals and effectiveness) and a significant public policy problem (because of the costs associated with hospitalization). Unfortunately, assessments of the effectiveness of particular settings are difficult to separate from the effectiveness of treatment modalities. Treatment setting is only one factor influencing effectiveness. The review below deals with research comparing outcomes by setting, although a more complete analysis requires parallel consideration of evaluative data for specific modalities.

There seems to be consensus across a number of literature reviews that inpatient treatment is not superior to outpatient care for alcoholism (see Emrick, 1982), but most of the available research is flawed because the effects of treatment variables cannot be distinguished from the effects of patient variables. Thus, more severely impaired patients, along with those of higher socioeconomic status, are more typically assigned to, or arrange to receive, inpatient treatment. Furthermore, a distinction is not often made between hospital- and nonhospital-based inpatient (i.e., residential) treatment, although, as noted (see also Tuchfeld et al., 1982), the nature of such settings may be very different. Not making this distinction results in the aggregating of results from different types of inpatient settings in literature reviews. Because alcoholism treatment takes place in a variety of hospital settings, it may be important to distinguish among their effects.

Reviews by Costello (1975a, 1975b; 1977) and Baekeland (1977) addressed the inpatient-outpatient issue, and the Rand analyses (Armor et al., 1978; Polich et al., 1981) compared inpatient and outpatient care. The reviews and several of the studies on which the reviews' conclusions are based are discussed below. Length of treatment as an outcome variable is also discussed.

Baekeland's (1977) review analyzed improvement rates and found that uncorrected improvement rates were essentially the same for inpatient and outpatient settings (41.5%). When the rates were corrected for sample attrition and spontaneous improvement, however, outpatient settings (with an average improvement rate of 36%) were slightly more effective than inpatient settings (with an improvement rate of 29.9%).

Costello's report (1975a, 1975b) concluded, on the other hand, that the inpatient unit was a valuable asset to a treatment program. However, the review also indicated that an inpatient setting without an intensive community milieu and aggressive outpatient follow-up would be of limited value. Ten of the studies characterized as having very good outcomes combined inpatient with outpatient treatment; two used outpatient only, and two, inpatient only. The studies reporting very good outcomes were also characterized by a variety of other characteristics associated with good outcomes: the use of screening procedures that eliminated high-risk clients, considerable use of Antabuse, social casework, family therapy, involvement of employers, and behavioral therapy. Costello's analysis is limited by the inclusion of both controlled and noncontrolled evaluation studies (cf. Baekeland, 1977, for a discussion of these limitations). Studies by Edwards (1966), Edwards and Guthrie (1967), and Ritson (1968, 1971), discussed below along with other specific studies, were included in the group with very good outcomes.

Ritson (1968, 1971) examined six-month and one-year outcomes in two groups of patients. He found no significant group differences between the group that received outpatient care (which consisted of individual therapy) and the one that received inpatient treatment (consisting of group therapy and AA). However, this study apparently confounded treatment modalities with settings. In addition, patients were not randomly assigned to experimental groups.

A series of studies by Edwards and colleagues has been well received critically because these studies randomly assigned patients to different settings for the same treatment modalities (Edwards, 1970; Edwards, 1966; Edwards and Guthrie, 1966). Matched patients were randomly assigned to either two months of "intensive" outpatient care followed by outpatient aftercare or to eight to nine weeks of inpatient treatment followed by outpatient aftercare. Outpatient care was found to be more efficacious with regard to global ratings, but not until 12 months after treatment. The populations differed somewhat in marital status (80% of the outpatients were married versus 60% of the inpatients), although the differences were probably of no consequence. The generalizability of findings are limited, however, by the exclusion of some treatment modalities (e.g., group therapy) and of alcoholics with severe mental or physical disease.

In apparent contradiction to Edwards' results, Wanberg et al. (1974)

found that two weeks of intensive inpatient treatment to be more effective than three or more in-community treatment sessions. In this study, both types of initial treatment were followed by outpatient group therapy. The Wanberg et al. study differed from the Edwards studies in that fewer (51%) of its patients were married, and the length of both intensive treatment and evaluation in this study was longer. In addition, outpatient treatment in the Edwards studies was intensive. It is possible that any short-term differences between the various Wanberg et al. groups might have disappeared or changed direction at a later point.

Gallant (1971) investigated a population of chronic offenders brought before a municipal court. Individuals convicted of an alcohol-related offense were randomly assigned to either one month of coerced inpatient treatment followed by five months of coerced outpatient treatment or six months of coerced outpatient treatment. Gallant found no differences between the inpatient and outpatient groups on outcome measures related to alcohol use; however, 44% of the offenders assigned to inpatient care received necessary medical attention.

The Rand 18-month follow-up study of patients treated at NIAAA ATCs (Armor et al., 1978) found only minor variations in outcomes among hospital, intermediate, and outpatient settings. Furthermore, these variations virtually disappeared when the analysis controlled for patient characteristics. The four-year follow-up by Polich et al. (1981) found no differences between outcomes for hospital and outpatient settings.

In addition to the issue of treatment setting, length of treatment in the various settings is an area of clinical controversy and policy importance. In general, controlled studies of psychotherapeutic treatments have not found any positive effects for lengthy intensive treatment received either by inpatients or outpatients (Emrick, 1982). An important methodological limitation of available controlled studies, however, is that none of these studies used an intensive treatment longer than 3.5 months of inpatient care; all of these studies used relatively brief treatments. The effects of long-term efforts, some of which are oriented to making character changes, have not been evaluated. Research subjects who receive differing amounts of treatment also receive different kinds of treatment, making it difficult to distinguish the type of therapy from its intensity or duration.

C. Specific Modalities

Within each treatment setting, a diverse set of modalities may be used. Some evidence on effectiveness exists for each, and evidence for behavioral treatments, aversion therapy, and AA is described below. Although not an exhaustive discussion of the research on each modality or the various forms of treatment, the discussion illustrates the range of research issues.

1. Behavioral Therapies

In the last 20 years, the most developed uses of psychotherapy for alcoholism problems have been in the application of behavioral conditioning techniques (see Nathan, 1978). Most behavioral therapies rely on positive reinforcement, although aversion conditioning is also employed (see below). Behavioral techniques include blood alcohol level (BAL) discrimination training, use of videotapes of patients when intoxicated, role playing, cognitive behavior therapy, and alternatives counseling. There has been some research interest, as well, in broad-spectrum approaches, and some of this work is also described.

The Individualized Behavior Therapy for Alcoholics (IBTA), developed by Sobell and Sobell (1972, 1973b) illustrates behavioral treatment. The IBTA approach attempts to provide treatment and drinking goals based on an assessment of what each patient needs. Initial stages of treatment focus on problem identification, identification of alternatives to drinking, and evaluation of those alternatives. A range of behavioral treatments, from assertiveness training to videotaped self-confrontation, is provided to help patients maintain their behavioral and drinking goals. Sobell and Sobell's findings indicated that regardless of whether the assigned treatment goal was "abstinence" or "controlled drinking," many of the patients who received treatment were drinking in a nonproblematic way compared to the patients in a control group. The investigators also found, ironically, that those patients who were assigned "controlled drinking" as a goal had more abstinent days than those assigned "abstinence." Another important aspect of this study was that the package prescribed a thorough analysis of each individual's behavioral determinants for drinking. A new repertoire of social behavior, designed to replace the old behavioral patterns, was carefully rehearsed. Changing attitudes toward drinking was a second major focus.

The Sobells' research has been criticized because it used the treatment goal of "controlled drinking"; recently, serious questions have been raised about the appropriateness of this goal, as well as their research procedures. A follow-up study by Pendery et al. (1982) of patients in the controlled drinking condition of the 1972 Sobell and Sobell study sharply contradicts the original study's findings. Pendrey et al. report that after 10 years, only 1 of 20 subjects was drinking "normally" and without problems. Four of the original subjects had died of alcohol-related causes, 8 were drinking excessively, 1 was not found for follow-up, and 6 were totally abstinent (although each had had serious drinking problems since the experiment). According to Pendery et al., learning how to control drinking is impossible for an alcoholic, and abstinence is the only workable treatment goal.

Three recent studies by Vogler and colleagues tested a treatment package similar to IBTA (Vogler et al., 1975, 1977a, 1977b). In one Vogler study, an overall success rate of about 65% was reported (i.e., 65% were not problem drinkers after a year according to Vogler et al. in 1975). There was no reported difference between the two matched groups of hospitalized chronic alcoholics. One group received the full broad-spectrum package, while the second group received only the educational component, counseling, and alternatives training. In another Vogler study (1977a), four groups of problem drinkers each received different combinations of treatments. Again, all groups showed improvements and there were no differences between groups. In this attempt to "unpackage" broad-spectrum treatment, Vogler found that groups with alcohol education alone did just as well as groups with more complex treatments. There was an 80% attrition rate in this study, however, limiting the weight that can be given the findings.

Pomerleau's (1978) study monitored middle-class alcoholics who were more motivated than subjects in other studies and who were functioning at higher levels. Of 18 patients treated with behavioral techniques, 16 continued in treatment. Of 14 treated with "traditional" methods, only 6 remained in the treatment. Because the numbers are so small, the conclusion that behavioral techniques may have advantages over some therapeutic approaches can be made only tentatively.

2. Aversion Therapy

Another controversial behavioral treatment approach is aversion-conditioning, based primarily on classical conditioning principles. Aversion conditioning approaches include the use of chemicals, electric shock, and imagined aversive stimuli. In the 1940s, Voegtlin and Broz (1949) described the use of chemical aversion therapy and reported that aversion was a successful treatment. Of over 4000 patients who received chemical aversion therapy, 42% had remained totally abstinent and 60% were abstinent for at least a year. Thimann (1949), in a study conducted at about the same time, reported a 51% success rate. More recently, Wiens et al. (1976), at the Raleigh Hills Portland Hospital, found that 63% who received the treatment were abstinent for a year. These relatively positive findings of the effectiveness of aversion therapy have been replicated at several hospitals.

Despite relatively high rates of reported abstinence, reviews of aversion therapy are cautious in their analysis of its effects based on nonexperimental studies. Nathan and Lipscomb (1979), for example, maintain that positive results are probably a function of the types of patients that enter these treatments. These investigators believe that patients at private hospitals, such as Raleigh Hills, have better prognoses at the beginning of treatment. The data of Neuberger et al. (1980, 1982) provide some support for Nathan and Libscomb's contention. In two samples from 1975 and 1976, these investigators found poorer results than typical (one-year post-treatment abstinence rates of 39% and 50%, respectively), and they attributed these to the fact that the samples included a larger number of Medicare, unemployed, and/or unmarried patients. Their most recent data indicate that disabled Medicare patients have relatively poor outcomes (36% abstinence rate, one-year posttreatment) but validate earlier findings of good outcomes for socially stable patients (up to 73% abstinence rate for married and employed patients according to Neuberger et al., 1982).

The principal question about evidence on aversion therapy is whether treatment outcomes can be attributed to demographic factors, to the use of a broad-spectrum treatment program, or to conditioning itself. Definitive answers to questions of efficacy will have to await controlled tests of components of programs that use aversion therapy. There is some basic research evidence of aversion therapy's usefulness (e.g., Cannon et al., 1981), as well as theoretical arguments to support its efficacy (Wilson, 1978). However, the mechanism may be more complicated than learned association, and cognitive factors may interfere with behavioral conditioning. The effectiveness of aversion therapy may also depend on the conditioning technique. Emetine-induced nausea is the most widely used stimulus, but there are many alternatives. Electric shocks have been used in some cases, although not very successfully (Nathan and Lipscomb, 1979). Some success has been reported with imagined aversive stimuli (Cautela, 1970), but this technique is not widely used.

3. Nonbehavioral Psychotherapies

Although there has been considerable research in recent years on the effectiveness of traditional psychotherapies (Office of Technology Assessment, 1980), their use for treating alcoholism has not been validated. In the first review of psychologically oriented treatments, Voegtlin and Lemere (1942) found little usable statistical information to indicate the success of psychoanalytically based therapy. Similarly, Hill and Blane (1967), in their review of psychotherapy outcome studies, found that methodological problems made conclusions about the effectiveness of psychotherapy difficult to support. Baekeland's (1977) and Emrick's (1979, 1982) reviews of controlled studies found no treatment effects for a variety of traditional outpatient psychotherapies compared with each other or with other treatments; only one study reviewed by Emrick found that traditional insight-oriented therapy resulted in better economic and legal outcomes than did a comparison treatment, in this case, contact with AA. Altogether, Emrick found only eight controlled studies, many of which varied aspects of treatment other than the type of therapy (e.g., abstinence versus controlled drinking as a goal of treatment).

In addition to methodological problems with existing studies, many approaches that are used widely with nonalcoholics (e.g., Gestalt therapy) have not been adequately investigated for use with alcoholics. Research comparing different lengths of treatment, from very brief (one to six sessions) to longer treatments (including extended aftercare), is also needed.

4. Drug Treatments

Pharmacological treatments for alcoholism have a long history of use, although the effectiveness of such drug treatments is not widely accepted (cf. Baekeland, 1977; Becker, 1979; Mottin, 1973; Voegtlin and Lemere, 1942). One reason for questioning their effectiveness is that research on drug treatments has been "careless" (Baekeland, 1977). In addition, the effects of drugs appear to be closely tied to patient compliance and the use of other therapies. Despite these problems, however, drugs are widely prescribed for alcoholics (as many as 90% of physicians in private practice report using medication in their treatment of alcoholism), and the use of drug therapies has been associated with positive treatment outcomes (Armor et al., 1978; Costello, 1975a, 1975b, 1979). Two major types of drugs for treating alcoholism are considered here: (1) sensitizing agents and (2) mood-altering drugs.

Treatment of alcoholism with drug agents such as Antabuse that sensitize (i.e., make ill) patients who ingest alcohol has become the most common form of drug treatment. Antabuse treatment is used as an adjunct in many inpatient and outpatient alcoholism treatment programs, and it is also used in conjunction with a number of therapies. The initial Rand report by Armor et al. (1971) indicated that 30% of all patients studied received Antabuse at some point in their treatment. Although there is substantial information about Antabuse, Becker (1979) notes that there is no consensus about its effectiveness. Studies that report effective outcomes with Antabuse tend to be uncontrolled. There seems to be clear evidence that older, more stable, and highly motivated people use Antabuse successfully, and this may explain positive outcomes.

If it is assumed that psychological factors are part of the alcoholism syndrome, it is reasonable to expect mood-altering drugs to have some benefit. In one large-scale and methodologically sophisticated study by

Overall et al. (1973), negative findings concerning the effectiveness of chlordizepoxide (Librium) in reducing symptoms of anxiety and depression were reported. Several studies, however, indicate that such medications are superior to placebos (Baekland, 1977). Studies of the efficacy of tricyclic antidepressants in the treatment of depressed alcoholics report contradictory results: Some fail to show beneficial effects from these drugs; others suggest a high rate of improvement with their usage (J. Solomon, 1982). As another example, the evidence regarding the use of lithium has been inconclusive (Kline et al., 1974; Merry et al., 1976).

5. Self-Help Groups

AA is regarded by some as the most effective form of treatment of alcoholism—more effective than any of the approaches that professionals offer. Various problems with specifying the population that uses AA and a lack of data make such conclusions regarding AA's effectiveness difficult to verify or discount. Baekeland (1977), in his review of literature about AA, reports a 34% success rate—much lower than some of the earlier figures. Other reviewers have reported abstinence rates from 45% to 75%, depending on the length of the reporting period (Leach and Norris, 1977). The problem in evaluating AA is that its members probably differ from the general population of alcoholics, but data supporting this statement as well as other data about AA are difficult to obtain (Baekeland, 1977). Although a substantial number of regular attendees are abstinent (AA, 1972), it is unclear how this relates to the number who try the program. Because nonabstainers may be subjected to ridicule and reproach by other members, it is probably more likely than not that those who remain in AA for long periods of time are those who have achieved sobriety. It seems clear that some aspects of AA programs have useful therapeutic roles (e.g., getting alcoholics to acknowledge their problem, providing a support system), but AA may only be applicable to some categories of alcoholics and alcohol abusers.

D. Conclusions

Research on treatments for alcoholism and alcohol abuse seems to be in transition. The 1970s saw a number of attempts to summarize conclusions of piecemeal research on treatment conducted during the last several decades. The conclusion of many of these reviews is that treatment seems better than no treatment, but that methodological problems render it difficult to conclude that any specific treatment is more effective than any other. Importantly, however, various treatments—such as aversion conditioning or AA—have been shown to be effective for some patients under some conditions. Given the diversity of alcohol problems and patients, what seems necessary are treatments tailored to specific patients.

Aside from questions of effectiveness, efficiency issues must also be addressed. As the costs for treatment increase, evidence is needed about which treatments offer the greatest value for the resources required. The research questions regarding such costs and benefits are described in the following section.

IV. ANALYSES OF COSTS AND BENEFITS

This section describes the costs and benefits of alcoholism treatment and the issues underlying the reimbursement debate about alcoholism treatment. The cost of treatment is an important focus for policymakers, as is the appropriateness of specific expenditures. Thus, for example, allegations of Medicare fraud and abuse in alcoholism treatment programs have generated considerable concern (U.S. Senate, 1982). In addition, cost-effectiveness has also been a focal point of debate. If, for example, halfway houses staffed by paraprofessionals are just as effective, but significantly less costly than a two-week stay in a medical facility, why should not alcoholics use the cheaper alternative? For researchers and practitioners, the important point is that if they are going to demonstrate that one treatment is more effective than any other treatment, they might also try to demonstrate which treatment is more cost-effective. In addition, the question of whether provision of treatment is beneficial to society is still at issue. Available tax dollars may be better spent preventing rather than treating alcoholism. As researchers and practitioners ponder the future of resource availability, an issue decided by policymakers, the cost context needs to be kept in mind.

In this section the costs of alcoholism are analyzed. The methods of cost-effectiveness and cost-benefit analysis (CEA/CBA) are described, and several extant CEA/CBA analyses of alcoholism treatment are reviewed. The discussion of the costs and benefits of alcoholism treatments extends the analysis of the effectiveness of alcoholism treatments. Many of the same methodological problems and caveats apply to analyses of the costs of treatment.

A. Cost Context

Evaluating treatments for alcoholism must be done in the context of costs of alcoholism. Cruze et al. (1981), in a report prepared for the Alcohol and Drug Abuse and Mental Health Administration (ADAMHA), estimated the cost of alcoholism to United States society in 1977 to be nearly $50 billion. As shown in Table 2, Cruze et al. divided total costs to society between "core costs" and "other related costs." "Core costs" were those costs most directly related to the alcoholism problem that are borne by some component of the health care system or are the indirect costs of morbidity and mortality. "Other related costs" included the direct costs of social programs other than those related to health accidents, and indirect costs of incarceration and noninjured time loss.

Cruze et al. also identified health care settings involved in the treatment of alcohol abusers and determined their alcohol-related expenditures. For example, it was estimated that to treat alcohol-specific illness (including cirrhosis), alcoholism specialty facilities expended about $700 million, and general health facilities spent $2 billion; another $3 billion was spent for alcohol-related illness and trauma.

Overall, lost productivity accounted for the greatest share of the economic costs of alcoholism, followed by costs for treatment, motor vehicle accidents, the criminal justice system, other, and social welfare administration—for a total of almost $50 billion. Using a 10% minimum for inflation since 1977, the current annual cost of alcoholism and alcohol abuse can be estimated at $72 billion.

Cruze et al.'s study, although it used a method that differs from earlier studies, yielded a total cost of alcoholism that, when adjusted to inflation, was similar to the estimate of the prior principal study. That study, by Berry et al. (1977), estimated the costs of alcoholism to be $43 billion in 1975. However, there were major differences in the two studies' costs by category; for present purposes, the most important of these differences was Berry et al.'s estimate of $12 million in health care costs owing to alcoholism and alcohol abuse and Cruze's estimate of $5 million.

The primary difference between the Cruze et al. and Berry et al. figures—and perhaps between any estimated and actual health care costs for alcohol abuse—can be accounted for by their differing estimates of the range of illnesses thought to be associated with alcohol abuse (cf. Eckardt et al., 1981). The analysis by Berry et al. comes closer to including costs associated with all such illnesses. However, the exclusion of data for family members and victims of accidents related to alcohol abuse, as well as the conservatism of the estimates, probably resulted in an underestimate. Support for the view that costs are underestimated by these analyses is provided by the IOM's (Institute of Medicine, 1980) report on alcoholism as a health problem. IOM's task force on the economics of alcoholism treatment (Schifrin et al., 1980) argued that each of Berry's categories underestimate the populations affected by alcoholism. In particular, the estimate of health costs did not include costs of related prob-

Table 2
Estimated Economic Costs of Alcoholism in 1977, in millions of dollars

Core costs:			
Direct:			
Treatment (for alcoholism and causally related illness)			$ 5,637
Support (research, education and training, construction, insurance administration)			735
Indirect:			
Lost productivity due to:			
Premature mortality		$10,715	
Morbidity resulting in:			
Reduced productivity and lost work time		23,593	
Lost employment		2,481	
		$36,789	
Total core costs		$36,789	36,789
			$43,161
Other Related Costs:			
Direct:			
Motor vehicle crashes (funeral, legal/court, insurance administration, accident investigation, vehicle damage)			$ 1,782
Criminal justice system			1,685
Social welfare program administration			142
Other (fire losses, fire protection, highway safety)			832
Indirect:			
Lost productivity due to:			
Alcoholics' incarceration			1,418
Others' lost worktime because of motor vehicle crashes			354
Total other related costs			$ 6,213
Total economic costs			$49,374

SOURCE: Adapted from A. M. Cruze, H. J. Harwood, P. L. Kristiansen, et al., *Economic Costs to Society of Alcohol and Drug Abuse and Mental Illness 1977*, final report prepared by the Research Triangle Institute for the Alcohol, Drug Abuse, and Mental Health Administration, Department of Health and Human Services, October, 1981.

lems (e.g., fetal alcohol syndrome) and of illnesses not directly related to the abuse of alcohol. The IOM indicates that Berry et al.'s estimate of the health care costs of alcoholism was understated by 40%. Nevertheless, it represented 12% of the total national health care expenditures by adults in 1975.

Noting the fact that both studies emphasized the conservative biases of almost all of their estimates, the IOM points out that disagreements over details should not obscure "the essential qualitative conclusion" that alcohol abuse imposes very large costs on society. The IOM study indicated that the 1975 total economic costs could be as high as $60 billion, which would make the 1982 economic costs of alcohol abuse approach $120 billion (Schifrin et al., 1980). Research that could contribute to a lessening of these costs is, in the view of the IOM's panel, seriously underfunded. The IOM notes by way of comparison that cancer research receives 70 times as much money as does alcoholism research in relation to the costs of the illnesses.

Assessment of the economic costs of alcoholism and alcohol-related problems is obviously limited by inability to identify clearly problems directly caused by, rather than merely associated with, alcohol use. The prevailing view seems to be that most estimates of these costs are too low because alcoholism's role in medical problems has not been fully explicated. One additional type of costs to which researchers invariably allude, but which is particularly difficult to measure, are the indirect psychological costs of alcoholism. Effects on children whose parents are alcoholic, including future losses in productivity, are also typically omitted from CBAs. Even if these psychological costs were identified, their effects on the future (e.g., for productivity) are often exceedingly difficult to measure.

B. Cost-Effectiveness and Cost-Benefit Analyses

Cost-effectiveness analyses are attempts to specify and compare systematically not only the effectiveness of particular treatments, but the costs of providing the treatments (e.g., therapist salaries, hospital stay costs). The goal of CEA is to assess which treatment gets the better results for the least expense. If inpatient and outpatient treatments, for example, are being compared and found to be equivalent in outcome, the clinically oriented effectiveness literature would judge the results to be ambiguous, but CEA would judge the less expensive of the treatments to be superior. Cost-benefit analyses also examine costs and effectiveness, but are more concerned with an entire realm of treatment provision. CBAs assess, for example, whether it would be more cost-beneficial to provide alcoholism treatment or to commit resources elsewhere, perhaps letting alcoholism run its course.

Conducting cost and outcome studies of alcoholism treatments is complex and potentially controversial. Clearly, it is desirable to conduct formal CEA/CBA analyses in order to determine definitively which of various treatment alternatives currently available are most effective at particular resource utilization levels. As the Office of Technology Assessment (1980) noted in its assessment of the methods of CEA and CBA, however, techniques of this type are probably most useful for structuring policy problems. Rarely is it possible to develop CEA/CBAs definitively.

CEAs and CBAs are difficult to conduct with precision because it is almost impossible to specify comprehensively the costs and benefits of alternative treatments. This is especially true in the area of alcoholism because of the lack of good data directly comparing alternative treatments and because of the difficulties in measuring and specifying outcomes of treatment. In CEA/CBA, the potential costs and benefits of alcoholism treatment can be assessed with varying degrees of comprehensiveness, although means for estimating costs and benefits vary. An analyst conducting a CBA must decide which benefits to measure, how to measure them, and what values to place on those measurements. It is also important to recognize that factors other than those that can be qualified in a CEA should be considered in making a policy decision (Office of Technology Assessment, 1980a).

Unemployment and lost productivity from alcoholism may be among the greatest costs of alcoholism, but limiting analyses to work-related measures underestimates the potential benefits of a program that aids individuals not currently in the labor force (e.g., the unemployed, full-time homemakers, adolescents in school). For example, Cicchinelli et al.'s (1978) output-value analysis (a simplified CEA/CBA) of an alcoholism treatment program indicated that the program was more efficient for men than for women. This finding was due to the average lower cost of treatment for men and the estimated lower salary rates for women. Another finding was that the program efficiency tended to decline with severity of impairment. If a choice had to be made concerning which program was more cost-beneficial, a decision based on an analysis which valued benefits either by income gained or by degree of impairment could foster inequities.

Despite problems, when CEA/CBA is done well, its use aids "the complete enumeration of expected costs and benefits as well as explicit consideration of assumptions underlying quantitative evaluations of the costs and benefits" (Swint and Nelson, 1977). Assuming such specification is possible, such analyses provide a solid scientific basis to aid in making decisions. Given the substantial variance in alcoholism program costs (e.g., inpatient versus outpatient) and the current policy debate over reimbursement policy, such information would obviously have great utility.

C. Studies of Cost-Effectiveness and Cost-Benefit

Led by state governments and private industry employers, a number of efforts to expand alcoholism treatment benefits have been developed and studied during the past 10 years. Jones and Vischi (1979), ADAMHA staff members, reviewed available literature with respect to alcoholism treatment's impact on medical care utilization. The settings of the studies they reviewed included a police department, a fire department, a Canadian General Motors plant, and an insurance program for California state employees. Their review, which included analyses of the dozen such studies then available, found surprisingly consistent results. Each of the investigations Jones and Vischi evaluated found that alcoholism treatment resulted in a significant reduction in medical care use and expenditures. The median reduction in sick days and accident benefits was 40%.

Unfortunately, methodological problems were present in each of the studies reviewed by Jones and Vischi. The principal difficulties were treatment design problems. Most studies were conducted in employee-based alcoholism programs or in organized health care settings, particularly health maintenance organizations (HMOs). Such programs and settings have particular economic incentives and tend to emphasize treatments that are low cost and do not take individuals away from their work. All of the studies were flawed by their failure to identify medical utilization outside of the study because they used nonequivalent comparison groups (i.e., quasi-experimental designs). The studies also failed to control or adjust for increases in pretreatment medical utilization caused by the referring visit. In general, the studies were of short duration (one year or less) and used limited treatment outcome measures. Nevertheless, the existence of positive results across 12 separate studies gives added weight to the conclusion that alcoholism treatment is cost-beneficial. Since the Jones and Vischi review appeared, additional cost-based analyses have been completed, with consistently positive results. Two such studies are further described below.

1. Group Health Association

The most extensive study of the cost effectiveness of providing alcoholism treatment benefits was a seven-year study conducted for the Group Health Association of America by Plotnick et al. (1982). This study evaluated the feasibility of providing comprehensive alcoholism treatment programs in four HMOs. The programs were outpatient oriented, but each attempted to provide comprehensive and continuous treatment services. The investigators collected and analyzed data on patient functioning, health status, and treatment use for over 2000 patients. Of the subjects in the study, 1000 were alcoholics in treatment; others were spouses, family members, and a group of nonalcoholic HMO members matched by age, gender, and length of membership in the HMO.

Plotnick et al. found that outpatient-oriented alcoholism treatment programs appeared to be both effective and cost beneficial. Patients in treatment over a 3-year period declined in their use of alcohol by 65% after 6 months and by approximately 70% after 2 years. Alcoholic patients also increased their length of abstinence from 8 days at intake to 19 days after 6 months, remaining at 19 or 20 days throughout the 3-year follow-up. Patients also showed improvement on work-related dimensions as measured through reduction in reprimands (75% to 90%) and days sick or absent from work (an average of 50%). These improvements paralleled improvements in measures of medical care use. Alcoholic patients reduced ambulatory health care service use between 11% (after 6 months) to 30% (after 4 years). These patients also showed an immediate decline in the percentage of emergency care visits (from 31% to 9% after 6 months) and an increase in the percentage of regularly scheduled visits (from 59% to 78% after 6 months). However, alcoholics used more ambulatory care services than did the members of the comparison group. Relative utilization went from seven times as many encounters with health care providers to three times as many encounters over 4 years of study.

Hospitalization experience was less positive. There were modest reductions relative to matched groups in three studies and an increase in a fourth site that was cautiously attributed to demographic characteristics of the sample. Furthermore, there was a substantial "peaking" phenomenon in one site at which utilization was measured frequently, with one increase in length of stay among alcoholics at 6 months before intake and another increase, though less dramatic, 24 months after intake. Plotnick and colleagues attribute this increase, and the high utilization rates overall, to the chronic and severe health problems generally experienced by alcoholics. Despite problems in interpreting results, it is noteworthy that all of the HMOs involved in the study have decided to continue providing alcoholism treatment services.

2. U.S. Air Force

Orvis et al. (1981) compared the cost-effectiveness of inpatient, outpatient, and education-only treatments for U.S. Air Force personnel in a nonexperimental clinical trial. Twenty-eight days of inpatient care at an Air Force Alcohol Rehabilitation Center cost $3000; 10 sessions of outpatient care cost $900; and a series of awareness seminars cost $60 per person. Much of the inpatient cost was attributable to lost work time. Direct costs were $1,705 for inpatient treatment, $649 for outpatient treatment, and $28 for alcohol awareness seminars.

The Orvis et al. CEA consisted of estimating the annual cost savings per capita for those severely and moderately impaired and comparing the savings to the cost of treatment. Calculations based on their analysis show that it would take 4 years for a 28-day inpatient treatment for the severely impaired to pay for itself, compared to a little less than 2 years for outpatient treatment to pay for itself. For nondependent alcoholics, it would take longer. These figures, based on the equivalent effectiveness of all treatment contexts, result in an average 50% reduction in problems for all participants and no statistical differences in remission rates, which were between 70% and 80%. However, while these figures are suggestive, the fact that patients were not randomly assigned to treatments and that most clients received a combination of all types of treatment limits the usefulness of the study.

D. Conclusions

There seems to be substantial evidence to support the hypothesis that alcoholism treatment is cost-beneficial. The benefits of alcoholism treatment, even if they fall short of what may be claimed, seem to be in excess of the costs of providing treatment. It is difficult from the available evidence to determine the relative effectiveness of inpatient versus outpatient treatment; it is also difficult to determine how changing the mix of providers or types of treatments would affect either effectiveness or cost-effectiveness. Because different groups receive different treatments, there is an inherent methodological difficulty in interpreting most of the available research.

It does seem clear, however, that many alcoholism treatment services are not cost-effective—that is, there are less expensive ways of providing treatment than are reflected in current reimbursement policy. However, reimbursement systems, particularly the Medicare and Medicaid programs, have overwhelmingly emphasized the most expensive treatment services—inpatient, medically based treatment. Questions about the wisdom of this approach have resulted in recent changes in private reimbursement systems as well as clarification of Medicare policy, and an attempt to evaluate systematically whether changes in policy would result in health care cost savings. These issues are addressed in the following section.

V. REIMBURSEMENT ISSUES

The development of the current system for treating alcoholics and alcohol abusers has been closely tied to funding and reimbursement policies of both private and governmental insurance programs. Since the acceptance of alcoholism as a disease over 25 years ago, an elaborate medically based treatment system for alcoholism has evolved. In some cases, development of treatment services has preceded reimbursement policy; in other cases, however, treatment seems to have developed around what is reimbursable.

In recent years, a number of private insurance companies, employers, and the federal government have expanded benefits for alcoholism treatment. Reimbursement for acute medical care, as well as inpatient treatment for alcoholism is currently available, although coverage is not universal. Nonhospital-based treatments, including outpatient care, aftercare, and nonmedically oriented residential care, are less frequently reimbursed, although there is a trend toward developing such benefits (Williams, 1981). Thirty-three states, as of 1983, mandate some form of coverage by health insurers for alcoholism treatment (Science Management Corporation, 1982).

Recent emphasis on expanding insurance benefits for alcoholism treatment (see, e.g., NIAAA, 1981) stems from a belief, supported by the evidence in the preceding section, that the costs of not providing alcoholism treatment are greater than the costs of providing such treatments (Archer, 1981; NIAAA, 1981; Sarvis, 1976). Whether alcoholism treatment should be reimbursed at all, therefore, does not seem to be at issue. The essential question seems to be whether current reimbursement policy supports the provision of the most cost-effective treatments. As already noted, several cost analyses have been conducted, yet some issues need to be addressed in greater depth. In particular, questions about whether ineffective treatments are being employed and concerns about whether lower-cost treatment alternatives are available to treat alcoholics but are not being used need to be examined.

The nation's health care budget has expanded to almost 10% of the gross national product, and although efforts have been made to improve benefits for alcoholism treatment, increasing such benefits conflicts with needs to reduce health care expenditures. There is an obvious need to develop a more efficient treatment system to deal with alcoholism—with such a system it is less likely that services will be denied to a large number of people or that costs will be prohibitive. The issues of reimbursement policy are complex, however, and changes in policy affect not only alcoholic patients, they have widespread implications for the costs and treatment of all health problems.

A. Funding of Alcoholism Services

Both the federal government and third-party private health insurers have a substantial stake in the funding of alcoholism treatment services. An estimated 66% of the direct costs of alcoholism treatment programs are paid for through federal, state, and local government programs. Another 20% of the costs are paid by private insurance carriers (NIAAA, 1981). The development of such benefits is relatively recent. A review of the current system and how it evolved may be useful for understanding the present policy debate about alcoholism treatment coverage under Medicare.

1. Medicare

Medicare is a nationwide, federally administered health insurance program authorized in 1965 to cover the costs of hospitalization, medical care, and some related services for eligible persons aver age 65. Since its inception, Medicare has not specifically provided benefits for the treatment of alcoholism. Rather, under the hospital insurance component of Medicare, alcoholism can be treated as a psychiatric disorder; hospitalization for a psychiatric disorder, in a psychiatric hospital, is limited to 190 days per lifetime. For treatment of alcoholism within a psychiatric ward of a general hospital, the standard (physical illness) Part A Medicare reimbursement and coverage provisions apply: 90 days of hospital care in each benefit period with $260 deductible (to be increased in January 1983), and 25% co-payment after 60 days, as well as a lifetime reserve of 60 days with a 50% co-payment. According to NIAAA (1978), the original limitation on psychiatric care was to avoid Medicare's reimbursing "custodial care," since Medicare was intended only to insure against illnesses that are being actively treated.

The supplementary medical insurance component of Medicare provides partial coverage for outpatient psychiatric services. The formula is complex, but it results (as of 1983) in a 50% co-insurance benefit with a maximum reimbursable of $250 per year. For physical illness, however, Medicare pays 80% of a physician's reasonable charge after a $75 deductible. Although outpatient psychiatric services are limited to a maximum reimbursement of $250 a year, there is no limit on reimbursement for medical or psychiatric care while a patient is in a psychiatric ward of a general hospital. The original limit on coverage of outpatient care was consistent with such limits by private insurers.

The Medicare program essentially funds providers who are physicians or who are under the direct supervision of a physician performing services incident to those of a physician. This has meant that many nonacute-care facilities and treatment centers that offer nonphysician-based care have not been eligible for reimbursement. Until recently, many such programs were funded directly by NIAAA. Medicare reimbursement policy is currently undergoing change. A series of studies found that medically based inpatient care was far more expensive than nonmedically-based inpatient or outpatient care (see reviews by Hallan, 1981; NIAAA, 1978). Furthermore, as shown in the review of treatment effectiveness literature, research evidence had not proven the superiority of the more expensive types of care. In 1983, the Health Care Financing Administration (HCFA) implemented new Medicare guidelines specifying treatment of alcoholism in outpatient facilities and placing limits on inpatient treatment and consultation with family members. Earlier guidelines had not specifically referred to hospital-based outpatient treatment; the new guidelines make it clear that such services are covered when reasonable and necessary. Outpatient treatment in free-standing clinics is also made available, with the same restrictions.

The rules for inpatient treatment have been relaxed somewhat in that patients need not be experiencing severe medical complications at the time of admission to be eligible for inpatient medical detoxification; however, the probability of such consequences occurring is necessary for reimbursement. The new Medicare guidelines also require that coverage of alcohol detoxification and rehabilitation be addressed separately (i.e., a patient who requires the hospital setting for detoxification may not necessarily require it for rehabilitation). Presumably, this requirement will reduce the number of patientdays spent in inpatient facilities.

The guidelines also require a closer look at the safety and feasibility of chemical aversion therapy in individual cases. Electrical aversion therapy has been excluded from coverage on grounds of safety and ineffectiveness, although the Public Health Service is coordinating an assessment of what is known about the technique. Another restriction is that family counseling is to be limited to those cases in which the primary purpose of the counseling is the treatment of the patient's condition.

2. Medicaid

The Medicaid program provides medical assistance to low-income individuals and families. Treatment costs are shared by the states and the federal government. Each participating state (all states except Arizona) must provide certain basic health services, according to Medicaid regulations. States, however, have substantial leeway concerning specific coverage and interpretation of regulations. According to NIAAA (1981), a major limitation in the Medicaid program is the exclusion of federal financial participation for care in psychiatric institutions for persons between the ages of 22 and 64. With respect to other treatment settings, Medicaid may theoretically provide more options for treatment, although Medicaid statutes do not specifically mention alcoholism treatment. For example, states have considerable latitude in defining physician participation. Services need not be those incident to a physician's, and clinics may be reimbursed for the services of paraprofessional rehabilitation counselors (HCFA, 1979).

In 1978, Medicaid provided 6% ($5 million) of the total funds of NIAAA-funded alcoholism treatment centers (Ferguson and Kirk, 1979). Information concerning how much Medicaid provided to other alcoholism treatment services is not readily available (HCFA, 1982). In one study (Booz-Allen and Hamilton, 1978), now several years old, the investigators found that 4 of the 45 state plans they reviewed referred specifically to treatment for alcoholism: 2 of the 4 allowed coverage, 1 explicitly excluded coverage, and 1 limited coverage to detoxification. Eight other states were found to have plans providing a relatively favorable environment for inpatient alcoholism treatment coverage, and 23 states were found to have plans providing a relatively favorable environment for outpatient services. Annual levels of reimbursement for alcoholism treatment, when reported, were generally low (e.g., in 1978: $45,000 in Mississippi, $800,000 in Maine, $1,409,000 in Washington), except in New York ($32.1 million). A survey conducted by NIAAA in 1978 indicated that all state Medicaid agencies reimbursed for inpatient care of organic illnesses related to alcoholism, and a majority reimbursed for outpatient care for such illnesses. However, a substantially lower proportion of state Medicaid agencies reimbursed for the treatment of alcoholism itself, especially when that treatment was not in a medical setting (HCFA, 1979).

There have been no changes in Medicaid regulations, but because of rescissions in formula grants, states have more latitude in deciding how federal funds are spent, yet they have fewer funds. In 1982, 35% of the sub-block grant for alcoholism, drug abuse, and mental health must be allocated to alcoholism; in 1983 and 1984, funds may be transferred by the states from alcohol and drug abuse to mental health (Califano, 1982). In 1981, block grant allocations for alcohol, drug abuse, and mental health services were found to be 20% lower than the levels of predecessor categorical programs; in the first six months of the new block grant program, 15% of alcoholism, drug abuse, and mental health grants had been drawn by the states (General Accounting Office, 1982).

3. Other Coverage

According to the National Drug and Alcoholism Treatment Utilization Survey (NDATUS), state governments provided $206 million to alcoholism treatment centers in 1980, or 21.9% of the total funds (NIAAA, 1978a). Local governments contributed $97 million, or 10.3% of the total. Although the states constitute the largest single source of funding for alcoholism services, they typically do not operate treatment programs directly; the states' role consists of allocating resources from various funding sources to local programs (NIAAA, 1978a). In addition, some states (e.g., California) have developed statewide alcoholism health insurance programs for their employees; and, increasingly, state legislatures are considering mandating, or requiring as an option, insurance coverage for alcoholism treatment. By 1981, such legislation had been enacted in 33 states, had been defeated in 14, was being considered in 2, and had not been considered in 1 (Science Management Corporation, 1982). The trend in private insurance coverage is toward increased coverage in free-standing centers, provision of treatment equal to that for other diseases, and provision of coverage for family counseling and care. Model legislation to provide this coverage has been developed, although it has not been enacted. Under terms of the model legislation, coverage would be a required option rather than a mandated inclusion.

Prior to 1972, the explicit exclusion of alcoholism treatment was standard in private insurance policies, although treatment was often covered under other diagnoses (Williams, 1981). Even though progress has been made, very few plans cover alcoholism on the same basis as other illnesses. Generally, outpatient care must be provided at a hospital, and is subject to a 50% co-payment provision as well as an annual maximum. There is often a lifetime maximum as well. These restrictions are reflected in the fact that while 21% to 85% of those served in NIAAA programs in 1976 had some form of health insurance, only 10% to 40% had coverage for alcoholism services (Cooper, 1979).

4. Research Developments

It is obviously impossible to determine the impact of the new Medicare regulations and other developments in treatment financing. The developments come, however, at the same time that HCFA and NIAAA are engaged in a joint alcoholism services demonstration project. The purpose of the project is to expand Medicare and Medicaid benefits to alcoholism treatment providers with the emphasis on less costly settings, such as free-standing inpatient and outpatient facilities and halfway houses. The demonstration has also been designed to test the effectiveness of using nonmedical personnel in the treatment of alcoholism.

The project is a four-year demonstration, with HCFA financing treatment costs and NIAAA providing administrative and evaluative services. Seven states are participating in the program, and approximately 120 providers are treating 5200 patients in the first year. Although the original intent of the demonstration was to fund programs not eligible under the Medicare and Medicaid formulas, there will be some overlap because of the recent changes in regulations. Independent evaluation of the demonstration program is being conducted. Because of the way in which the demonstration projects were funded, the design will necessarily be quasi-experimental—that is, patients will not be randomly assigned to facilities, service providers, or treatment modalities. The research, instead, will track patients from their entry in the programs for a two- to three-year period. The design calls primarily for collecting cost information about the use of medical services. Program experience for two years prior and two years subsequent to the demonstration project will be assessed. Other research developments consist of increased use of randomized clinical trials (Institute of Medicine, 1980), attempts at patient-treatment matches (see Emrick, 1982, for a review of four such studies), and quantitative syntheses of the literature.

B. Implications of Current Developments

Reimbursement formulae have emphasized inpatient, medically based treatment for alcoholism. Although there may be some patients for whom such intensive treatment is necessary and appropriate, it is also true that there are many for whom it is not appropriate. In fact, because of the stigma and time required to be treated in an acute facility, many will not seek such treatment. The evidence does not seem strong enough, however, to support further restricting benefits for inpatient services. Because it would not be possible to restrict acute care admissions, the likely result of not funding residential or free-standing treatment settings would probably be to increase use of acute care facilities. This might result if alcoholic patients were admitted under other primary diagnoses.

The best strategies would seem to be ones that encourage early outpatient treatment and continuing aftercare service on an outpatient basis (Regan, 1981). Given both research evidence that does not clearly indicate the necessity of inpatient care and the lower cost of outpatient treatment, such a strategy might lead to better use of health care resources. The recent changes in Medicare guidelines appear to be consistent with this direction (see also Diesenhaus, 1982). Reimbursement criteria for inpatient services are tightened, while the availability of reimbursement for outpatient treatment and involvement of nonmedically trained personnel has been increased.

Although it appears that the new guidelines will have positive effects in making the treatment system more efficient, it may be difficult to determine the impact of these changes. They are being introduced nationwide and at a time when the health care system and the economy are undergoing major changes. There will be no comparative data on whether and how they are effective. In addition, because responsibility for alcoholism treatment services has been transferred from the federal government to the states, national data may no longer be available. It may be unclear whether the new regulations simply make possible the treatment of a larger group of alcoholics and alcohol abusers, whether their use of the benefit represents changes in the diagnostic labels given patients, and whether they achieve the intended effect of the legislation.

C. Conclusions

Alcoholism treatments have evolved steadily over the last 30 years. The last decade, in particular, has witnessed a dramatic increase in the availability of treatment as government, industry, and private insurers have made health resources available to treat alcoholism. Recent expansion of the alcoholism treatment system and increased use of public funds has, however, raised a series of important public policy questions about the efficacy and benefits of treatment. Unfortunately, evaluation of alcoholism treatment is relatively new, and neither the alcoholism problem nor evidence about treatment effects are clear-cut. Because the effects of alcoholism are so diverse and the treatments multivariant, attributing effectiveness is extremely difficult. Nevertheless, despite this and a number of other methodological problems, it seems clear from our review that alcoholism treatment has demonstrable benefits. The hypothesis that alcoholism treatment is beneficial seems more strongly supported than any alternative hypothesis.

Interestingly, although it is often difficult to identify the benefits (especially monetary) of health and mental health treatments, for alcoholism, the issue is relatively clear. The costs of alcoholism are staggering and, in comparison, costs of providing treatment are minimal. With respect to federal health policy, recent changes in Medicare guidelines (which permit greater use of outpatient services) seem a useful step. They should, at the very least, increase the number of individuals who receive alcoholism treatment services and make the system more efficient. However, it should be recognized that alcoholism is a systemic problem—changes in any aspect of the system will have reverberations (across the health system, the social service system, the criminal justice system, etc.). Whatever further changes are made should be made cautiously. Perhaps most important from our perspective as researchers, we must develop currently lacking information about treatment effectiveness (cf. General Accounting Office, 1982; Institute of Medicine, 1980). Only with such information can reimbursement and treatment decisions be made with more confidence, and only then will we be able to develop a more effective treatment system.

REFERENCES

Aaron, P., and Musto, D., 1981, Temperance and prohibition in America: A historical review, in *Alternative Policies Affecting the Prevention of Alcohol Abuse and Alcoholism,* National Academy of Sciences, Washington, D.C.

Alcocer, A. A., 1975, Chicano alcoholism, unpublished paper, California State University.

Alcoholics Anonymous, 1972, Profile of an AA Meeting, Alcoholics Anonymous World Service, Inc., New York.

American Medical Association, 1977, *Manual on Alcoholism,* AMA, Chicago.

Archer, L., 1981, A Review of Progress in Development of Health Insurance Coverage for Alcoholism Treatment, *Al. Health & Res. World,* 5:4.

Armor, D., Johnson, P., Polich, S., et al., 1977, Trends in U.S. adult drinking practices, contract no. (ADM) 281-76-0020, summary report prepared by the Rand Corporation for the National Institute on Alcohol Abuse and Alcoholism, Alcohol, Drug Abuse, and Mental Health Administration, Santa Monica, Calif.

Armor, D., Polich, J. M., and Stambul, H. B., 1978, *Alcoholism and Treatment,* John Wiley & Sons, New York.

Baekeland, F., 1977, Evaluation of treatment methods in chronic alcoholism, in *Treatment and Rehabilitation of the Chronic Alcoholic* (B. Kissin and H. Begleiter, eds.), Plenum Press, New York.

Baekeland, F., Lundwall, L., and Kissin, B., 1975, Methods for the treatment of chronic alcoholism: A critical appraisal, in *Research Advances in Alcohol and Drug Problems,* vol. II (Y. Israel, ed.), John Wiley & Sons, New York.

Becker, C. E., 1979, Pharmacotherapy in the treatment of alcoholism, in *The Diagnosis and Treatment of Alcoholism* (J. H. Mendelson and N. K. Mello, eds.), McGraw-Hill Book Company, New York.

Beckman, C. J., and Kocel, K. M., 1982, The treatment-delivery system and alcohol abuse in women: Social policy implications, *J. Soc. Issues,* 38:139.

Berry, R. E., Jr., Boland, J. P., Smart, C. N., et al., 1977, The economic costs of alcohol abuse and alcoholism—1975, contract no. (ADM) 281-76-0016, final report prepared by Policy Analysis for National Institute on Alcohol Abuse and Alcoholism, Boston.

Blane, H. T., and Hewitt, L. E., 1977, Mass media, public education and alcohol: A state of the art review, contract NIA-76-12, prepared by the University of Pittsburgh for National Institute on Alcohol Abuse and Alcoholism, Pittsburgh, Pa.

Booz-Allen & Hamilton, Inc., 1978, Alcoholism funding study: Evaluation of sources of funds and barriers to funding alcoholism treatment programs, Booz-Allen, Washington, D.C.

Bourne, P. G., and Light, E., 1979, Alcohol problems in blacks and women, in

The Diagnosis and Treatment of Alcoholism (J. H. Mendelson and N. K. Mello, eds.), McGraw-Hill Book Company, New York.

Brandsma, J. M., 1980, *Outpatient Treatment of Alcoholism: A Review and Comparative Study*, University Park Press, Baltimore.

Braucht, M. G., 1981, Problem drinking among adolescents: A review and analysis of psychosocial research, in *Special Population Issues, Alcohol and Health Monograph No. 4*, National Institute on Alcohol Abuse and Alcoholism, Rockville, Md.

Bromet, E., Moos, R., and Bliss, F., 1976, The social climate of alcoholism treatment programs, *Arch. Gen. Psychiat.*, 33:910.

Caddy, G. R., 1980, Problems in conducting alcohol treatment outcome studies: A review, in *Evaluating Alcohol and Drug Treatment Effectiveness* (L. C. Sobell, M. B. Sobell, and E. Ward, eds.), Pergamon Press, New York.

Caddy, G. R., 1978, Toward a multivariate analysis of alcohol abuse, in *Alcoholism: New Directions in Behavior Research and Treatment* (P. E. Nathan, G. A. Marlatt, and T. Lorberg, eds.), Plenum Press, New York.

Cahn, S., 1970, *The Treatment of Alcoholics: An Evaluative Study*, Oxford University Press, New York.

Califano, J. A., Jr., 1982, *The 1982 Report on Drug Abuse and Alcoholism*, Warner Books, New York.

Camp, J. M., and Kurtz, N. R., 1982, Redirecting manpower for alcoholism treatment, in *Prevention, Intervention and Treatment: Concerns and Models, Alcohol and Health Monograph No. 3*, National Institute on Alcohol Abuse and Alcoholism, Alcohol, Drug Abuse, and Mental Health Administration, Rockville, Md.

Cannon, D. S., Baker, T. B., and Wehl, C. K., 1981, Emetic and electric shock alcohol aversion therapy: Six- and twelve-month follow-up, *J. Cons. Clin. Psychol.*, 49:360.

Cautela, J. R., 1970, The treatment of alcoholism by covert sensitization, *Psychotherapy: Theory, Research, and Practice*, 7:86.

Cicchinelli, L. F., Binner, P. R., and Halpern, J., 1978, Output value analysis of an alcoholic treatment program, *J. Stud. Alc.*, 39:435.

Cochrane, A. L., 1972, *Effectiveness and Efficiency: Random Reflections on Health Services*, Burgess, London.

Cook, T. D., and Campbell, D. T., 1979, *Quasi-Experimentation: Design and Analysis Issues for Field Settings*, Rand McNally Company, Chicago.

Cooper, M. L., 1979, *Private Health Insurance Benefits for Alcoholism Drug Abuse and Mental Illness*, The George Washington University, Intergovernmental Health Policy Project, Washington, D.C.

Costello, R. M., 1975a, Alcoholism treatment and evaluation, I. In Search of Methods, *Int. J. Addict.*, 10:251.

———, 1975b, Alcoholism treatment and evaluation, II. Collation of two year follow-up studies, *Int. J. Addict.*, 10:857.

Costello, R. M., Biever, P., and Baillargeon, J. G., 1977, Alcoholism treatment programming: Historical trends and modern approaches, *Alcoholism: Clin. Exp. Res.*, 1(4):311.

Costello, R. M., Baillargeon, J. G., Biever, P., et al., 1979, Second-year alcoholism treatment outcome evaluation with a focus on Mexican-American patients, *Am. J. Drug Alcohol Abuse*, 6(1):97.

Crawford, J. J., and Chalupsky, A. B., 1977, The reported evaluation of alcoholism treatments, 1968–1971: A methodological review, *Addict. Behav.,* 2:63.

Cruze, A. M., Harwood, H. J., Kristiansen, P. L., et al., 1981, *Economic Costs to Society of Alcohol and Drug Abuse and Mental Illness 1977,* final report prepared by the Research Triangle Institute for the Alcohol, Drug Abuse, and Mental Health Administration, Department of Health and Human Services, Rockville, Md.

Diesenhaus, H., 1982, Current trends in treatment programing for problem drinkers and alcoholics, in *Prevention, Intervention, and Treatment: Concerns and Models,* Alcohol and Health Monograph No. 3, National Institute on Alcohol Abuse and Alcoholism, Alcohol, Drug Abuse, and Mental Health Administration, Rockville, Md.

Donovan, J. E., and Jessor, R., 1978, Adolescent problem drinking: Psychosocial correlates in a national sample study, *J. Stud. Alc.,* 39(9):1506.

Dunn, J. H., and Clay, M. L., 1971, Physicians look at the general hospital alcoholism service, *Q. J. Stud. Alc.,* 32:162.

Eckardt, M. H., Harford, T. C., Kaelber, C. T., et al., 1981, Health hazards associated with alcohol consumption, *JAMA,* 246(6):648.

Edwards, G., 1970, Alcoholism: The analysis of treatment, in *Alcohol and Alcoholism* (R. E. Popham, ed.), University of Toronto Press, Toronto.

Edwards, G., 1966, Hypnosis in treatment of alcohol addiction: Controlled trial, with analysis of factors affecting outcome, *Q. J. Stud. Alc.,* 27:221.

Edwards, G., and Guthrie, S., 1966, A comparison of inpatient and outpatient treatment of alcohol dependence, *Lancet,* 1:467.

Edwards, G., and Guthrie, S., 1967, A controlled trial of inpatient and outpatient treatment of alcohol dependency, *Lancet,* 1:555.

Emrick, C. D., 1982, Evaluation of alcoholism therapy methods, in *Encyclopedic Handbook of Alcoholism* (E. M. Pattison and E. Kaufman, eds.), Gardner Press, New York.

Emrick, C. D., 1979, Perspectives on clinical research: Relative effectiveness of alcohol abuse treatment, *Fam. Comm. Health,* 2:71.

Emrick, C. D., 1974, A review of psychologically oriented treatment of alcoholism: I. The use and interrelations of outcome criteria and drinking behavior following treatment, *Q. J. Stud. Alc.,* 35:523.

Emrick, C. D., 1975, A review of psychologically oriented treatment of alcoholism: II. The relative effectiveness of different approaches and the effectiveness of treatment versus no treatment, *J. Stud. Alc.,* 36:88.

Emrick, C. D., and Stilson, D. W., 1977, The Rand Report: Some comments and a response, *J. Stud. Alc.,* 38(1):152.

Federal Register, 1982, Notices, 47:38837, Sept. 1, 1982.

Ferguson, L., and Kirk, J., 1979, *Statistical Report: National Institute on Alcohol Abuse and Alcoholism-Funded Treatment Programs, Calendar Year 1978* National Institute on Alcohol Abuse and Alcoholism, Alcohol, Drug Abuse, and Mental Health Administration, Rockville, Md.

Fine, E. W., and Steers, R. A., 1976, The relationship between alcoholism and depression in black men, paper presented at the National Council on Alcoholism Conference, Washington, D.C., May, 1976.

Foster, F. M., Horn, J. L., and Wanberg, K. W., 1972, Dimensions of treatment outcome: A factor analytic study of alcoholics' response to a follow-up questionnaire, *Q. J. Stud. Alc.,* 33:1079.

Fusillo, M., and Skoch, E. M., 1981, The psychiatric hospital treatment of alcoholism: A multidisciplinary approach, *J. Nat. Assn. Priv. Psych. Hosp.,* 12:97.

Gallant, D. M., 1971, Evaluation of compulsory treatment of the alcoholic municipal court offender, in *Recent Advances in Studies of Alcoholism: An Interdisciplinary Symposium* (N. K. Mello and J. H. Mendelson, eds.), National Institute on Alcohol Abuse and Alcoholism, Rockville, Md.

General Accounting Office, U.S. Congress, 1982, Early observations on block grant implementation, report to the Congress by the Comptroller General of the United States, GAO IGGD-82-79, Washington, D.C., August 24, 1982.

Gerard, D. L., and Saenger, G., 1966, *Out-patient Treatment of Alcoholism: A Study of Outcome and Its Determinants,* Brookside Monograph No. 4, University of Toronto Press, Toronto.

Gerard, D. L., Saenger, G., and Wile, R., 1962, The abstinent alcoholic, *Arch. Gen. Psychiat.,* 6:83.

Gomberg, E. S., 1982, Historical and political perspectives: Women and drug use, *J. Soc. Iss.,* 38(2):9.

Goodwin, D. W., Othmer, E., and Halikas, J. A., 1970, Loss of short-term memory as a predictor of the alcoholic "black-out," *Nature,* 227:201.

Hall, D. C., Chaikan, K., and Piland, B., 1977, A review of the problem drinking behavior literature associated with the Spanish-speaking population group, contract no. 281-76-0025, final report prepared by the Stanford Research Institute for the National Institute on Alcohol Abuse and Alcoholism, Menlo Park, Calif.

Hallan, J. B., 1981, Health insurance coverage for alcoholism: A review of costs and utilization, *Alc. Health & Res. World,* 5(4):16.

Health Care Financing Administration, 1979, Coverage of alcoholism treatment services Titles XVIII and XIX, August 24, 1979, HCFA, Department of Health, Education, and Welfare, Washington, D.C.

Health Care Financing Administration, 1982, Medicare intermediary manual, part 3—claims process, Transmittal No. 992, HCFA Publication No. 13-3, August, 1982, HCFA, Department of Health and Human Services, Washington, D.C.

Heather, N., and Robertson, I., 1981, *Controlled Drinking,* Methuen & Co., Ltd., London.

Hill, M. J., and Blane, H. T., 1967, Evaluation of psychotherapy with alcoholics, *Q. J. Stud. Alc.,* 28:76.

———, 1977, Issues in the evaluation of alcoholism treatment, *Profess. Psychol.,* 28:593.

Institute of Medicine, National Academy of Sciences, 1980a, *Alcoholism and Alcohol Abuse Related Problems: Opportunities for Research,* National Academy Press, Washington, D.C.

———, 1980b, *Reliability of Hospital Discharge Abstracts,* National Academy of Sciences, Washington, D.C.

Jellinek, E. M., 1960, *The Disease Concept of Alcoholism,* Yale University Press, New Haven, Conn.

———, 1952, Phases of alcohol addiction. *Q. J. Stud. Alc.,* 13:673.

Jessor, R., and Jessor, S. L., 1975, Adolescent development and the onset of drinking, *J. Stud. Alc.,* 36:27.

————, 1977, *Problems in Behavior and Psychsocial Development: A Longitudinal Study of Youth*, Academic Press, New York.

Johnson, P. B., 1982, Sex differences, women's roles and alcohol data, *J. Soc. Issues*, 38:93.

Jones, K. R., and Vischi, T. R., 1979, Impact of alcohol, drug abuse and mental health treatment on medical care utilization: A review of the research literature, *Med. Care*, 17(Suppl.):1.

Justin, R. G., 1979, Use of routine breath alcohol tests in the diagnosis of alcoholism in a primary care practice, *J. Stud. Alc.*, 40(1):145.

Kane, G. P., 1981, *Inner-City Alcoholism*, Human Sciences Press, New York.

Kasl, S., and Colb, S., 1979, Some mental health consequences of plant closing and job loss, in *Mental Health and the Economy* (L. Ferman and J. Gordus, eds.), W. E. UpJohn Institute, Kalamazoo, Mich.

Kissin, B., and Hanson, M., 1982, The bio-psycho-social perspective in alcoholism, in *Alcoholism and Clinical Psychiatry* (J. Solomon, ed.), Plenum Press, New York.

Klerman, G. L., 1982, Prevention of alcoholism, in *Alcoholism and Clinical Psychiatry* (J. Solomon, ed.), Plenum Press, New York.

Kline, N. S., Wren, J. C., Cooper, T. B., et al., 1974, Evaluation of lithium therapy in chronic alcoholism, *Clin. Med.*, 81:33.

Leach, B., and Norris, F. L., 1977, Factors in the development of Alcoholics Anonymous (A.A.), in *Treatment and Rehabilitation of the Chronic Alcoholic* (B. Kissin and H. Begleiter, eds.), Plenum Press, New York.

Leatham, R. C., 1978, A report on the etiology of American Indian/Alaskan Native alcoholism and an evaluation of the National Institute on Alcohol Abuse and Alcoholism supported American Indian/Alaskan Native alcoholism projects, paper submitted to the National Advisory Council on Alcohol Abuse and Alcoholism, National Institute on Alcohol Abuse and Alcoholism, and the Department of Health, Education, and Welfare.

Leland, J., 1976, *Firewater Myths: North American Indian Drinking and Alcohol Addiction*, Monograph No. 11, Rutgers Center of Alcohol Studies, New Brunswick, N.J.

Leland, J., 1977, North American Indian drinking and alcohol abuse, contract no. NIA-77-08(P), report prepared for National Institute on Alcohol Abuse and Alcoholism, Alcohol, Drug Abuse, and Mental Health Administration.

Leon, R. L., 1965, Maladaptive interaction between Bureau of Indian Affairs, staff and clients, *Am. J. Orthop.*, 35:723.

Ludwig, A. M., Levine, J., and Stark, L. H., 1970, *LSD and Alcoholism: A Clinical Study of Treatment Efficacy*, Charles C. Thomas, Springfield, Ill.

MacAndrew, D., and Garfinkel, H., 1962, A consideration of changes attributed to intoxication as common-sense reasons for getting drunk, *Q. J. Stud. Alc.*, 23:252.

Maccoby, M., 1972, Alcoholism in a Mexican village, in *The Drinking Man* (D. C. McClelland, W. N. Davis, R. Kalin, et al., eds.), The Free Press, New York.

Madsen, W., 1964, The alcoholic agringado, *Am. Anthropol.*, 66:355.

Mandell, W., 1979, A critical overview of evaluations of alcoholism treatment, *Alcoholism: Clin. Exp. Res.*, 3(4):315.

Medical Times, 1975, An alcohol abuse manual for family physicians, Special Issue, 103(6).

Mendelson, J. H., and Mello, N. K., 1979, The diagnosis of alcoholism, in *The Diagnosis and Treatment of Alcoholism* (J. H. Mendelson and N. K. Mello, eds.), McGraw-Hill Book Company, New York.

Merry, J., Reynolds, C. M., Bailey, J. et al., 1976, Prophylactic treatment of alcoholism by lithium carbonate, *Lancet,* 2:481.

Moore, R. A., 1982, The involvement of private psychiatric hospitals in alcoholism treatment, in *Encyclopedic Handbook of Alcoholism* (E. M. Pattison and E. Kaufman, eds.), Gardner Press, New York.

Moore, R. A., 1977, Ten years of inpatient programs for alcoholic patients, *Am. J. Psychiat.,* 134:542.

Moore, R. A., and Buchanan, T. K., 1966, State hospitals and alcoholism: Nationwide survey of treatment techniques and results, *Q. J. Stud. Alc.,* 27:459.

Moos, R. H., and Bliss, F., 1978, Difficulty of follow-up and outcome of alcoholism treatment, *J. Stud. Alc.,* 39:473.

Mottin, J. L., 1973, Drug-induced attenuation of alcohol consumption: A review and evaluation of claimed, potential, and current therapies, *Q. J. Stud. Alc.,* 34:444.

Nathan, P. E., 1978, Overview of behavioral treatment approaches, in *Behavioral Approaches to Alcoholism* (G. Marlatt and P. E. Nathan, eds.), Rutgers Center of Alcohol Studies, New Brunswick, N.J.

Nathan, P. E., and Lipscomb, T. R., 1979, Behavior therapy and behavior modification in the treatment of alcoholism, in *The Diagnosis and Treatment of Alcoholism* (J. H. Mendelson and N. K. Mello, eds.), McGraw-Hill Book Company, New York.

National Institute on Alcohol Abuse and Alcoholism, Alcohol, Drug Abuse, and Mental Health Administration, 1978, Excerpts: Medicare coverage for the treatment of alcoholism, National Institute on Alcohol Abuse and Alcoholism, Department of Health, Education, and Welfare, Rockville, Md.

———, 1981a, Fourth special report to the U.S. Congress on alcohol and health, National Institute on Alcohol Abuse and Alcoholism, Department of Health and Human Services, Rockville, Md.

———, 1981b, National drug and alcoholism treatment utilization survey, National Institute on Alcohol Abuse and Alcoholism, Department of Health and Human Services, Rockville, Md.

———, 1982, Statistical report on National Institute on Alcohol Abuse and Alcoholism-funded treatment programs for calendar year 1980: Data from NAPIS, contract no. ADM 281-81-0004, National Institute on Alcohol Abuse and Alcoholism, Department of Health and Human Services, Rockville, Md.

Neuberger, O. W., Matarazzo, J. D., Schmitz, R. E., et al., 1980, One year follow-up of total abstinence in chronic alcoholic patients following emetic counterconditioning, *Alcoholism: Clin. Exper. Res.,* 4:306.

Neuberger, O. W., Miller, S. I., Schmitz, R. E., et al., 1982, Replicable abstinence rates in an alcoholism treatment program, *JAMA* 248:960.

Office of Technology Assessment, U.S. Congress, 1980a, The implications of cost-effectiveness analysis of medical technology, GPO stock No. 052-003-00765-7, U.S. Government Printing Office, Washington, D.C.

———, 1980b, The efficacy and cost-effectiveness of psychotherapy, NTIS order No. PB81-144 610, National Information Service, Washington, D.C.

————, 1980c, Strategies for medical technology assessment, GPO stock No. 052-003-00887-4, U.S. Government Printing Office, Washington, D.C.

Orvis, B. R., Armor, D. J., Williams, C. E., et al., 1981, Effectiveness and cost of alcohol rehabilitation in the United-States Air Force, The Rand Corporation, Santa Monica, Calif.

Overall, J. E., Brown, D., Williams, J. D., et al., 1973, Drug treatment of anxiety and depression in detoxified alcoholic patients, *Arch. Gen. Psychiat.*, 29:218.

Pattison, E. M., 1966, A critique of alcoholism treatment concepts: With special reference to abstinence, *Q. J. Stud. Alc.*, 247:49.

————, 1977a, Management of alcoholism in medical practice, *Med. Clin. N. A.*, 61:797.

————, 1977b, Ten years of change in alcoholism treatment and delivery, *Am. J. Psychiat.*, 134(3):261.

————, 1979, The selection of treatment modalities for the alcoholic patient, in *The Diagnosis and Treatment of Alcoholism* (J. H. Mendelson and N. K. Mello, eds.), McGraw-Hill Book Company, New York.

————, 1980, The NCA diagnostic criteria: Critique, assessment, alternative, *J. Stud. Alc.*, 41(9):965.

Pattison, E. M., Coe, R., and Rhodes, R. J., 1969, Evaluation of alcoholism: A comparison of three facilities, *Arch. Gen. Psychiat.*, 20:478.

Pattison, E. M., Sobell, M. B., and Sobell, L. C., 1977, *Emerging Concepts of Alcohol Dependence*, Springer, New York.

Pendery, M. L., Maltzman, I. M., and West, L. J., 1982, Controlled drinking by alcoholics? New findings and a revaluation of a major affirmative study, *Science*, 217:169.

Plotnick, D. E., Adams, K. M., Hunter, H. R., et al., 1982, *Alcoholic treatment programs within prepaid group practice HMOs: A final report*, contract No. ADM 281-80-004, prepared by the Group Health Association of America for National Institute on Alcohol Abuse and Alcoholism, Alcohol, Drug Abuse, and Mental Health Administration, Rockville, Md.

Polich, J. M., Armor, D. J., and Braiker, H. B., 1981, *The Course of Alcoholism: Four Years After Treatment*, John Wiley & Sons, New York.

Pomerleau, O. F., Pertschuk, M., Adlans, D. et al., 1978, A comparison of behavioral and traditional treatment methods for middle-income, problem drinkers, *J. Behav. Med.*, 1:187.

Public Health Service, Office of the Assistant Secretary for Health and Surgeon General, 1979, Healthy people: The Surgeon General's report on health promotion and disease prevention, GPO stock. No. 017-001-00416-2, U.S. Government Printing Office, Washington, D.C.

Rachal, J. V., Maisto, S. A., Guess, L. L., et al., 1981, Alcohol use among adolescents, in *Alcohol Consumption and Related Problems*, Alcohol and Health Monograph No. 1, National Institute on Alcohol Abuse and Alcoholism, Alcohol, Drug Abuse, and Mental Health Administration, Rockville, Md.

Ritson, B., 1971, Personality and prognosis in alcoholism, *Br. J. Psychiat.*, 118:79.

————, 1968, The prognosis of alcohol addicts treated by a specialized unit, *Br. J. Psychiat.*, 114:1019.

Sarvis, K. C., 1976, Insurance cost savings due to an adequate alcoholism health benefit, prepared for the State of Florida Department of Health and Rehabilitation Services.

Saxe, L., and Fine, M., 1981, *Social Experiments: Methods for Design and Evaluation,* Sage Publications, Beverly Hills, Calif.

Saxe, L., Dougherty, D., Esty, K., and Fine, M., 1983, The Effectiveness and Costs of Alcoholism Treatment, prepared by the Office of Technology Assessment, U.S. Government Printing Office, Washington, D.C.

Schifrin, L. G., Hartzog, C. E., and Brand, D. H., 1980, Costs of alcoholism and alcohol abuse and their relation to alcohol research, in *Alcoholism and Related Problems: Opportunities for Research,* National Academy of Sciences, Washington, D.C.

Schuckit, M. A., and Miller, P. L., 1975, Alcoholism in elderly men: A survey of a general medical ward, *Ann. N.Y. Acad. Sci.,* 273:558.

Schuckit, M. A., Pitts, F. M., Reich, T., et al., 1969, Alcoholism: I. Two types in women, *Arch. Gen. Psychiat.,* 20:301.

Science Management Corporation, 1982, Status of state legislation and research on health insurance coverage for alcoholism treatment, contract No. ADM 281-81-0008, report prepared for the National Institute on Alcohol Abuse and Alcoholism, Rockville, Md.

Sellers, E. M., and Kalant, H., 1982, Alcohol withdrawal and delirium tremens, in *Encyclopedic Handbook of Alcoholism* (E. M. Pattison and E. Kaufman, eds.), Gardner Press, New York.

Smart, R. G., 1976, Spontaneous recovery in alcoholics: A review and analysis of the available literature, *Drug & Al. Depend.,* 1:227.

Smith, J. W., 1982, Treatment of alcoholism in aversion conditioning hospitals, in *Encyclopedic Handbook of Alcoholism* (E. M. Pattison and E. Kaufman, eds.), Gardner Press, New York.

Sobell, L. C., and Sobell, M. B., 1972, Individualized behavior therapy for alcoholics: Rationale, procedures, preliminary results, and appendix State of California Department of Mental Hygiene, Sacramento, Calif.

————, 1982, Alcoholism treatment outcome evaluation methodology, in *Prevention, Intervention and Treatment: Concerns and Models,* Alcohol and Health Monograph No. 3, National Institute on Alcohol Abuse and Alcoholism, Rockville, Md.

Sobell, M. B., and Sobell, L. C., 1973, Alcoholics treated by individual behavior therapy: One year treatment outcome, *Behav. Res. & Ther.,* 11:599.

————, 1978, *Behavioral Treatment of Alcohol Problems,* Plenum Press, New York.

Solomon, J., 1982, The role of drug therapies in the context of alcoholism, in *Encyclopedic Handbook of Alcoholism* (E. M. Pattison and E. Kaufman, eds.), Gardner Press, New York.

Solomon, S. D., 1982, Bias in exposure of outpatient therapy to different alcoholism client types, presented at the meeting of the American Psychological Association, Washington, D.C.

Solomon, S. D., 1982, Measures of alcoholism treatment outcome, *Alc. Health & Res. World* 6(4):44.

Solomon, S. D., 1981, *Tailoring Alcoholism Therapy to Client Needs,* National Institute on Alcohol Abuse and Alcoholism, Rockville, Md.

Stack, C., 1974, Sex roles and survival strategies in an urban black community, in

Women, Culture and Society (M. Z. Rosaldo and L. Lamphere, eds.), Stanford University Press, Stanford, Calif.

Stuckey, R. F., and Harrison, J. S., 1982, The alcoholism rehabilitation center, in *Encyclopedic Handbook of Alcoholism* (E. M. Pattison and E. Kaufman, eds.), Gardner Press, New York.

Swint, J. M., and Nelson, W. B., 1977, Prospective evaluation of alcoholism rehabilitation efforts: The role of cost-benefit and cost-effectiveness analyses, *J. Stud. Alc.,* 38:1386.

Thimann, J., 1949, Conditioned reflex treatment of alcoholism: II. The risk of its application, its indications, contraindications and psychotherapeutic effects, *N. Eng. J. Med.,* 241:408.

Torres de Gonzalez, B., 1973, Treating the inner city young Spanish speaking alcohol abuser, paper presented on behalf of the East Harlem Tenants Council (New York, N.Y.) and the Puerto Rican Inter-Agency Council, Dec. 5.

Tuchfeld, B. S., 1981, Spontaneous remission in alcoholics: Empirical observations and theoretical implications, *J. Stud. Alc.,* 42:626.

Tuchfeld, B. S., and Lipton, W. L., 1982a, *Alcoholism Treatment Research Study: An Evaluation of Treatment Outcomes 18 Months Post-Admission to Schick-Shadel Hospital of D/FW, Inc.,* Texas Christian University, Fort Worth.

Tuchfeld, B. S., and Marcus, M. S., and Lipton, W. L., 1982b, *Salient Issues in Evaluating Alcoholism Treatment Effectiveness,* Texas Christian University, Fort Worth.

Valentine, B. L., 1978, *Hustling and Other Hard Work: Lifestyles in the Ghetto,* Free Press, New York.

Vischi, T. R., Jones, K. R., Shank, E. L., et al., 1980, *The Alcohol, Drug Abuse, and Mental Health National Data Book,* Alcohol, Drug Abuse, and Mental Health Administration, Rockville, Md.

Vitols, M. M., 1968, Culture patterns of drinking in Negro and white alcoholics, *Dis. Nerv. Syst.,* 29:391.

Voegtlin, W. L., and Broz, W. R., 1949, The conditioned reflex treatment of chronic alcoholism: X. An analysis of 3125 admissions over a period of ten and a half years, *Ann. Int. Med.,* 30:580.

Voegtlin, W. L., and Lemere, F., 1942, The treatment of alcohol addiction: A review of the literature, *Q. J. Stud. Alc.,* 2:717.

Vogler, R. E., Compton, J. V., and Weissbach, J. A., 1975, Integrated behavior change techniques for alcoholism, *J. Consul. Clin. Psych.,* 43:233.

Vogler, R. E., Weissbach, T. A., and Compton, J. V., 1977a, Learning techniques for alcohol abuse, *Behav. Res. Ther.,* 15:31.

Vogler, R. E., Weissbach, T. A., and Compton, J. V., et al., 1977b, Integrated behavior change techniques for problem drinking in the community, *J. Consult. Psychol.,* 45:267.

Wanberg, K. W., Horn, J. L., and Fairchild, D., 1974, Hospital versus community treatment of alcoholism problems, *Int. J. Ment. Health,* 3:160.

Wiens, A. N., Montague, J. R., Manaugh, T. S., et al., 1976, Pharmacological aversive counterconditioning to alcohol in a private hospital, *J. Stud. Alc.,* 37:1320.

Williams, W. G., 1981, Nature and scope of benefit packages in health insurance coverage for alcoholism treatment, *Al. Health & Res. World,* 5(4):5.

Wilson, G. T., 1978, Alcoholism and aversion therapy approaches, in *Behavioral Approaches to Alcoholism* (G. A. Marlatt and P. E. Nathan, eds.), Rutgers Center of Alcohol Studies, New Brunswick, N.J.

Wiseman, J. P., 1970, *Stations of the Lost: The Treatment of Skid Row Alcoholics,* Prentice-Hall, Englewood Cliffs, N.J.

Wortman, P. M., and Saxe, L., 1982, Assessment of medical technology: Methodological considerations, in *Strategies for Medical Technology Assessment,* prepared by the Office of Technology Assessment, U.S. Government Printing Office, Washington, D.C.

Zylman, R., 1974, Fatal crashes among Michigan youth following reduction of legal drinking age, *Q. J. Stud. Alc.,* 35:293.

————, 1976, Collision behavior of young drivers: Comment on the study by Whitehead et al., *J. Stud. Alc.,* 37:393.

Index

ABOUT THE EDITORS

Dr. Jack H. Mendelson and Dr. Nancy K. Mello have collaborated in research on alcoholism for the past 20 years. They were, respectively, Chief of the first federal program on alcoholism and Chief of the Intramural Laboratory of Alcohol Research between 1967 and 1974. At present, Dr. Mendelson is a Professor of Psychiatry at Harvard Medical School and Codirector of the Alcohol and Drug Abuse Research Center at McLean Hospital. Dr. Mello is Professor of Psychology in the Department of Psychiatry at Harvard Medical School and Codirector of the Alcohol and Drug Abuse Research Center at McLean Hospital. Widely acclaimed for their work, Dr. Mendelson and Dr. Mello were awarded the prestigious Jellinek Award for research in alcoholism by an international committee of experts in 1978. In 1983, Drs. Mendelson and Mello became editors of the Journal of Studies on Alcohol, America's oldest and most widely read journal devoted to advances in research on alcohol abuse and alcoholism.